Afoot & Afield
Inland Empire

256 Spectacular Outings in Southern California

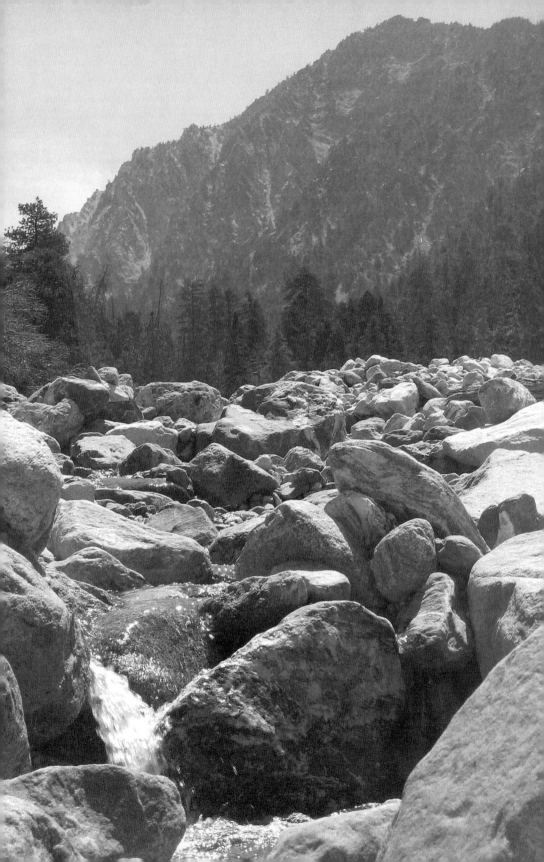

Afoot & Afield

Inland Empire

256 Spectacular Outings in Southern California

SECOND EDITION

David Harris

WILDERNESS PRESS ... *on the trail since 1967*

In memory of Alfred Kwok, who died in the mountains he loved best

Afoot & Afield Inland Empire: 256 Spectacular Outings in Southern California

Second edition, first printing

Copyright © 2018 by David Harris

Editor: Lady Vowell Smith
Project editor: Ritchey Halphen
Cover and interior photos: copyright © 2018 by David Harris, except where noted
Maps: David Harris
Cover design: Scott McGrew
Text design: Andreas Schüller, with updates by Annie Long
Proofreaders: Laura Franck, Rebecca Henderson
Indexer: Galen Schroeder/DakotaIndexing.com

Library of Congress Cataloging-in-Publication Data

Names: Harris, David, author.
Title: Afoot & afield, Inland Empire : 256 spectacular outings in Southern California /
    David Harris.
Description: Third edition. | Birmingham, AL : Wilderness Press, [2017]
Identifiers: LCCN 2017031825 | ISBN 9780899978154 (pbk.)
Subjects: LCSH: Hiking—California—Inland Empire—Guidebooks. | Inland Empire (Calif.)—
    Guidebooks.
Classification: LCC GV199.42.C22 I555 2017 | DDC 796.5109794/97—dc23
LC record available at lccn.loc.gov/2017031825

Manufactured in the United States of America

Distributed by Publishers Group West

Published by: 🏔 **WILDERNESS PRESS**
     An imprint of AdventureKEEN
     2204 First Ave. S, Ste. 102
     Birmingham, AL 35233
     800-443-7227; FAX 205-326-1012

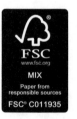

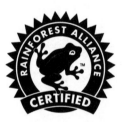

Visit wildernesspress.com for a complete listing of our books and for ordering information. Contact us at info@wildernesspress.com, facebook.com/wildernesspress1967, or twitter.com /wilderness1967 with questions or comments. To find out more about who we are and what we're doing, visit blog.wildernesspress.com.

Cover photos: (Front, clockwise from top) Cycling the Skyline Trail above Big Bear Lake (Trip 4.11, page 88); Big Split Rock Canyon, Mecca Hills (Trip 13.2, page 318); Deep Creek, Western San Bernardino Mountains (Trip 3.6, page 62). (Back) Sycamore Canyon, Riverside (Trip 7.7, page 159).

Frontispiece: Galena Peak above Mill Creek (see Trip 5.3, page 107)

Safety Notice Although Wilderness Press and the author have made every attempt to ensure that the information in this book is accurate at press time, they are not responsible for any loss, damage, injury, or inconvenience that may occur to anyone while using this book. You are responsible for your own safety and health while in the wilderness. The fact that a trail is described in this book does not mean that it will be safe for you. Be aware that trail conditions can change from day to day. Always check local conditions, and know your own limitations.

Contents

Acknowledgments

I am grateful to many people for their help with this project.

Hiking is safer and more enjoyable with companions. I'd particularly like to thank the following friends and family for their company on the trail: Tony Condon, Sian Davies-Vollum, Brian Elliot, Emile Fiesler, Tobias Georg, Rick Graham, Daniel Harris, Mark Headricks, Alex Honnold, Alfred Kwok, David Lee, Charlie Marquart, Aaron Money, Melissa Money, Cidney Scanlon, Joe Sheehy, John Spruce, and Elizabeth Thomas.

I've also enjoyed the company of several hiking clubs, including Delta H, On the Loose, the Sierra Club, and the Coachella Valley Hiking Club.

Above all, my three sons, Abraham, Samuel, and Benjamin, have accompanied me on the majority of the fieldwork for this book, including more than 188 days for the first edition and 75 days for this edition.

Many reviewers have helped improve this book. They include the following: Ashley Adams, Amanda Allen, Sharon Barfknecht, James Bryant, Doug Chudy, Kimberly Cobb, Tony Condon, Caroline Conway, Buford Crites, Don Davidson, Brad Eells, Meg Foley, Jim Foote, Phillip Gomez, Jeanette Granger, Frazer Haney, David Harris (what a great name!), Sally Harris, Mike Herman, Andre Herndon, Tim Hough, Dan Kasang, Sherli Leonard, Bradley Mastin, Paul Melzer, David Miller, Christina Mills, Bart O'Brien, Erin Opliger, Karen Pope, Gina Richmond, Bob Romano, Charles Russell, April Sall, Audrey Scranton, Joe Sheehy, Ginny Short, Andy Smith, Kevin Smith, Wayne Steinmetz, Paula Taylor, Jack Thompson, Rocky Toyama, Pam Tripp, Carol Underhill, Laura Verdugo, Richard Wilkerson, Richard Wismer, and Betty Zeller.

Lady Vowell Smith's editing greatly improved the manuscript. The remaining errors are my own.

Wildlands are a precious resource. Each trip in this book owes its existence to the vision and effort of many people, from grass-roots volunteers to conservation organizations to civil servants to forward-thinking political leaders, who have protected the land and constructed and maintained the trails that we now enjoy.   —David Harris

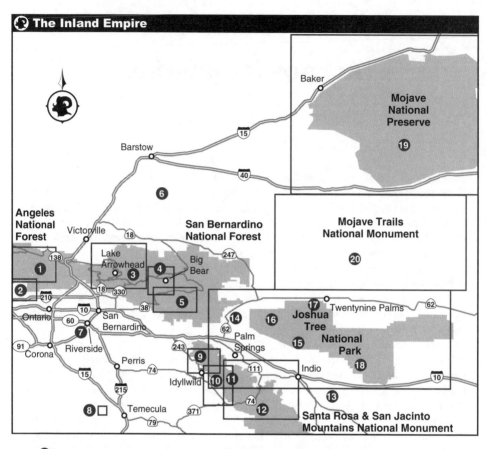

The Inland Empire

1 Mount Baldy Area
2 San Gabriel Foothills
3 San Bernardino Mtns.: West
4 San Bernardino Mtns.: Big Bear
5 San Bernardino Mtns.: San Gorgonio
6 High Desert
7 Urban Parks
8 Santa Rosa Ecological Reserve

11 Palm Springs & Indian Canyons
12 Santa Rosa National Monument
13 Colorado Desert
14 Desert Preserves
15 Joshua Tree: Park Blvd.
16 Joshua Tree: Black Rock
17 Joshua Tree: Indian Cove
18 Joshua Tree: East

Preface

This book covers more than 250 hikes around the Inland Empire. While the region is too large to include every trail worth hiking, I personally enjoyed each of the selected trips.

For the second edition, I revisited more than 99% of the trailheads and reviewed the text with rangers responsible for nearly all of the areas. I rehiked any trip where there was reason to suspect changes. Furthermore, I added more than 60 great new trips spanning nearly every chapter of the book.

I removed four obscure trips that have become too brushy for my tastes—Arrowhead Peak, Six Peaks of the Western San Bernardinos, Cone Peak, and Leatherneck Ridge—along with California Citrus State Historic Park, which is an interesting destination but not much of a hike. Finally, I eliminated several urban hikes that I felt fit better in *Afoot & Afield Los Angeles County.*

My eldest son was born near the start of the first edition and is 12 years old at the completion of the second edition. I now have three sons who have accompanied me on hundreds of days of fieldwork. The greatest pleasure of this project has been spending time with the boys outdoors, scrambling on rocks, splashing in creeks, looking for acorns and crystals, and camping under the stars. I hope that these experiences nurture in them a lifelong love of wild places, and I've selected a diverse collection of trips so that readers of all ages and experience levels can find their own perfect hikes.

These trips are constantly changing. Roads and trails get rerouted. Wildfire scours the mountains, and chaparral grows over seldom-visited tracks. Property owners deny access to trails, and forward-thinking leaders open new areas. Authors have even been known to make mistakes, writing "left" when they mean "right," among other things. When the facts on the ground seem inconsistent with the trip descriptions, use your best judgment and err on the side of safety.

Overview of Hikes

OVERVIEW OF HIKES (continued)

HIKE NUMBER	HIKE	DISTANCE (miles)	ELEVATION GAIN (feet)	TRAIL TYPE	BACKPACKING	MOUNTAIN BIKING	EQUESTRIANS	DOGS	KIDS
Chapter 3: SAN BERNARDINO MOUNTAINS: WEST (Continued)									
3.4	Rock Camp/Metate Interpretive Trail	0.8	100	loop				🐕	🧒
3.5	Little Bear Creek	4	800	out-and-back				🐕	
3.6	Deep Creek	6	600	out-and-back	🚶			🐕	
3.7	Fisherman's Camp	5	700	out-and-back	🚶	🚲	🐎	🐕	
3.8	Deep Creek Canyoneering	6.5	1,300	loop					
3.9	Holcomb Crossing Trail Camp	5	900	loop	🚶		🐎	🐕	
3.10	Cox Creek	10	1,100	out-and-back	🚶		🐎	🐕	
3.11	Heaps Peak Arboretum	0.8	100	loop					🧒
3.12	Exploration Trail	4	1,300	point-to-point		🚲	🐎	🐕	
3.13	Little Green Valley	2.5	700	out-and-back		🚲	🐎	🐕	
Chapter 4: SAN BERNARDINO MOUNTAINS: BIG BEAR LAKE AREA									
4.1	Grays Peak	7	1,200	out-and-back		🚲	🐎	🐕	
4.2	Delamar Mountain	5.5	800	out-and-back				🐕	
4.3	Cougar Crest (and Bertha Peak)	5+	700+	out-and-back			🐎	🐕	🧒
4.4	Alpine Pedal Path	4	200	loop		🚲		🐕	🧒
4.5	Woodland Trail	1.7	300	loop				🐕	🧒
4.6	Gold Mountain	8	1,400	out-and-back				🐕	
4.7	Sugarloaf Mountain	7	1,300	out-and-back	🚶	🚲	🐎	🐕	
4.8	Wildhorse Creek	8	1,400	out-and-back	🚶	🚲	🐎	🐕	
4.9	Grand View Point	6.5	1,100	out-and-back		🚲		🐕	
4.10	Castle Rock	1.6	700	out-and-back				🐕	🧒
4.11	Skyline Trail	15	1,700	point-to-point		🚲		🐕	
4.12	Seven Oaks Trail	4.6	1,600	out-and-back		🚲	🐎	🐕	
4.13	Champion Lodgepole Pine	0.6	50	out-and-back		🚲	🐎	🐕	🧒
4.14	Siberia Creek Trail Camp from Champion Lodgepole Pine	14	2,900	out-and-back	🚶			🐕	
4.15	Siberia Creek Trail Camp from Snow Valley	5.5	2,200	out-and-back	🚶			🐕	
4.16	Siberia Creek Trail Camp from Seven Pines	8	1,300	out-and-back	🚶			🐕	
4.17	Butler Peak	0.25	100	out-and-back					🧒
4.18	Granite Peaks	6	1,800	out-and-back					
Chapter 5: SAN BERNARDINO MOUNTAINS: SAN GORGONIO WILDERNESS									
5.1	San Gorgonio via Vivian Creek	17	5,500	out-and-back	🚶			🐕	
5.2	Little San Gorgonio Peak	5	3,100	out-and-back					
5.3	Galena Peak	8	3,400	out-and-back	🚶				

TRAIL TYPE LEGEND: ○ = loop   = out-and-back   = point-to-point

OVERVIEW OF HIKES (continued)

HIKE NUMBER	HIKE	DISTANCE (miles)	ELEVATION GAIN (feet)	TRAIL TYPE	BACKPACKING	MOUNTAIN BIKING	EQUESTRIANS	DOGS	KIDS
Chapter 5: SAN BERNARDINO MOUNTAINS: SAN GORGONIO WILDERNESS *(Continued)*									
5.4	Big Falls	0.6	100	out-and-back				dogs	kids
5.5	Alger Creek or Dobbs Trail Camp	7+	2,100+	out-and-back	backpacking			dogs	
5.6	Momyer to Falls Creek Loop	20	5,900	loop	backpacking			dogs	
5.7	Aqueduct Trail	4.5	700	loop				dogs	
5.8	Mountain Home Flats	3.5	1,100	out-and-back	backpacking			dogs	
5.9	San Bernardino Peak	16	4,700	out-and-back	backpacking			dogs	
5.10	Whispering Pines and Ponderosa Vista Nature Trails	0.7	200	loop				dogs	kids
5.11	Johns Meadow	6	800	out-and-back	backpacking			dogs	
5.12	San Bernardino Peak via Forsee Creek	17	4,000	loop	backpacking			dogs	
5.13	South Fork Meadows	8	1,400	out-and-back				dogs	
5.14	San Gorgonio via Dollar and Dry Lakes	21	4,700	loop	backpacking			dogs	
5.15	Jenks Lake	3	600	loop		mountain biking	equestrians	dogs	kids
5.16	Santa Ana River Trail	38	2,800	point-to-point	backpacking	mountain biking	equestrians	dogs	
5.17	Aspen Grove	1.8	350	out-and-back				dogs	kids
5.18	Fish Creek Meadows	4	650	out-and-back				dogs	
5.19	San Gorgonio via Fish Creek	19	3,600	out-and-back	backpacking			dogs	
5.20	San Gorgonio Nine Peaks Challenge	25	8,000	point-to-point	backpacking			dogs	
5.21	Ten Peaks of the Yucaipa Ridge	19	6,700	point-to-point					
Chapter 6: HIGH DESERT									
6.1	Mormon Rocks Nature Loop	1	200	loop				dogs	kids
6.2	East Ord Mountain	2.5	2,000	out-and-back				dogs	
6.3	Owl Canyon	4	1,000	out-and-back				dogs	kids
Chapter 7: URBAN PARKS									
7.1	Pacific Electric Trail	20	300	point-to-point		mountain biking	equestrians	dogs	
7.2	Prado Lake	2.5	50	loop		mountain biking	equestrians	dogs	kids
7.3	Mount Rubidoux	3.0	450	loop		mountain biking		dogs	
7.4	Box Springs: Two Trees Trail	2.6	1,000	point-to-point		mountain biking	equestrians	dogs	
7.5	Box Springs: Skyline Trail	3+	600+	loop		mountain biking	equestrians	dogs	
7.6	Box Springs: Towers Loop	3.5	800	loop		mountain biking	equestrians	dogs	
7.7	Sycamore Canyon Wilderness Park	2+	varies	loop		mountain biking		dogs	kids
7.8	Olive Mountain	2.4	900	out-and-back		mountain biking		dogs	
7.9	Terri Peak	4	800	out-and-back		mountain biking	equestrians		
7.10	South Hills Preserve: Jedi Trail	5	800	out-and-back		mountain biking	equestrians		
7.11	San Timoteo Nature Sanctuary	3.4	200	loop		mountain biking	equestrians	dogs	

TRAIL TYPE LEGEND: ◯ = loop   ⬈ = out-and-back   ➚ = point-to-point

OVERVIEW OF HIKES (continued)

HIKE NUMBER	HIKE	DISTANCE (miles)	ELEVATION GAIN (feet)	TRAIL TYPE	BACKPACKING	MOUNTAIN BIKING	EQUESTRIANS	DOGS	KIDS
Chapter 7: URBAN PARKS *(Continued)*									
7.12	Oakmont Park	3.4	400	Loop		✓	✓	✓	✓
7.13	Wildwood Canyon State Park	2.6	500	Loop		✓	✓		✓
7.14	Crafton Hills: Park-to-Peak Loop	5	1,100	Loop		✓		✓	
7.15	Crafton Hills: Grape Avenue Trail	4.7	1,000	Loop		✓	✓	✓	
7.16	Crafton Hills: Hilltop Trail	7	1,200	Out-and-back		✓	✓	✓	
7.17	El Dorado Ranch Park	3.5	500	Loop		✓	✓	✓	✓
7.18	Bogart Park Loop	3.5	600	Loop			✓	✓	✓
7.19	Simpson Park	3.6	900	Loop		✓	✓	✓	
Chapter 8: SANTA ROSA PLATEAU ECOLOGICAL RESERVE									
8.1	Granite Loop	1.2+	100	Loop					✓
8.2	Sylvan Meadows Loop	4.5	300	Loop		✓	✓	✓	
8.3	Oak Tree Trail	2	100	Loop					✓
8.4	Los Santos Loop	5	500	Loop					
8.5	Vernal Pool	1.5	100	Out-and-back					✓
8.6	Historic Adobes	3.5	300	Out-and-back					
8.7	Santa Rosa Plateau Loop	11	700	Loop					
Chapter 9: SAN JACINTO MOUNTAINS									
9.1	Black Mountain	7	2,700	Out-and-back	✓			✓	
9.2	Indian Mountain	5.5	1,300	Out-and-back				✓	
9.3	San Jacinto Peak via Fuller Ridge	15	4,100	Out-and-back	✓			✓	
9.4	North Fork of the San Jacinto River	1.4	400	Out-and-back					
9.5	Seven Pines Trail	7	2,400	Out-and-back					
9.6	San Jacinto Peak via the Marion Mountain Trail	12	4,500	Out-and-back	✓				
9.7	Panorama Point	0.8	100	Loop				✓	✓
9.8	Webster Trail	5	2,000	Out-and-back				✓	
9.9	Idyllwild Nature Center Loop	2.1	600	Loop				✓	✓
9.10	Suicide Rock	7	1,900	Out-and-back					
9.11	Tahquitz Rock	2.2	1,600	Out-and-back					
9.12	Ernie Maxwell Scenic Trail	5	700	Out-and-back				✓	
9.13	Skunk Cabbage Meadow	6.5	1,700	Out-and-back	✓			✓	
9.14	Tahquitz Peak via Saddle Junction	8.5	2,400	Out-and-back	✓			✓	
9.15	Caramba	14	3,300	Out-and-back	✓			✓	
9.16	Strawberry Valley Loop	10	2,600	Out-and-back	✓			✓	
9.17	Idyllwild–Round Valley Loop	14	3,600	Loop	✓				
9.18	San Jacinto Peak from Humber Park	18	4,500	Loop	✓				
9.19	Tahquitz Peak via the South Ridge Trail	7	2,400	Out-and-back				✓	
9.20	Desert View Loop	1.6	350	Loop					✓

OVERVIEW OF HIKES (continued)

HIKE NUMBER	HIKE	DISTANCE (miles)	ELEVATION GAIN (feet)	TRAIL TYPE	BACKPACKING	MOUNTAIN BIKING	EQUESTRIANS	DOGS	KIDS
Chapter 9: SAN JACINTO MOUNTAINS (Continued)									
9.21	Round Valley	4.5	700	➚	🥾				🧒
9.22	Cornell Peak	6	1,400	➚	🥾				
9.23	San Jacinto Peak from the Palm Springs Aerial Tramway	10	2,600	➚	🥾				
9.24	Seven Peaks of the San Jacinto Wilderness	14	5,400	⟳					
Chapter 10: DESERT DIVIDE									
10.1	Antsell Rock	4	2,300	➚					
10.2	Apache Peak	6+	2,100	➚	🥾				
10.3	Palm View Peak	8	2,100	➚				🐕	
10.4	Cedar Spring	6.5	1,700	➚	🥾			🐕	
10.5	Northern Desert Divide	11	2,000	➚	🥾				
10.6	Nine Peaks of the Desert Divide	27	9,000	➚	🥾				
10.7	Thomas Mountain	12	2,400	➚	🥾	🚲	🐎	🐕	
10.8	Cahuilla Mountain	6	1,400	➚	🥾			🐕	
10.9	Hurkey Creek	8	900	⟳		🚲	🐎	🐕	
10.10	South Fork of the San Jacinto River	5	800	➚	🥾		🐎	🐕	
Chapter 11: PALM SPRINGS AND THE INDIAN CANYONS									
11.1	South Lykken Trail	4.5	1,100	➚					
11.2	North Lykken Trail	4	1,500	➚					
11.3	Museum Trail	2	1,000	➚					
11.4	Cactus-to-Clouds	10	8,000	➚					
11.5	Tahquitz Canyon	2	350	⟳					
11.6	Desert Angel	1.6	1,200	➚					
11.7	Vargas Palms	4.4	500	➚				🐕	
11.8	Snow Creek	12	10,000	➚					
11.9	Andreas Canyon	1	200	⟳					🧒
11.10	Maynard Mine	5.5	2,400	➚					
11.11	Murray Canyon	4	500	➚			🐎		
11.12	Lower Palm Canyon	2.6	500	⟳					🧒
11.13	Fern Canyon	6.5	1,000	⟳			🐎		
11.14	Pines-to-Palms	15	3,500	➚	🥾		🐎		
11.15	Jo Pond Trail	16	6,200	➚	🥾		🐎		
Chapter 12: SANTA ROSA MOUNTAINS									
12.1	Garstin Trail	3.6	1,000	⟳			🐎		
12.2	Murray Hill	7	1,700	➚			🐎		
12.3	Araby Trail	4.6	1,400	⟳			🐎		
12.4	Jane's Hoffbrau Oasis	2	700	➚		🚲	🐎		
12.5	Magnesia Spring Falls	2.5–9	varies	➚					

OVERVIEW OF HIKES (continued)

HIKE NUMBER	HIKE	DISTANCE (miles)	ELEVATION GAIN (feet)	TRAIL TYPE	BACKPACKING	MOUNTAIN BIKING	EQUESTRIANS	DOGS	KIDS
Chapter 12: SANTA ROSA MOUNTAINS (Continued)									
12.6	Bump and Grind Trail	4	1,100	loop		✓	✓		
12.7	Art Smith Trail	6+	1,300+	out-and-back		✓	✓		
12.8	Randall Henderson Loop	1.2+	300+	loop					✓
12.9	Living Desert Zoo and Gardens	5	800	loop					✓
12.10	Bear Creek Oasis	9	2,400	out-and-back			✓		
12.11	Boo Hoff Loop	12	2,200	loop			✓		
12.12	Stone Sentinel	4.4	1,000	out-and-back					
12.13	Guadalupe Trail	14	5,100	out-and-back	✓				
12.14	Sawmill Trail	16	3,900	out-and-back	✓			✓	
12.15	Horsethief Creek	4.5	900	out-and-back	✓		✓	✓	
12.16	Cactus Spring Trail	21	3,000	out-and-back	✓				
12.17	Martinez Mountain	17	4,300	out-and-back	✓				
12.18	Pinyon Trail	8.5	1,400	out-and-back		✓	✓	✓	
12.19	Rabbit Peak from the Salton Sea	16	6,800	out-and-back	✓				
12.20	Rabbit and Villager Peaks	21	7,900	out-and-back	✓				
12.21	Rabbit Peak from Clark Lake	15	6,100	out-and-back					
Chapter 13: COLORADO DESERT									
13.1	Ladder and Big Painted Canyons	4	750	loop					✓
13.2	Big Split Rock Canyon	2	400	out-and-back					✓
13.3	Never Ending Canyon	3.5	500	loop				✓	
13.4	Utah Canyon	4	500	out-and-back				✓	
13.5	The Grottos	7	1,500	loop				✓	
13.6	Black Butte	3	1,600	out-and-back					
13.7	Chuckwalla Mountain	2.8	1,600	out-and-back					
13.8	Stepladder Mountain	10	1,300	out-and-back					
13.9	Mopah Point	8	2,000	out-and-back					
Chapter 14: DESERT PRESERVES									
14.1	McCallum Nature Trail	2	100	out-and-back					✓
14.2	Pushwalla, Horseshoe, and Hidden Palms Loop	6	1,000	loop					
14.3	Moon Country–Willis Palms Loop	8	1,100	loop					
14.4	Big Morongo Canyon Preserve	0.6+	100	loop					✓
14.5	Pioneertown Mountains Preserve: Pipes Canyon Loop	6	1,100	loop				✓	
14.6	Pioneertown Mountains Preserve: Sawtooth Loop	5+	500+	loop			✓	✓	
14.7	Oak Glen Preserve	1.8	300	loop				✓	✓

TRAIL TYPE LEGEND: ⟳ = loop   ↗ = out-and-back   ↗ = point-to-point

OVERVIEW OF HIKES (continued)

HIKE NUMBER	HIKE	DISTANCE (miles)	ELEVATION GAIN (feet)	TRAIL TYPE	BACKPACKING	MOUNTAIN BIKING	EQUESTRIANS	DOGS	KIDS
Chapter 14: DESERT PRESERVES *(Continued)*									
14.8	Whitewater Preserve to Mission Creek Preserve	7	900	point-to-point			🐎	🐕	
14.9	Whitewater Preserve: Canyon View Loop	3.7	600	loop				🐕	
14.10	Whitewater Preserve: San Gorgonio Overlook	11+	1,500+	point-to-point/loop				🐕	
14.11	Dos Palmas Preserve	1	flat	loop				🐕	🧒
Chapter 15: JOSHUA TREE NATIONAL PARK: PARK BOULEVARD									
15.1	Maze and Window Rock Loop	6.5	1,100	loop					
15.2	Boy Scout Trail	8	−1,300	point-to-point	🥾				
15.3	Willow Hole	7	200	out-and-back					
15.4	Wonderland Traverse	6	−1,300	point-to-point					
15.5	Barker Dam Nature Trail	1.5	100	loop					🧒
15.6	Garrett's Arch	4.2	300	out-and-back					🧒
15.7	Wall Street Mill	1.4	100	out-and-back					🧒
15.8	Lost Horse Mine and Mountain	4	500	out-and-back					🧒
15.9	Ryan Mountain	3	1,000	out-and-back					
15.10	Queen Mountain	4	1,200	out-and-back					
15.11	Desert Queen Mine	1	300	out-and-back					🧒
15.12	Negro Hill	1.2	400	out-and-back					
15.13	Malapai Hill	1.5	500	out-and-back					🧒
15.14	Mount Inspiration	1.5	700	out-and-back					🧒
15.15	Mount Inspiration from the Coachella Valley	14	4,600	out-and-back					
15.16	Mount Minerva Hoyt	7	1,900	out-and-back					
15.17	Quail Mountain	13	1,800	point-to-point	🥾				
15.18	Skull Rock Nature Trail	1.7	200	loop					🧒
15.19	Split Rock	2	500	loop					🧒
15.20	Eagle Cliffs and Mine	3	900	out-and-back					🧒
15.21	Arch Rock Nature Trail	0.3	50	loop					🧒
15.22	Joshua Mountain	2.8	1,200	out-and-back					
15.23	California Riding and Hiking Trail	37	2,500	point-to-point	🥾		🐎		
Chapter 16: JOSHUA TREE NATIONAL PARK: BLACK ROCK AND COVINGTON									
16.1	Black Rock Canyon Panorama Loop	6.5	1,200	semiloop			🐎		
16.2	Eureka Peak	9	1,800	loop	🥾				
16.3	West Side Loop	4.5	900	loop			🐎		
16.4	High View Nature Trail	1.4	400	loop					🧒
16.5	Covington Crest	3	100	out-and-back			🐎		
16.6	Covington Loop	6	800	semiloop					

TRAIL TYPE LEGEND: ◯ = loop   C = semiloop   ↗ = out-and-back   ↗ = point-to-point

OVERVIEW OF HIKES (continued)

HIKE NUMBER	HIKE	DISTANCE (miles)	ELEVATION GAIN (feet)	TRAIL TYPE	BACKPACKING	MOUNTAIN BIKING	EQUESTRIANS	DOGS	KIDS
Chapter 17: JOSHUA TREE NATIONAL PARK: INDIAN COVE									
17.1	Indian Cove Nature Trail	0.6	100	loop					✓
17.2	Gunsight Loop	3	800	loop					
17.3	Rattlesnake Canyon	2.5	400	out-and-back					
17.4	Fortynine Palms Oasis	3	600	out-and-back					✓
Chapter 18: JOSHUA TREE NATIONAL PARK: EAST									
18.1	Pinto Mountain	9	2,700	out-and-back					
18.2	Fried Liver Wash	15	−1,500	out-and-back	✓				
18.3	Bernard and Little Berdoo Peaks	6	2,200	loop					
18.4	Mastodon Peak Loop	2.6	400	loop					✓
18.5	Lost Palms Oasis	7.5	700	out-and-back					
18.6	Eagle Mountain	10	2,500	out-and-back					
18.7	Munsen Palms	8	1,200	out-and-back					
18.8	Carey's Castle	8	1,200	out-and-back					
18.9	Spectre Point	13	3,200+	out-and-back					
Chapter 19: MOJAVE NATIONAL PRESERVE									
19.1	Kelso Dunes	3	500	out-and-back					
19.2	Hole-in-the-Wall	1.5	200	loop				✓	✓
19.3	Barber Peak Loop	5	800	loop				✓	
19.4	Mid Hills to Hole-in-the-Wall	8	600	out-and-back			✓	✓	
19.5	Table Mountain	4	1,100	out-and-back				✓	
19.6	Mitchell Caverns	1	100	out-and-back					✓
19.7	Edgar Peak	4.2	3,000	out-and-back					
19.8	Old Dad Mountain	5	2,000	out-and-back					
19.9	Lava Tube	0.5	100	out-and-back					✓
19.10	Teutonia Peak	3.2	700	out-and-back				✓	
19.11	Kessler Peak	4	1,100	loop					
19.12	Fort Piute	6	1,000	loop				✓	
19.13	Caruthers Canyon	2	400	out-and-back				✓	✓
19.14	New York Mountain	6	2,200	out-and-back					
19.15	Castle Peaks	2.2+	200+	out-and-back				✓	
19.16	Clark Mountain	2.8	1,500	out-and-back					
Chapter 20: MOJAVE TRAILS NATIONAL MONUMENT									
20.1	Afton Canyon	3.6	200	out-and-back			✓	✓	✓
20.2	Sheephole Mountain	4.5	2,300	out-and-back					
20.3	Pisgah Lava Tubes	2	300	out-and-back					✓
20.4	Amboy Crater	3	400	out-and-back				✓	✓
20.5	Cadiz Dunes	1	120	out-and-back					✓

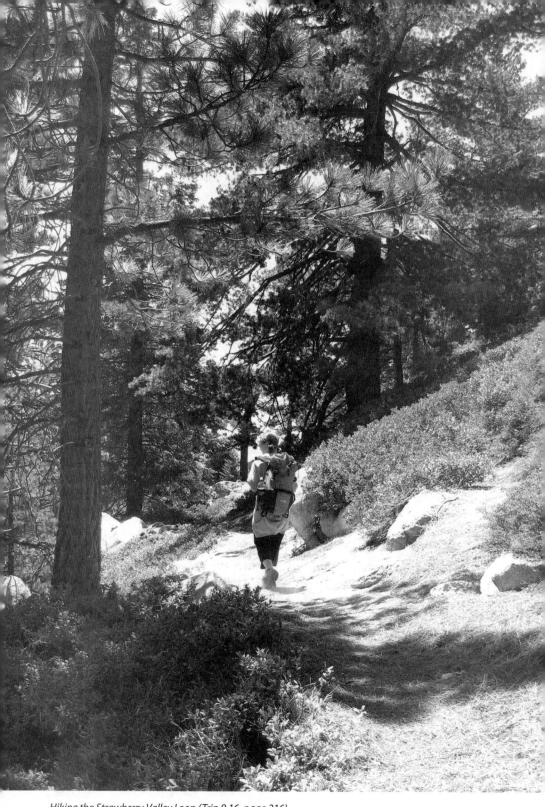

Hiking the Strawberry Valley Loop (Trip 9.16, page 216)

Introducing the Inland Empire

The origin of the name Inland Empire is shrouded in the mists of history, but one theory says it was coined by real estate developers to lure buyers to this purported paradise. The boundaries of the Inland Empire are even murkier. One definition, adopted in this guide, is that the Inland Empire spans Riverside and San Bernardino Counties. Though these boundaries are inexact, few would dispute that the Inland Empire is a hiker's paradise.

The Inland Empire is home to California's best and most diverse hiking south of the Sierra Nevada. The area encompasses Southern California's three tallest mountains along with six national parks and preserves. Hundreds of lesser-known but tremendously enjoyable hikes can be found just about anywhere you live or visit in this area. It's remarkable that these hikes, many of them within the peaceful tranquility of the mountains or desert, are located in the fastest-growing region of California, within a short drive of more than 15 million residents.

Before European invaders arrived, the Inland Empire was lightly populated by Native Americans who were keenly adept at living in the unforgiving deserts and mountains. The Spanish came in the late 16th century, established a few missions and ranches, and named the major geographical features, but considered the region poorly suited for colonization. A hardy band of Mormon settlers were the first white Americans to arrive in numbers, coming by wagon over Cajon Pass in 1851; they established an outpost near present-day San Bernardino but soon returned to Salt Lake City.

The development of railroads and irrigation drastically changed the Southern Californian landscape. The citrus industry took root in the 1870s, and soon industrious farmers (one of the author's great-grandparents included) flocked to the area to seek their fortune growing oranges and shipping them back to the East Coast.

California joined the United States in 1850 in the wake of the Gold Rush, and the government moved promptly to survey the new state. In November of 1852, Colonel Henry Washington and a team of surveyors made the arduous ascent of San Bernardino Peak, where they established the initial point from which all of Southern California was measured. Curious hikers can take in the expansive views where his survey monument still stands on the shoulder of the peak. Base Line Road loosely follows his survey line from Highland to San Dimas.

When explorers and miners first set foot in the San Bernardino Mountains, they found a vast forest of great pines, firs, and cedars. The lumber potential wasn't overlooked and, starting in 1852, wagon roads were painstakingly carved up the foothills and the huge trees were felled to build the burgeoning cities of Los Angeles and San Bernardino. The loggers worked with great diligence, and by the end of the 19th century most of the forest had been chopped to the ground. By this point, the interests of the cities began to conflict with the interests of the lumber companies: residents and ranchers were dependent on the

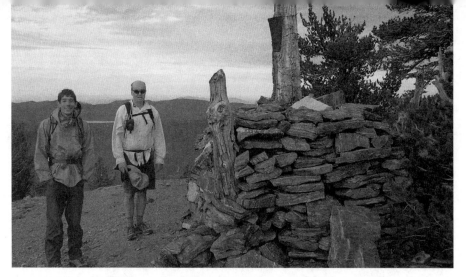

Colonel Washington's Monument on San Bernardino Peak (Trip 5.9, page 115)

mountain streams for their water, and the mountain watersheds, denuded of timber, were becoming polluted and drying up.

Intensive lobbying led to the Forest Reserve Act of 1891, which gave the president authority to protect forests on public lands. In the next two years, Benjamin Harrison established Forest Reserves in the San Gabriel, San Bernardino, and Santa Ana Mountains. At first, protections were lax, but in 1905, the reserves were reorganized under the leadership of Gifford Pinchot. He renamed them National Forests and laid the foundation of today's Forest Service.

More-recent stories of the Inland Empire are chronicled in each chapter of this book. A recurring theme is the tension between development and conservation—the same threads continue to play out today as we balance the benefits of access with the threat of loving our wilderness to death. Please tread lightly so that our grandchildren can enjoy the same special places that we do today.

Geography and Weather

The greater Los Angeles Basin is cut off from the vast Mojave and Colorado Deserts by three tall mountain ranges: the San Gabriels, San Bernardinos, and San Jacintos. The San Jacintos form the northern end of the Peninsular Ranges that stretch all the way to the tip of Baja California. The San Gabriels and San Bernardinos are part of the Transverse Ranges, an anomalous mountain group running east and west rather than the prevailing southeast to northwest direction. These complex mountains were pushed up by the San Andreas Fault at a bend along the interface of the Pacific and North American Plates. The topography of Southern California strongly influences the weather patterns that hikers will encounter.

The Los Angeles Basin exhibits a classic Mediterranean climate, with rainy winters and dry summers. In the summer, a high-pressure system over the eastern Pacific dominates the weather patterns, ensuring warm, dry weather. The high-pressure system also creates an inversion layer over the cooler ocean, forming a marine layer of low clouds known as "June gloom." Moreover, this inversion layer traps the pollution produced by Southern California's factories and freeways, resulting in notorious smog. While aggressive air-quality management has led to a gradual improvement over the past four decades, there are still days when the air in the basin is unhealthy for vigorous activity. On these days, climbing above 5,000 feet dramatically improves air quality and views.

The Inland Empire experiences hot summers, routinely over 100°F. In the winter, the high-pressure system shifts, and Southern California is exposed to intermittent Pacific storms that carry the bulk of the year's rain. Occasional cold fronts can bring subfreezing temperatures, which were the bane of the citrus farmers.

The San Bernardinos and San Jacintos present a formidable barrier to moisture moving in from the Pacific, so the lands to the east and north receive far less rainfall. (For example, Riverside averages 10 inches of rain a year.) The exposed western slopes of the San Bernardino Mountains receive 40 inches or more of rain and snow, while Palm Springs, in the rain shadow, averages just 6 inches annually. Beyond these mountains lie the legendary deserts of the American Southwest, which stretch all the way to the Rocky Mountains.

The deserts are divided into two major regions. The Sonoran Desert is the lower and hotter, extending south and east from Joshua Tree National Park to Mexico and central Arizona. The portion of the Sonoran Desert in California is called the Colorado Desert; it receives the occasional Pacific storm, which can lead to outstanding wildflowers in the spring. Nevertheless, when the town of Ontario is cloudy on a dreary February morning, you can likely drive to Palm Springs and find clear blue skies and temperatures perfect for hiking. The Mojave Desert is higher and cooler, extending from Joshua Tree northward toward the Great Basin. Winter snowfall is not uncommon at the higher elevations. However, hiking any of the deserts on a summer afternoon is an activity only for the perversely masochistic.

Not surprisingly, the interfaces between these climate zones experience unusual weather. In particular, hot, dry winds exceeding 70 miles per hour blow through Cajon and Banning Passes several times a year. These winds—called *Santa Ana winds* and occurring most often in the spring and fall—form when a high-pressure region develops over the Great Basin, forcing warm air down through the narrow passes and out to the ocean. Santa Ana winds have been known to topple big rigs on the 15 Freeway and have fanned the flames of the most devastating wildfires in Southern California. Banning Pass has some of the most consistently strong winds; the famous wind farm along the 10 Freeway converts some to electricity. Hiking in these strong winds tends to be unpleasant, but the wind speed drops dramatically as soon as you get away from the mouths of the passes.

Safety

Hiking is a relatively safe activity. As an example, fewer than one in a million Yosemite National Park visitors have a fatal hiking accident in a typical year. When you compare this statistic with those for car accidents—approximately one fatality per 100 million miles driven—the risk of getting killed while driving to the hike apparently exceeds the risk of dying in the outdoors.

Nevertheless, hiking does have its own special risks, and prudent hikers manage these risks through preparation and awareness. Always be prepared for an emergency, even on a short hike. The bare essentials to have along include the following:

- Water
- Map and compass or GPS (and knowledge of how to navigate)
- Headlamp
- Matches or lighter
- Extra food
- Extra clothing (enough to survive an unplanned night out)

Other items that can be very helpful:

- Whistle
- Sunscreen, sunglasses, hat
- Toilet paper
- First aid kit
- Cell phone (*note:* don't count on a signal in the wilderness)

Outdoor perils include weather extremes, slippery footing, getting lost, old mine shafts, hazardous animals and plants, and contaminated drinking water. The best way to learn about safety in the outdoors is to travel with smart and experienced hikers.

Get a weather report before you go, but also come prepared for any unexpected change in the weather. Winter and early spring are the rainy season in the Inland Empire, and snow is common at higher elevations. Hypothermia is a particular risk if your clothes get wet; carry warm, waterproof clothes. The summer can be dangerously hot in the desert, leading to heat exhaustion and heatstroke—temperatures can exceed 100°F as early as April and as late as October—so carry a generous supply of water, even on short hikes. Summer afternoons are also the most common time for thunderstorms over the mountains; don't get caught exposed on a mountaintop in an electrical storm or in a canyon during a flash flood.

Cross-country hiking often involves walking on unstable boulders, where it's easy to slip and twist an ankle. The best way to develop cross-country travel skills is through practice on easier hikes. Many hikers find that a trekking pole (or two) helps with balance and relieves one's knees on downhill trails.

Ice is a much more serious threat—highly experienced hikers have died in falls on Mount Baldy and San Gorgonio in recent years. Ice can remain in north-facing gullies long after most of the mountain appears free of snow; under these conditions, carry an ice ax and crampons, and know how to use them. If you're unfamiliar with these tools, take a mountaineering class before you try them on your own.

Always let somebody know where you're going and when you expect to return. If you do get lost, the best advice is to stay in one spot. If search-and-rescue teams know where

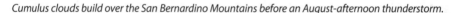

Cumulus clouds build over the San Bernardino Mountains before an August-afternoon thunderstorm.

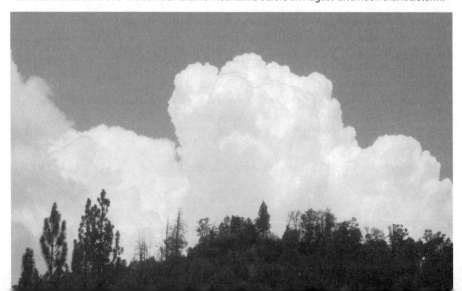

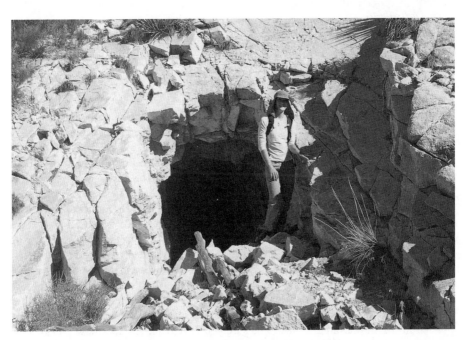

Adit (horizontal mine shaft) on Silver Peak near Holcomb Valley

to look for you, they're almost certain to find you. Make yourself easy to spot by wearing brightly colored clothes (red, for example, is a better choice than green).

With sufficient water and clothing, an unplanned night out is inconvenient but not catastrophic. A fire is helpful in an emergency for warmth and visibility, but be sure to thoroughly clear the area first. (In 2003, a lost hunter set a fire in the Cleveland National Forest to signal rescuers. Unfortunately, it got out of control, fanned by Santa Ana winds. The Cedar Fire ended up burning more than a quarter-million acres and 2,000 homes and killing 15 people.)

Because hiking alone is statistically more dangerous than hiking with a group, the cautions about letting somebody know where you're going are even more important when hiking solo. Ask your friend or family member to notify law enforcement if you're not back by an agreed-upon time.

On the other hand, being lost is partly a matter of perspective. Henry David Thoreau wrote, "If a person lost would conclude that after all he is not lost, he is not beside himself, but standing in his own old shoes on the very spot where he is, and that for the time being he will live there; but the places that have known him, they are lost,—how much anxiety and danger would vanish." With proper navigation equipment and careful attention to one's surroundings, experienced hikers may not always be certain exactly where they are, but they should certainly be able to get to a known destination.

Many trips in this book lead to old mines or through areas of historical or active mining. Resist the temptation to enter these places—hikers have died while exploring some of the mines near trails in this book. Besides the obvious risks of structural collapse and hikers falling down shafts, mines carry other hazards, including hantavirus from rodents, poison gas, and even radiation. Keep an especially close eye on children near mines.

Rattlesnakes, scorpions, bees, ticks, bears, and mountain lions are occasionally encountered in the wilds. Rattlesnakes want to stay away from you at least as much as you want to stay away from them. About 75% of snakebites happen to men between the ages of 19 and

30 years, and most of these bites occur when the victim is drunk and/or playing with the snake. Don't put your feet or hands anywhere that you can't see. If you have to cross dense grass or brush, make plenty of noise to warn away any snakes. In the unlikely event that you get bitten, seek medical attention as quickly as possible.

Scorpions sting with their barbed tails. The only dangerous scorpions in California live near the Colorado River; the stings of scorpions encountered on hikes in this book are painful but no more poisonous than bee stings. If you leave your boots outside while camping, turn them over and shake them first in the morning in case a critter has crawled in overnight.

Africanized bees, popularly known as killer bees, migrated to California and elsewhere in the US after escaping from a botched agricultural experiment in Brazil in the 1950s. Some have established hives in Joshua Tree National Park. Africanized bees are aggressive and tend to attack in large numbers when disturbed. The best way to avoid trouble with bees is to not disturb them. If you're pursued by a swarm, run away as fast as possible and seek shelter. Seek medical attention if you get stung, particularly if you're allergic to bee venom.

Ticks are found in the brush in California. They range in size from poppy seeds to sesame seeds. Ticks drop onto hikers and like to crawl to a protected spot before they attach themselves and suck blood. If you must walk through brush, wearing long pants and gaiters (worn over the boot and lower leg) eliminates many opportunities for ticks to reach your skin. Bug repellents, such as those containing DEET, are also effective at deterring ticks. Be sensitive to slight sensations that might be a clue that a tick is crawling on you, and check yourself in the shower after a hike to be sure you haven't picked up a tick. The greatest problem with tick bites is that deer ticks sometimes carry Lyme disease. They usually must be attached for at least 36 hours to convey the disease to a human. Symptoms of Lyme disease include rashes, fever, headache, fatigue, and joint pain. Lyme disease is treated with antibiotics and is readily curable if treated when symptoms first appear.

Grizzly bears, once common enough to be celebrated on the California state flag, were hunted to extinction in the state by 1922. Fortunate hikers might still see evidence of black bears: scat, footprints, or even the back end of a bear shambling into the woods. Black bears seldom cause trouble for day hikers in Southern California, but it's prudent to store your food in a bear-proof canister while backpacking in bear habitat such as the San Gorgonio Wilderness. Canisters are available for rent at the Mill Creek Ranger Station and the Barton Flats Visitor Center (see Appendix B, page 463). Bears are usually more afraid of people than the other way around; thus, attacks are extremely rare. Don't get between a mother bear and her cubs, though. If you do see a bear on the trail, stop and let it pass.

Mountain lions, also called cougars, are North America's largest cats. They're notoriously shy, and hikers should consider themselves lucky if they see one in a lifetime. Mountain lion attacks were almost unheard of before 1986, but the encroachment of humans on their habitat has increased pressure on the cats and made them more aggressive. Fourteen verified attacks, three of them fatal, have occurred in the US and Canada over the last three decades. If you do encounter a mountain lion, shout loudly, wave your hands, throw rocks, and make a point of not looking like cat food. If attacked, *fight back*—don't run or play dead. Children and petite women have been the predominant victims. Hiking in groups is always safer. Don't allow young children to run out of sight, especially in areas where mountain lions are known to live.

Hazardous plants include poison oak, cactus, and yucca. Poison oak, not a true oak, is a plant all hikers should learn to identify. It has shiny green or red leaflets in clusters of three. It grows as a vine in shady canyons and as a bush or dense thicket in direct sun. Moist, shady canyon bottoms are the most common place that you'll encounter poison oak on trips in this book. Poison oak secretes an oil called urushiol that causes a highly irritating

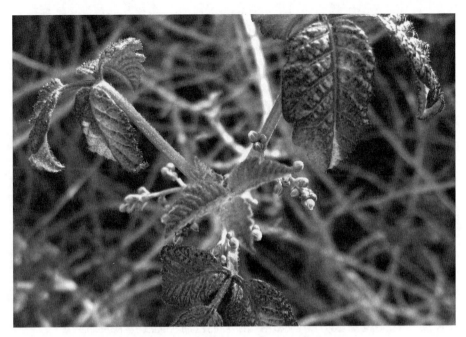

"Leaves of three, let it be": poison oak thicket in the San Gabriel foothills

rash in more than 80% of people. The rash is occasionally serious enough to require hospitalization. In winter, the leafless stalks still carry the oil and cause skin irritation.

Even if you're lucky enough to be immune to urushiol, your immunity can wear off after repeated exposure. Wearing long pants helps reduce your risk of contact. If you do come in contact with poison oak, wash with soap and cold water as soon as possible after exposure. Also, take care when handling clothes that might have been exposed, and wash the clothes thoroughly in hot water. A rash usually develops about 24 hours after exposure and lasts up to two weeks. Antihistamines can help treat severe rashes.

Yucca and cactus have sharp tips or barbs that can inflict nasty jabs to the unwary hiker. Long pants and gaiters can help, especially when hiking cross-country through the desert, but a direct hit by a yucca will penetrate even the sturdiest of clothes. The best defense is alertness.

Cactus barbs tend to lodge in your skin. Jumping cholla cactus get their name because of their propensity to latch onto anyone who comes nearby. Don't try to remove a cactus barb with your hands; you'll only get it embedded in your fingers. Tweezers, pliers, or a wide-toothed comb are helpful, but a pair of rocks will do in a pinch.

Unfortunately, untreated water in Southern California should generally be considered unsafe to drink. Thoroughly boil it first, or use a pump or chemical treatment kit available from outdoor equipment stores. The availability of water is also a problem; springs and creeks can dry up. Never get in a situation where you depend on finding water in a spring or creek but can't locate a reliable source if the first is dry.

Vehicle break-ins, while rare, do occur in Southern California. Don't leave valuables in your vehicle. Report incidents to law enforcement.

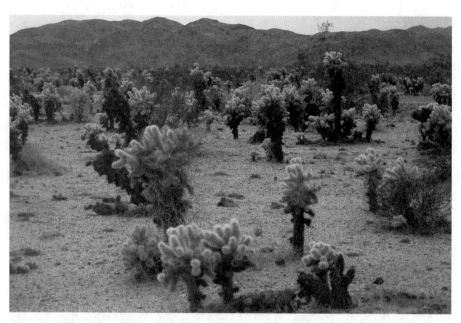

Cute but not-so-cuddly teddy bear cholla cactus in Pinto Basin, Joshua Tree National Park. Fallen stem joints are a common desert hazard.

Courtesy

While you enjoy yourself afoot and afield, follow simple courtesies so that others will enjoy themselves too, and so that the wilderness will be there for future generations to discover.

The general rule is to *leave no trace*. It's common sense not to litter or vandalize our wild places, and it's even better form to pick up litter when you come across it. Don't cut switchbacks; this causes erosion. Deposit human waste in a cathole at least 200 feet from water. Limit campfires to already existing fire rings—when practical, cook on a gas stove, which doesn't consume wood or scar the rocks. (Some wilderness areas have more specific campfire rules.) Collecting rocks, pinecones, wildflowers, Native American artifacts, and so forth is forbidden in many areas. Leave these things for the next visitors to enjoy too. If you must smoke, do so seated in an area cleared of flammable materials. Serious wildfires have been caused by cigarettes. In areas where dogs are allowed, they should be well behaved and generally must be leashed. Leave loud and aggressive dogs at home.

Each jurisdiction has its own specific regulations, and visitors are responsible for knowing them.

Camping

There are many established campgrounds in the Inland Empire. To assure yourself a site, make reservations. Many of the most popular campgrounds fill up well ahead of time in high season; for example, Joshua Tree is heavily visited in the spring and fall. Camping fees have been on the rise and are approaching $20 in some locations.

The best deals in the National Forests are the so-called yellow-post campsites. These dispersed primitive sites are mostly sprinkled along dirt roads in the San Gabriel, San Bernardino, and San Jacinto Mountains and are marked with numbered yellow posts. They charge no fees, and you rarely have to deal with noisy neighbors. You can't reserve these sites, but it's rare for all of the sites in an area to be occupied. Keep your eyes out as you explore the back roads, or call the local ranger station (see Appendix B, page 463, for a list) to get more information.

Yellow-post sites in locations covered here include the areas northwest of Lytle Creek off Forest Road 3N06, Keller Peak Road near Running Springs, the ridge south above Big Bear off Forest Road 2N10, the Coon Creek Jumpoff area northeast of San Gorgonio on Forest Road 1N02, and Fuller Ridge Road (4S01) on San Jacinto above Black Mountain Campground.

Backpackers may camp at established sites along many trails. Regulations regarding backcountry camping vary from area to area, so check with one of the information sources in Appendix B for details.

Using This Book

This book is organized into 20 chapters, each covering a different region of the Inland Empire. It's not intended to be read cover to cover—instead, browse for trips that look interesting, or turn to a specific chapter when you're looking for hikes in an area that you plan to visit.

TRIP SUMMARIES

Each trip begins with a summary of key information to help you choose the right hiking adventure. Here's a quick rundown.

DISTANCE

The total distance of the trip is given. For out-and-back trips, both directions are included. Some trips have alternative paths that change the distance. Your mileage may vary.

Decimal distances such as 2.3 miles are generally accurate to within a tenth of a mile, while integer distances such as 7 miles are accurate to within a half mile. I measured distances with a GPS, but two different GPS units carried along the same trail by the same person simultaneously can report substantially different distances, so accuracy should not be overestimated. Total trip distance is generally rounded to the nearest mile for longer trips.

HIKING TIME

An estimate of the hiking time is given. Note that this is just the time spent walking: it doesn't include breaks, lunch, or time to smell the flowers. Plus, the time is only an average; trail runners will clearly be faster, and many hikers prefer a more leisurely saunter. If you're carrying a heavy backpack, the times may double. The very strenuous trips in this book assume that you are exceptionally fit and will be walking faster than on the more moderate trips.

ELEVATION GAIN

Elevation gain accounts for the entire elevation a hiker must climb. For example, if a trail starts at 500 feet and climbs to a 2,500-foot summit but has a 400-foot dip in the middle, the elevation gain for the round-trip is 2,800 feet because the hiker must climb out of the dip in both directions. You can reduce the elevation gain for some one-way trips by hiking in the downhill rather than uphill direction.

DIFFICULTY

The difficulty depends on the terrain as well as the distance and elevation. There are four general categories, each roughly twice as difficult as the previous:

EASY Suitable for families with young hikers

MODERATE Suitable for anyone of ordinary fitness

STRENUOUS Suitable for strong and highly motivated hikers

EXTREMELY STRENUOUS Profoundly long and difficult—harder than a marathon

Extremely strenuous trips are not recommended unless you are already intimately familiar with an area and highly skilled at navigation, are in excellent physical condition, and are equipped to spend an unplanned night in the wilderness. Descriptions of extremely strenuous trips tend to be less detailed.

Some trips in this book involve what rock climbers refer to as **third-class climbing:** scrambling up rocks using your hands and feet. The handholds and footholds covered here are large and fairly obvious, but be aware that a fall could cause serious injury or death. *Such climbing is not advisable for hikers who are uncomfortable with heights or unsure of their balance.* If your group includes a competent rock climber and some inexperienced hikers, the climber might belay the novices on a rope.

Fourth- and fifth-class climbing involve smaller holds and more-severe consequences for a fall, so even experienced climbers will likely want a rope. None of the main trips in this book require fourth- or fifth-class climbing, but interesting rock climbs near the trips are mentioned occasionally.

TRAIL USE

All trips are open to hikers. I've also noted if the trip is well suited for dogs, equestrians, mountain bikers, families with kids, or backpackers.

BEST TIMES

The best times listed are generally those where the trailhead can be reached and the trail isn't excessively hot or covered in snow. If you have the proper equipment and experience, however, many of these trips are great fun in the snow on skis or snowshoes.

AGENCY

The office of the agency that manages the area is listed. Contact information for the agencies appears in Appendix B.

PERMITS

Many wilderness areas require permits for entry. Some popular areas have quotas that fill up long in advance on summer weekends, so plan ahead.

Most of the popular trailheads in Angeles and San Bernardino National Forests require parked cars to display a **National Forest Adventure Pass.** These passes cost $5 for a day or $30 for a year. You may also use an **America the Beautiful Pass,** which covers admission to national parks and most other federal lands.

In the 2014 *Fragosa et al. v. U.S. Forest Service* decision, the California Central District Court ruled that people who do not use facilities and services such as restrooms, picnic tables, and trash cans cannot be required to buy a pass to park in or enter a National Forest. The Forest Service has agreed to designate free parking close to developed trailheads, but signage is still in flux.

National Forest Wilderness Permits are different from Adventure Passes. The latter cost money and are required to park your car at developed sites; Wilderness Permits are free, sometimes subject to quota limits, and required to enter many wilderness areas. For more information on both, visit www.fs.fed.us/visit/passes-permits.

Anyone 16 years of age or older must possess and wear a **California Sport Fishing License** while angling. Licenses, good for one calendar year, can be purchased from the California Department of Fish and Wildlife or from authorized agents. See wildlife.ca.gov/licensing /fishing for more information.

Access and permit fees are subject to change, so check the resources in Appendix B for the latest information before you set out on your hike.

MAPS

Locator maps for the trails appear in each chapter. These maps may be sufficient for easy trips and are also helpful for newer trails and cross-country routes that don't appear on published maps. But for many trips, there's no substitute for a good topographic map and knowing how to use it. Most of the maps described below can be purchased from local outdoor equipment stores, ranger stations, and rei.com, as well as directly from the publishers.

For trips in this book, maps are categorized as *optional, recommended,* or *required.* If you already know an area well, you may be able to do without a recommended map. Required maps, however, are essential for successful navigation.

Tom Harrison Maps (tomharrisonmaps.com) publishes the best maps for many popular regions in California. The maps highlight the critical features, are waterproof, and are significantly more affordable than buying the equivalent set of U.S. Geological Survey (USGS) quad maps. Harrison's relevant maps in the Inland Empire include the following:

Map Legend			
Freeway	════════	Stream or canyon	
Highway	────────		
Paved road	────────	Body of water	
Dirt road	============		
Trail	------------	Trip number	**1**
Cross-country route	··············	Range of trips	**1-3**
Ranger station/ visitor center	⌂	Point of interest	•
Picnic area	⊞	Peak	▲
Campground	◭	Spring	∿
Fire lookout	⌺	Oasis	⍓
Mine	✕		
Gate	•—•	North arrow	

- *Angeles High Country*
- *Mount Baldy & Cucamonga Wilderness*
- *San Gorgonio Wilderness*
- *San Jacinto Wilderness*
- *Mojave National Preserve*

The **Santa Rosa & San Jacinto Mountains National Monument** trail map, published in 2008, is by far the best map for hikes in this area. This large, waterproof map shows trails that are not depicted anywhere else and covers a vast amount of territory. It can be purchased through the monument visitor center at desertmountains.org. **Note:** Don't mix this up with the less-detailed monument brochure.

National Geographic publishes **Trails Illustrated**–series maps of Joshua Tree National Park and Mojave National Preserve showing many trails (including several described in this book) that don't appear on the Tom Harrison map. Trails Illustrated maps can be purchased from natgeomaps.com.

The entry fee to the **Indian Canyons** trail complex south of Palm Springs includes a helpful trail guide. A larger trail map with contour lines is available at the Trading Post at the trailhead, but this map is unnecessary unless you plan to hike some of the more obscure trails. Free digital maps and downloadable GPS tracks are available at the websites for the Indian Canyons and Tahquitz Canyon (see page 250).

In other regions, **USGS** 7.5-minute topographic maps are the next best choice. Each map covers approximately 7 by 9 miles and has contours at 40-foot or 80-foot intervals. USGS maps are sold at some hiking stores or can be ordered from store.usgs.gov; they're also available in electronic format. For example, you can print free maps from natgeomaps.com/trail -maps/pdf-quads or buy them on CD with National Geographic TOPO!

The **San Bernardino National Forest Atlas** contains 42 USGS 7.5-minute maps shrunk to fit on 8.5- by 11-inch pages and covers the entire San Bernardino National Forest, including the Mount Baldy area, the western San Bernardino Mountains, the Big Bear area, the San Gorgonio Wilderness, and the San Jacinto area. The atlas is the most cost-effective way to obtain maps covering the trails in this national forest. It can be purchased from national foreststore.com.

Finding some of the trailheads can be challenging, especially on the maze of ever-changing dirt roads. **AAA** maps provide good general coverage of the area and are free to members. The *San Bernardino Mountains Guide* map covers the western San Bernardinos, Big Bear, and San Gorgonio areas. The *San Diego Region* map covers Palm Springs, the Santa Rosa Mountains, and the Mecca Hills. The *San Bernardino County* map covers the vast county at a coarse level of detail, and includes Mojave National Preserve.

The U.S. Forest Service's **San Bernardino National Forest** map covers the roads through the entire forest.

Finally, the book **San Bernardino Mountain Trails** (Wilderness Press) includes a detailed foldout map covering the National Forest and the San Gorgonio and San Jacinto areas.

DRIVING DIRECTIONS

Many of these trips are reached by dirt roads, described in this book as **excellent, good, fair,** or **four-wheel-drive (4WD)**. Conventional passenger vehicles should have no trouble with excellent and good roads. Driven slowly and carefully, they can often navigate fair dirt roads too, but high clearance makes driving on such roads easier. 4WD roads have large rocks, serious ruts, or sandy sections that make the appropriate vehicle advisable, but an experienced driver in a 2WD pickup truck can likely handle these roads as well.

Forest Service roads and trails are identified by a four-character code, such as **7W02**, that appears on some maps and signposts. These codes are listed in parentheses after the road or trail name to help identify the route.

Mountain and desert roads are constantly changing. Roads get washed out and covered with debris. New roads are constructed and old ones are rerouted. Use your discretion.

Hiking with a GPS

GPS technology has revolutionized hiking. While navigational skills, a map and compass, and experience will always be critical, a GPS unit can make finding the trailhead or following the trail significantly easier. Properly used, a GPS also adds a level of safety by helping you find your way home even through darkness, fog, or snow. The locator maps include GPS waypoints for trailheads, destinations, and critical points along the hikes. Entering coordinates and receiving turn-by-turn driving directions to an unfamiliar trailhead is especially convenient. That said, all of the hikes in the book can be done without a GPS.

GPS tracks and waypoints can be downloaded from the web into many GPS units and also displayed on a map using software such as Google Earth, MapSource, or National Geographic TOPO! Be sure to use the WGS84 datum.

The GPS coordinates listed in this book include latitude and longitude, followed by altitude. Latitude and longitude are listed in degrees and decimal minutes. For the purposes of estimating distances on a map, 1 minute equals approximately 1 mile.[1]

Note that GPS data isn't foolproof—it often contains errors of up to 50 feet horizontally and even more vertically—so don't worry if your position varies slightly from a coordinate in this book. Also, note that GPS units have poor or nonexistent reception under trees and in canyons, have limited battery life, and occasionally lock up during normal use. Carry spare batteries, and know how to navigate on your own if your GPS fails. Smartphone apps such as Gaia GPS and BackCountry Navigator are sufficient for much hiking and have better-quality maps than conventional GPS units, but these apps will deplete your battery quickly and presently can't be relied upon to track your hike for a full day.

Electronic Supplements

The free **eTrails** app for iOS complements this book. It contains high-quality maps and waypoints for the trips in this guidebook, as well as for the Pacific Crest Trail and several other books. It also helps automate driving directions from your present position to the trailheads. Download eTrails from the Mac App Store; in the app, go to the menu tab, select "AAIE2e" as the book, and then pick the hike(s) that interests you.

GPS tracks and waypoints for most of the trips in this book can also be downloaded from eTrails.net.

---

1 A minute of latitude is technically 1 nautical mile, or 1.15 ordinary (statute) miles. A minute of longitude varies with your distance from the equator but is almost exactly 1 statute mile in the Inland Empire.

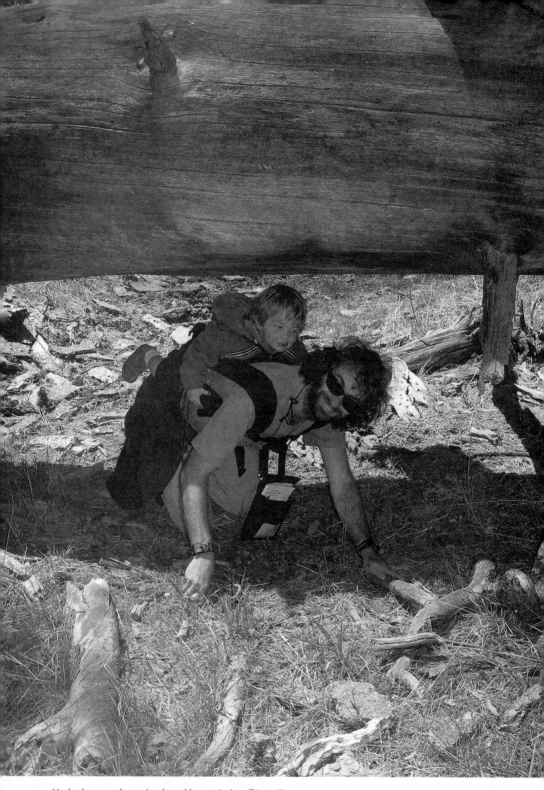

Under-log crawl near Lookout Mountain (see Trip 1.6)

chapter 1

San Gabriel Mountains National Monument: Mount Baldy Area

Mount Baldy, also known as Mount San Antonio, is one of the four towering saints standing watch over the Inland Empire. At 10,064 feet, it stands well above any other summit in the San Gabriel Mountains and is taller than the Zugspitze, Germany's highest peak. The bare, snowcapped top is readily recognizable from great distances in Southern California and constantly reassures tens of millions of suburban residents that wilderness is within sight. In 1923, Charles Francis Saunders wrote of Baldy in *The Southern Sierras of California,* "If you have anything of the Californian in you, you mark it for the objective of an outing sometime." The summit has been a Southern California hiker's favorite for more than a century now.

Numerous tall peaks surrounding Mount Baldy also offer superb hiking opportunities. The 44,000-acre Sheep Mountain Wilderness to the west is the largest roadless area in the San Gabriel Mountains. The 12,000-acre Cucamonga Wilderness to the southeast protects many of the best hiking opportunities in Southern California. Between the two wilderness areas are the quiet mountain resort of Mount Baldy Village and a small ski area that offers excellent runs immediately after good winter storms.

San Gabriel Mountains National Monument, designated by President Obama in 2014, encompasses the western portion of the area in this chapter as well as much of the Angeles National Forest to the west. Monument status has not yet brought much more resources to the understaffed rangers in this popular area.

Sheep Mountain Wilderness is named for the desert bighorn sheep (*Ovis canadensis nelsoni*) that once roamed these mountains in large herds. Their numbers plummeted from about 750 in 1982 to about 90 in 1995, most likely because of predation by mountain lions, but they've slowly recovered and number almost 300 due to conservation efforts. Sightings are not uncommon near the Mount Baldy Bowl and in the more remote parts of the wilderness.

A wilderness permit is required to enter the Cucamonga Wilderness and can be obtained, at no charge, in person or by mail from the Mount Baldy Visitor Center or Lytle Creek Ranger Station (see Appendix B, page 463). Most hikers enter this area via the Icehouse Canyon Trail. Campfires are not allowed at any backcountry campsites; bring a camp stove. A fire permit is required for the use of a stove. Dogs are permitted on a leash no longer than 6 feet. Leave vicious or noisy dogs at home.

A wilderness permit is required to enter Sheep Mountain Wilderness from the East Fork Trailhead only. The only trip that this affects is Iron Mountain (Trip 1.13). A free self-issue permit can be obtained at the trailhead.

Continued on page 18

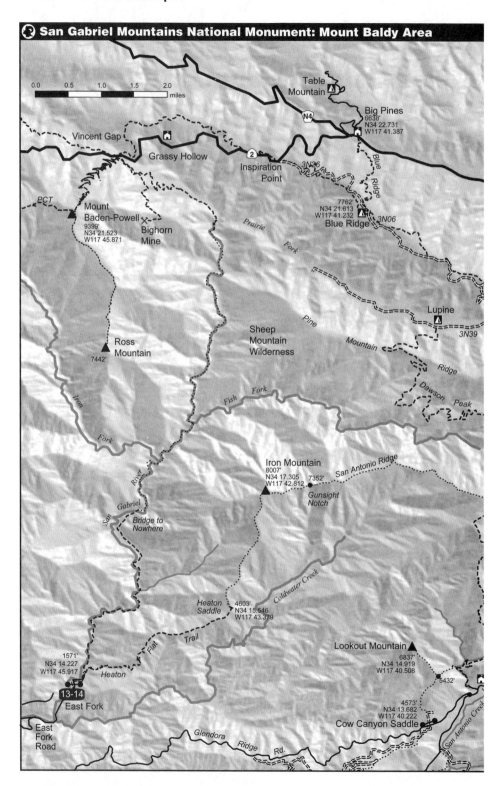

San Gabriel Mountains National Monument: Mount Baldy Area

Table Mountain

Big Pines
6638'
N34 22.731
W117 41.387

N4

Vincent Gap

Grassy Hollow

2

Inspiration Point

3N26

Blue Ridge

PCT

Mount Baden-Powell
9399'
N34 21.523
W117 45.871

Bighorn Mine

7762'
N34 21.613
W117 41.232

Blue Ridge

3N06

Prairie

Fork

Lupine

3N39

Ross Mountain
7442'

Sheep Mountain Wilderness

Pine

Mountain

Ridge

Iron

Fork

Fish

Fork

Dawson   Peak

River

Iron Mountain
8007'
N34 17.305
W117 42.812

7352'

San Antonio Ridge

Gunsight Notch

Gabriel

San

Bridge to Nowhere

Coldwater Creek

Heaton Saddle

4603'
N34 15.546
W117 43.379

Flat

Trail

1571'
N34 14.227
W117 45.917

Heaton

Lookout Mountain
6837'
N34 14.919
W117 40.508

5432'

13-14

East Fork

4573'
N34 13.682
W117 40.222

Cow Canyon Saddle

San Antonio Creek

East Fork Road

Glendora   Ridge   Rd.

0.0   0.5   1.0   1.5   2.0
miles

(Trips 1.1–1.16)

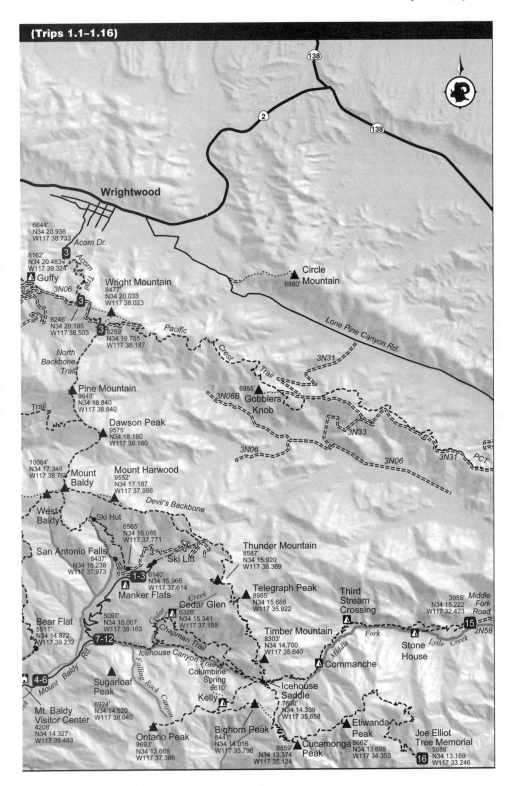

138

2

138

Wrightwood

6644'
N34 20.936
W117 38.733 Acorn Dr.

8162'
N34 20.483 3
W117 39.324

Guffy   Acorn Trail
3N06   Wright Mountain
           8477'
           N34 20.033
           W117 38.023

3

8246'
N34 20.195   3 8259'
W117 38.503   N34 19.755
                W117 38.187   Pacific

North
Backbone   Crest
Trail   3N31

Pine Mountain   6955'
9648'   Gobblers
N34 18.840   3N06B   Knob
W117 38.640

Trail   Dawson Peak
               9575'
               N34 18.180   3N33
               W117 38.160

                                3N06
10064'
N34 17.348   3N06   3N31   PCT
W117 38.762 Mount   Mount Harwood
             Baldy   9552'
                      N34 17.187
                      W117 37.986   Devil's Backbone

West
Baldy   Ski Hut
                6565'
                N34 16.085
San Antonio Falls W117 37.771
           6437'   Thunder Mountain
           N34 16.238 Ski Lift 8587'
           W117 37.973   N34 15.920
                    6140'   W117 36.369
                    N34 15.966
                    W117 37.614
            1-3   Third   3955' Middle
           Manker Flats Creek   Stream   N34 15.222 Fork
                    Cedar Glen   Telegraph Peak Crossing W117 32.423 Road
           5097'   6326'   8985'
           N34 15.007 N34 15.341 N34 15.688
Bear Flat W117 38.163 W117 37.188 W117 35.922   15
5511'   Cedar   2N58
N34 14.872 Chapman Trail Timber Mountain   Fork
W117 39.232 7-12   8303'   Stone   Lyle Creek
            Icehouse Canyon Trail N34 14.700 House
                          W117 35.640 Middle Fork
                     Columbine
                     Spring   Commanche
4-6   6610'
  Mount Baldy Rd.   Kelly   Icehouse
           Sugarloaf   Saddle
           Peak   7600'
           6924'   N34 14.339
Mt. Baldy N34 14.520 Falling Rock Canyon W117 35.658
Visitor Center W117 38.040
4208'   Etiwanda
N34 14.327   Ontario Peak   Bighorn Peak Peak   Joe Elliot
W117 39.483   8693'   8441'   8662' Tree Memorial
                  N34 13.668   N34 14.016   8859' N34 13.699 5888'
                  W117 37.386   W117 35.796   Cucamonga W117 34.353 N34 13.169
                                 N34 13.374 Peak   16 W117 33.246
                                 W117 35.124

Circle
6880' Mountain

Lone Pine Canyon Rd.

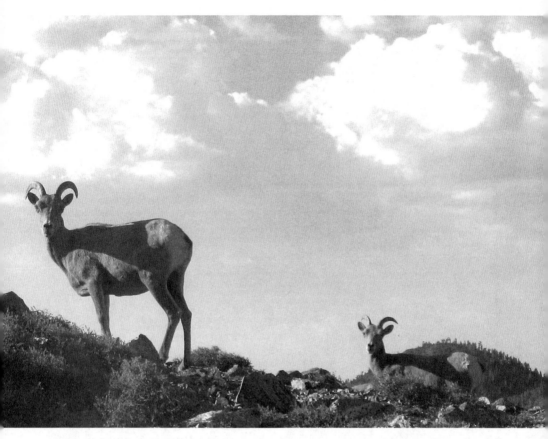

Nelson bighorn sheep

Continued from page 15

Directions to Mount Baldy Visitor Center

Many trips in this chapter start from Mount Baldy Road, near Mount Baldy Village. The road can be reached from either the 210 Freeway (I-210/SR 210) or the 10 Freeway (I-10) by taking the Mountain Avenue exit in Upland—Exit 50 from the 10 or Exit 54 from the 210—and driving north. The top of Mountain Avenue turns right and then back left (west); passes San Antonio Dam to your left; then leads north to the Lower San Antonio Fire Station, across San Antonio Creek, and back south and west to a T-junction with Mount Baldy Road—about 4.6 miles total from Exit 54 off the 210. Turn right and drive 5 miles up to Mount Baldy Village. The Mount Baldy Visitor Center (ranger station) is on the left (west) side of the road, just past Mount Baldy Lodge.

Alternatively, if you're coming from west of Claremont, take Exit 52 off the 210 onto Base Line Road. Go west 0.1 mile, and then turn right (north) onto Padua Avenue. At the top of Padua, turn right onto Mount Baldy Road and follow it 7.5 miles up to Mount Baldy Village.

trip 1.1 Mount Baldy Loop

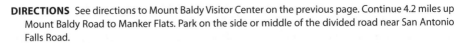

see
map on
p. 17

Distance	10 miles (loop)
Hiking Time	6 hours
Elevation Gain	3,900'
Difficulty	Strenuous
Trail Use	Dogs allowed
Best Times	June–October
Agency	Angeles National Forest (Mount Baldy Visitor Center)
Recommended Map	Tom Harrison *Angeles High Country* or USGS *Mount San Antonio* 7.5' (trail not depicted fully)

DIRECTIONS See directions to Mount Baldy Visitor Center on the previous page. Continue 4.2 miles up Mount Baldy Road to Manker Flats. Park on the side or middle of the divided road near San Antonio Falls Road.

Mount Baldy is one of the most popular hikes in Southern California. Its high summit offers breathtaking views, yet the route is straightforward for a hiker of average ability. There are many routes on the mountain, but this one is especially enjoyable because it makes a loop up past the Baldy Bowl and down along the stunning Devil's Backbone to the ski area at the Baldy Notch. From here, one can follow a dirt service road back to Manker Flats.

Note: *This is a deceptively dangerous route when it's icy. Only experienced mountaineers with ice ax, crampons, and sufficient knowledge should attempt it under winter- or springtime conditions.*

Alternatively, you can do the loop in reverse and ride the chairlift up, saving 1,300 feet and 3.5 miles of climbing. The lift begins 0.4 mile above Manker Flats at the top of Mount Baldy Road. At this writing, the chairlift is open summer weekends and holidays 8 a.m.–5 p.m. Call Mount Baldy Ski Lifts at 909-982-0800 for more information.

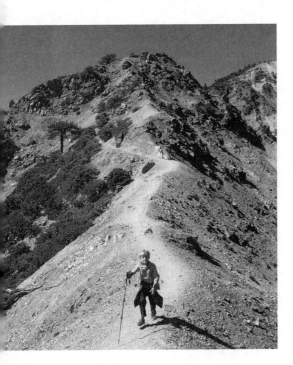

From Manker Flats, you walk west through a gate and then up a service road. In 0.5 mile, the road makes a hairpin turn, and you have an excellent view of San Antonio Falls (see Trip 1.2). In another 0.3 mile, look for the Baldy Bowl Trail switchbacking up the slope to the left. It's easy to miss—if you get to a point directly overlooking Manker Flats, you've gone too far.

Follow the trail 1.6 miles through an open forest up to a Sierra Club ski hut, built by volunteers in 1937, located off the right side of the trail. This marks the halfway point in distance and elevation gain. Just beyond, cross the head of San Antonio Creek beneath the scree-filled Baldy Bowl. This area is a backcountry

Devil's Backbone Trail

skier's paradise in the winter and early spring. On a rare quiet day, it's also a good place to look for bighorn sheep.

The trail continues around the southwest edge of Baldy Bowl, crossing a field of talus and switchbacking up to the ridge in 0.6 mile. Shady spots along this north-facing part of the trail remain icy long after most of the mountain has melted out. Expert mountaineers have suffered serious and even fatal slips on this seemingly innocuous stretch of trail.

Now follow the ridge north. In 0.5 mile, at a sign labeled BALDY BOWL TRAIL, look for a use trail dropping into the canyon. On October 5, 1945, a Curtiss C-46 Commando grazed the cloud-socked ridge of Mount Baldy and tumbled down the canyon. You can find wreckage strewn down the gully, with the largest wing section 0.1 mile below the trail. Our trip, however, climbs 0.6 mile farther to the windswept summit above treeline.

After taking in the magnificent scenery, descend east along the Devil's Backbone Trail. Beware that five trails depart the summit ridge and that many hikers have headed the wrong way, especially when visibility is poor. This spectacular 3-mile trail passes along the south side of Mount Harwood and then follows a knife-edge ridge down to the ski area at Baldy Notch. Again, be extremely careful here—a slip down one of the steep chutes has repeatedly proved fatal.

From the lodge at Baldy Notch, follow the service road descending to the southwest. In 2.4 miles, reach the original junction with the Baldy Bowl Trail and, in another 0.8 mile, arrive back at Manker Flats.

VARIATION

Baldy Bowl is a popular winter snow climb and ski descent. The couloirs at the top reach an angle of 35–40 degrees and can be icy; bring crampons and an ice ax. Sierra Club members and the general public can stay at the ski hut. See angeles.sierraclub.org/san_antonio_ski_hut for details and reservations.

---

trip 1.2   San Antonio Falls

see map on p. 17

Distance	1.2 miles (out-and-back)
Hiking Time	1 hour
Elevation Gain	200'
Difficulty	Easy
Trail Use	Dogs allowed, good for kids
Best Times	April–November
Agency	Angeles National Forest (Mount Baldy Visitor Center)
Optional Map	Tom Harrison *Angeles High Country* or USGS *Mount San Antonio* 7.5'

DIRECTIONS See the directions to Mount Baldy Visitor Center on page 18. Continue 4.2 miles up Mount Baldy Road to Manker Flats. Park on the side or middle of the divided road near San Antonio Falls Road.

San Antonio Creek begins as a snow-fed trickle high up on the east face of Mount Baldy. It gains strength as it descends the canyon and then cascades down a series of steep drops. The final and most impressive three-level drop is called San Antonio Falls. This short hike leads to a viewpoint near the falls. Go on a warm spring day, when the creek is in full flow and the chaparral is in bloom.

From Manker Flats, walk west through a gate and up a service road past some cabins. In 0.5 mile, the road makes a hairpin turn. This is the best viewpoint for San Antonio Falls.

If you want a closer view, you can follow a narrow and tenuous dirt trail 150 yards to the base of the falls. Rock climbers sometimes practice alongside the falls.

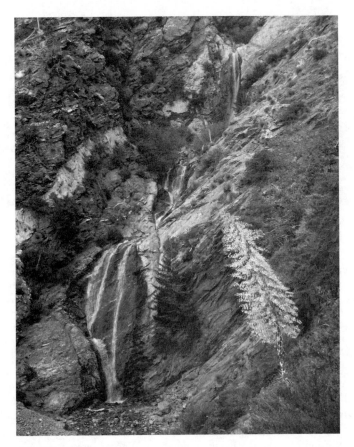

San Antonio Falls

VARIATION

You could follow San Antonio Creek up the falls all the way to the Sierra Club ski hut, but this involves some fourth-class climbing (see page 10), and a rope is advisable. Stay left of the first waterfall and then right of the next ones. The walking then eases until you reach another waterfall just below the ski hut. Climb loose rock on the left side or bushwhack up the steep slope farther left.

---

trip 1.3   **North Backbone Traverse**

see map on p. 17

Distance	11 miles (one-way)
Hiking Time	7 hours
Elevation Gain	5,100'
Difficulty	Strenuous
Trail Use	Dogs allowed
Best Times	June–October
Agency	Angeles National Forest (Mount Baldy Visitor Center)
Recommended Map	Tom Harrison *Angeles High Country* or USGS *Mount San Antonio* 7.5'

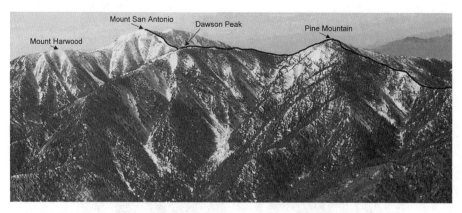

Mount Baldy's North Backbone from the northeast

DIRECTIONS This trip requires a lengthy car shuttle. From Exit 131 off the 15 Freeway (I-15) south of Cajon Pass, drive northwest on Highway 138 for 8.8 miles and then west on Highway 2 for 5.3 miles to Wrightwood. Turn left onto Spruce Street, immediately right onto Apple Avenue, and then immediately left again onto Acorn Drive. Follow Acorn Drive 0.6 mile to where it becomes a private road, and park off the pavement. (See below for directions to the alternative finish on Blue Ridge Road.)

Drive the other car back down to the 15 Freeway; then drive about 16 miles south to the 210 Freeway, heading west and then north to Mount Baldy Village (see directions on page 18). Then continue 4.2 miles up Mount Baldy Road to Manker Flats.

This trip traverses the San Gabriel Mountains from south to north, climbing over Mount Baldy and following its rugged north backbone over Dawson Peak and Pine Mountain down to Wrightwood. It features grand views from the rarely visited north face of Baldy down into the remote Fish Fork of the San Gabriel River. The long drive is justified by the fantastic scenery and seclusion of Sheep Mountain Wilderness. With an early start, you can reach Wrightwood in time for lunch with a friend who picks you up. Beware: these north slopes hold snow and ice in the spring long after the south face snow has completely melted.

Follow the Baldy Bowl Trail 4 miles to the summit of Mount Baldy (see Trip 1.1). Descend the steep North Backbone Trail on the north side to a saddle of 8,800 feet; then follow the trail that climbs steeply up to Dawson Peak, 1.5 miles from Baldy. Descend the far ridge 0.5 mile past a junction with the Dawson Peak Trail, which drops westward into Fish Fork Canyon. Continue north on the Backbone Trail over Pine Mountain; a 100-foot detour is necessary to reach the true summit. Then drop back down to a saddle and up to an unmarked trailhead on Forest Road 3N06 (Blue Ridge Road), 3.8 miles from Baldy.

ALTERNATIVE FINISH ———————————————————————————

End the hike here if you wish. Instead of using the Acorn Drive trailhead, park your car at this trailhead, which is reached from Inspiration Point on Highway 2 by driving 7.2 miles east on fair dirt Blue Ridge Road—labeled 3N26 at the start but soon becoming 3N06—to the point above the prominent saddle between Pine and Wright Mountains. The driving time may exceed the time you save hiking, but the views of the North Backbone, Iron Mountain, the San Antonio Ridge, and the San Gabriel River Canyon are breathtaking.

VARIATION ———————————————————————————

Peak baggers may choose to make a short excursion to the summit of Wright Mountain. Cross the road and continue, very steeply for the first few yards, straight up the toe of the ridge. Soon, cross the Pacific Crest Trail (PCT) and look for traces of an old jeep trail. In 0.1 mile, the slope levels out under the Jeffrey pines and white firs. In another 0.2 mile, the jeep trail dips and climbs back up to reach a T-junction on top of the ridge. Turn left and walk 100 yards to a yellow triangular sign. Look for a faint climber's trail on the right leading north 100 feet to the indistinct summit, which is marked with a large cairn. Then continue west on the jeep trail to rejoin the PCT. This option adds 200 feet of climbing and negligible distance.

Find the PCT on the north side of 3N06 and follow it west as it contours around Wright Mountain. In 0.8 mile, turn north onto the Acorn Trail and follow it 2.1 miles down to the top of Acorn Drive. Continue 0.2 mile to a gate; then go another 0.4 mile down the paved private road to your vehicle.

trip 1.4 Bear Flat

see map on p. 17

Distance	4 miles (out-and-back)
Hiking Time	2 hours
Elevation Gain	1,200'
Difficulty	Moderate
Trail Use	Dogs allowed, suitable for backpacking
Best Times	All year
Agency	Angeles National Forest (Mount Baldy Visitor Center)
Recommended Map	Tom Harrison *Angeles High Country* or USGS *Mount Baldy* 7.5'

DIRECTIONS See directions to Mount Baldy Village, page 18. Then, from Mount Baldy Village, continue up Mount Baldy Road past the Mount Baldy Visitor Center and find a legal place to park on the shoulder of the road. You'll definitely find parking across from the Mount Baldy Trout Pools, and perhaps some on the street near Buckhorn Lodge.

Bear Flat is actually a sloping valley at the head of Bear Canyon and is only flat in comparison to the rugged slopes of Mount Baldy. The short but steep trail leads along Bear Creek and past numerous cabins, through forest and chaparral. It's enjoyable either for a quick workout or for a leisurely tour of the canyon live oaks, bigcone Douglas-firs, cedars, and spring wildflowers. Lucky and patient observers might catch sight of bighorn sheep roaming the mountainside nearby. Ambitious hikers may continue from the flat all the way to the summit of Mount Baldy (see Trip 1.5).

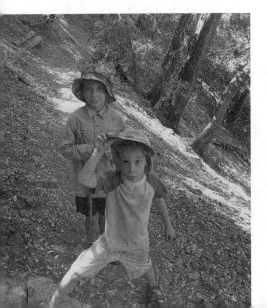

Walk back down Mount Baldy Road and turn right onto Bear Canyon Road just below the visitor center. Hiker parking is prohibited along this road. Walk up Bear Canyon Road past numerous cabins. Watch for a sign on the left about Old Glory, the world's largest known bigcone Douglas-fir. The tree stands 173 feet tall and 91 inches in diameter, and is an estimated 600–700 years old.

Hiking up to Bear Flat

When the road ends in 0.4 mile, turn right onto the Bear Canyon Trail (7W12). The Bear Canyon Trail was washed out in the floods of 2014 but has been repaired. In 0.2 mile, reach a sharp switchback. The old Bear Canyon Loop Trail continued into the creek, but was mostly destroyed, so ascend the switchbacks staying on the main trail.

Eventually our trail switchbacks across the sunbaked slope with fine views of San Antonio Canyon, and then it reenters the shady canyon. In 0.9 mile, it passes a small clearing beneath an oak tree, not far from the east fork of Bear Creek, shortly before it arrives at signed Bear Flat. The clearing is large enough for a tent, but campfires are not allowed.

Bear Flat is an ecological anomaly. The stream issues from a spring a few hundred yards upstream from the trail, and rarely dries up. Ferns grow profusely in an area exposed to the sun. Geologists offer an explanation: the water table is unusually high here because of the San Antonio Fault.

In May 2008, the Bighorn Fire charred 500 acres of chaparral from the edge of Bear Flat up to the ridge. The vegetation has largely recovered, but skeletal remains of the larger shrubs serve as a reminder of the blaze. An old path to Lookout Mountain once departed west from here, but the regrowth after the fire obliterated the path.

trip 1.5   Bear Ridge

Distance	12 miles (out-and-back)
Hiking Time	7 hours
Elevation Gain	5,800'
Difficulty	Strenuous
Trail Use	Dogs allowed
Best Times	June–October
Agency	Angeles National Forest (Mount Baldy Visitor Center)
Recommended Maps	Tom Harrison *Angeles High Country* or USGS *Mount Baldy* and *Mount San Antonio* 7.5'

see map on p. 17

DIRECTIONS See directions to Mount Baldy Visitor Center, page 18; then find a legal place to park on the shoulder of the road. You'll definitely find parking across from the Mount Baldy Trout Pools, and perhaps some on the street near Buckhorn Lodge.

Bear Ridge from the south

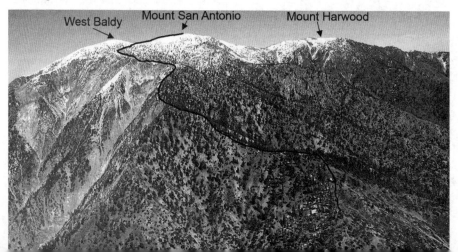

West Baldy   Mount San Antonio   Mount Harwood

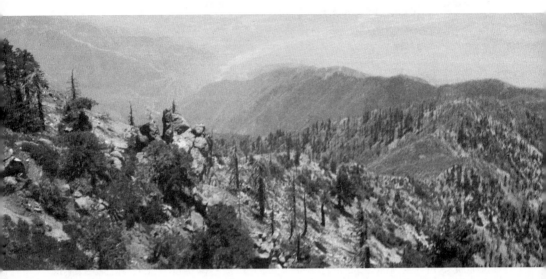

Bear Ridge   Photo: Wayne Steinmetz

The great south ridge of Mount Baldy rises directly from Mount Baldy Village to the summit, and climbs nearly 6,000 feet in 3.5 horizontal miles. The trail offers the greatest sustained elevation gain of any in the San Gabriel Mountains. This is a tough climb, but the views are fantastic and you avoid the usual Baldy crowds until reaching the summit. Start early in summer because the switchbacks above Bear Flat are long and shadeless.

Walk back down Mount Baldy Road and turn right onto Bear Canyon Road just below the visitor center. Hiker parking is prohibited along this road. Walk up Bear Canyon Road past numerous cabins. When the road ends in 0.4 mile, turn right onto the Bear Canyon Trail (7W12). Switchback up through the canyon live oaks and bigcone Douglas-firs; then traverse a sunbaked slope and head back into the canyon to reach Bear Flat.

The 2008 Bighorn Fire burned from Bear Flat up to the ridge. The trail makes 16 long, steep switchbacks through the burn zone before reaching the first intact Jeffrey pines. Enjoy views of Icehouse Canyon and the surrounding peaks. Another 20 or so shorter switchbacks bring you to Bear Ridge, the halfway point on the trip and 1,800 feet up from Bear Flat.

Hike up the ridge, enjoying more great views. In another 1,000 feet of climbing, near the 8,400-foot contour, the ridge merges with a second ridge to the east rising from Lookout Mountain and dramatic views open into Cattle Canyon. In another 600 feet of climbing, cross a section known as the Narrows where the ridge drops steeply on both sides.

The last 1.6 miles are gentler, climbing the upper ridge and traversing across the southeast side of West Baldy to reach the high point of the San Gabriel Mountains. The forest gives way to lodgepole pines, which become ever more stunted by wind and ice as you climb until they vanish entirely on the bald summit. This is a good place to watch for elusive desert bighorn sheep. The trail passes close by West Baldy before reaching the true summit. Return the way you came.

ALTERNATIVE FINISH

If you left a car or bike at Manker Flats, descend the Devil's Backbone or Baldy Bowl Trail (see Trip 1.1). These options are highly recommended because they're spectacular, you avoid retracing your steps, and you save your knees from the brutal descent.

see
map on
p. 17

trip 1.6   Lookout Mountain

Distance	4 miles (out-and-back)
Hiking Time	4 hours
Elevation Gain	2,400'
Difficulty	Strenuous
Trail Use	Dogs allowed
Best Times	March–November
Agency	Angeles National Forest (Mount Baldy Visitor Center)
Required Maps	Tom Harrison *Angeles High Country* or USGS *Mount Baldy* and *Mount San Antonio* 7.5'

DIRECTIONS See directions to Mount Baldy Visitor Center, page 18; then find a legal place to park on the shoulder of the road. You'll definitely find parking across from the Mount Baldy Trout Pools, and perhaps some on the street near Buckhorn Lodge.

Lookout Mountain, a seemingly minor bump on the south ridge of Mount Baldy, plays an important role in the history of science. In 1915, a fire lookout was constructed on the summit to take advantage of the commanding views. In 1926, Albert Michelson conducted a groundbreaking experiment here to measure the speed of light. He placed a prism on Mount Wilson and a large mirror on Lookout Mountain. The United States Geodetic Survey team surveyed the distance between the two peaks with unprecedented accuracy. By bouncing a beam of light from the prism off the mirror and cleverly measuring the round-trip travel time, he determined that the speed of light is nearly 300,000 kilometers per second or about 670 million miles per hour. In 1927, a windstorm destroyed the fire lookout, and now all that remains are some concrete pilings.

The historic trail from Bear Flat was wiped out in the 2008 Bighorn Fire and is now overgrown. The firebreak trail from Cow Canyon Saddle was gated off around 2016. Now the most reasonable approach is to climb the southwest ridge from a saddle reached from Bear Canyon. This steep and rough route is recommended only for adventurous mountaineers. As you hike through the rugged terrain, imagine the struggles that Michelson and the lookout builders must have overcome. Bighorn sheep frequent this area, so don't camp here—just enjoy it as a day hike.

Walk back down Mount Baldy Road and turn right onto Bear Canyon Road just below the visitor center. Hiker parking is prohibited along this road. Walk up Bear Canyon Road past numerous cabins. When the road ends in 0.4 mile, either turn right onto the Bear Canyon Trail (7W12) or continue up the rough but interesting creek bed. In 0.2 mile, reach a tributary canyon (locally known as Erv Bartel Canyon) on the left where the main canyon bends right (**N34° 14.607' W117° 39.815'; 4,800'**). If you're on the Bear Canyon Trail, this is where the trail switchbacks and the old Bear Canyon Loop Trail departs.

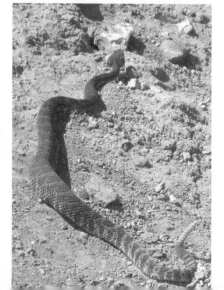

Rattlesnakes favor the south-facing slopes on Lookout Mountain.

Climb the tributary canyon for about 100 yards until you see footprints exiting the canyon on the left. You might find blue tape, ducks, or other evidence of the path. Some switchbacks soon establish you in the next canyon to the left (**N34° 14.578' W117° 39.895'**), trending west-southwest up to a saddle (**N34° 14.469' W117° 40.098'; 5,480'**) just northwest of Peak 5,896'.

Two ducked trails depart the saddle; the one on the left drops toward Cow Canyon Saddle, but this trip takes the one on the right directly up the ridge to the summit.

On a clear day, you can enjoy views in all directions. Nearby are Ontario, Timber, Telegraph, Thunder, Baldy, and Iron Mountains. To the west are Mount Wilson and the rest of the San Gabriels.

trip 1.7   Icehouse Canyon

Distance	7 miles (out-and-back)
Hiking Time	4 hours
Elevation Gain	2,600'
Difficulty	Strenuous
Trail Use	Dogs allowed
Best Times	May–November
Agency	Angeles National Forest (Mount Baldy Visitor Center)
Recommended Maps	Tom Harrison *Angeles High Country* or USGS *Mount Baldy* and *Cucamonga Peak* 7.5'
Permit	Cucamonga Wilderness Permit required

see map on p. 17

DIRECTIONS See directions to Mount Baldy Visitor Center, page 18. Get your free self-issue Cucamonga Wilderness Permit at the Mount Baldy Visitor Center; then continue up Mount Baldy Road 1.5 miles. Turn right into Icehouse Canyon, and park at the trailhead on the left.

Icehouse Canyon is the most accessible hike in the beautiful Cucamonga Wilderness. Formed by earthquake fault activity, the canyon is part of a larger system of east–west running canyons that stretches along the southern San Gabriel Mountains out to the west fork of the San Gabriel River. The shady recesses remain cool well into the summer, and the canyon gets its name from purveyors of ice that supplied Southern California residents in the 1850s or 1860s. This trip climbs through a forest of incense cedars to the saddle at the head of the canyon. A five-way junction on the saddle tempts the ambitious hiker with numerous ways to continue exploring (see Trips 1.8–1.10 and 1.14).

Hike east along the popular Icehouse Canyon Trail past numerous cabins along the north side of the creek. Icehouse Canyon had its heyday during the great age of hiking and mountain resorts in the 1920s and 1930s. The devastating floods of 1938 wiped out many cabins. Fires and avalanches have also taken their toll.

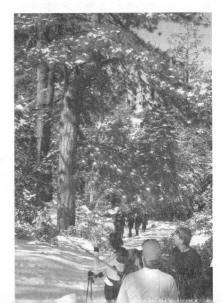

Winter wonderland in Icehouse Canyon
Photo: Emile Fiesler/BioVeyda

In 0.5 mile, pass the mouth of the first tributary canyon carved between steep cliffs on the right (south). This is Falling Rock Canyon, and is a possible descent route from Ontario or Sugarloaf Peaks (see Trips 1.9 and 1.12). In another 0.5 mile, pass an intersection with the Chapman Trail to the left (see Trip 1.8).

In the summer and fall, the rabbitbrush and boulders alongside the stream are frequently clothed with vast numbers of ladybugs, more formally known as convergent lady beetles or *Hippodamia convergens*. Their antifreeze-like blood enables them to survive the winter buried by snow, and their bright-red coloration indicates "toxic and distasteful" to would-be predators.

As you ascend, the canyon bottom becomes dry. Pass the wilderness boundary, and then watch for Columbine Spring on the downhill side of the trail, 2.4 miles from the start. The spring is located immediately before a series of switchbacks and is often surrounded by a patch of columbine in the summer. In 0.5 mile of serious climbing, pass the second junction with the Chapman Trail, and then saunter up the last 0.6 mile to Icehouse Saddle.

---

trip 1.8 ### Cedar Glen

see map on p. 17

Distance	4.5 miles (out-and-back), 7.5 miles (loop)
Hiking Time	2.5–4 hours
Elevation Gain	1,200'/2,100'
Difficulty	Moderate
Trail Use	Dogs allowed, suitable for backpacking
Best Times	May–November
Agency	Angeles National Forest (Mount Baldy Visitor Center)
Recommended Maps	Tom Harrison *Angeles High Country* or USGS *Mount Baldy, Cucamonga Peak,* and *Telegraph Peak* 7.5'
Permit	Cucamonga Wilderness Permit required

DIRECTIONS See directions to Mount Baldy Village, page 18. Get your free self-issue Cucamonga Wilderness Permit at the Mount Baldy Visitor Center; then continue up Mount Baldy Road 1.5 miles. Turn right into Icehouse Canyon, and park at the trailhead on the left.

Cedar Glen Trail Camp is perched on a bench overlooking Icehouse Canyon. This beautiful trip up to the glen follows the shady Icehouse Canyon Trail to the Chapman Trail, and then climbs the wall of the canyon, alongside Cedar Creek, passing chaparral and wildflowers. Cedar Glen has one of the most diverse conifer groves in Southern California, with most of the local species growing together. This trip can be done as a short out-and-back jaunt or, better yet, as a loop continuing on to rejoin Icehouse Canyon and returning via the canyon floor. It's also an enjoyable destination for a short backpacking trip. The climb to Cedar Glen is steep and shadeless. If you're going in the summer, start in the morning before it gets too hot.

From the popular Icehouse Canyon Trailhead, hike east up the canyon past cabins. The dirt road soon narrows to a trail and continues along the north bank of the rushing creek beneath oaks, incense cedars, and broad-leaf trees. In the summer, expect to pass a field of exquisite red- and yellow-flowered columbines growing along the trail.

In 1.0 mile, reach a trail junction with the Chapman Trail; at this writing, the sign was damaged. Turn sharply left and follow the Chapman Trail up the north slope of the canyon along Cedar Creek. This slope is exposed to the searing sun and is covered with yuccas, buckthorns, manzanitas, and other chaparral adapted to the harsh conditions. Watch for

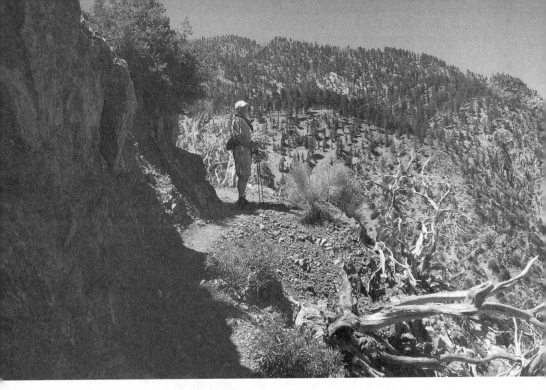

Chapman Trail with Ontario Peak in the background

rattlesnakes, especially in the summer. The trail crosses to the west side of Cedar Creek and then crosses back east again in a lush field of vines and wildflowers. This is the best place to get water if you're camping. Follow one more switchback and arrive at Cedar Glen, 1.3 miles up from Icehouse Canyon.

The small grove on the bench includes Jeffrey, ponderosa, and sugar pines; bigcone Douglas-firs; white firs; and, of course, incense cedars. It's a great place to study the trees and learn to identify the different species. Incense cedars have distinctive scalelike leaves instead of needles. White firs and bigcone Douglas-firs have short needles, which grow individually rather than in bundles. White fir cones are rarely seen at the base of the tree; the barrel-shaped cones grow near the top of the tree and decompose on the branch rather than falling. Bigcone Douglas-fir, also called bigcone spruce, is neither a fir nor a spruce. Its cones grow up to 7 inches long. Pines have longer needles growing in bundles. Sugar pines have bundles of five needles, about 4 inches long, and are easily recognized by their long, skinny cones; sugar pine cones are the world's longest, usually exceeding 12 inches. Jeffrey and ponderosa have long needles in bundles of three and are much more difficult to distinguish. The size of the cones is your best clue: Jeffrey pine cones grow up to 10 inches, while ponderosa pine cones are 3–5 inches long.

Return the way you came.

ALTERNATIVE FINISH

You can make a wonderful loop by continuing 2.2 miles up the Chapman Trail to where it rejoins the Icehouse Canyon Trail. This stretch offers fantastic views of the north wall of Ontario Peak across the canyon, and out to Sunset Peak and Bear Ridge to the west. Reach the Icehouse Canyon Trail at a switchback beneath some sugar pines. You can also head uphill 0.6 mile to Icehouse Saddle and then on to any of several terrific peaks (see Trips 1.9–1.11)—for now, though, turn right and follow the switchbacks downhill 0.6 mile. At the base of the last switchback is Columbine Spring, whose clear, cold waters gush forth beneath the trail in a patch of columbine and scarlet monkeyflowers. Continue down the trail past the wilderness boundary into a talus field, and soon reach the stone foundations of old cabins. Icehouse Creek begins flowing strongly again. In 1.3 miles from Columbine Spring, reach the lower junction with the Chapman Trail; then hike the final mile down to the trailhead.

---

trip 1.9   Ontario Peak

see map on p. 17

Distance	12 miles (out-and-back)
Hiking Time	7 hours
Elevation Gain	3,600'
Difficulty	Strenuous
Trail Use	Dogs allowed, suitable for backpacking
Best Times	June–October
Agency	Angeles National Forest (Mount Baldy Visitor Center)
Recommended Maps	Tom Harrison *Angeles High Country* or USGS *Mount Baldy* and *Cucamonga Peak* 7.5'
Permit	Cucamonga Wilderness Permit required

DIRECTIONS See directions to Mount Baldy Visitor Center, page 18. Get your free self-issue Cucamonga Wilderness Permit at the Mount Baldy Visitor Center; then continue up Mount Baldy Road 1.5 miles. Turn right into Icehouse Canyon, and park at the trailhead on the left.

Ontario and Cucamonga Peaks form an imposing wall overlooking the western end of the Inland Empire. They rise more than a vertical mile from the endless subdivisions at the 2,000-foot base to the summits at almost 9,000 feet. Ontario Peak is one of the classic climbs of Southern California. It's named for the town of Ontario, which in turn was named by the founding Chaffey brothers for their home province of Ontario, Canada. The easiest way to the summit is to ascend the Icehouse Canyon Trail and then turn southwest and hike up past Kelly Camp along the long ridge to the summit. The north side of the ridge can be deceptively icy in early summer and after the first storms of the fall.

Ontario Peak from Sunset Peak

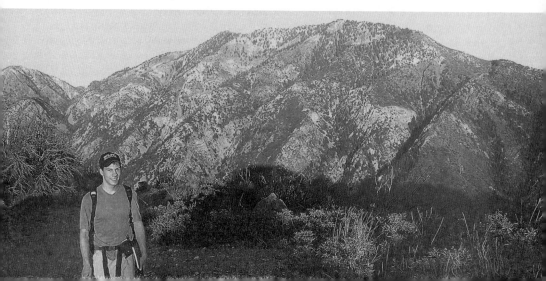

Follow the Icehouse Canyon Trail 3.5 miles to the signed five-way junction at Icehouse Saddle (see Trip 1.7). Turn sharply right and take the Ontario Peak Trail 0.9 mile to Kelly Camp. John Kelly began prospecting here in 1905 and Henry Delker turned the site into a backcountry resort in 1922. It's now a simple trail camp and an excellent place to stay if you're backpacking. In the early summer, you may find water trickling from a small spring by the camp. It's always prudent to treat water before you drink it.

Beyond Kelly Camp, continue 0.4 mile to the ridge, where there are breathtaking views down into Cucamonga Canyon and out over the Inland Empire. Continue west along the undulating ridge. This area is in a burn zone, and travel is hampered by the occasional need to scramble over large fallen timber. Most of the annoying deadfalls across the trail have been removed by enterprising Boy Scouts. In a seemingly endless 1.2 miles, reach the 8,693-foot summit, which is readily recognizable by a granite spire.

ALTERNATIVE FINISH

Most parties descend the way they came. You can also take cross-country routes down Falling Rock Canyon or Shortcut Ridge, but these routes are recommended only for experienced cross-country travelers. Yet another option is to follow the ridge east over Bighorn Peak and then down and up to Cucamonga Peak (see Trips 1.10 and 1.12).

Falling Rock Canyon is accessed from the broad bowl beneath the trail 0.3 mile east of Ontario Peak. Pick a way down to the north through the fallen timber. The canyon steepens and passes a small saddle next to Sugarloaf Peak. It then veers right and descends through talus fields before reaching the bottom of Icehouse Canyon 0.5 mile east of the trailhead. This route saves substantial distance but not much time because of the difficult terrain. Be careful not to be lured down the wrong canyon because some of the canyons have cliff bands of decomposing rock.

Shortcut Ridge descends from Kelly Camp and reaches Icehouse Canyon 0.1 mile east of the wilderness-boundary sign. It's flanked by Delker Canyon to the east and Lost Creek Canyon to the west. Descending the ridge on the return from Ontario Peak saves distance but likely increases time and effort. The upper part of the ridge is brushy in places, while the lower section involves easy scrambling on loose metamorphic rock.

---

trip 1.10 Cucamonga Peak

Distance	12 miles (out-and-back)
Hiking Time	7 hours
Elevation Gain	3,800'
Difficulty	Strenuous
Trail Use	Dogs allowed
Best Times	June–October
Agency	Angeles National Forest (Mount Baldy Visitor Center)
Recommended Maps	Tom Harrison *Angeles High Country* or USGS *Mount Baldy* and *Cucamonga Peak* 7.5'
Permit	Cucamonga Wilderness Permit required

see map on p. 17

DIRECTIONS See directions to Mount Baldy Visitor Center, page 18. Get your free self-issue Cucamonga Wilderness Permit at the Mount Baldy Visitor Center; then continue up Mount Baldy Road 1.5 miles. Turn right into Icehouse Canyon, and park at the trailhead on the left.

Ontario and Cucamonga Peaks form an imposing wall overlooking the western end of the Inland Empire. They rise more than a vertical mile from the endless subdivisions

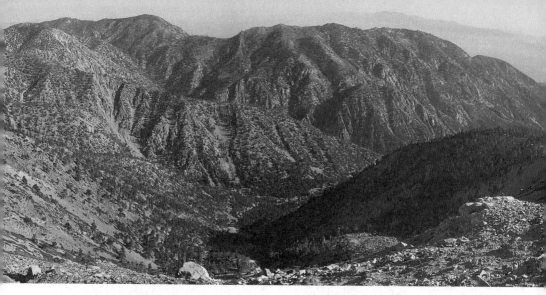

Ontario-Cucamonga Ridge from above Baldy Bowl

at the 2,000-foot base to the summits at almost 9,000 feet. Cucamonga Peak is another of the classic climbs of Southern California. It's named for the Cucamonga Rancho, established in the valley below in 1839 by Tiburcio Tapia. The ranch, in turn, got its name from the Tongva–Shoshonean word *kukill-mongo,* whose meaning is uncertain. The easiest way to the summit is to hike to Icehouse Saddle and then follow a good trail to the summit. The north-facing leg beyond Icehouse Saddle traverses a steep slope and holds unconsolidated snow late into the spring, rendering it nearly impassable long after the snow has melted away on the surrounding mountains.

Follow the Icehouse Canyon Trail 3.5 miles to the signed five-way junction at Icehouse Saddle (see Trip 1.7). Cross the saddle and follow the trail southeast 0.9 mile as it contours around the steep east slope of Bighorn Peak. It reaches another saddle separating the rugged drainages of Cucamonga Canyon and Lytle Creek; then it switchbacks steeply up through a forest of lodgepole pines and white firs to Cucamonga Peak. Reach the 8,859-foot peak in 1.4 strenuous miles. The last 0.2 mile of trail on the flattish top can be faint and confusing, but aim for the highest point with unobstructed views south over the Inland Empire.

trip 1.11 The Three T's

Distance	13 miles (one-way, with short shuttle)
Hiking Time	8 hours
Elevation Gain	5,000'
Difficulty	Strenuous
Trail Use	Dogs allowed
Best Times	June–October
Agency	Angeles National Forest (Mount Baldy Visitor Center)
Recommended Maps	Tom Harrison *Angeles High Country* or USGS *Mount Baldy, Cucamonga Peak,* and *Telegraph Peak* 7.5'
Permit	Cucamonga Wilderness Permit required

see map on p. 17

DIRECTIONS This trip requires a short car or bicycle shuttle. See directions to Mount Baldy Visitor Center, page 18. Get your free self-issue Cucamonga Wilderness Permit; then continue up Mount Baldy Road 4.2 miles to Manker Flats, where you leave one vehicle. Drive or pedal 2.7 miles down the hairpin turns, and turn left into Icehouse Canyon; then park at the trailhead on the left.

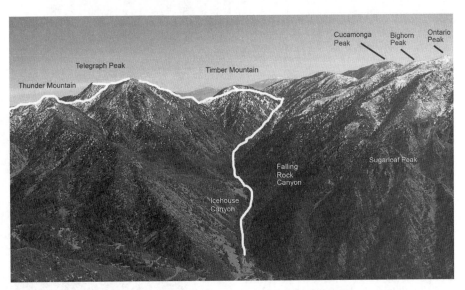

Aerial view of Ontario-Cucamonga Ridge and the Three T's from the northwest

Timber, Telegraph, and Thunder Mountains form the undulating northeast wall of San Antonio Canyon. This superb romp over the Three T's begins up Icehouse Canyon and descends through the ski resort at Baldy Notch. For an easier hike with only 9.5 miles of distance and 2,100 feet of elevation gain, take the ski lift from the top of Mount Baldy Road up to the notch and do the trip in reverse.

Follow the Icehouse Canyon Trail 3.5 miles to the signed five-way junction at Icehouse Saddle (see Trip 1.7). Turn left and climb north 0.7 mile toward Timber Mountain. The trail curves around the west side, so you'll have to make a 0.2-mile detour to reach the true summit. Follow the trail 2.0 miles down to a saddle and up to Telegraph Peak. Again, make a short detour on a use trail to the northeast to reach the summit, which is the highest point of the trip. Return to the trail and drop steeply to a third saddle, and then climb back up to the final summit, reaching Thunder Mountain in 1.2 miles. From here, the Gold Ridge ski road leads 1.5 miles back down to Mount Baldy Notch.

From the notch, hike down the service road 3.2 miles to Manker Flats. Alternatively, the ski lift runs on weekends and is a tempting way to save the wear and tear on your knees.

trip 1.12   **Nine Baldy Area Peaks**

Distance	26 miles (one-way, with short shuttle)
Hiking Time	15 hours
Elevation Gain	10,600'
Difficulty	Very strenuous
Trail Use	Suitable for backpacking, dogs allowed
Best Times	June–October
Agency	Angeles National Forest (Mount Baldy Visitor Center)
Recommended Maps	Tom Harrison *Angeles High Country* or USGS *Mount Baldy, Mount San Antonio, Cucamonga Peak,* and *Telegraph Peak* 7.5'
Permit	Cucamonga Wilderness Permit required

see map on p. 17

DIRECTIONS This trip requires a short car or bicycle shuttle. See directions to Mount Baldy Visitor Center, page 18. Get your free self-issue Cucamonga Wilderness Permit at the Mount Baldy Visitor Center; then continue up Mount Baldy Road 4.2 miles to Manker Flats, where you leave one vehicle. Drive or bike 2.7 miles down the hairpin turns, and turn left into Icehouse Canyon; then park at the trailhead on the left.

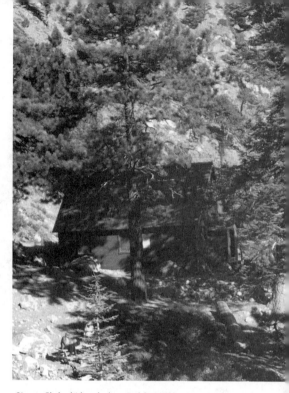

Sierra Club ski hut below Baldy Bowl

The mother of all hikes in Southern California, this trek tours nine major summits around San Antonio Canyon: Ontario, Bighorn, Cucamonga, Timber, Telegraph, Thunder, Harwood, Baldy, and West Baldy. There is substantial elevation gain and loss between most of the peaks, making this the toughest of the multi-mountain challenges in this book. As you stand atop Ontario Peak at dawn, mighty Mount Baldy beckons from across the deep canyon separating the peaks. Standing atop Baldy at dusk, you look back at the dramatic ridges of Ontario. This is a great trip to do when there's a full moon, because the extra light may be helpful. Bring a headlamp, a generous supply of water, and boundless enthusiasm.

Hike 3.5 miles up Icehouse Canyon to Icehouse Saddle. Turn sharply left and hike up past Kelly Camp to the ridge; then follow the trail along the ridge to Ontario Peak. Return along the ridge; when the main trail begins descending to Kelly Camp, stay on the ridge and follow a use trail east to Bighorn Peak. Make a cross-country descent of the southeast ridge of Bighorn Peak to a saddle, where you join the Cucamonga Peak Trail and switchback up to the summit. Then return via the trail to Icehouse Saddle.

At this point, you have climbed 5,700 feet and toured three magnificent peaks. If time or energy is waning, follow the Icehouse Canyon Trail back to your vehicle. Otherwise, continue north up to the Three T's (see Trip 1.11) and on to the Mount Baldy Notch.

If you reach the top of the notch before 5 p.m., you may be able to get water or snacks at the Top of the Notch Restaurant. This is also your next escape route. You can either hike down the service road to Manker Flats or take the chairlift if it's running.

Again, if energy permits, begin climbing west up the Devil's Backbone. Before making the final push up Baldy, take a short detour from the trail to the summit of Mount Harwood. Then top out on Mount Baldy before you take an easy 0.5-mile jaunt to West Baldy. Return to Baldy and descend via the Baldy Bowl Trail to Manker Flats.

VARIATIONS————————————————————————————————

If you're in supremely good condition and you know the trails of this region well, consider adding even more peaks. Climb Ontario by way of Falling Rock Canyon to scale Sugarloaf Peak. Follow the Cucamonga Peak Trail a mile east to the 8,662-foot Etiwanda Peak (not named on most maps). Descend from Baldy by way of Pine and Dawson Peaks or, even more boldly, down the grueling San Antonio Ridge to Iron Mountain.

trip 1.13 **Iron Mountain**

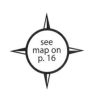

see map on p. 16

Distance	14 miles (out-and-back)
Hiking Time	8 hours
Elevation Gain	6,200'
Difficulty	Strenuous
Trail Use	Dogs allowed
Best Times	October–November, April–May
Agency	Angeles National Forest (Mount Baldy Visitor Center)
Required Maps	Tom Harrison *Angeles High Country* or USGS *Glendora, Mount Baldy,* and *Mount San Antonio* 7.5'
Permit	Sheep Mountain Wilderness Permit required

DIRECTIONS From the 210 Freeway in Azusa, take Exit 36 north onto Azusa Avenue (Highway 39) and drive up into San Gabriel Canyon. In 11.9 miles, turn right (east) onto East Fork Road. At a hairpin turn in 5.3 miles, stay straight (east) on a minor road that crosses a bridge and ends in 0.9 mile at a parking lot and closed gate. Get a free self-issue wilderness permit at a box near the entrance to the lot.

Big Bad Iron Mountain stands west of Mount Baldy, towering over the headwaters of the San Gabriel River. It's the toughest single-peak hike in the San Gabriel Mountains, and the second hardest (after Rabbit Peak) in this book. The hike begins near the river at 2,000 feet and climbs to the 8,007-foot summit. The first half is on good trail to Heaton Saddle, but the second half follows a steep climber's path up the interminable south ridge of Iron Mountain. The mountain is defended by sharp yuccas, so wear sturdy pants and gaiters. Most people will want at least 4 quarts of water on a cool day; don't even *think* about this shadeless climb on a hot day. This is also a popular conditioning hike and gets regular use by a number of sturdy mountaineers. The route is south-facing and lower than many others in the region, so it can often be done in the winter months if snowfall has been light.

Hike north past the gate along the dirt road to Heaton Flat Campground. At a sign near the outhouse, turn right and follow the Heaton Flat Trail 3.9 miles to Allison Saddle. The maintained trail ends here, but a surprisingly good climber's path leads up the crest of the south ridge for 2.5 intense miles with 3,500 feet of elevation gain. The route is distinct and straightforward to follow, even on a foggy day.

Return the way you came. Or, if you have plenty of time and are feeling extremely strong, follow the great San Antonio Ridge east to Mount Baldy (see Trip 1.14).

trip 1.14 **San Antonio Ridge**

see map on p. 16

Distance	16 miles (one-way)
Hiking Time	14 hours
Elevation Gain	10,200'
Difficulty	Very strenuous
Best Times	October–November
Agency	Angeles National Forest (Mount Baldy Visitor Center)
Required Maps	Tom Harrison *Angeles High Country* or USGS *Glendora, Mount Baldy,* and *Mount San Antonio* 7.5'
Permit	Sheep Mountain Wilderness Permit required (for entry from East Fork only)

DIRECTIONS This trip requires a 1-hour car shuttle. Follow the directions to Mount Baldy Visitor Center (see page 18). Continue up Mount Baldy Road 4.2 miles, and leave a vehicle at the Manker Flats Trailhead.

Return to the 210 Freeway and drive 13 miles west to Azusa. Take Exit 36 north onto Azusa Avenue (Highway 39), and drive up into San Gabriel Canyon. In 11.9 miles, turn right (east) onto East Fork Road. At a hairpin turn in 5.3 miles, stay straight (east) on a minor road that crosses a bridge and ends in 0.9 mile at a parking lot and closed gate. (Those familiar with the area can shortcut between the trailheads via Glendora Ridge Road if it's open.) Get a free self-issue wilderness permit at a box near the entrance to the lot.

The great San Antonio Ridge connects Iron Mountain to Mount Baldy. This is a monster hike: strenuous, with interesting rock scrambling, completely devoid of water, and absolutely spectacular. It should be done when temperatures in the canyons have cooled but while Baldy is still free of ice. This is most common in late fall, but sometimes conditions are still good in early winter during a light snow year. It's good to know the Baldy area well so you can find the descent trail in the dark. Headlamps are usually necessary and some parties have spent an unplanned night (or two!) on the ridge. Most climbers will want at least 6 quarts of water on a cool day. The trip is easier if you do it in reverse, but it still involves more than 5,000 feet of climbing. It's theoretically possible to backpack this trip and camp on Iron Mountain, the San Antonio Ridge, or Mount Baldy, but there's no water on the route and you may need to carry 10 quarts or more.

Follow the Heaton Flat Trail and south ridge to Iron Mountain (see Trip 1.13). Look east along the San Antonio Ridge and pick out Mount Baldy, only 4 miles away and 2,000 feet higher. Despite appearances, getting there is at least as hard as the climb of Iron Mountain that you have just completed. Unless it's still early in the day and you're bubbling with energy, this is the last good place to turn around.

Pick a path down the dramatic trailless knife-edge ridge to the east through rocks and brush. Cross the aptly named Gunsight Notch, which involves exposed third-class moves

San Antonio Ridge

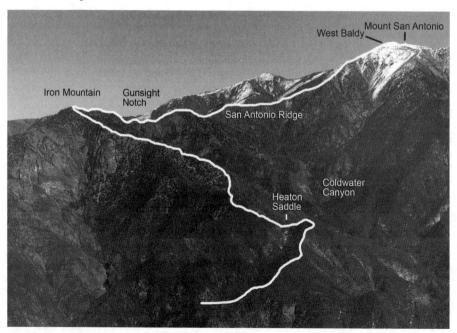

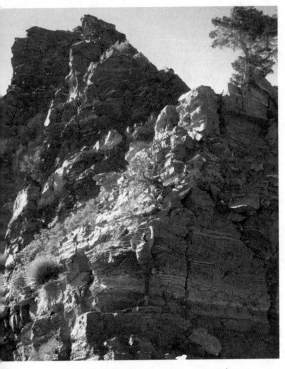

on poor-quality rock. There is little benefit in bringing a rope along, because it would be hard to establish a trustworthy anchor. Eventually reach the low point on the ridge, 1 mile from Iron Mountain. Follow the undulating ridge 1.5 miles over two bumps to the eastern saddle before the steep rise to Mount Baldy. There are a few manzanita patches along the way, but you can stay on bighorn sheep trails to avoid the worst of the chaparral. Then make the final 2,200-foot climb up the west ridge of Baldy, going over West Baldy to the true summit of Mount Baldy.

Descend via the Baldy Bowl Trail to Manker Flats. Remember that this trail is prone to ice on the switchbacks above the ski hut; take special care as this area is especially treacherous in the dark.

Climbing shattered metamorphic rock out of Gunsight Notch

see map on p. 17

trip 1.15   Icehouse Saddle from Lytle Creek

Distance	12 miles (out-and-back, with a possible overnight camp)
Hiking Time	6 hours
Elevation Gain	3,600'
Difficulty	Strenuous
Trail Use	Dogs allowed, suitable for backpacking
Best Times	June–October
Agency	San Bernardino National Forest (Lytle Creek Ranger Station)
Recommended Maps	Tom Harrison *Angeles High Country* or USGS *Telegraph Peak* and *Cucamonga Peak* 7.5'
Permit	Cucamonga Wilderness Permit required

DIRECTIONS From the 15 Freeway between the 210 and 215 (I-215) Freeways, take Exit 119 north onto Sierra Avenue, which becomes Lytle Creek Road. Proceed 4.6 miles to the Lytle Creek Ranger Station, where you can pick up your free Cucamonga Wilderness Permit. Continue 1.7 miles and turn left onto Middle Fork Road, which soon becomes fair dirt Forest Road 2N58 (high clearance may be required). In 2.9 miles, reach the trailhead parking at the end of the road beside an outhouse, at 3,955 feet.

This trip takes the back way up to Icehouse Saddle. It follows the middle fork of Lytle Creek past three pleasant trail camps before making the steep climb to the saddle. A herd of bighorn sheep roam the crumbling canyon walls. Chickadees sing from the trees and wildflowers decorate the trail. You're much more likely to find solitude on this side of

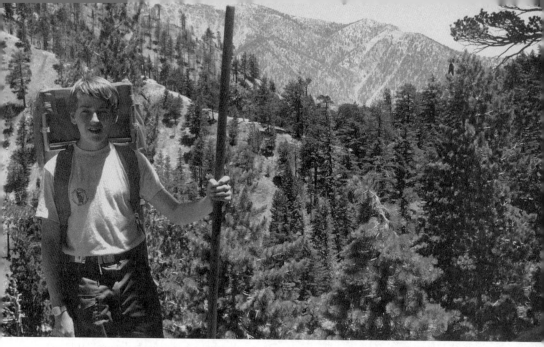
Boy Scout backpacking on the Lytle Creek Trail

Photo: Wayne Steinmetz

Icehouse Saddle, though the trail camps are favored by Boy Scout troops. The Cucamonga Wilderness has a quota for permits from the San Bernardino side; you can apply for a permit in advance at cucamongawilderness.org.

The trail leads west, climbing onto the slope north of the creek, passing yuccas and scrub oak. This part of the canyon burned in the Grand Prix Fire of 2003. The chaparral is growing back on the north side of the creek, but the toothpick forest on the south side will take decades to recover. After climbing some switchbacks, round a corner and reach an unmarked junction in 0.6 mile. The old trail to the left descends to Stone House Trail Camp at 4,403 feet. In another 0.8 mile, reach a second junction with the old trail leading back to Stone House. By now, you have passed the end of the burn area and entered a forest of live oak and bigcone Douglas-fir.

In 1.1 miles, turn left and cross the Middle Fork to reach Third Stream Crossing Trail Camp at 5,194 feet. (This would have been your third creek crossing if you'd taken the old trail.) The section near the creek crossing is somewhat indistinct; look for a rock-lined trail resuming at the campsite.

The trail now switchbacks up onto a ridge and joins a southern tributary of the Middle Fork above a spectacular section of narrows. (Some canyoneers enjoy making a technical descent of this gorge.) It crosses some scree and talus slopes with poor tread and reaches Commanche Trail Camp in 1.5 miles, at 6,132 feet. The camp is beautifully situated beneath oaks, firs, incense cedars, and ponderosa pines. The choice and spelling of the camp name are curious as the Comanche Indians lived east of the Rockies.

The last part of the trail is the toughest, climbing 1.7 miles to Icehouse Saddle. Along the way, you can enjoy the dramatic views of the rugged canyons as they abruptly drop to the San Andreas Fault. Return the way you came, or follow any of the other four trails radiating from Icehouse Saddle (see Trips 1.7–1.11).

VARIATION

The three trail camps along the way are great backpacking destinations.

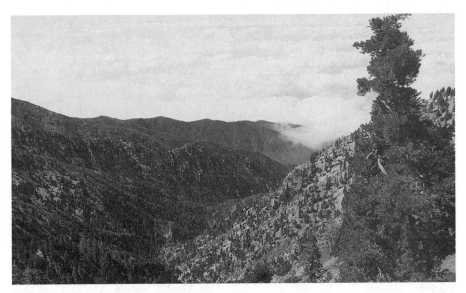

Looking down Icehouse Canyon from Icehouse Saddle

trip 1.16   **Etiwanda Peak**

Distance	10 miles (out-and-back)
Hiking Time	6 hours
Elevation Gain	2,800'
Difficulty	Strenuous
Trail Use	Dogs allowed, suitable for backpacking
Best Times	September–November
Agency	San Bernardino National Forest (Lytle Creek Ranger Station)
Required Map	Tom Harrison *Angeles High Country* or USGS *Cucamonga Peak* 7.5'
Permit	Cucamonga Wilderness Permit required

see map on p. 17

DIRECTIONS This trip involves a long drive on dirt Forest Road 1N34, which is typically open from Labor Day until the first winter storms; it may also be closed during Santa Ana wind conditions. Call the Lytle Creek Ranger Station (909-382-2851) for current status. A moderate- to high-clearance vehicle is required.

From the 15 Freeway between the 210 and 215 Freeways, take Exit 119 north onto Sierra Avenue, which immediately becomes Lytle Creek Road. Follow Lytle Creek Road 1.5 miles; then turn left onto signed San Sevaine Road (1N34). Proceed 12 miles up the road—this may take well over an hour depending on road conditions and your vehicle. At a signed T-junction, veer right into Joe Elliot Campground, and continue 0.2 mile to the top of the campground.

Etiwanda Peak is the informal name given to Peak 8,662' east of Cucamonga Peak. It's named for the community below, which was in turn named in 1881 by the founding Chaffey brothers for a Native American chief from Lake Michigan who had been a family friend. This hike takes the scenic but unmaintained and lightly used Cucamonga Peak Trail (7W04) up to Etiwanda and optionally on to Cucamonga Peak. The initial segment ascends through the burn zone of the 2003 Old Fire. The trail is rocky and has many downed trees and slumping portions across scree slopes, but it's generally easy to follow and clear of brush. Long pants and boots are advisable. Several flat spots on ridges are good for dry camping,

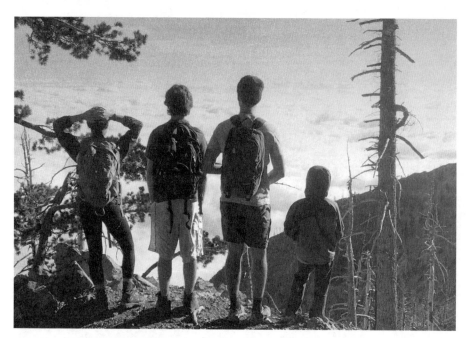

Above the clouds on Etiwanda Peak Trail

weather permitting. Because of the seasonal access and long drive, Etiwanda Peak is lightly visited compared with other peaks in the region. Nevertheless, this is an enjoyable hike with varied scenery, well worth the effort for those who love the Mount Baldy high country.

The Joe Elliot Tree Memorial Campground burned in the Old Fire and is now largely overgrown, but two free yellow post sites are still available. The tree itself was once recognized as the largest in Southern California, but fell sometime around 1970 and was burned in the fire.

The hike begins at an unsigned gap in a fence and passes through stands of buckthorn and yerba santa growing between fallen trees. The trail enters the Cucamonga Wilderness above a switchback and then crosses the rocky washes that form the headwaters of the South Fork of Lytle Creek. At 2.0 miles, the trail reaches a point on a ridge where you'll see evidence of a burned-down miner's cabin beside the Blew Jordam mine. The prospect, also known as the Cucamonga Zinc Mine, was first discovered in the 1920s and was worked during the 1940s to produce lead, zinc, and some silver, but was never particularly successful.

Switchbacks lead out of the burn zone and onto a scenic narrow ridge forested with sugar pines and white fir. The trail then detours north before switchbacking into a lodgepole pine forest and passing around Peak 8,386'. Cross a small saddle; then traverse the north slopes of Etiwanda Peak. When you're west of the peak, look for a cairn marking a well-used climber's trail on the left that ascends steeply to the summit.

VARIATION

You can continue 1.0 mile west along the trail to reach Cucamonga Peak. Similarly, Etiwanda Peak can be reached from Cucamonga Peak (see Trip 1.10).

trip 1.17 Bonita Falls

Distance	1.6 miles (out-and-back)
Hiking Time	1.5 hours
Elevation Gain	300'
Difficulty	Easy
Trail Use	Dogs allowed, good for kids
Best Times	January–May
Agency	San Bernardino National Forest (Lytle Creek Ranger Station)
Recommended Maps	USGS *Cucamonga Peak* and *Devore* 7.5' (trail not shown)

DIRECTIONS From the 15 Freeway between the 210 and 215 Freeways, take Exit 119 north onto Sierra Avenue, which immediately becomes Lytle Creek Road. Follow Lytle Creek Road 4.6 miles to the ranger station and another 1.2 miles farther. Park on the shoulder near the mouth of the South Fork of Lytle Creek, the major canyon on the left.

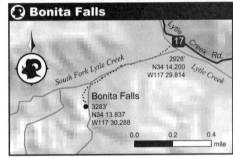

Bonita Falls, the second tallest waterfall in San Bernardino National Forest, consists of three levels. The lowest and most impressive, Lower Bonita Falls, plunges 160 feet straight down. It lives up to its beautiful name after a heavy rainfall, but drains a small watershed and disappears by early summer. Although the hike is short, it involves rock-hopping along the trailless South Fork of Lytle Creek, followed by scrambling over slippery rocks near the base of the falls. The canyon has become extremely popular but suffers from graffiti and litter left by thoughtless visitors; consider bringing a trash bag to carry out some of the cans and bottles. Be aware that Lytle Creek can be dangerous to cross after a heavy rain.

Descend to the broad wash and ford Lytle Creek; then walk southwest into the major canyon, which is the South Fork of Lytle Creek. The easiest path through the rocks may be on the north side of the creek. In 0.6 mile, reach the first small canyon on the left. Follow a well-used path 0.2 mile up this canyon to Bonita Falls.

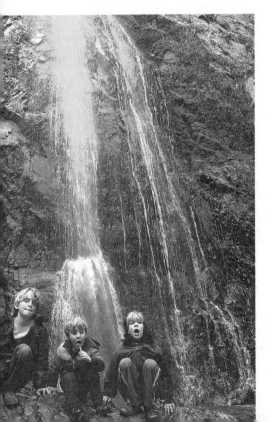

Bonita Falls

chapter 2

San Gabriel Foothills

Residents of Inland Empire communities around Claremont, Upland, and Rancho Cucamonga enjoy remarkable hiking, biking, running, bird-watching, and equestrian opportunities at the base of the foothills on the northern edge of their towns.

This chapter focuses on the higher country. The extremely popular trails of Marshall Canyon Regional Park and Claremont Hills Wilderness Park are covered in *Afoot & Afield Los Angeles County.*

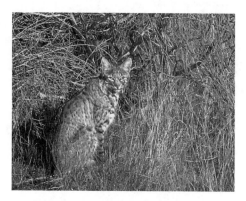

A blasé bobcat stares down the camera.

trip 2.1 Sunset Peak

Distance	5 miles (loop)
Hiking Time	2.5 hours
Elevation Gain	1,300'
Difficulty	Moderate
Trail Use	Dogs allowed
Best Times	All year
Agency	Angeles National Forest (Mount Baldy Visitor Center)
Recommended Map	Tom Harrison *Angeles High Country* or USGS *Mount Baldy* 7.5'

see map on p. 45

DIRECTIONS From the 210 (I-210/SR 210) Freeway, take Exit 52 onto Base Line Road and drive west to the first intersection, Padua Avenue. Turn right (north) onto Padua and, in 1.8 miles, turn right on Mount Baldy Road. In 7 miles, on the outskirts of Mount Baldy Village, turn left onto Glendora Ridge Road. Travel 0.8 mile up the road to Cow Canyon Saddle. If the gate at the bottom of Glendora Ridge Road is closed, park outside the gate and hike the road.

Sunset Peak offers the perfect hike for stepping out of city life for an afternoon. It's a quick drive into the mountains, and the hike is relatively short, yet the trail travels through the rugged and picturesque San Gabriel Mountains.

You have two options for hiking Sunset Peak. One is a steep and rough firebreak that follows the ridge 1.6 miles up to the peak. The other is a dirt service road that switchbacks 3.6 miles up the mountain. From the summit one can see miles of the San Gabriel Mountains, as well as great views of the cities below. A recommended loop is to climb the firebreak, enjoy a picnic at sunset, and descend the dirt road by headlamp.

Sunset over the San Gabriel Mountains from Sunset Peak Photo: Mark Hendricks

The firebreak and the road both start on the south side of the paved Glendora Ridge Road. The firebreak starts very steeply and follows the ridge over one major crest and a couple of minor bumps before passing a bend in the fire road at 1.2 miles. Continue up the ridge another 0.4 mile to rejoin the road just before reaching the summit. The chaparral encroaches on the trail at points, so wearing long pants is a good idea.

If you choose to take the road instead, walk past the gate near the parking area. Follow the road southwest 1.9 miles until reaching the first junction; take a sharp left at this junction. Hike another 0.6 mile and pass the firebreak trail at a hairpin turn. Hike another 0.7 mile until reaching a final junction; take a sharp left here and reach the summit in 0.4 mile.

trip 2.2   Sunset Ridge

Distance	13–15 miles (one-way)
Hiking Time	7 hours
Elevation Gain	1,500'
Difficulty	Strenuous
Trail Use	Dogs allowed, suitable for mountain biking
Best Times	September–May
Agency	Angeles National Forest (Mount Baldy Visitor Center)
Recommended Maps	Tom Harrison *Angeles High Country* or USGS *Mount Baldy* and *Glendora* 7.5'

see map on p. 45

DIRECTIONS This is a one-way hike and is described in the mostly downhill direction. Leave one vehicle at the end of the hike and then take another to the start.

To reach the end from the 210 Freeway, take Exit 47 onto Foothill Boulevard. Drive west 0.3 mile; then turn right (north) onto San Dimas Canyon Road. Follow it 2.0 miles to a stop sign at the corner of Golden Hills; then continue up the canyon. Park at a wide spot in the road just above mile marker 1.32, shortly before you reach the top of the San Dimas Dam.

Continued on page 46

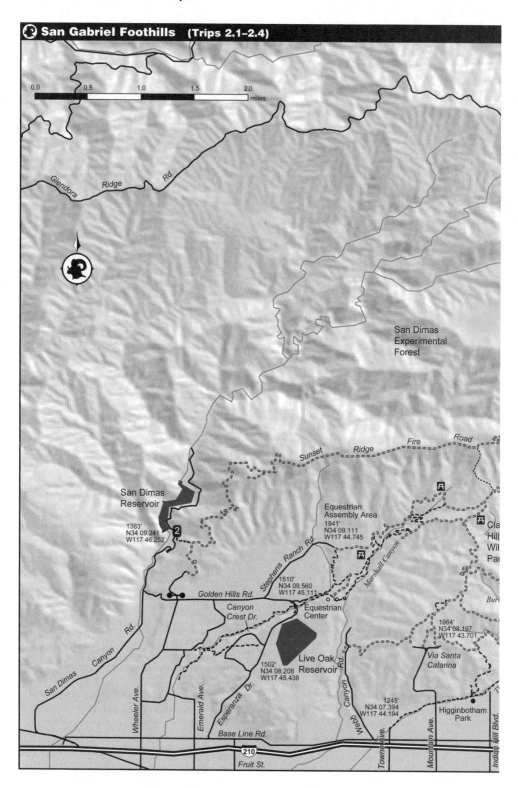

San Gabriel Foothills (Trips 2.1–2.4)

0.0   0.5   1.0   1.5   2.0
miles

Glendora Ridge Rd.

San Dimas Experimental Forest

Sunset Ridge Fire Road

San Dimas Reservoir

1383'
N34 09.241
W117 46.252
②

Equestrian Assembly Area
1941'
N34 09.111
W117 44.745

Cla
Hill
Wil
Pai

Marshall Canyon

Stephans Ranch Rd.

1510'
N34 08.560
W117 45.111

Golden Hills Rd.

Equestrian Center

Canyon Crest Dr.

1964'
N34 08.197
W117 43.701

Buri

San Dimas Canyon Rd.

1502'
N34 08.208
W117 45.438

Live Oak Reservoir

Via Santa Catarina

Webb Canyon Rd.

Wheeler Ave.

Emerald Ave.

Esperanza Dr.

1245'
N34 07.394
W117 44.194

Higginbotham Park

Towne Ave.

Mountain Ave.

Indian Hill Blvd.

Base Line Rd.

210

Fruit St.

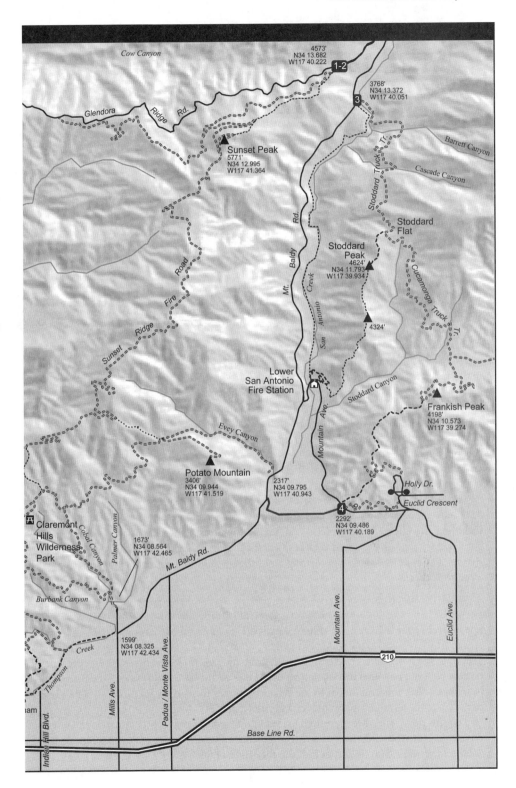

Cow Canyon

4573'
N34 13.682
W117 40.222

1-2

3768'
N34 13.372
W117 40.051

3

Glendora

Ridge Rd.

Barrett Canyon

Cascade Canyon

Stoddard Truck Tr.

Sunset Peak
5771'
N34 12.995
W117 41.364

Stoddard
Flat

Mt. Baldy Rd.

Stoddard
Peak
4624'
N34 11.793
W117 39.934

Cucamonga Truck Tr.

San Antonio Creek

4324'

Road

Fire

Ridge

Sunset

Lower
San Antonio
Fire Station

Stoddard Canyon

Frankish Peak
4198'
N34 10.573
W117 39.274

Evey Canyon

Potato Mountain
3406'
N34 09.944
W117 41.519

2317'
N34 09.795
W117 40.943

Mountain Ave.

Holly Dr.

Euclid Crescent

4

2292'
N34 09.486
W117 40.189

Claremont
Hills
Wilderness
Park

1673'
N34 08.564
W117 42.465

Mt. Baldy Rd.

Cobal Canyon

Palmer Canyon

Burbank Canyon

Creek

1599'
N34 08.325
W117 42.434

Thompson

am

Indian Hill Blvd.

Mills Ave.

Padua / Monte Vista Ave.

Mountain Ave.

Euclid Ave.

210

Base Line Rd.

Continued from page 43

To reach the start, return the way you came to the 210 Freeway and drive east to Base Line Road. Take Exit 52 and drive west to the first intersection, Padua Avenue. Turn right (north) onto Padua and, in 1.8 miles, turn right on Mount Baldy Road. In 7 miles, on the outskirts of Mount Baldy Village, turn left onto Glendora Ridge Road. Travel 0.8 mile up the road to Cow Canyon Saddle and park. If the gate at the bottom of Glendora Ridge Road is closed, park outside the gate and hike the road.

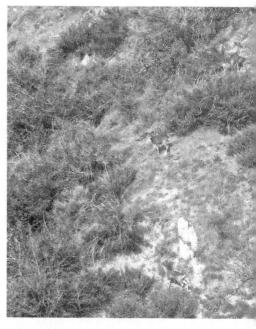

Deer graze near Sunset Ridge.

Sunset Ridge is an island in the sky extending from Mount Baldy Village to San Dimas Reservoir. A fire road runs the length of the ridge and makes for a good, long, and mostly downhill hike with views of Mount Baldy, the San Gabriel Mountains, and the Inland Empire. In the spring after good winter rains, the chaparral slopes burst into color with wildflowers. For a more strenuous alternative with 4,700 feet of elevation gain, take this trip in the opposite (uphill) direction.

The start from Cow Canyon Saddle has two options: a 3.6-mile dirt road or a much steeper 1.6-mile firebreak (see Trip 2.1). Both options lead to the top of Sunset Peak, a 1,300-foot climb. Beyond, the fire road is almost all downhill.

Along the more open and exposed ridgeline, look for western bluebirds and Townsend's solitaires among the more common juncos and chickadees. With luck, you may also encounter a family of mountain quail. The males announce their presence in the spring with a piercing, far-carrying *keeear* call.

The road leads south along the eastern edge of the San Dimas Experimental Forest. This 32-square-mile parcel of land is closed to public access and is used for scientific research, including the effects of erosion, air pollution, and fire in the chaparral ecosystem. In 3 miles, pass beneath the antenna farm called the Sunset Ridge Electronic Site. To the west, Browns Flat is an unusual level clearing amid the steep hills. The road descends, making large switchbacks.

ALTERNATIVE FINISH

Below the last switchback, you can take a shortcut by dropping down steep ridges into the upper reaches of the Claremont Hills Wilderness Park or Marshall Canyon. The trail in this area mostly has vistas to the south, but look for a "window" on Sunset Ridge where you can peer onto the north side. A yellow box with a fire hydrant is located here. Just beyond, the narrow path can be found hidden among the bushes on the left (south) side of the fire road. It follows a slick firebreak down to the saddle at the northernmost point of the wilderness park, where the terminus is also hidden in brush. The USGS topographic map shows an old trail on this ridge. The lower part used to lead into Marshall Canyon but now takes the more direct route into the wilderness park. Arrange to meet a vehicle at one of these trailheads. Yet another firebreak connects Sunset Ridge to the saddle at the head of Evey Canyon.

The fire road continues west along the ridge above Marshall Canyon and then switchbacks down to a point just above the reservoir. Beware of poison oak, which grows in large stands along the edge of the road. Pass a collapsed old water tank. Shortly beyond, at an elevation of 1,700 feet, the road turns south. Look for a trail on the right, easy to miss, descending steeply westward. If you reach a large white water tank beside the road, you've gone 0.2 mile too far. Descend the trail 0.3 mile to where your vehicle awaits.

trip 2.3   Stoddard Peak

Distance	6 miles (out-and-back)
Hiking Time	3 hours
Elevation Gain	1,000'
Difficulty	Moderate
Trail Use	Dogs allowed
Best Times	All year
Agency	Angeles National Forest (Mount Baldy Visitor Center)
Recommended Map	Tom Harrison *Angeles High Country* or USGS *Mount Baldy* 7.5'

see map on p. 45

DIRECTIONS To reach the start from the 210 Freeway, take Exit 52 onto Base Line Road and drive west to the first intersection, Padua Avenue. Turn right (north) onto Padua and, in 1.8 miles, turn right on Mount Baldy Road. In 2.7 miles, pass the turnoff on the right for Mountain Avenue. Continue 3.7 miles. Just after you pass over the dirt hogback blocking San Antonio Canyon, turn right at the sign for Barrett–Stoddard Road and park in the small lot before the bridge crossing.

Stoddard Peak (4,624') is located on the shoulder of Ontario Peak overlooking San Antonio Canyon. Despite its diminutive stature among the huge peaks circling the canyon, Stoddard offers excellent views of Mount Baldy and is an enjoyable exercise hike or half-day excursion. The peak and nearby canyon were named for William Stoddard, who, in 1880, founded the first of many mountain resorts in this area. These resorts were immensely popular before the development of air-conditioning. Ranchers sent their families up into the high country to escape the oppressive heat that blankets the Inland Empire during the summer months.

Mount Baldy from Stoddard Peak

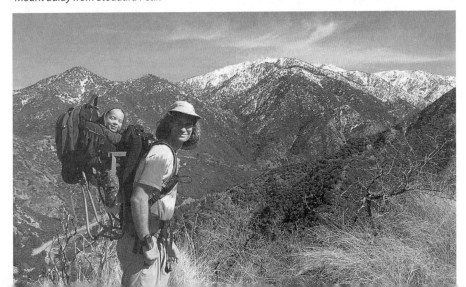

From the trailhead, hike east down the road, and cross the bridge over San Antonio Creek. On the west side of the creek, you can see traces of the old Mount Baldy Road that once ran along the creek before being washed out one too many times. Follow Barrett–Stoddard Road past some private residences near Barrett Canyon and, in 0.8 mile, pass a gate. Continue, generally southward, past the mouth of Cascade Canyon and above the flat-topped Spring Hill, where traces of an old farm can still be seen. In another 1.7 miles, cross a saddle to reach Stoddard Flat. Look to the right (west) for a trail chopped through the chaparral. Follow it up the hill and then along the rocky crest of a ridge. Hike 0.4 mile, passing two false summits before you reach the true summit of Stoddard Peak at the south end of the ridge. Return the way you came.

ALTERNATIVE FINISH ———————————————————————

For a substantially longer adventure, continue following the Cucamonga Truck Trail south from Stoddard Flat 5.6 miles down to Cucamonga Canyon and out to the top of Skyline Road in Alta Loma. Beware of washouts and poison oak along the route.

To leave a shuttle before you head to the start, take Exit 57 north off the 210 Freeway onto Carnelian Street; then take the first left onto Highland Avenue and, in 0.5 mile, turn right on Sapphire Street. In 1.8 miles, turn left on Almond Street. Skyline Road is the first right off Almond, but you can't park there—you must park in the designated area stretching along the left (south) side of Almond, and you must pay for a parking permit (go to parkrancho .com for details).

Another option is to descend 2.2 miles cross-country along Stoddard's south ridge over Peak 4,324' to the Lower San Antonio Fire Station on Mountain Avenue beside San Antonio Creek. The fire station is about 4.5 miles north of Exit 54 off the 210; park along the road.

---

trip 2.4   Frankish Peak

Distance	4 miles (out-and-back)
Hiking Time	3 hours
Elevation Gain	1,900'
Difficulty	Strenuous
Trail Use	Dogs allowed
Best Times	September–May
Agency	Angeles National Forest (Mount Baldy Visitor Center)
Recommended Map	USGS *Mount Baldy* 7.5'

see map on p. 45

DIRECTIONS From the 10 Freeway (I-10), take Exit 51 north onto Euclid Avenue in Upland. Drive all the way to the north end of Euclid, following it as it curves west to join Mountain Avenue 5.3 miles from the freeway. Continue west 0.4 mile, passing two turnouts beneath a hilltop water tank on the right; then park at a third turnout almost directly opposite the San Antonio Dam.

While the Claremont Hills Wilderness Park teems with hikers, nearby Frankish Peak rarely sees any visitors. It's steep and brushy, but it offers an outstanding workout in a short distance and provides fabulous views over the valley on a clear day. Long pants and shoes with good tread are recommended.

From the turnout, find the steep trail to the left of a gated service road, and follow this trail as it climbs a ridge to a dirt road in 0.6 mile. Turn right, proceed 0.1 mile, and then turn left and head up 0.2 mile to the end of the road atop a small hill, where you have a bird's-eye view of planes approaching Cable Airport. From here, a trail climbs steeply. It turns right and levels out briefly before ascending an even steeper knife-edge dirt ridge. At the top, turn

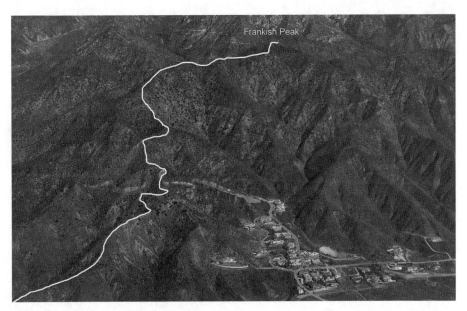

Aerial view of Frankish Peak route

right and follow the use trail, faint in places, through head-high chaparral over a false summit. Continue east and join a fire road, which leads 0.2 mile on to the true summit. From here, enjoy the close-up views of Ontario Peak looming to the north and the expansive views of the Inland Empire spread out below.

ALTERNATIVE FINISH

For a substantially longer trip, descend northeast from Frankish Peak on a fire road 1.3 miles to the Cucamonga Truck Trail, which you take 2.3 miles down Cucamonga Canyon; then turn right and hike 1.1 miles to the edge of Alta Loma, at the top of Skyline Road. This requires a car shuttle and a good map. Beware of washouts and poison oak along the Cucamonga Truck Trail.

To leave a shuttle before you head to the start, take Exit 57 north off the 210 Freeway onto Carnelian Street; then take the first left onto Highland Avenue and, in 0.5 mile, turn right on Sapphire Street. In 1.8 miles, turn left on Almond Street. Skyline Road is the first right off Almond, but you can't park there—you must park in the designated area stretching along the left (south) side of Almond, and you must pay for a parking permit (go to parkrancho .com for details).

---

trip 2.5   Etiwanda Falls and Preserve

see map on next page

Distance	3.5 miles (out-and-back), 5.0 miles (loop)
Hiking Time	2–3 hours
Elevation Gain	800'/1,000'
Difficulty	Moderate
Trail Use	Good for kids
Best Times	All year, but hot in summer; best flows in the spring

Agency San Bernardino County Special Districts
Recommended Map Tom Harrison *Angeles High Country* or USGS *Cucamonga Peak 7.5'* (not all locations of dirt roads are accurate)

DIRECTIONS From the 210 Freeway, take Exit 61 onto Day Creek Boulevard in Rancho Cucamonga. Drive north and then east 2.1 miles; then turn left onto Etiwanda Avenue and proceed 0.4 mile to the end of the road, where you'll find the trailhead parking. Pay close attention to parking restrictions—the city has aggressively towed vehicles.

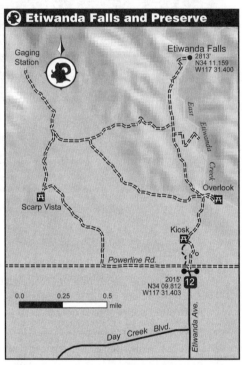

One of the Inland Empire's rare accessible waterfalls is hidden near the mouth of East Etiwanda Canyon just out of sight of millions of commuters. This moderate hike to the falls follows a good dirt road all the way.

The route passes through the North Etiwanda Preserve, which protects an area of diverse habitats and significant cultural history. Part of the 1,200-acre preserve was initially set aside in 1998 to offset the impact of 210 Freeway development, and the preserve formally opened in 2009. Situated on an alluvial fan between two washes and bisected by the Sierra Madre Fault, this alluvial sage scrub and fragile riparian habitat is home to 15 animal species and two plants that are endangered, threatened, or of other special concern, including the San Bernardino kangaroo rat and the southwestern willow flycatcher. It's a great place to watch for lizards, birds, and wildflowers. Remember that all of the plants and animals in the preserve are protected.

The area was long used by the Tongva and Serrano peoples. The Spanish established Mission San Gabriel in 1771, then granted the 13,000-acre Rancho Cucamonga to Tiburcio Tapia in 1839. George Day purchased a parcel at the mouth of the canyon in 1867 and built a ditch and then a flume for irrigation; the area is now crisscrossed with numerous historic and modern irrigation systems. This hike can be done as an out-and-back to the falls, but if you have time, it's even better to loop back and see more of North Etiwanda Preserve.

From the parking area, gated dirt roads lead north and west into Etiwanda Preserve. Head north toward the mountain. The alluvial fan sage scrub community along the trail was once plentiful, but is now endangered by heavy development north of the 210 Freeway and by containment of the creeks. Common species include California sagebrush and buckwheat, white sage, ceanothus, and scale broom. In 0.2 mile, pass the main kiosk on the left, where you can learn more about the preserve. In another 0.4 mile, come to a four-way junction. The preserve loop turns left. If you walk 500 feet to the right, you'll come to a picnic area overlooking East Etiwanda Wash. This trip heads straight north on the unsigned road to the falls.

The path soon exits the preserve and enters the San Bernardino National Forest. In 0.5 mile, continue straight at another four-way junction. Pass another gate and continue on the flank of the deep wash. In 0.6 mile, the road ends at the top of the falls, which usually run year-round. Enjoy the overlook, but take care on the slick rock.

You can return the way you came, or make a loop by hiking back to the northernmost four-way junction and turning west to reenter Etiwanda Preserve in a burn zone near mile marker 1.5. The May 2014 Etiwanda Fire scorched 2,190 acres after an illegal campfire got out of control. Fortunately, sage scrub is adapted to recover rapidly from wildfires. Continue counter-clockwise on the preserve loop. At the highest point along the route, a spur forks right to visit a gaging station on Day Creek, but your path turns south toward a prominent scarp with two trees beside a picnic bench and restroom. From here you can enjoy magnificent views over the Inland Empire to San Gorgonio, San Jacinto, and Santiago Peaks.

Continuing on the loop, come to a board-walk overlooking a freshwater bog. This sag pond, the vista point you just came from, and another scarp ahead are all products of the Cucamonga Fault Zone, which relieves the tremendous pressures produced as the San Gabriel Mountains have thrust upward. Your path, now a deteriorating asphalt road, drops down to meet a power-line road. Turn left (west) and soon emerge at the trailhead where you began.

VARIATION

Another option is to skip the falls and simply hike the 3.2-mile loop through North Eti-wanda Preserve. This option involves 700 feet of elevation gain.

Etiwanda Falls

chapter 3

San Bernardino Mountains: West

The San Bernardino Mountains are part of California's unusual Transverse Ranges, running east to west rather than north to south. They've long attracted the attention of humans, at first for hunting, logging, and gold, but now most of all for recreation. The range is so large that trips for this area are divided into three chapters. This chapter describes the western end, especially around Lake Arrowhead and the alluring creeks at the interface of forest and desert. Chapter 4 focuses on the eastern end, where richly forested hills circle the jewel-like Big Bear Lake. Chapter 5 explores the steep and rugged San Gorgonio Wilderness on the southeast side of the range, cut off from Big Bear by the deep trench of the Santa Ana River.

The southern side rises abruptly from the endless concrete and asphalt of suburbia to the tall forests nearly a mile above sea level. This dramatic escarpment is the work of the infamous San Andreas Fault, which is likely to thrust the mountains even higher in the near geological future. The northern edge rolls off more gradually into the Mojave Desert. Numerous streams carve canyons on the north slopes and then flow together until they merge into the Mojave River and sink beneath the shifting sands. The hills and canyons are laced with a variety of mostly short trails.

The low western end of the San Bernardino Mountains is the most heavily populated, with significant communities at Lake Arrowhead, Crestline, Running Springs, Arrowbear, and Green Valley Lake. Lake Arrowhead was originally constructed as part of an ambitious project to divert the headwaters of the Mojave River southward to irrigate San Bernardino. The efforts began in 1892. After decades of effort and vast sums of money spent, the diversion project was defeated. A 1913 court ruling favored the desert residents who would have lost access to their water. However, the real estate and recreational value of the alpine lake became obvious, and mountain-goers have flocked to the region for a century now to enjoy its charms.

The western San Bernardinos have been hit by a succession of disastrous forest fires. Forests and chaparral have evolved to withstand naturally occurring fires from time to time. In a healthy environment, the mature trees generally survive these low-intensity fires; in fact, chaparral needs periodic burns in order to reproduce. Fire plays an essential role in clearing out the undergrowth and keeping the ecosystem healthy. As the population in the forest increased during the 20th century, the government began aggressively fighting fires to protect property. Years of fire suppression have led to overcrowded forests with large amounts of flammable debris on the forest floor. Ozone pollution and drought have further weakened the trees, rendering them susceptible to outbreaks of bark beetles that have killed many of the trees. The combination of heavily packed dead trees and dense ground cover has left the forest extremely vulnerable to high-intensity fires. The 1999 Willow Fire burned 64,000 acres north of Lake Arrowhead and was the largest fire in the San Bernardino National Forest in the past 80 years. Then, in October 2003, 14 major fires

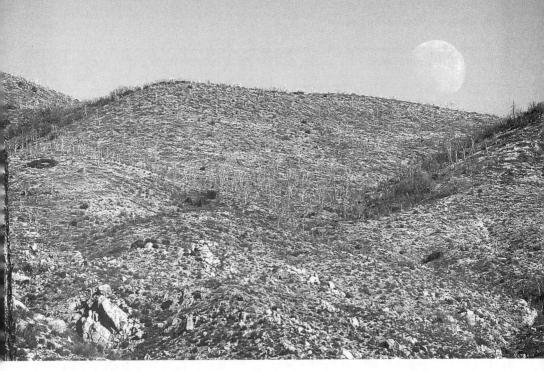

Moonrise over the burnt hills above Deep Creek

simultaneously swept across California. The Grand Prix and Old Fires hit the Lake Arrowhead area, charring 59,000 acres and destroying 135 residences. The Cedar Glen area was particularly hard hit, with whole neighborhoods of cabins reduced to their foundations. The Slide Fire in October 2007 burned another 12,000 of the remaining acres and 272 homes around Running Springs and Green Valley Lake. Many of the trails in this chapter offer a sobering reminder of the power of wildfire and a fascinating glimpse into the ecological recovery process. The historic policy of fire suppression is obviously untenable and land managers are struggling to find a better approach and to reconcile the need for natural wildfires with people's desire to live in these fire-prone areas.

The best time to visit this area is in the fall or the late spring. Summers can be uncomfortably warm, although hiking early in the day or along shady creeks is still enjoyable. In the winter, access to higher trails is blocked by snow.

An extensive network of dirt roads has been carved through the San Bernardino Mountains, providing easy access to otherwise remote areas. These same roads draw throngs of ATV riders, especially on the northwestern slopes. The ceaseless roar of engines is detrimental to good hiking. Most of these trails are set back from the worst ATV traffic, but a few, especially around Holcomb Creek, can be a problem. Moreover, hunters flock to these hills in deer season (October and November), so it's prudent to dress brightly and stay especially alert to your surroundings in the fall.

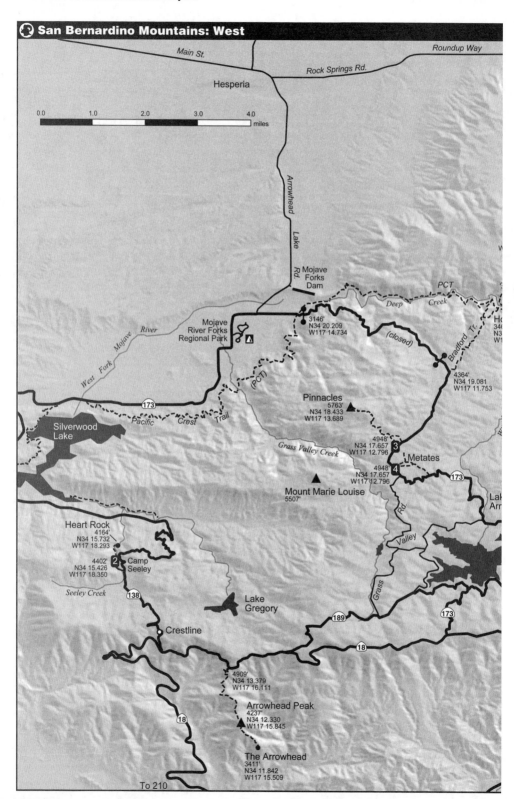

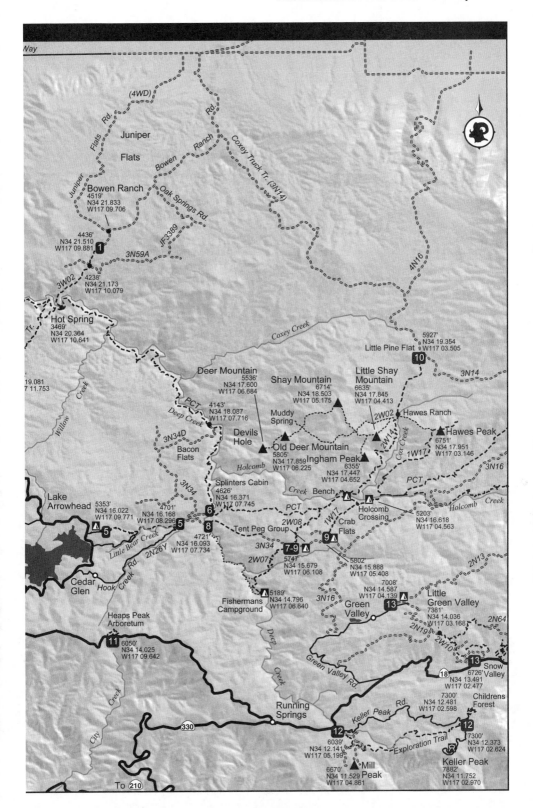

trip 3.1	**Deep Creek Hot Springs**

Distance	4 miles (out-and-back)
Hiking Time	2 hours
Elevation Gain	900'
Difficulty	Moderate
Best Times	September–May
Agency	San Bernardino National Forest (Big Bear Discovery Center)
Recommended Map	USGS *Lake Arrowhead* 7.5'
Permit	Day-use fee required

see map on p. 55

DIRECTIONS From the 15 Freeway (I-15), 6 miles north of Cajon Pass in Hesperia, take Exit 143 east onto Main Street. In 7.2 miles, bear left (east) onto Rock Springs Road where Main Street curves south. Cross the dry bed of the Mojave River, and follow Rock Springs Road east 2.8 miles to a junction where the name of the road changes to Roundup Way. Continue east on Roundup Way for 4.4 miles; then turn right (south) onto good dirt Bowen Ranch Road. Stay right at a junction with Coxey Truck Trail at 2.1 miles, and right again in 1.9 miles at a junction with Oak Springs Road; then continue 1.4 miles to Bowen Ranch. Register at the ranch house and pay a modest use fee; then continue 0.5 mile through the ranch to the trailhead, at the road's end on top of a hill.

High-clearance 4WD vehicles can reach a free alternate trailhead a half mile closer, although the drive is slow enough that the shortcut is unlikely to save time. To reach this point, veer left onto Oak Springs Road at the junction mentioned above. In 1.4 miles, turn right onto a road signed JF3389 and pass through a gate. In 1.0 mile, stay right at a pair of junctions onto Forest Road 3N59A (marked JF3381 in some places). Drive 2.0 miles to a sign on the left for trail 3W02, which leads southwest to Deep Creek Hot Springs. 3N59A continues west and eventually joins an intricate maze of jeep trails that connect back to Bowen Ranch Road, but navigating in this area is quite difficult.

Deep Creek pours down a rugged canyon through the desert slopes of the San Bernardino Mountains before emptying into the Mojave River. The best hot spring in the Inland Empire is found on the cliffs above Deep Creek; it pours through a series of pools down into

Deep Creek Hot Springs

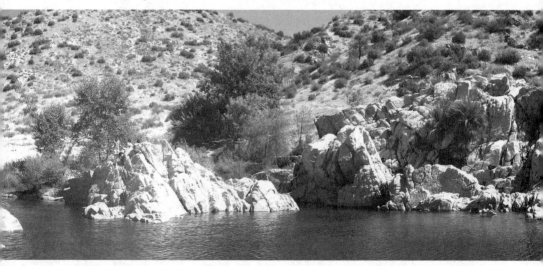

the cool creek. This popular spot draws hikers to soak in the warm water during the winter and frolic in the creek on warmer days. Camping is allowed at the trailhead on Bowen Ranch but not at the hot spring. Do not bring glass, and take care to leave the place cleaner than you found it. Don't submerge your head in the pools, which contain high levels of fecal coliform bacteria. A bather died in 1991 after becoming infected here with *Naegleria fowleri,* a brain-eating amoeba that lives in warm waters and enters through the nose.

If you plan to do this hike in the summer, be aware that the trail leads across shadeless desert where temperatures commonly exceed 100°F. Bring plenty of water and remember that the return is all uphill. Avoid Deep Creek during thunderstorms because the narrow canyon presents a flash flood risk.

Follow the trail south, and then pass through a gate onto Forest Service land. In 0.5 mile, reach a junction with the 4WD road, 3N59A. This is the alternate starting point, locally known as the Freedom Trailhead, and is the last legal place to camp. Turn left, walk down the road 200 feet, and then turn right at another sign where trail 3W02 continues southwest. The next section of trail, nicknamed the Goat Trail, traverses onto a ridge that drops steeply down to Deep Creek. Turn left and walk upstream to a bend in the creek. There is a sandy beach on the north side, but you must ford the cold waters to reach the hot springs on the south side.

VARIATION

The unofficial Bradford Ridge Trail from the south avoids the cold ford and the dirt road and fees at Bowen Ranch. A 5.5-mile round-trip with 1,900 feet of elevation gain—600 feet on the way to the creek and 1,300 feet on the steep, shadeless return—this hike is not recommended in summer.

The trail starts at the bridge where Highway 173 crosses Kinley Creek, 2.5 miles north of the Rock Camp Forest Service Station (note that Highway 173 is closed north of here). Take the trail on the northeast side of the road and pass through a gate. Round a corner and look left for a waterfall on Kinley Creek; then follow the creek. The 1999 Willow Fire ravaged more than 60,000 acres including almost everything along this trail, but look for the "Unburned Acre," where you can still see mature oaks as they once stood.

In 0.7 mile, the trail begins climbing steeply out of Kinley Creek. In another 0.7 mile, cross a minor saddle and start descending into a drainage leading down toward Deep Creek. In 0.4 mile, reach a junction by a gap in an old fence. A very steep side trail to the right shortcuts down, but the main trail leads straight down the ridge to the north and intersects the Pacific Crest Trail (PCT) in 0.4 mile at the toe of the ridge. Turn right and follow the PCT 0.5 mile to Deep Creek Hot Springs.

The hot springs can be reached from the Mojave River Forks Reservoir dam via a 6.1-mile (each way) hike up the PCT with 800 feet of elevation gain. The trailhead is on Highway 173 0.6 mile east of Arrowhead Lake Road. Follow the PCT northeast 0.8 mile; then, after passing Point 3,353', ford Deep Creek. The crossing can be difficult because the creek is, well, er, deep. Continue east 0.4 mile up onto the dam to the spillway at the east end, where the trail switchbacks up into the canyon. In 1.8 miles, watch for Hesperia Falls, a cliff-jumping site that draws rowdy kids and distressing amounts of graffiti. In April 2015, a local teen died while jumping here. The PCT crosses Deep Creek on an arched bridge, passes the unsigned Bradford Trail, and reaches the hot springs.

trip 3.2 | Heart Rock

Distance	1 mile (out-and-back)
Hiking Time	1 hour
Elevation Gain	200'
Difficulty	Easy
Trail Use	Dogs allowed, good for kids
Best Times	All year, but waterfall is best in the spring
Agency	San Bernardino National Forest (Big Bear Discovery Center)
Recommended Map	USGS *Silverwood Lake* 7.5'

see map on p. 54

DIRECTIONS From the 10 (I-10) or 210 (I-210/SR 210) Freeway in San Bernardino, take Exit 73B or 76, respectively, onto Waterman Avenue, which becomes Rim of the World Scenic Byway (Highway 18). At the top of the ridge (11.5 miles from the 210 exit), exit onto Highway 138. Proceed north 1.2 miles to the stop sign in the middle of Crestline, and then continue 1.5 miles down to the Camp Seely entrance road at mile marker 138 SBD 35.00. Turn left and then left again just outside the gate to Camp Seely, and follow the narrow paved road across Seely Creek to a gate, 0.4 mile from the highway. Park outside the gate on the right, next to the 4W07 trail post.

The cool waters of Seely Creek flow down the north slope of the San Bernardino Mountains beneath incense cedars and oaks. Through a fortuitous quirk of geology, they've carved a remarkable heart-shaped basin in the rock alongside a waterfall. Beyond, they rush down the granite slabs into an alluring pool. This short hike follows the bank of Seely Creek to the Heart Rock overlook and the pool. The best times for this trip are in the spring when the waterfall is most dramatic and in the early summer when the water is tempting for a dip.

The creek and camp are named for David and Wellington Seely, brothers who established a sawmill here in the 1850s to provide for the Mormon outpost in San Bernardino. Their name has been misspelled "Seeley" on many official documents, including the USGS topographic map.

Follow the shady trail as it leads north from the parking area. Soon you'll enjoy views of the creek as the trail follows above it. In 0.5 mile, look for an unmarked three-way fork in the trail. From here, the route devolves into a maze of footpaths. To the right, descend a rocky path to a boulder overlooking Heart Rock and the waterfall. Keep a close eye on young children because the overlook is perched above a sheer cliff.

The path straight from the fork joins up with another path descending from the overlook to reach the base of the falls and a pleasant pool slightly farther downstream. This is a good place for a picnic. Unfortunately, thoughtless visitors leave their trash here; if you bring a garbage bag and pack out some of the litter, the site will be better for everyone.

The left fork leads back up to the paved road, which parallels the trail. However, the trail you arrived by is more scenic, so return the way you came.

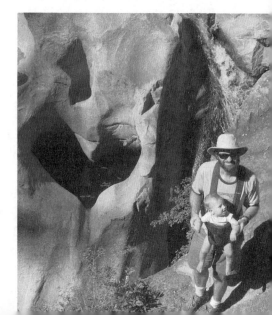

Bonding time at Heart Rock

trip 3.3   The Pinnacles

Distance	4 miles (out-and-back)
Hiking Time	2.5 hours
Elevation Gain	1,000'
Difficulty	Moderate
Trail Use	Dogs allowed, good for kids
Best Times	October–May
Agency	San Bernardino National Forest (Big Bear Discovery Center)
Recommended Map	USGS *Lake Arrowhead* 7.5'

see map on p. 54

DIRECTIONS From Lake Arrowhead, follow Highway 173 north to the Rock Camp Forest Service Station; then continue 0.5 mile north to a turnout on the west side of the road. If you reach the old trailhead at the Arrowhead Shooting Range, you've gone 0.2 mile too far.

The granite Pinnacles sit atop a hill on the desert slopes northwest of Lake Arrowhead. Rock climbers flock to the impressive boulders to test their skills. A trail leads to the high point, where you can scramble up some boulders for an outstanding view.

Walk through an opening in the fence and follow the trail north, crossing a dry wash. If the path seems to fork at times, follow the most-used branch. In 0.3 mile, reach an unsigned junction with the old trail coming in on the right from the Arrowhead Shooting Range. Veer left and meander up a wash through chaparral and boulders until you can climb the steep hill to the Pinnacles.

The most prominent tower to the north of the trail, called The Bong, features routes to challenge even the extreme rock climber (rated at 5.10–5.12). The trail continues to the summit boulder pile on the northwest end of the plateau. Some easy third-class scrambling is necessary to reach the airy perch.

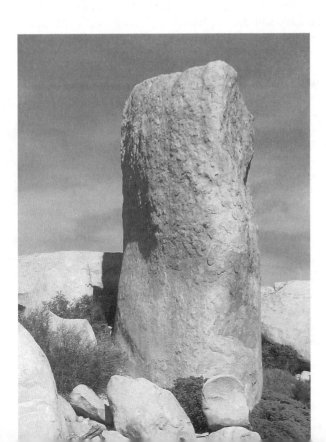

Bong Rock
Photo: Evan Harris

trip 3.4   Rock Camp/Metate Interpretive Trail

Distance	0.8 mile (loop)
Hiking Time	30 minutes
Elevation Gain	100'
Difficulty	Easy
Trail Use	Dogs allowed, good for kids
Best Times	March–November
Agency	San Bernardino National Forest (Big Bear Discovery Center)
Required Map	USGS *Lake Arrowhead* 7.5' (trail not shown)

see map on p. 54

DIRECTIONS From Lake Arrowhead, follow Highway 173 north to the Rock Camp Forest Service Station; then continue 0.5 mile north to a turnout on the west side of the road. If you reach the old trailhead at the Arrowhead Shooting Range, you've gone 0.2 mile too far.

In bygone days, the Serrano Indians gathered each fall to collect acorns and grind them into flour. One of their favored foraging grounds can be visited just north of the present-day Lake Arrowhead. This site was ideal because of the plentiful acorns, mild weather, nearby stream, and convenient rocks. Over the centuries, the Serrano wore deep holes, called *metates*, into the bedrock where they ground their food. A loop trail visits some of these metates and offers a pleasant easy walk. The trail is designated 3W15 by the Forest Service but isn't shown on the USGS map. It would benefit from directional and interpretive signage, but it's not hard to follow.

Cross Highway 173 and pass a gate into the Rock Camp Forest Service Station. Continue straight ahead to a sign reading INTERPRETIVE AREA. A wide trail leads east and immediately forks. Take the left fork, marked with another Interpretive Area sign. The trail enters a lovely open forest of pine and oak.

In 0.2 mile, reach an unmarked junction. The left fork leads north 0.2 mile to an ATV track, but this trip takes the right fork. Immediately after the junction, look for a stone monument with a plaque placed by the Woman's Club of Lake Arrowhead to mark this historic site. Climb onto some granite slabs behind the sign to look for a number of prominent metates. With some imagination, you can conjure the sights and sounds of families camped beneath the tall trees, racing against the squirrels to gather a fine crop of acorns. Explore the area and see if you can find more metates.

You could return the way you came, but for an enjoyable loop, continue east and cross a seasonal tributary of Willow Creek. The trail abruptly turns right. A faint unmarked

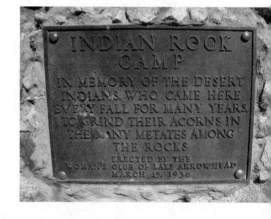

spur on the left leads southwest up a hill 0.4 mile to a gate alongside Highway 173, but the main trail continues through a small meadow and turns right to recross the creek and return to the Forest Service station through a green metal gate.

see
map on
p. 55

trip 3.5   Little Bear Creek

Distance	4 miles (out-and-back)
Hiking Time	3 hours
Elevation Gain	800'
Difficulty	Moderate
Trail Use	Dogs allowed
Best Times	March–June, October–December
Agency	San Bernardino National Forest (Big Bear Discovery Center)
Recommended Map	USGS *Lake Arrowhead* 7.5' (inaccurate near North Shore Campground)

DIRECTIONS From Highway 173, 2.8 miles northeast of the junction with Highway 189 at Lake Arrowhead Village, turn right (east) onto Hospital Road. Follow this road 0.25 mile to the North Shore Campground entrance, opposite the hospital. If you park in the campground, you must pay a day-use fee. You may park for free in a small lot just outside the campground, but you may not park in the hospital lot without permission.

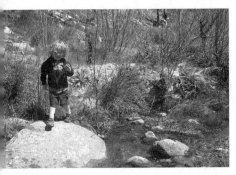

Little Bear Creek

The campground amazingly escaped the 2003 Old Fire. The campground is open between May 1 and September 30.

If you wish to make an even shorter one-way trip with a car or bicycle shuttle, arrange a ride at the lower trailhead. (The 4.3-mile bicycle shuttle involves significant elevation gain in both directions and is more strenuous than simply walking back up the trail.) To reach the lower trailhead, go back south on Highway 173 for 1.2 miles, and then turn left (east) onto Hook Creek Road. Pass through the village of Cedar Glen for 2.3 miles to a gate at Forest Road 2N26Y. Continue 0.8 mile down the winding one-lane road and cross Hooks Creek. Look for a 3W12 trail marker on the left. If you reach a junction with 3N34 in 0.1 mile, you just missed the lower trailhead.

Little Bear Creek rolls playfully down the hill from Lake Arrowhead into Hooks Creek and onward into Deep Creek. It once cavorted beneath a delightful forest of pines, oaks, and incense cedars, but the 2003 Old Fire incinerated the entire canyon, along with countless cabins in Cedar Glen. Now, this hike is a sobering reminder of the power of wildfire and a fascinating opportunity to watch the forest regenerate itself.

The North Shore National Recreation Trail (3W12) begins at the far eastern end of the campground. It descends into a grove of black oaks, passing a spur leading over to a maintenance yard. In 0.1 mile, cross a dirt road and continue down along the north fork of Little Bear Creek. Follow the switchbacks down the hill and cross the tributary to reach a trail junction on the north bank of the main creek in 0.9 mile.

The right branch leads 0.1 mile to an alternate trailhead shaded under the cedars on Big Tree Drive, but this trip takes the left branch, which follows Little Bear Creek down the canyon past ghostly hulks of charred trees and through the manzanita, buckthorn, and other brush that comes first in the plant succession after fire. In 0.3 mile, climb 50 feet over a low ridge to bypass a bend in the creek. In another 0.7 mile, cross Little Bear Creek on a large log or some rocks and emerge at the 3W12 trailhead marker at the junction of Forest Roads 2N26Y and 3N34.

Return the way you came unless you've set up a car or bicycle shuttle.

see map on p. 55

trip 3.6 **Deep Creek**

Distance	6 miles (out-and-back)
Hiking Time	3 hours
Elevation Gain	600'
Difficulty	Moderate
Trail Use	Dogs allowed, suitable for backpacking
Best Times	March–June, October–November
Agency	San Bernardino National Forest (Big Bear Discovery Center)
Recommended Maps	USGS *Lake Arrowhead* and *Butler Peak* 7.5'

DIRECTIONS From Highway 173 on the east shore of Lake Arrowhead, 1.6 miles northeast of the junction with Highway 189 at Lake Arrowhead Village, drive east on Hook Creek Road through the village of Cedar Glen 2.3 miles to a gate at Forest Road 2N26Y. Continue 0.8 mile down the winding one-lane road and cross Hooks Creek. Continue 0.1 mile on a good dirt road; then stay left at the junction with 3N34. Cross the creek again and make a right turn at 3N34C after 0.2 mile. Pass another gate and proceed 0.4 mile to the Splinters Cabin Trailhead, where the hike begins. If the 3N34C gate is locked, park outside and walk from the gate, taking care not to block access. This parking area has seen a rash of vandalism, so don't leave valuables in your vehicle.

Deep Creek carves a dramatic canyon through the desert slopes of the northern San Bernardino Mountains before emptying into the Mojave River. Although it flows through parched country, the creek and its many tributaries drain such a broad watershed that the water runs reliably year-round. This hike follows a section of the PCT overlooking Deep Creek and then dips down to reach a pool. Deep Creek is a designated Wild Trout Stream.

The 2003 Old Fire wiped out the forest along the southern end of this hike and incinerated many cabins in Cedar Glen. A burning pine crushed the steel bridge across Deep Creek, but the bridge has been repaired.

From the end of the road at the site of Splinters Cabin, follow a path north to ford Hooks Creek and reach the PCT in 0.2 mile at the bridge over Deep Creek. You'll find a large and easily accessible swimming hole beneath the bridge. Follow the PCT as it gently descends along the wall of the canyon. The dramatic trail clings to the canyon wall above

The author's oldest son at Deep Creek in 2006 (left) and 2017 (right)

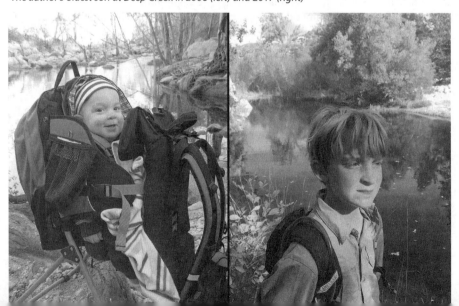

a sheer drop at times. Watch for a number of use trails down to the water. In 0.6 mile, a prominent path drops to Aztec Falls, a cliff-jumping site that attracts a party crowd and their associated litter.

Pass the confluence with Holcomb Creek and, in 3 miles, reach a jeep trail coming down from Bacon Flats. Turn right and follow the path down to a large pool in Deep Creek.

ALTERNATIVE FINISH ────────────────────────────────────

Return the way you came. Alternatively, follow the jeep road (3N34D) up to Bacon Flats; then turn left and follow 3N34 back to the Splinters Cabin Trailhead. This route is a mile longer but offers a change of scenery. Yet another option with a long car shuttle is to continue down the PCT 6.8 miles to Deep Creek Hot Springs, and emerge at Bowen Ranch (see Trip 3.1).

VARIATION ──

If time permits, it's well worth visiting another beautiful nearby section of Deep Creek. Drive back to the junction of Forest Roads 3N34 and 2N26Y, and turn east onto 3N34. The road is posted as 4WD, but the first part is usually passable by low-clearance vehicles. In 0.7 mile, reach a concrete bridge over Deep Creek and park on the far side. The section of Deep Creek leading upstream (see Trip 3.8) is one of the most rugged and beautiful streams in the San Bernardino Mountains, carving a course through granite cliffs. There is a fine sandy beach, and you can explore along the ledges upstream for a short distance before the going gets difficult. Forest Road 3N34 continues east but promptly deteriorates into an extremely rocky and difficult jeep road with serious risk of body damage to stock SUVs.

---

trip 3.7 **Fisherman's Camp**

Distance	5 miles (out-and-back)
Hiking Time	3 hours
Elevation Gain	700'
Difficulty	Moderate
Trail Use	Dogs allowed, suitable for backpacking, suitable for mountain biking, suitable for equestrians
Best Times	March–November
Agency	San Bernardino National Forest (Big Bear Discovery Center)
Recommended Maps	USGS *Butler Peak* and *Keller Peak* 7.5'

see map on p. 55

DIRECTIONS From the Rim of the World Scenic Byway (Highway 18), 2.9 miles northeast of the intersection with Highway 330 at the town of Running Springs and just past mile marker 018 SBD 34.50, turn left (north) onto Green Valley Lake Road. After 2.6 miles—just before you reach Green Valley Lake—turn left again onto Forest Road 3N16 (Crab Flats Road). Descend on this good dirt road toward Crab Flats Family Campground, passing several side roads and crossing Crab Creek (impassable in high water). Reach the junction with Big Pine Flat Road after 3.8 miles. Stay left on 3N34, passing Crab Flats Campground after 0.2 mile. Continue 1.1 miles along the deteriorating road (high clearance recommended) to park at a clearing and a large VISITORS TO DEEP CREEK sign just beyond Tent Peg Group Campground.

F isherman's Camp sits on the bank of Deep Creek in the rolling hills northwest of Green Valley. This trip involves an enjoyable tour of the backcountry roads and trails down to the rushing creek. It can be done as a day hike or an easy backpacking trip. Anglers should bring a rod and try their luck at coaxing the trout from their hiding spots.

Note that all of Deep Creek is a Wild Trout Stream, which means a daily limit of two fish with a minimum size of 8 inches; use of bait and hooks with barbs is prohibited. As always, a valid California fishing license must be displayed by anyone fishing who is 16 years of age or older.

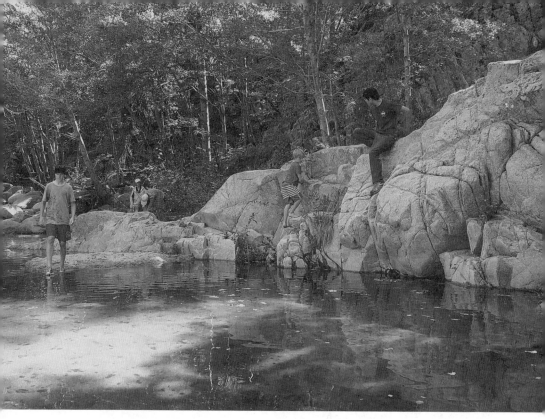

Pool in Deep Creek near Fisherman's Camp

The Crab Creek Trail (2W07) heads west and climbs gently around a low hill. The tall Jeffrey and Coulter pines that once graced the slopes were incinerated by the October 2007 Slide Fire and have shown no signs of regrowth. The tough black oaks are sprouting from their root burls, but much of the slope has been replaced by chaparral and this change might be permanent if the hot, dry climate persists.

The trail climbs gently and then contours west before switchbacking down the burnt slope. In 1.2 miles, the Crab Creek crossing marks the halfway point. Walk up Crab Creek a few yards to find a 30-foot cascade flowing down a granite step. The Crab Creek drainage escaped the ravages of the fire and hosts a diverse forest including alder, dogwood, incense cedar, white fir, Jeffrey pine, Coulter pine, and sugar pine.

Beyond, the trail becomes more gently graded, paralleling Crab Creek southwestward. In 0.5 mile, it gains a low ridge and turns south away from Crab Creek. Look for an unsigned use trail on the right, described in Trip 3.8. This trip continues on the main trail 0.7 mile to the bank of Deep Creek. Look for the trail continuing on the far side, leading 200 yards upstream to Fisherman's Campground. Fording the vigorous stream can be dangerous during times of high water. Watch for striking scarlet monkeyflower along the creek.

Those who wish to camp at Fisherman's Group Campground must make reservations through recreation.gov at least 24 hours in advance. The campground has a solar toilet and four sites with picnic tables. A service road reaches the campground from the west, but the sites are walk-in only. You can rock-hop or wade 0.2 mile upstream from the campground to a swimming hole on Deep Creek lined with low granite cliffs. Before the Slide Fire, the hole was much deeper and one could jump off the cliffs into the water, but erosion has carried sand down the creek and the hole is far too shallow at this writing.

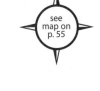

trip 3.8 **Deep Creek Canyoneering**

Distance	6.5 miles (loop)
Hiking Time	6 hours
Elevation Gain	1,300'
Difficulty	Strenuous
Best Times	August–October
Agency	San Bernardino National Forest (Big Bear Discovery Center)
Required Maps	USGS *Butler Peak, Keller Peak,* and *Lake Arrowhead* 7.5' (trail not shown)

see map on p. 55

DIRECTIONS From Highway 173 on the east shore of Lake Arrowhead, 1.6 miles northeast of the junction with Highway 189 at Lake Arrowhead Village, drive east on Hook Creek Road through the village of Cedar Glen 2.3 miles to a gate at Forest Road 2N26Y. Continue 0.8 mile down the winding one-lane road and cross Hooks Creek. Continue 0.1 mile on a good dirt road to a junction with 3N34 on the right. If you have a low-clearance vehicle, park near here. Follow 3N34 for 0.7 mile to the T6 Bridge where it crosses Deep Creek. The last quarter mile can be very rocky, but you'll find plenty of places to park earlier if you don't want to risk banging up your vehicle.

The section of Deep Creek between Fisherman's Camp and Forest Road 3N34 is one of the most beautiful canyons in the San Bernardino Mountains. Cut through granite walls, the narrow canyon is full of pools and cascades. Two waterfalls grace the upper section. During much of the year, the raging creek is impassable, but by late summer, it may offer an outstanding canyoneering experience. The easiest way to make a loop is to hike up rugged 3N34 to the Fisherman's Camp Trailhead, descend the trail, cut off down to the waterfalls, and wade the creek back to your starting point.

This is a strenuous trip suitable for experienced cross-country hikers who are comfortable negotiating a slippery creekbed. Check Deep Creek at the trailhead, and don't do this hike if the flow is strong. Likewise, avoid this trip if thunderstorms raise the risk of flash flooding. Bring at least a gallon of water in the summer.

From the Deep Creek T6 Bridge, hike east up Forest Road 3N34 (Dishpan Springs Road) 3 miles to the Fisherman's Camp Trailhead. This rugged road has rock gardens that thrill dirt bikers but exceed the clearance of most unmodified 4WD vehicles. The road traverses the burn area from the 2003 Old Fire, and the exposed uphill slog can be a hot affair in the

Wading through Deep Creek Canyon

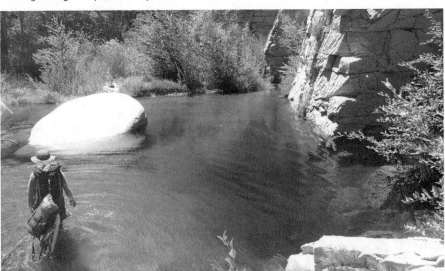

summer. You can avoid this road walk with a car shuttle by way of Little Green Valley (see Trip 3.7 driving directions), but the drive is more than an hour each way.

When you top out at a clearing near Tent Peg Group Campground, take the signed 2W07 Crab Creek Trail to Fisherman's Camp. This area burned in the 2007 Slide Fire. The trail descends to cross Crab Creek in 1.1 miles and then contours southwest above the creek. When the trail turns left in 0.5 mile, look for a use trail dropping 200 feet over 0.2 mile to the top of the falls in Deep Creek. You could also stay on the trail down to Fisherman's Camp and then walk 0.6 mile down the creek to the falls, but this portion of the canyon is full of downed trees, stinging nettle, and wild-rose thickets, and it's very slow-going.

The upper falls drop about 10 feet into a deep pool. One can jump directly into the pool (beware of a submerged ledge nearby), or scramble up and around granite blocks to the left. Shortly beyond, reach a second cascade with a bigger drop into a larger pool. This waterfall is most easily bypassed via a third-class crack on the left.

These obstacles behind you, embark on the gorgeous 2.2-mile canyoneering descent of Deep Creek. This stretch will take a fast group at least 2.5 hours under good conditions. Expect all sorts of obstacles, including smaller waterfalls, log jams, deep pools, algae-covered rocks, and occasional bushwhacking. Scarlet monkeyflower blooms into the fall, and you're likely to find trout in the creek.

trip 3.9 Holcomb Crossing Trail Camp

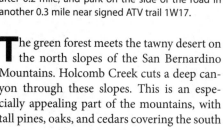
see map on p. 55

Distance	5 miles (loop)
Hiking Time	3 hours
Elevation Gain	900'
Difficulty	Moderate
Trail Use	Dogs allowed, suitable for backpacking, suitable for equestrians
Best Times	March–June, September–November
Agency	San Bernardino National Forest (Big Bear Discovery Center)
Recommended Map	USGS *Butler Peak* 7.5'

DIRECTIONS From the Rim of the World Scenic Byway (Highway 18), 2.9 miles northeast of the intersection with Highway 330 in Running Springs and just past mile marker 018 SBD 34.50, turn left (north) onto Green Valley Road. After 2.6 miles—just before you reach Green Valley Lake—turn left again onto Forest Road 3N16 (Crab Flats Road). Descend this good dirt road toward Crab Flats Family Campground, passing several side roads and crossing Crab Creek (impassable in high water). Reach the junction with Big Pine Flat Road after 3.8 miles. Stay left on 3N34, passing Crab Flats Campground after 0.2 mile, and park on the side of the road in another 0.3 mile near signed ATV trail 1W17.

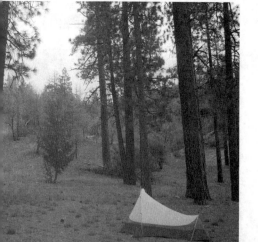

The green forest meets the tawny desert on the north slopes of the San Bernardino Mountains. Holcomb Creek cuts a deep canyon through these slopes. This is an especially appealing part of the mountains, with tall pines, oaks, and cedars covering the south

Holcomb Crossing Trail Camp

side of Holcomb Creek. Growing on the sunbaked north side are pinyon pines, junipers, and desert scrub, while riparian woodland shades the stream bottom. Two trail camps are situated beneath shady pines on the banks of the creek. When the desert is sizzling and the high peaks are blanketed in snow, Holcomb Creek is an ideal destination for this hike or short backpacking trip. This area also attracts large numbers of off-roaders and hunters, so the constant whine of engines and occasional crack of rifles interrupts the tranquility of the setting. Wear bright clothing so that you're easily visible.

This trip makes a loop, first following the dirt road west to Tent Peg Group Campground and then following a trail north down to the Pacific Crest Trail (PCT). It then turns east on the PCT and follows Holcomb Creek to the trail camps before returning up a steep trail to where you parked. The return trail may not be obvious from the parking area, but don't worry—finding your vehicle won't be difficult.

Hike west along 3N34 for 0.8 mile to a large sign reading VISITORS TO DEEP CREEK, near Tent Peg Group Campground. Take the signed 2W08 trail leading north through the forest. Soon views open into the Holcomb Creek canyon below. The Willow Fire swept through this area in 1999, and evidence of the damage is still clearly visible.

In 1.5 miles, the trail ends at the PCT near the canyon bottom. Turn right (east) and walk upstream. In 0.6 mile, reach Bench Camp. In another 0.3 mile, pass ATV trail 1W17, leading back up to where you parked. Before taking it, however, continue another 0.3 mile on the PCT to Holcomb Crossing Trail Camp, shaded beneath the magnificent pines.

If time permits, consider exploring farther upstream along the PCT. When you're done, return to 1W17 and follow it southwest back to your vehicle.

trip 3.10   Cox Creek

see map on p. 55

Distance	10 miles (out-and-back)
Hiking Time	5 hours
Elevation Gain	1,100'
Difficulty	Moderate
Trail Use	Dogs allowed, suitable for backpacking, suitable for equestrians
Best Times	September–May
Agency	San Bernardino National Forest (Big Bear Discovery Center)
Recommended Map	USGS *Butler Peak* 7.5'

DIRECTIONS From the Rim of the World Scenic Byway (Highway 18), 2.9 miles northeast of the intersection with Highway 330 in Running Springs and just past mile marker 018 SBD 34.50, turn left (north) onto Green Valley Lake Road. After 2.6 miles—just before you reach Green Valley Lake—turn left again onto Forest Road 3N16 (Crab Flats Road). Descend 3N16 for 3.8 miles, passing several small side roads and crossing Crab Creek (impassable in high water) to a signed junction with 3N34. Stay right on 3N16 and proceed 8.3 more miles northeast to Big Pine Flat, watching the transition from forest to desert vegetation. Then turn left (west) onto the Coxey Truck Trail (3N14) and follow it 3.4 miles to Little Pine Flat. Turn left onto Hawes Ranch Road (3N41) and park in the clearing outside the locked gate.

Alternatively, the trailhead can be reached from the north. From the 15 Freeway, 6 miles north of Cajon Pass, turn right (east) at Exit 143 in Hesperia. Follow Main Street east 7.2 miles until it begins to curve south; then bear left (east) onto Rock Springs Road. Cross the Mojave River. In 3 miles, Rock Springs Road becomes Roundup Way. Continue 4.4 miles; then turn right (south) onto good dirt Bowen Ranch Road. In 2.1 miles, veer left onto good dirt Coxey Truck Trail (3N14/JF3255). Follow this road as it climbs through the desert wonderland of Joshua trees and jumbo granite boulders, passing numerous side roads. In 9.3 miles, turn right onto Hawes Ranch Road (3N41) and park in the clearing outside the locked gate.

The north slopes of the San Bernardino Mountains are visited more often by hunters and ATV riders than by hikers. However, this region offers seclusion and unique scenery in the transition zone between forest and desert. The drive to the trailhead is an enjoyable backroad experience in itself, as you explore the maze of dirt roads that lace the range. An old path from Little Pine Flat leads past the defunct Hawes Ranch and down Cox Creek to its junction with Holcomb Creek. Two trail camps along Holcomb Creek make ideal destinations for a weekend backpacking trip. Be alert for hunters, especially during deer season in October and November. Large swaths of this area burned in the 1999 Willow Fire and this is a good place to watch nature regenerate. The trail is now unmaintained and starting to become overgrown in places because it receives little use, so long pants or gaiters may be helpful.

From Little Pine Flat, follow the gated jeep road south 0.5 mile until it deteriorates into a trail. Continue along the upper reaches of Cox Creek and pass another stand of pines. Overhead you're likely to see numerous aircraft descending into the Los Angeles Basin because this trail is directly under Victor 283, one of the major airways used by jet traffic.

In another mile, descend a small slope and pass a clearing on your left where all that remains of Hawes Ranch is a stone foundation and some barbed wire. Reach a signed junction 0.2 mile farther where Cox Creek begins to cut a deeper canyon. Trail 2W02 once led west toward Muddy Spring, but it has been obliterated by a jumble of downed trees left by the 1999 Willow Fire. Our route leads south on 2W14 (labeled 2W03 on the *Butler Peak* quadrangle).

The trail rounds the shoulder of Little Shay Mountain and passes the bushy draw that marks Chipmunk Spring (no reliable water). Keep your eyes out for a small waterfall and some pools down in Cox Creek. In 2.6 miles, the trail crosses an ATV path, which is the best and most direct way down to Holcomb Creek. The former hiking trail, 2W14, turns west and contours above Holcomb Creek for some distance before descending, but it's overgrown and difficult to follow in places. On a warm day, Holcomb Creek invites you to relax in its cool waters. You can walk upstream to spend a night at the pleasant Holcomb Crossing PCT Trail Camp.

Hawes Ranch Trail

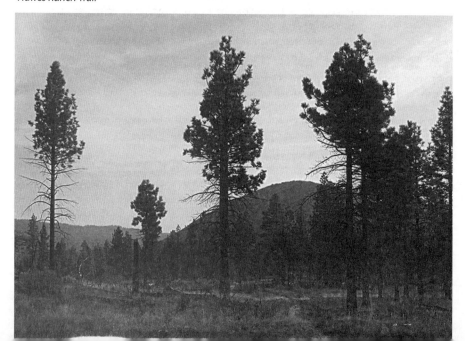

ALTERNATIVE FINISH ─────────────────────────

Just east of Holcomb Crossing PCT Trail Camp, another ATV trail climbs the ridge to Hawes Peak. If you choose to explore this route on your return, beware that the north and west sides of the peak have dense brush and trees, making for an awkward cross-country descent to Hawes Ranch or Little Pine Flat.

---

trip 3.11 Heaps Peak Arboretum

Distance	0.8 mile (loop)
Hiking Time	1 hour
Elevation Gain	100'
Difficulty	Easy
Trail Use	Good for kids, wheelchair accessible
Best Times	March–November
Agency	Rim of the World Interpretive Association
Map	None

see map on p. 55

DIRECTIONS Heaps Peak Arboretum is located on the north side of the Rim of the World Scenic Byway (Highway 18) near mile marker 18 SBD 27.3, 2 miles east of Highway 173 and 4.5 miles west of the junction with Highway 330 in Running Springs.

The Heaps Peak Arboretum is one of the best places to learn how to recognize trees commonly found in the San Bernardino Mountains. The wheelchair-accessible trail makes a short loop through the forest, stopping at interpretive signs identifying Coulter, sugar, Jeffrey, and knobcone pines; black oak; white fir; and incense cedar, ending at a grove of giant sequoias. Open year-round 24 hours a day, it's well worth a stop while driving between Lake Arrowhead and Big Bear. Volunteer staff are usually available to answer questions on weekends 11 a.m.–3 p.m. There is no admission fee, but an Adventure Pass (see page 10) is required to park, and donations are appreciated.

Fred Heaps built a ranch near the site in the late 1800s. After a fire swept through the area in 1922, the Lake Arrowhead Women's Club and students from the elementary school replanted a diverse forest on the site. In the middle of the 20th century, the land was abandoned and became an illegal dumping ground, but in 1982, volunteers led by George Hesemann restored the site and reestablished the arboretum. The 2003 Old Fire swept along the perimeter and thinned some of the seedlings, but it left most of the trees healthier than ever.

The gently graded Sequoia Trail leads clockwise from the kiosk, passing the restroom before making the pleasant loop.

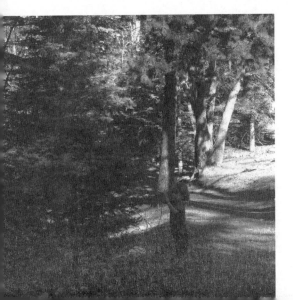

Heaps Peak Arboretum is an easy hike for families.

trip 3.12   Exploration Trail

Distance	4 miles (one-way), 8 miles (out-and-back)
Hiking Time	4 hours (out-and-back)
Elevation Gain	1,300'
Difficulty	Moderate
Trail Use	Dogs allowed, suitable for mountain biking, suitable for equestrians
Best Times	April–November
Agency	San Bernardino National Forest (Big Bear Discovery Center)
Recommended Map	USGS *Keller Peak* 7.5'

see map on p. 55

DIRECTIONS From Highway 18 at a bend just east of Running Springs at mile marker 18 SBD 32.81, turn east onto Keller Peak Road and drive 0.1 mile. Park your vehicle at the signed Exploration Trail Trailhead, on the right. If you want to do a one-way hike, leave another car or bicycle at the upper end of the trail, 4 miles up paved Keller Peak Road. The upper trailhead is just beyond the right-hand fork in the road, on your right; the left fork leads to the National Children's Forest Interpretive Trail.

The Exploration Trail was completed in August 2005 as part of the Forest Service Centennial Project to celebrate the 100th birthday of the U.S. Forest Service. It parallels Keller Peak Road through beautiful open oak and pine forest to the top of the road where the road meets the National Children's Forest Interpretive Trail. For an easier trip, follow the trail in reverse, downhill all the way. While you're in the area, consider visiting the historic Keller Peak Fire Lookout, where volunteer firespotters may be able to give you a tour. Keller Peak Road is an excellent route for cross-country skiing when the snow level is low enough.

Two trails depart from the lower trailhead; take the one on the right. The trail crosses Dry Creek, and then climbs alongside it 0.6 mile through an open forest past huge granite boulders to a dirt road. Cross the road; then hike another 0.2 mile and cross a second road.

VARIATION

Mill Peak is located just south of this point, and you can make an easy detour up to the summit if you like. The jaunt adds 1 mile and 300 feet of elevation gain to your hike. To get there, turn right onto the road, staying right at an immediate branch. In 0.4 mile, reach a gully on the north side of the peak, where you may see footprints. Hike up the last steep 0.1 mile to the top. The highest point is a boulder on the east lip of the peak. From here, you have expansive views down into the valley and out to the fire lookouts on Keller and Butler Peaks. Return the way you came.

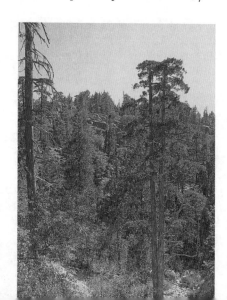

The Exploration Trail continues climbing, roughly parallel to Keller Peak Road but out of sight of traffic. It passes through fields of manzanita before returning to open sugar pine forest and contouring across the northwest slopes of Keller Peak to its upper terminus, at the paved road.

The National Children's Forest Interpretive Trail is an unremarkable half-mile loop through the chaparral across the road from the upper end of the Exploration Trail.

Conifer forest along the Exploration Trail

trip 3.13 Little Green Valley

Distance	2.5 miles (out-and-back)
Hiking Time	1.5 hours
Elevation Gain	700'
Difficulty	Moderate
Trail Use	Dogs allowed, suitable for mountain biking, suitable for equestrians
Best Times	April–November
Agency	San Bernardino National Forest (Big Bear Discovery Center)
Recommended Map	USGS *Keller Peak* 7.5'

see map on p. 55

DIRECTIONS Drive up the Rim of the World Scenic Byway (Highway 18) to mile marker 038 SBD 37.24, 0.3 mile west of the Snow Valley parking area and 5 miles east of Running Springs. A dirt road forks left (north) to some cabins; turn up this road and turn left immediately again to park in the clearing where you see the 2W10 GREEN VALLEY TRAIL sign.

Nestled on the ridge between Green Valley Lake and the Snow Valley Mountain Resort is a small meadow in Little Green Valley. The Little Green Valley Trail climbs from Highway 18 up to the meadow. Along the way, it passes an extensive network of roads and trails that are popular among mountain bikers and cross-country skiers.

This short trip can be extended by returning via these trails or by continuing on to Green Valley Lake. This is a particularly beautiful area in the autumn when the black oaks are losing their leaves.

In October 2007, much of Southern California went up in flames. Twenty major fires raged across the state from Malibu to San Diego, fed by drought and unusually strong winds. The Slide Fire burned 12,000 acres and 200 homes in this area. It cleared the brush and some small trees near Little Green Valley, but left most of the mature trees intact. Unfortunately, the same fire completely incinerated the forest farther north, including massive pines that had stood there since before the American Revolution.

Hike up the trail (2W10) northwest, crossing a small brook. In 0.2 mile, reach a dirt road. Turn right onto the dirt road, go a few yards, and then turn left and rejoin the trail on

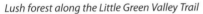

Lush forest along the Little Green Valley Trail

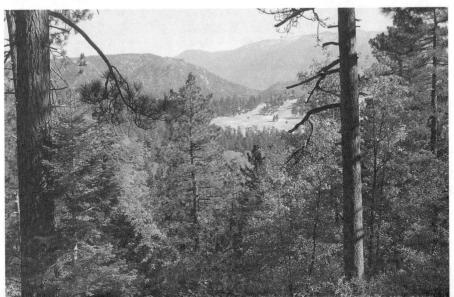

the other side. In another 0.4 mile, the trail crosses the road again. Beyond, the steepening trail follows switchbacks through the lightly burned zone.

In 0.4 mile, reach an unmarked and easily missed junction near some power lines. A bicycle trail forks off to the right and starts descending, while the main trail continues up along the power lines. This area might change as the Forest Service cleans up the fire damage; with luck the trail will become better marked.

Stay left and continue 0.1 mile up to the top of the ridge, where you reach Little Green Valley. This is a good spot to have a snack and enjoy the wildflowers. Beware of snakes in the tall grass. You have several options from here that are explained in the following paragraphs. You can return the way you came. You can continue on to Green Valley Lake. Or you can return on the bicycle trail.

ALTERNATIVE FINISH

To reach Green Valley Lake, you cross the lower end of the meadow and the creek to reach Forest Road 2N19A. The path across the meadow can be indistinct, but the road picks up near the power lines. This road soon joins the main road, 2N19. Turn right and follow it 1.4 miles to the end of Meadow Lane in the resort town of Green Valley Lake. Numerous unmarked roads fork off of 2N19, and they change frequently because of logging. Try staying on what appears to be the main road, but keep in mind that navigation may be challenging.

A better option is to make a return loop on the south side of Little Green Valley. This is a popular area for bicycle races and you may be able to follow the arrows marking the racecourse. Return to the unmarked junction that you passed earlier just below Little Green Valley, and turn east. The trail contours along the hillside and then crosses the North Fork of Deep Creek before reaching a hairpin turn on Forest Road 2N64 in 1.3 miles. Turn right onto Forest Road 2N64, and follow the road 0.8 mile down to Highway 18 by Lakeview Point. Just before you reach the highway, turn right onto another singletrack bicycle trail. This area is a maze with countless forks and variations, but as long as you pick a path that leads downhill and doesn't cross Highway 18, you'll eventually find your way back to the trailhead in less than 2 miles, making this a 5-mile loop. If you get completely disoriented, hike downhill to the highway and follow it down instead.

chapter 4

San Bernardino Mountains: Big Bear Lake Area

The San Bernardino Mountains are part of California's unusual Transverse Ranges, which run east to west rather than north to south. They've long attracted the attention of humans, at first for hunting, logging, and gold, but now primarily for recreation.

The range is so large that trips for this area are divided into three chapters. This chapter focuses on the eastern end, where richly forested hills circle the jewel-like Big Bear Lake. Chapter 3 describes the western end, especially around Lake Arrowhead and the alluring creeks at the interface of forest and desert. Chapter 5 explores the steep and rugged San Gorgonio Wilderness on the southeast side of the range, cut off from Big Bear by the deep trench of the Santa Ana River.

When ranchers, loggers, and miners first explored the San Bernardino Mountains, they found a long alpine meadow tucked between two ridges at the head of a creek. A seasonal lake, now called Baldwin Lake, sat at the east end of the valley. Benjamin Wilson and his posse stormed into the valley in 1845 in pursuit of Indians who had been rustling cattle from ranches in Riverside. Instead of locating the marauders, Wilson's gang discovered swarms of grizzly bears. He later wrote of the experience: "Twenty-two Californians went out in pairs, and each pair lassoed one bear, and brought the result to camp, so that we

Big Bear Lake

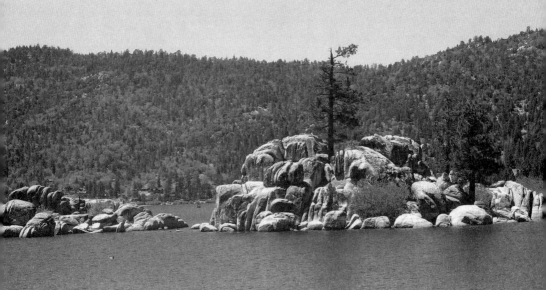

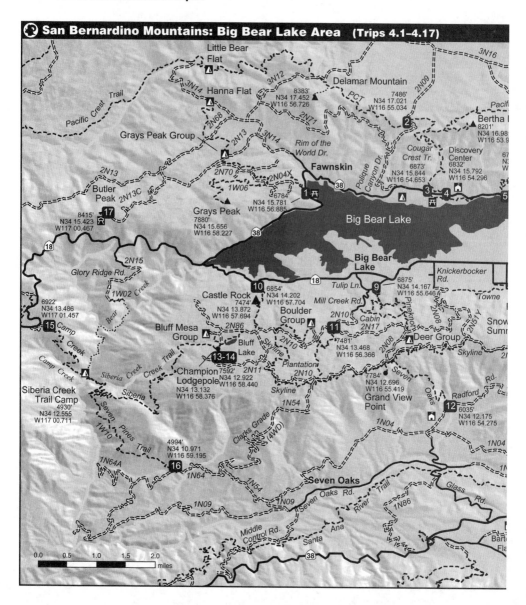

San Bernardino Mountains: Big Bear Lake Area (Trips 4.1–4.17)

had at one and the same time eleven bears. That prompted me to give the Lake the name it now bears." Wilson's story didn't end here; he went on to become the first mayor of Los Angeles, a California state senator, and a wealthy philanthropist. A prominent mountain overlooking Pasadena also bears Wilson's name.

Big Bear Lake, as we know it, didn't exist at the time Wilson named it. In 1884, citrus ranchers in Redlands began to build a dam across the mouth of Bear Valley to create a reservoir. In 1910, the dam was expanded to its present height, forming, at the time, the world's largest man-made lake.

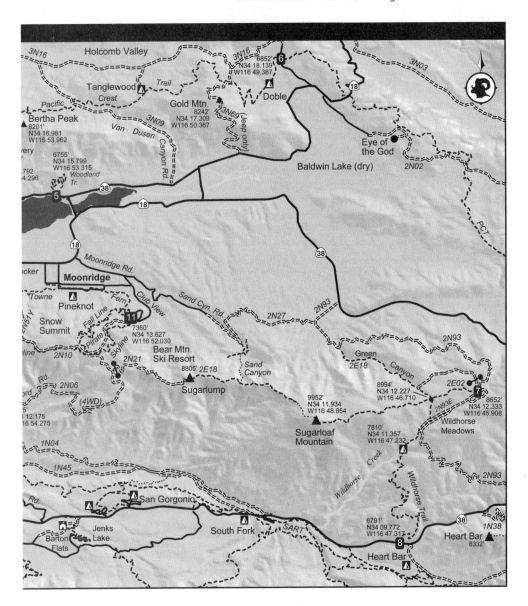

Hunters flocked to the San Bernardino Mountains in search of grizzly pelts. By 1906, the majestic beast was hunted to extinction in this range. In 1860, while tracking a wounded grizzly, Bill Holcomb discovered gold. Miners flocked to the valley north of Big Bear, which became known as Holcomb Valley, and soon a boomtown of 2,000 sprung up, becoming the most populous place in San Bernardino County. Within two years, it became evident that the visions of riches were overblown and the prospectors drifted away. The colorful Elias "Lucky" Baldwin started a second boom in 1874 at the nearby Gold Mountain, but it, too, proved disappointing.

Although gold prospectors were unsuccessful, entrepreneurs soon realized the lumber potential in the rich forestlands. Approximately 22 sawmills were built in the vicinity of Big Bear. The intensive timber harvesting proved unsustainable and the environmental catastrophes that followed led President Roosevelt to establish a reserve in 1906 to protect the remaining forests in the San Bernardino Mountains.

In the first part of the 20th century, winter-sports enthusiasts began developing the slopes around the lake. By the 1950s and 1960s, skiing became a big business, and now Big Bear is best known among Southern Californians for the ski slopes. In the 1940s, developers pushed hard to establish a massive downhill ski area in the San Gorgonio wilderness south of Big Bear. Conservationists put up a fierce battle and ultimately prevailed when chief forester Lyle Watts ruled that the mountains had "a higher public value as a wilderness and a watershed than as a downhill ski area." Threats of development continue to resurface from time to time.

Big Bear is now a popular mountain resort community. Skiers and snowboarders flock to the lifts during the winter, while boaters and anglers come in droves during the summer. The community of Big Bear Lake on the south side along Highway 18 offers every amenity that a visitor might desire. The ridges on all sides are laced with easy and moderate trails to tempt hikers up from the lake to the refreshingly cool ridges of the mountains. The Sierra Club has a summer tradition of hiking the Five Peaks of Big Bear: Bertha, Grays, Delamar, Gold, and Sugarloaf.

Cross-country skiers enjoy the dirt roads around Big Bear in the winter. Some particularly suitable roads include 2N93 to Wildhorse Meadows, with great views of San Gorgonio, Polique Canyon Road (2N09) near Fawnskin, and the gently graded Van Dusen Canyon Road (3N09).

---

trip 4.1 **Grays Peak**

see map on p. 74

Distance	7 miles (out-and-back)
Hiking Time	3 hours
Elevation Gain	1,200'
Difficulty	Moderate
Trail Use	Dogs allowed, suitable for mountain biking, suitable for equestrians
Best Times	April–October
Agency	San Bernardino National Forest (Big Bear Discovery Center)
Recommended Map	USGS *Fawnskin* 7.5'

DIRECTIONS Follow Highway 38 along the north shore of Big Bear Lake to the Grays Peak parking area, just west of mile marker 038 SBD 56.41, 2.7 miles northeast of Bear Valley Dam and Highway 18, and a half mile southwest of Fawnskin. There are restrooms and picnic tables here, along with many spaces for parking.

Grays Peak is named for Alex Gray, who founded Gray's Landing on the north shore of Big Bear Lake in 1918. The 7,952-foot summit is heavily forested, making for an enjoyable walk through the woods. This is one of the most popular moderate hikes in the Big Bear area and you should expect to have plenty of company on a pleasant summer day. Grays Peak is a winter habitat for recently reestablished bald eagles, and the trail is closed November 1–April 1.

From the signed trailhead, follow the trail north overlooking the highway and Grout Bay. The trail soon begins switchbacking northwest up the Jeffrey pine-, white fir-, and black oak–clad slopes. After cresting the low ridge, the trail abruptly turns left and reaches

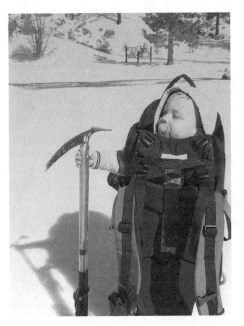

Forest Road 2N04X in 0.7 mile. Turn right. In 0.3 mile, turn right again at a T-junction with Forest Road 2N70.

In 0.1 mile, reach a sign on the left (south) for the Grays Peak Trail. Take this trail as it climbs through the forest. The Butler 2 Fire burned 14,000 acres on the northwest side of Big Bear Lake in September 2007. It singed the northwest side of Grays Peak and incinerated most of the forest around Hanna Flat and Butler Peak. You'll have occasional glimpses through the trees down to the lake below. After 2 miles of climbing, the trail circles around the summit and ends 100 feet below the top. You'll have to scramble through buckthorns and over fallen logs if you wish to reach the true high point.

VARIATION

Grays Peak can also be reached from Grays Peak Group Camp. A 1.4-mile trail leads east from the camp to a point lying immediately northwest of the junction of the Grays Peak Trail with Forest Road 2N70. Pick up the Grays Peak Trail on the south side of 2N70 and follow the directions above for 2 miles to the summit.

Young mountaineer with ice ax and binky

A 1.5-mile trail also connects Grays Peak Group Camp to Hanna Flat Campground.

---

trip 4.2   **Delamar Mountain**

see map on p. 74

Distance	5.5 miles (out-and-back)
Hiking Time	3 hours
Elevation Gain	800'
Difficulty	Moderate
Trail Use	Dogs allowed
Best Times	May–October
Agency	San Bernardino National Forest (Big Bear Discovery Center)
Recommended Map	USGS *Fawnskin* 7.5'

DIRECTIONS From Highway 38, 2 miles east of Fawnskin at mile marker 038 SBD 54.04, turn north onto good dirt Polique Canyon Road (2N09). At a fork in 1.5 miles with 2N71, stay right on 2N09 toward Holcomb Valley. Continue 0.8 mile to the top of the divide, where you'll see the signed Holcomb View Trail, part of the Pacific Crest Trail (PCT). Park here or on the side of the road where it becomes wider just beyond.

Delamar Mountain (8,398') is the high point on the ridge between Big Bear Lake and Holcomb Valley. The summit boulders stand clear of the dense forest, granting hikers panoramic views in all directions. This trip reaches the mountain from the east by way of the PCT.

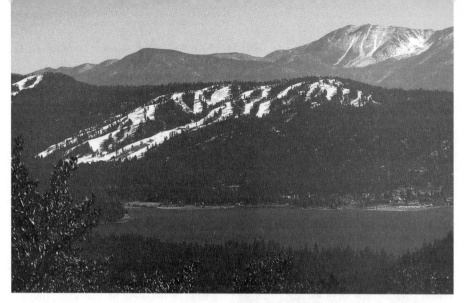
Big Bear Lake and San Gorgonio Mountain from Delamar Mountain

Hike west along the PCT through the open forest of pines, oaks, and firs. In 1.4 miles, the trail crosses to the north side of the ridge, where snow may sometimes linger late in the spring. Holcomb Valley, to the north, is named for Bill Holcomb, a prospector who found gold in the area while hunting grizzly bears in 1859. Within two years, 1,400 people had flocked to the area seeking their fortune, but the placer gold was rapidly depleted and the valley was soon abandoned.

In another 0.8 mile, where the trail begins to descend after passing a ravine, arrive at a good spot to leave the trail and strike uphill for the mountaintop. Thread a steep 0.3-mile path northwestward through the trees to reach the granite summit boulders.

ALTERNATIVE FINISH

Alternatively, the PCT intersects Forest Road 3N12 to the west, 0.4 mile from where you left the trail. With a car or bicycle shuttle, you can descend to the road and loop back to the start. From the junction of the PCT with 3N12, go west and then southwest 1.2 miles on 3N12. Turn left onto 2N71 and follow it east around the south side of Delamar Mountain for 4.2 miles back to Polique Canyon Road. Turn left again and go 0.7 mile north to the initial trailhead.

---

trip 4.3   Cougar Crest (and Bertha Peak)

see map on p. 74

Distance	5–7 miles (out-and-back)
Hiking Time	2.5–4 hours
Elevation Gain	700'/1,400'
Difficulty	Moderate
Trail Use	Dogs allowed, good for kids (to Cougar Crest), suitable for equestrians
Best Times	April–November
Agency	San Bernardino National Forest (Big Bear Discovery Center)
Recommended Map	USGS *Fawnskin* 7.5'

DIRECTIONS This trail starts on the north side of Highway 38, on the north shore of Big Bear Lake near mile marker 038 SBD 53.50, a half mile west of the Big Bear Discovery Center.

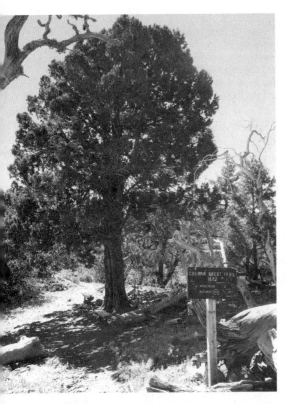

Western juniper at Cougar Crest

A thousand-foot-tall forested ridge separates Big Bear Lake from Holcomb Valley to the north. The Cougar Crest Trail climbs from the north shore of Big Bear Lake up to a low point on this ridge, where it meets the Pacific Crest Trail (PCT). The Cougar Crest Trail offers a family-friendly hike through the forest, with occasional views down to the lake and across to the San Gorgonio Wilderness. It's extremely popular on the weekends, so don't expect to find solitude here. Peak baggers may choose to continue farther to Bertha Peak, though dense forest obscures the views from the summit and a cluster of antennas detracts from the natural ambience.

From the north end of the large parking lot, hike north up a paved path. In 0.1 mile, the path veers right (east) toward the Big Bear Discovery Center, but this trip continues straight onto the Cougar Crest Trail, which leads north through a forest of pines, cedars, and western junipers. Small stands of manzanitas dot the open forest floor.

The Cougar Crest Trail climbs gradually but steadily. Look for the antenna-studded Bertha Peak to the north. In 2 miles, shortly before you reach the crest, look out for the best views back over the lake. Also, you can make out the fire lookout dramatically situated atop Butler Peak to the west. After crossing the first crest, the trail turns east and in another 0.3 mile reaches a signed junction with the PCT. Some magnificent western junipers and pinyon pines grow near this junction. Most hikers turn back here.

VARIATIONS

To reach Bertha Peak, turn right (east) and follow the PCT 0.4 mile to its junction with a road on the ridge. Continue east up this steep service road to the antennas atop Bertha Peak. This adds 800 feet of elevation gain and 1.2 miles each way.

Alternative trailheads for Bertha Peak include Polique Canyon Road (see Trip 4.2) and Van Dusen Canyon Road at their intersections with the PCT.

---

trip 4.4 **Alpine Pedal Path**

Distance	Up to 4 miles (semiloop)
Hiking Time	2 hours
Elevation Gain	200'
Difficulty	Easy
Trail Use	Dogs allowed, good for kids, suitable for mountain biking, wheelchair accessible

see map on p. 74

Best Times   April–November
Agency   San Bernardino National Forest (Big Bear Discovery Center)
Optional Map   USGS *Fawnskin* 7.5'

DIRECTIONS This trail starts at the Big Bear Discovery Center, at 40971 Highway 38 on the north shore of Big Bear Lake just west of mile marker 038 SBD 53.00. The gate at the parking area closes early (5 p.m. in the summer), so park outside if you don't think you'll be back in time.

A flat trail along the north shore of Big Bear Lake links the Big Bear Discovery Center, popular Cougar Crest Trail, Serrano Campground, and Meadows Edge Picnic Area. Though this trail isn't much of a destination in itself, it makes for a pleasant lakeside excursion on foot or bicycle for those visiting the area. It's also accessible to strollers and wheelchairs.

The trail begins at the bicycle racks in front of the Discovery Center and leads west through a forest of Western junipers and pinyon pines 0.5 mile to a junction with the Cougar Crest Trail (see Trip 4.3). It descends to the Cougar Crest parking lot, and then crosses under Highway 38 to a junction in another 0.2 mile. Turn right to reach the Serrano Campground, but the main trail turns left (east) and leads 0.4 mile through more junipers and pines to the Meadows Edge Picnic Area on the shore of Big Bear Lake, where you can enjoy views of the ski areas on the ridge to the south and of Sugarloaf Mountain to the southeast. It continues 1.2 miles along the shore of the lake to the eastern terminus at the Stanfield Cutoff bridge.

On the return, when you reach Meadows Edge, you can take a shortcut back by following the access road up to Highway 38 just west of the Discovery Center.

Sugarloaf Mountain and the Big Bear ski areas from the Alpine Pedal Path

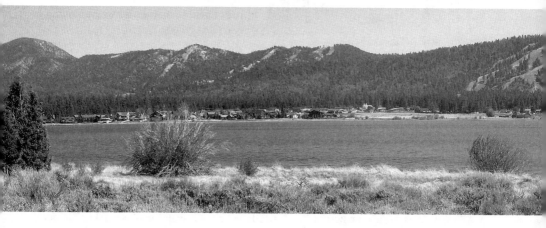

trip 4.5   **Woodland Trail**

Distance   1.7 miles (loop)
Hiking Time   1 hour
Elevation Gain   300'
Difficulty   Easy
Trail Use   Dogs allowed, good for kids
Best Times   April–November
Agency   San Bernardino National Forest (Big Bear Discovery Center)
Optional Map   USGS *Fawnskin* 7.5' (trail not shown)

see map on p. 75

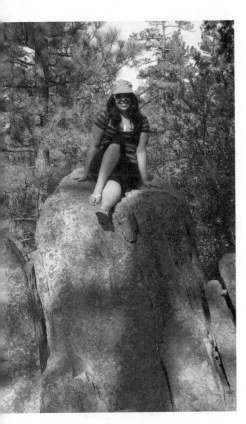

A hiker poses on a boulder along the Woodland Trail.

DIRECTIONS This trailhead is located on the north shore of Big Bear Lake, off Highway 38 immediately opposite the East Boat Ramp on the north side of the road. It's 1 mile east of the Big Bear Discovery Center at mile marker 038 SBD 52.11.

The Woodland Trail tours a particularly fine portion of the forest on the north shore of Big Bear Lake in the transition region between the conifer and pinyon–juniper zones of the San Bernardino Mountains. The trail was constructed by volunteers in 1986, and features 20 numbered posts around the loop. Pick up a brochure at the trailhead, which provides historic, botanical, and geological information keyed to the signposts. The Woodland Trail is ideal for families with young children looking for a good place to take a walk while visiting the Big Bear area.

The signed trail starts on the east side of the large parking area. It makes a counterclockwise loop. Watch for the Western juniper trees. Unlike their bushlike brethren common in the desert, the Western juniper stands tall and is sometimes confused with incense cedar. However, they're readily recognized as junipers by their characteristic needles. As you proceed, watch for oaks, stately 400-year-old Jeffrey pines, and pinyon pines. There are also good views of Big Bear Lake and the ski areas on the far side.

---

trip 4.6 **Gold Mountain**

see map on p. 75

Distance	8 miles (out-and-back)
Hiking Time	4 hours
Elevation Gain	1,400'
Difficulty	Moderate
Trail Use	Dogs allowed
Best Times	May–October
Agency	San Bernardino National Forest (Big Bear Discovery Center)
Required Map	USGS *Big Bear City* 7.5'

DIRECTIONS From Highway 18 at mile marker 18 SBD 58.15, about 2.2 miles east of the Big Bear water-treatment plant, turn north onto Holcomb Valley Road. In 0.8 mile, look for an easy-to-miss sign marking the Pacific Crest Trail (PCT) on the left. Park here along the roadside.

Gold Mountain (8,235') was at the center of the 1860–1875 Holcomb Valley gold rush. In May 1860, Billy Holcomb was hunting grizzly bear when he came across gold-bearing quartz ledges. By the end of the summer, nearly 1,000 prospectors, merchants, prostitutes, and assorted ne'er-do-wells had made camp in Holcomb Valley. Competent prospectors could extract $2–$10 of gold dust a day—a decent wage back then—using pans or primitive tools.

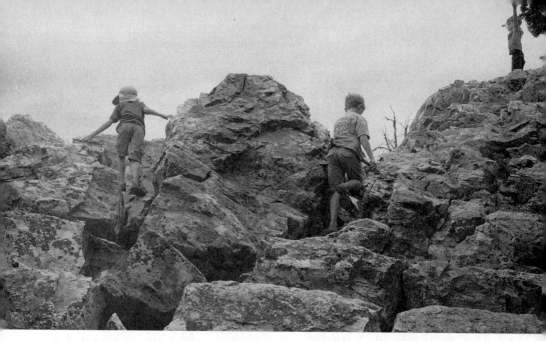

Prospecting on the Gold Mountain summit rocks

Disputes broke out regularly and were settled by gunfights; an estimated 40–50 bodies rest in unmarked graves around the valley. In August 1861, placer gold was running low and Francis Mellus installed a steam-driven eight-stamp mill to pulverize gold-bearing quartz ore. Soon after this hard-rock mining began, unrelenting winter blizzards drove miners from the valley. In 1873, Carley Carter found gold in the quartz atop Gold Mountain. Elias "Lucky" Baldwin, having made his fortune at the Nevada Comstock Lode, acquired a controlling interest in the new mine and invested heavily by installing a 40-stamp mill. This time, Baldwin wasn't so lucky. The quartz was less rich than he hoped, and the mine shut two years later. Various others sought their fortunes here in the subsequent decades, but none had much success.

Follow the PCT west from the trailhead. Looking right (northwest) up the slope, you may notice the timbers from the rundown mill at Doble Mine. In 0.5 mile, reach Doble PCT Trail Camp, the least-attractively situated of the five trail camps along the PCT in the San Bernardino Mountains. This hot camp unfortunately has power lines running right past it, spoiling the wilderness ambience. You can find an outhouse, corral, and spigot here; treat the water before using it. The 2017 Holcomb Fire burned 1,500 acres around the camp.

The trail soon starts climbing the east slope of pinyon-clad Gold Mountain. Traverse colorful screelike tailings from the mining activity. In 2.1 miles, reach unsigned Forest Road 3N69, a rough jeep road. Turn left here and follow the road 1.3 miles up to the rather flat mountaintop. The road is strewn with bolts, hooks, and other components that have fallen off jeeps and trucks over the years. The forest is predominantly Western juniper, pinyon pine, and Jeffrey pine, with large shrubs of curl-leaf mountain mahogany. Just before you start downhill, veer left (east) off the road to the colorful quartz boulder pile that marks the true summit. From here, you can enjoy excellent views of the other Seven Summits, as well as the ski resorts and eastern end of the lake. On your return, don't miss the junction with the PCT.

VARIATION

For a shorter but less scenic route, drive 1.2 miles up 3N16; then hike up the steep and rocky 3N69 jeep road 1.7 miles to the summit.

trip 4.7 Sugarloaf Mountain

Distance	7 miles (out-and-back)
Hiking Time	4 hours
Elevation Gain	1,300'
Difficulty	Moderate
Trail Use	Dogs allowed, suitable for backpacking (but no water available), suitable for mountain biking, suitable for equestrians
Best Times	May–October
Agency	San Bernardino National Forest (Big Bear Discovery Center)
Recommended Map	USGS *Moonridge* 7.5'

see map on p. 75

DIRECTIONS From Redlands, drive east on Highway 38 through Barton Flats to the beginning of Forest Road 2N93, near mile marker 038 SBD 35.7. The fair dirt road is easy to miss, so keep a sharp eye out for it on your left (north), immediately past a small wash. Drive 5.5 miles up 2N93 to Wildhorse Meadows. Continue up 2N93 for 0.6 mile beyond the meadow, to a fork on your left with a gated jeep road (again, easy to miss). Park your vehicle at the clearing on the east side of 2N93.

Alternatively, the trailhead can be reached from the north. From Highway 38, 3 miles southeast of Big Bear City near mile marker 038 SBD 45.75, drive 5.6 miles up Forest Road 2N93 to a fork on your right.

The rounded Sugarloaf Mountain (9,952') is the tallest summit in the San Bernardino Mountains outside the San Gorgonio Wilderness. Located at the interface of two vegetation zones, it supports both the rich forests of Jeffrey pines and white firs common in the San Bernardino high country, and the juniper and pinyon pine woodland of the desert slopes. In late August and early September, lucky hikers may see the rare black swallowtail butterfly (*Papilio bairdii*). Fine trails scale the mountain from all four directions. This trip

Sugarloaf Mountain from the San Bernardino Divide

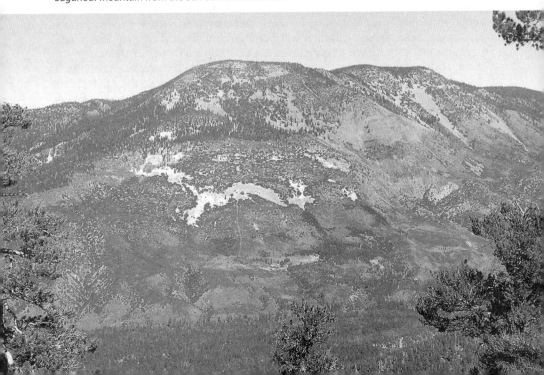

is the shortest route, taking advantage of a forest service road leading high onto the east shoulder of the mountain. From the south, one can make the long and strenuous climb via Wildhorse Creek (see Trip 4.8). Variations at the end of this trip describe the approaches from Green Canyon to the north and Sand Canyon to the west.

Hike west through a wooden gate immediately left of the gated road and follow the ducked (ducks are rock piles marking the trail) path up onto the ridge. This area is home to some of the largest Western junipers in California. Unlike the bushlike California junipers found in the Mojave Desert, the Western junipers are mighty trees with reddish ropelike bark. The pines in this part of the forest are mostly ponderosas, rather than the similar-looking Jeffreys, as you can tell by the smaller cones.

From the gated jeep road, come to a four-way trail junction in 0.9 mile. The right fork leads down Green Canyon to a lower trailhead on Forest Road 2N93 and the left fork leads down to Wildhorse Creek, but this hike continues straight along the ridge. In 1.5 miles, reach Bump 9,775'. Descend to a saddle, and then climb again, reaching the cairn on top of Sugarloaf Mountain in 1 more mile after the bump.

VARIATIONS————————————————————————————————————

Sugarloaf can be reached from Green Canyon, as shown on the map. This is a fine 10-mile round-trip with 2,700 feet of elevation gain. The trailhead is reached from Highway 38 about 3.7 miles southeast of Big Bear City. At mile marker 038 SBD 45.75, turn southwest onto Forest Road 2N93, directly across from Hatchery Road. Follow 2N93 for 1.3 miles as it passes multiple side roads. Park at the signed Sugarloaf Trail, on your right by the Green Creek crossing.

A jeep road once led up Green Canyon, but the track has deteriorated into a rocky trail. Follow the trail southeast along the creek 1.8 miles to a cairn and sign. A jeep road leads east to rejoin 2N93 at the gate mentioned in the main driving directions, but this trip continues southeast 0.4 mile to the four-way junction mentioned in the main trip description. Turn right (west) and join the main trail, which leads 2.5 miles to the summit.

Sugarloaf can also be reached by an obscure route from the west. The old trail from Bear Mountain is shown on the Moonridge topo map and is passable but now requires permission from the ski resort. Local hikers now bypass the resort via Sand Canyon. This route is only 5 miles round-trip, but it involves 2,400 feet of climbing on steep use trails.

From Highway 18 near the east end of Big Bear, turn southeast onto Moonridge Road. In 1.9 miles, turn left onto Sand Canyon Road. Follow the road (making three left turns to stay on Sand Canyon) 1.1 miles until it turns into good dirt Forest Road 2N27. Continue 0.8 mile to a hairpin turn and park at a small turnout.

Before starting, look south and identify the lowest saddle on the ridge at the head of Sand Canyon. Your goal is to navigate the unsigned paths to reach this saddle. A trail leads south up the canyon through a gap in a fence. In 0.2 mile, reach a T-junction with an old road/trail. Turn right, go 15 yards, and then turn left at a cairn. A well-used trail continues south, paralleling the draw. You could also walk directly up the draw, but the path is cluttered with vegetation. As the canyon steepens and narrows, the use trail merges into the dry creekbed. Stay right at a fork in the canyon near the top and work your way up to the ridge, 0.9 mile from the trailhead. Turn left and follow the old ridgeline trail until it becomes too faint at about 9,200 feet; then walk straight up the steep slopes to the summit.

trip 4.8	**Wildhorse Creek**

Distance	8 miles (out-and-back)
Hiking Time	4 hours
Elevation Gain	1,400'
Difficulty	Moderate
Trail Use	Dogs allowed, suitable for backpacking, suitable for mountain biking, suitable for equestrians
Best Times	April–October
Agency	San Bernardino National Forest (Big Bear Discovery Center)
Recommended Map	USGS *Moonridge* 7.5'

see map on p. 75

DIRECTIONS From Redlands, drive east on Highway 38 to the turnoff for the Wildhorse Creek Trail, on your left just before mile marker 038 SBD 33.40 and 0.2 mile before Heart Bar Campground Road on your right. Turn left (north) and drive about 20 yards up a dirt road to a signed parking area.

Wildhorse Creek carves a canyon along a fault line down from the shoulder of Sugarloaf Mountain. The well-built Wildhorse Trail switchback takes you up to Wildhorse Creek Trail Camp, located at a spring near the top of the creek. This is an enjoyable backpacking trip or day hike in the spring when San Gorgonio is clad in deep snow, and also in the summer when San Gorgonio permits are difficult to obtain.

The first mile of the Wildhorse Creek Trail is an old logging road. It climbs through

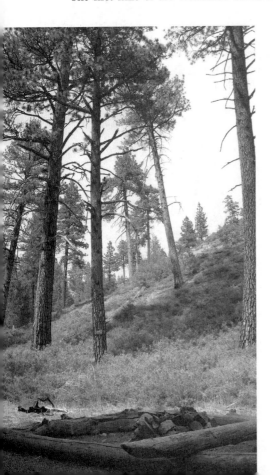

Jeffrey pines, pinyons, and junipers. The trail switchbacks take you onward for 2 miles, and views steadily improve as you ascend. The last mile passes around a bump on the ridge and descends into the richly forested Wildhorse Creek, where you'll find the trail camp in a clearing beside the stream beneath Jeffrey pines. Water is usually available in the creek.

VARIATION

If you want a longer hike or a side trip after camping, the Wildhorse Creek Trail continues up the canyon on the opposite side of the creek. You can take it to Wildhorse Meadows or all the way to Sugarloaf Mountain. This part of the trail is steep, but your efforts are rewarded by wild roses, Indian paintbrush, spectacular Western juniper trees, and the meadow full of ferns and corn lilies. In 0.7 mile, the trail reaches an old closed jeep track (2N93E) that follows the west side of Wildhorse Meadows. In another 0.2 mile up the road, a trail on the left is marked with a sign reading SUGARLOAF MOUNTAIN. This trail climbs 0.4 mile to the four-way junction on

Wildhorse Trail Camp

the Sugarloaf Mountain Trail. From here, you can turn left and hike another 2.5 miles to the summit.

Return the way you came. An old trail once descended Wildhorse Creek, but it crossed private property. The Forest Service has closed the trail and allowed it to return to nature.

trip 4.9   Grand View Point

Distance	6.5 miles (out-and-back)
Hiking Time	3 hours
Elevation Gain	1,100'
Difficulty	Moderate
Trail Use	Dogs allowed, suitable for mountain biking, horseback riding permitted but not recommended
Best Times	May–October
Agency	San Bernardino National Forest (Big Bear Discovery Center)
Recommended Map	USGS *Big Bear Lake* 7.5' (not all trails and roads shown)

see map on p. 74

DIRECTIONS From westbound Highway 18 in Big Bear Lake Village at mile marker 018 SBD 47.43, where a sign points to Mill Creek Road and picnic grounds, turn right (south) onto Tulip Lane. Proceed 0.5 mile to the Aspen Glen Picnic Area, on your right.

Grand View Point, high on the ridge above Big Bear Lake, offers an unobstructed view across the Santa Ana River Canyon to the tall summits of the San Gorgonio Wilderness. A network of trails leads up from the Aspen Glen Picnic Area to the point. Take this popular hike on a clear day when you can fully appreciate the vistas. This whole ridge south of Big Bear is laced with fire roads and singletrack trails that draw mountain bikers from across Southern California. The bottom portion of this trail was rerouted in 2013 and the path is now much easier to follow.

Follow the Pineknot Trail (1E01) from the trailhead sign at the south end of the picnic area. The trail climbs through a forest of black oak, white fir, and Jeffrey pine, with an understory of boulders, buckthorn, and wildflowers. This area is particularly appealing in the late spring when the flowers are in bloom and in October when the oak leaves turn golden.

In a quarter mile, come to a junction with the Cabin Trail (1E24). Both trails rejoin in 1.5 miles, but the Pineknot Trail has better views and is more popular, while the Cabin Trail draws mountain bikers seeking a loop ride.

Pineknot Trail climbs, crosses a ridge, and then drops to cross the creek in Red Ant Canyon. Watch for traces of the old trail here,

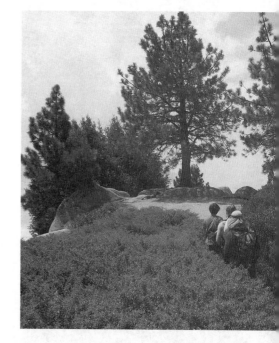

Hikers approach Grand View Point.

but stay on the rerouted path to protect the riparian area. Climb back up to a ridge and turn south. When the trail comes close to the creek again, watch for an unsigned junction with the Cabin Trail on the right.

The main trail continues straight (south) and crosses Forest Road 2N08 in 0.5 mile. It then levels out, passes Deer Group Campground, and parallels 2N08 to reach Forest Road 2N10 at the top of the ridge. Cross the road to meet the Skyline Trail; then follow the signed Grand View Point Trail 0.3 mile southeast to the clearing on Grand View Point.

VARIATION

The unsigned Cabin Trail loops around from the junction near the start to the junction before 2N08. It offers an alternative path on the return trip, or a 3.6-mile family-friendly loop with 700 feet of climbing from the picnic area.

---

trip 4.10 **Castle Rock**

Distance	1.6 miles (out-and-back)
Hiking Time	1.5 hours
Elevation Gain	700'
Difficulty	Moderate
Trail Use	Dogs allowed, good for kids
Best Times	May–October
Agency	San Bernardino National Forest (Big Bear Discovery Center)
Recommended Map	USGS *Big Bear Lake* 7.5' (incorrectly shows the trail climbing west of Castle Rock)

see map on p. 74

DIRECTIONS From Highway 18 across from mile marker 018 SBD 45.50, 1.2 miles east of Big Bear Dam or 3 miles west of Big Bear Lake Village, marked trail 1W03 starts up a forested gully. Park 100 yards east of the trailhead, in a clearing on the north side of the highway.

The ridge south of Big Bear Lake is studded with granite outcrops. Castle Rock is the largest and most interesting, regularly drawing rock climbers to its steep walls. A scrambling route around the back side leads agile hikers to the summit. Castle Rock offers some of the most spectacular views of Big Bear Lake because it towers above the trees that obstruct views from most points around the lake.

The steep and rocky trail climbs through a lush forest of Jeffrey pines and white firs. Watch for old false trails and take care not to cut switchbacks. In 0.6 mile, the trail reaches Castle Rock. Be sure to stay on the main trail rather than veering off on some of the climbers' trails that lead up to the steep walls of the rock. The main trail curves around the south side of the

Big Bear Lake from Castle Rock

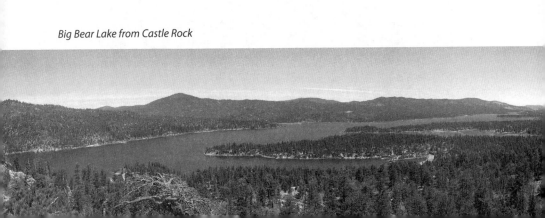

outcrop and crosses a dry creekbed. On the far side of the creek, the main trail starts leading south up the hill away from Castle Rock, but an access trail heads back north across the creek to the west end of the rock. Follow this access trail around to the north side of the rock and look for an obvious notch on the north side of the rock west of the highest point. Scramble up boulders toward the notch, but before you reach it, turn left up a gigantic "stairway" that leads to the eastern summit. This involves third-class climbing and those uncomfortable with rock scrambling will prefer to stop at the base. After enjoying the view, return the way you came.

VARIATION

Alternatively, the Castle Rock Trail (1W03), faint in places, continues south from Castle Rock 0.6 mile through beautiful open forest dotted with boulders and manzanita patches to a signed trailhead on Forest Road 2N86 near its junction with 2N10.

---

trip 4.11 Skyline Trail

see map on p. 75

Distance	15 miles (one-way)
Hiking Time	7 hours
Elevation Gain	1,700'
Difficulty	Strenuous
Trail Use	Dogs allowed, suitable for mountain biking
Best Times	May–October
Agency	San Bernardino National Forest (Big Bear Discovery Center)
Optional Maps	USGS *Big Bear Lake* and *Moonridge* 7.5' (trail not shown)

DIRECTIONS To do a one-way trip from west to east, pre-position a getaway vehicle at the Club View Trailhead. From Highway 18, at the east end of Big Bear Lake Village, turn southeast onto Moonridge Road. In 1.0 mile, veer right onto Club View Road. Proceed 1.4 miles to the Club View Trailhead parking, where the road turns to dirt and becomes Forest Road 2N10.

A trail map is posted at the junction of Forest Roads 2N10 and 2N17.

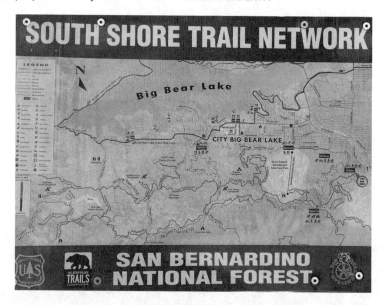

Return to Highway 18 and follow it back 2.6 miles to 018 SBD 48.0; then turn left (southwest) onto Mill Creek Road. Mill Creek Road eventually becomes good dirt Forest Road 2N10. In 1.9 miles, reach a trail map at the junction of 2N10 and 2N17. Just beyond, look for an unobtrusive post labeled SKYLINE TRAIL 1E12 on the left marking the trailhead. Find a place to park nearby.

The Skyline Trail (1E12), developed through a partnership between the Big Bear Valley Trails Foundation and the U.S. Forest Service, has become an instant classic since its completion in 2015. Particularly popular as an intermediate-level mountain biking trail because of its flowing course, fun technical obstacles, gentle grades, and fine scenery, it's also used by trail runners. Hikers seeking shorter loops find options along any segment of the trail, although hikers who don't like sharing trails with cyclists will prefer going elsewhere.

The easy-to-miss Skyline Trail begins at a post and starts a long nonmonotonic climb through open forest to the 8,000-foot ridgeline. In 1.1 miles, it returns to Forest Road 2N10 at the signed start of the Plantation Trail (1W12). Continue a few more yards; then cross 2N10 and follow a spur road (2N10B) 0.2 mile to the Boulder Group Camp, where the Skyline Trail resumes. In 1.4 miles, cross back to the southeast side of 2N10; then in another 1.6 miles, cross back to the southwest. In 0.7 mile, top out on the ridgeline, where views open up southward across the Santa Ana River to the San Gorgonio Wilderness and east toward Sugarloaf Mountain.

The next leg of the trail makes a long traverse east along the skyline ridge. The environmental impact assessment of the trail was simplified by following a firebreak bulldozed south of 2N10 during the 2003 Old Fire. However, this constrained the trail to a narrow ribbon of land, resulting in tight switchbacks as the path traverses the many bumps along the ridge. The forest is mostly Jeffrey pine, with an understory of manzanita, chinquapin, buckthorn, and granite boulders. Penstemon, prickly poppies, and other seasonal wildflowers dot the ridge.

In 0.8 mile, join the upper end of Bellyache Spring Road. In 0.1 mile, the trail resumes eastbound at an intersection with Clarks Grade Road (1N54). (If you take Clarks Grade Road north 0.1 mile, you'll reach the top of the Plantation Trail.) In 2.5 miles, cross the Grand View Point/Pineknot Trail (see Trip 4.9). The Grand View Point Trail climbs a quarter mile south to a viewpoint, but the views are no better than those you've been enjoying from the ridge. Just beyond, the Seven Oaks Trail descends to Converse Flats (see Trip 4.12), but again, continue on Skyline. In 1.6 miles, come to a large clearing with another viewpoint to the south. In 2.9 miles, reach a junction with the Radford Truck Trail (2N06) and the Pirate Trail (1E29). From here, the descent begins in earnest and the trail soon passes through a burn area. In 1.0 mile, cross Bear Mountain Road and, in another 1.0 mile, reach the Club View Trailhead.

VARIATIONS

Here are three options for shorter hikes:

• Park at the bottom of the Plantation Trail (0.7 mile up 2N10 from the 2N10/2N17 junction), hike up the road to Boulder Group Camp, follow the Skyline Trail up to Clarks Grade Road, and descend via the Plantation Trail (6 miles, 800' gain).

• Park at the top of Clarks Grade Road, hike 2.5 miles on the Skyline Trail to Grand View Point, and return via bicycle or foot along 2N10 (4 miles, 500' gain).

• The Pirate and Fall Line Trails offer an enjoyable alternative descent, especially for mountain bikers who enjoy rock gardens, jumps, and steep terrain. These trails and the eastern part of the Skyline Trail can also be reached using the Snow Summit ski lift.

trip 4.12   Seven Oaks Trail

Distance	4.6 miles (out-and-back)
Hiking Time	3 hours
Elevation Gain	1,600'
Difficulty	Moderate
Trail Use	Dogs allowed, suitable for mountain biking, suitable for equestrians
Best Times	October–June
Agency	San Bernardino National Forest (Big Bear Discovery Center)
Optional Map	USGS *Big Bear Lake* 7.5'

see map on p. 74

DIRECTIONS From Highway 38 between Jenks Lake Road and Barton Flats near mile marker 038 SBD 26.54, turn north onto Glass Road and descend 2.2 miles to Seven Oaks Road. In 0.1 mile, make an immediate left and follow a road to Converse Station. Several roads diverge here; continue onto Radford Road (2N06), signed BIG BEAR at the junction. In 0.8 mile, reach the well-marked trailhead.

The Seven Oaks Trail (0E01) makes a no-nonsense climb from Converse Flats in the Santa Ana River Canyon up to Skyline Drive overlooking Big Bear Lake. The Forest Service established the Converse Flats experimental station in 1913 to research reforestation following wildfires, and the popular Camp Radford opened nearby in 1918. The Seven Oaks Trail was depicted on a 1928 Auto Club map, but had become overgrown in recent years. In 2010, the Big Bear Valley Trails Foundation and the U.S. Forest Service cut back the oak thickets and reopened the trail. Go on a cool, clear day when you can enjoy the views and vigorous climb.

The signed trail leads north-northwest up a valley through majestic canyon live oaks. Upon crossing Converse Creek, it makes a pair of switchbacks and crosses a ridge into the Hamilton Creek drainage. The trail continues up steep slopes until it reaches a shallower valley at the head of the second fork of Hamilton Creek. The trail ends on the crest at a junction with the Skyline Trail, just yards from a trailhead parking area. Those seeking more views here can pick up the Grand View Point Trail and take it an additional 0.3 mile south to the vista point. Return the way you came.

VARIATIONS

The upper end of this trail starts on Forest Road 2N10 by Grand View Point. If you're coming from Big Bear, you could go down and back up. You could also consider a downhill trip with a car shuttle or grueling bicycle shuttle back up 2N06 and 2N10. 2N06 above the Seven Oaks Trailhead is poorly maintained and rocky; a high-clearance vehicle is required. Clarks Grade Road (1N54) is equally rough.

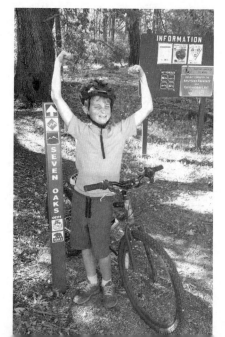

Proud to descend the Seven Oaks Trail

trip 4.13 **Champion Lodgepole Pine**

Distance	0.6 mile (out-and-back)
Hiking Time	30 minutes
Elevation Gain	50'
Difficulty	Easy
Trail Use	Dogs allowed, good for kids, suitable for mountain biking, suitable for equestrians
Best Times	June–October
Agency	San Bernardino National Forest (Big Bear Discovery Center)
Optional Map	USGS *Big Bear Lake* 7.5'

see map on p. 74

DIRECTIONS From eastbound Highway 18 in Big Bear Lake Village at mile marker 018 SBD 47.43, where a sign points to Mill Creek Road and picnic grounds, turn right (south) onto Tulip Lane. Proceed 0.4 mile; then turn right onto Mill Creek Road, which becomes good dirt Forest Road 2N10 in 0.7 mile. Proceed 3.8 miles, and turn right onto 2N11 at a sign pointing to Champion Lodgepole. Proceed 1.0 mile to a signed parking area on the right for the Lodgepole Pine Trail (1W11).

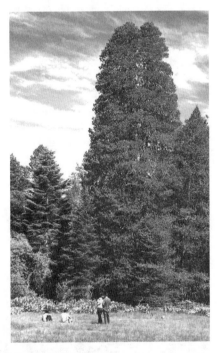

Champion Lodgepole Pine

Lodgepole pines (*Pinus contorta*) are so named because saplings were used by Native Americans to build their dwellings. They're common in the Sierra Nevada and also live above 8,000 feet in the cool upper reaches of the San Gorgonio Wilderness. Lodgepole pines are easily recognized by their thin gray scaly bark, golf ball–sized cones, and pairs of needles. A small stand of lodgepoles, likely left over from a colder bygone era, can be found perched on Bluff Mesa at about 7,600 feet. One of these, a double-trunked behemoth, is the largest known lodgepole in the world. It stands 110 feet tall and is 20 feet in circumference. Biologists estimate that the Champion germinated in 1560, four years before Shakespeare's birth. It's reached by way of a scenic drive on a good dirt road followed by a short nature walk.

Look for an interpretive pamphlet at the trailhead. Fourteen numbered posts point out features along the route that are explained in the pamphlet. The trail (1W11) leads down along a seasonal creek through a forest of white firs and Jeffrey pines. It then curves left and comes to a fork in 0.3 mile. The left fork is the Siberia Creek Trail, which leads 7 miles down to Siberia Creek Trail Camp (see Trip 4.14). Stay right and promptly arrive at the Champion Lodgepole beside a lush meadow. The Forest Service has fenced off the tree; keep your distance so that the Champion isn't loved to death.

Return the way you came.

VARIATIONS

Alternatively, you can explore the trail as it continues north 300 yards; then turn right and walk 0.1 mile to the low dam on Bluff Lake. Bluff Lake Reserve is owned by The Wildlands Conservancy and is open to the public for day use. Trails circle the small lake, and this is a good destination for a picnic.

---

trip 4.14 Siberia Creek Trail Camp from Champion Lodgepole Pine

Distance	14 miles (out-and-back)
Hiking Time	7 hours
Elevation Gain	2,900'
Difficulty	Strenuous
Trail Use	Dogs allowed, suitable for backpacking
Best Times	September–October, April–June
Agency	San Bernardino National Forest (Big Bear Discovery Center)
Required Maps	USGS *Big Bear Lake* and *Keller Peak* 7.5'

see map on p. 74

DIRECTIONS From westbound Highway 18 in Big Bear Lake Village at mile marker 018 SBD 47.43, where a sign points to Mill Creek Road and picnic grounds, turn right (south) onto Tulip Lane. Proceed 0.4 mile; then turn right onto Mill Creek Road, which becomes good dirt Forest Road 2N10 in 0.7 mile. Proceed 3.8 miles, and turn right onto 2N11 at a sign pointing to Champion Lodgepole. Proceed 1.0 mile to a signed parking area on the right for the Lodgepole Pine Trail (1W11).

The Siberia Creek Trail (1W04) from Champion Lodgepole to Siberia Creek Trail Camp is a long, strenuous, beautiful, and lightly used trail cloaked in mystery because of insufficient maintenance and unreliable condition reports. The trail traverses gorgeous forested country on Bluff Mesa before plunging down chaparral-covered slopes to the lovely Siberia Creek Trail Camp on Bear Creek. Hewn from dense chaparral, the trail can become overgrown unless cut back regularly. As of 2017, the Forest Service website indicates that the trail is overgrown and impassable. Actually, however, the path is in decent shape at this writing, and those who love solitude will enjoy this hike.

From the trailhead, follow the Champion Lodgepole Trail north 0.3 mile to a signed junction with the Siberia Creek Trail on the left. It's worth a very short detour on the right to enjoy the Champion Lodgepole (see Trip 4.13); then return to the junction and hike west on the Siberia Creek Trail.

The trail follows Siberia Creek across Bluff Mesa through an attractive forest of lodgepole, Jeffrey, and sugar pines and white firs. In 0.9 mile, reach the edge of the bluff where Siberia Creek plunges into a boulder-choked ravine. The trail begins a gradual descent across

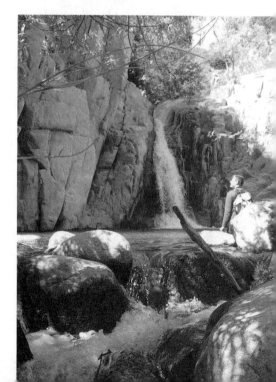

Waterfall along Bear Creek

slopes clad in chinquapin, buckthorn, and manzanita. Enjoy the views of Slide Peak across Bear Creek's deep gorge. In 0.3 mile, pass through the Gunsight, an unimposing gap between two angular rocks. This is a good turnaround point if you're looking for a casual outing or if the trail ahead is overgrown.

Otherwise, begin the long drop into Bear Creek. In 0.6 mile, be sure to make a switchback. If you miss this switchback and continue onto an abandoned section of trail, the brush will get progressively worse until the path vanishes. Coulter pines and eventually bigcone Douglas-fir join the mix as you lose altitude. In 1.5 miles, the trail turns west below a saddle. Watch for gooseberry bushes. In 0.8 mile, it gains a ridge. Switchbacks hewn from the tall chaparral take you down the ridge 1.5 miles to a junction with Trail 1W10 from Seven Pines (see Trip 4.16).

Turn right and hike into the Siberia Creek drainage. Cross the creek; then descend to Siberia Creek Trail Camp at its confluence with Bear Creek in 0.8 mile. The forest of black oak, incense cedar, and bigcone Douglas-fir is especially attractive around here, but the leaf litter often obscures the rocky trail and makes it difficult to follow.

You might stay a night down here and spend some time exploring Bear Creek. Wading upstream will take you to countless trout-filled holes. In a little over an hour, you can reach a section of narrows with a 30-foot waterfall pouring into a pool. Fishermen should be aware that Bear Creek is a California Wild Trout Water. There is a limit of two fish, and no bait or hooks with barbs may be used. Unless you've arranged a shuttle at one of the other trailheads, a long climb back awaits.

trip 4.15   Siberia Creek Trail Camp from Snow Valley

see map on p. 74

Distance	5.5 miles (out-and-back)
Hiking Time	4 hours
Elevation Gain	2,200'
Difficulty	Strenuous
Trail Use	Dogs allowed, suitable for backpacking
Best Times	September–November, April–June
Agency	San Bernardino National Forest (Big Bear Discovery Center)
Required Map	USGS *Keller Peak* 7.5'

DIRECTIONS From Highway 18 at mile marker 18 SBD 38.00 (5.5 miles east of Running Springs and 0.5 mile east of Snow Valley), turn south onto the first dirt road, 2N97. Drive 0.4 mile, staying left at a fork, to the trailhead parking on the right.

The Camp Creek Trail (1W09) drops abruptly down a ridge from Snow Valley to the confluence of Bear and Siberia Creeks, where a secluded trail camp attracts fishermen, picnickers, and campers in search of wilderness (see Trip 4.16). The descent is easy, but the climb back out is grueling, especially on a hot day. The trail is lightly maintained; often branches of scrub oak and thickets of buckthorn intrude into the narrow path. The rangers at the Big Bear Discovery Center don't always have accurate information about the conditions of this lightly used trail, but it's worth asking before you venture forth. Wear protective clothing; exposed flesh is likely to be ripped by the bushes. A heavy-duty pruner would help you cut back the worst of the vegetation. Beware of ticks, especially in the spring. Fishermen should be aware that Bear Creek is a California Wild Trout Stream. There is a limit of two fish, and no bait or

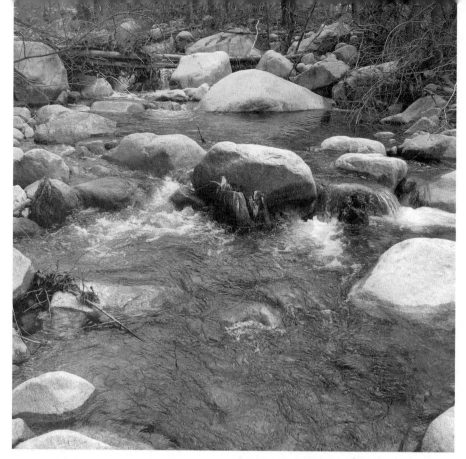

Bear Creek

barbed hooks may be used. Also beware of the confusing names: Siberia Creek Trail Camp is on Bear Creek (near the confluence with Siberia Creek), and is reached from the west via the Camp Creek Trail, which comes near but never crosses Camp Creek!

The path starts behind a sign for the Camp Creek Trail and initially traverses to the east. Don't be tempted by a false path that seems to lead straight down from the sign. The sign indicates that it's 4 miles to Bear Creek, but the trail is actually only 2.8 miles. It leads through Jeffrey pines, white firs, buckthorn, and manzanita. As you begin to switchback downward, you reach sugar and Coulter pines and scrub oak. Occasional breaks in the vegetation give views into the wild canyon cut by Bear Creek and the steep cliffs of Bluff Mesa. Camp Creek is the minor tributary north of the trail. Shortly before you reach the bottom, pass a good overlook into another unnamed tributary of Bear Creek and reach a zone of bigcone Douglas-firs.

The trail becomes hard to see in spots when it reaches the canyon floor and crosses Bear Creek. Watch for occasional cairns and ribbons. Cross to the east side of the creek and follow a washed-out path southward along the base of some cliffs, arriving at the small signed trail camp in about 100 yards.

Return the way you came or, with a 2-hour car shuttle, explore the trail (1W10) leading south to Seven Pines (Trip 4.16). The long, strenuous, and lightly maintained 1W04 Siberia Creek Trail to Champion Lodgepole offers another way to make an interesting shuttle trip (Trip 4.14).

VARIATION ———

Yet another option for experienced and adventurous explorers is to hike up Bear Creek to the Glory Ridge Trail (1W02). This involves about 3.5 hours of cross-country travel up the canyon, mostly wading in the beautiful creek to avoid heavy vegetation on the banks. Easy scrambling is necessary to ascend two waterfalls along the route. Watch for stinging nettle, rattlesnakes, and lots of wild trout. At a fishermen's campsite at the bottom of the Glory Ridge Trail (**N34° 13.905' W117° 0.052'; 5,711'**), climb the steep trail (800' gain over 0.6 mile) to Forest Road 2N15. This road climbs 1.9 miles to Highway 18 at mile marker 18 SBD 42.4. The road is 2WD accessible if it has been recently maintained. Arrange a car or bicycle shuttle to close the loop.

———

trip 4.16 **Siberia Creek Trail Camp from Seven Pines**

Distance	8 miles (out-and-back)
Hiking Time	4 hours
Elevation Gain	1,300'
Difficulty	Moderate
Trail Use	Dogs allowed, suitable for backpacking
Best Times	October–April
Agency	San Bernardino National Forest (Big Bear Discovery Center)
Recommended Maps	USGS *Big Bear Lake* and *Keller Peak* 7.5'

DIRECTIONS From Redlands, drive east on Highway 38 to the town of Angelus Oaks. At a dirt turnout just beyond the north end of town, turn left (north) and descend Middle Control Road (1N06), a good dirt road. (If it's closed for the winter, continue east to the paved Glass Road, follow Glass Road down to Seven Oaks Road, and then backtrack to the bottom of Middle Control Road.)

In 0.5 mile, pass a waterfall at a bend in the road. Continue down to reach the Santa Ana River Road (1N09), 3.8 miles from the highway. Turn left (west) and drive 0.2 mile to a junction with fair dirt Clarks Grade Road (1N54). Turn right and ascend Clarks Grade 1.8 miles to a junction with Forest Road 1N64. Turn left (west) and descend. Past Clark's Ranch Yellow Post Site camp, cross Deer Creek twice, but note that it may be impassable in high water. After 1.7 miles, you'll arrive at the easily missed Siberia Creek Trailhead (1W10) on the right.

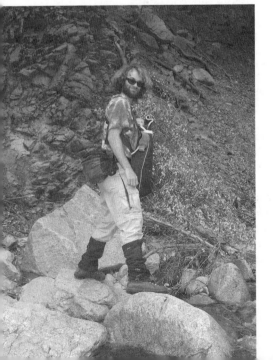

Siberia Creek Trail Camp is a small campsite nestled in the forest at the confluence of Siberia and Bear Creeks southwest of Big Bear Lake. It's accessed by three rugged and lightly maintained trails, one from Snow Valley, a second from Champion Lodgepole above Big Bear, and a third from Seven Pines on the Santa Ana River to the south. Beware that ticks can be plentiful here, especially in the spring. Long pants, long sleeves, gaiters, and even a garden pruner are recommended if the trail has not been recently maintained. At this writing, the trail was damaged by landslides and

Fording Bear Creek

isn't recommended for casual hikers. However, this trip is an enjoyable adventure for those willing to brave the dirt roads and brush to see a little-visited corner of the San Bernardino Mountains. Check with the Big Bear Discovery Center for updated conditions.

The trail cuts west through the dense south-facing chaparral, especially scrub oak, manzanita, sage, buckthorn, and yucca. This section can be brutally hot in summer months. In 1.3 miles, the trail rounds the bend and turns north on the slopes overlooking Bear Creek. The west-facing chaparral is subtly different in character, but possibly even denser. The bare slopes of Slide Peak across the canyon are impressive to behold. If you're watchful, you may notice an abandoned mine shaft adjacent to the trail. Old mine shafts are extremely dangerous. Some hikers asphyxiated while exploring this one.

In another 1.7 miles, pass a junction with the Siberia Creek Trail (1W04) coming from the Champion Lodgepole tree above Big Bear. Your trail drops abruptly, enters a splendid forest, crosses Siberia Creek, and arrives in a mile at Siberia Creek Trail Camp, a small clearing above the roaring Bear Creek. The last part of the trail before the camp can be hard to find in the autumn because of the fallen leaves. However, cross-country travel in the canyon is difficult, so it's worth searching out the correct trail.

After enjoying the creek and possibly spending a night at the secluded camp, return the way you came.

---

trip 4.17   **Butler Peak**

Distance	0.25 mile (out-and-back)	
Hiking Time	15 minutes	
Elevation Gain	100'	
Difficulty	Easy	
Trail Use	Good for kids	
Best Times	May–October	
Agency	San Bernardino National Forest (Big Bear Discovery Center)	
Optional Map	USGS *Butler Peak* 7.5'	

see map on p. 74

DIRECTIONS From Highway 38 in Fawnskin, turn northwest at the sign for Butler Peak onto Rim of the World Drive, which becomes Forest Road 3N14. In 1.3 miles, turn left onto Forest Road 2N13 at a sign pointing to the lookout. Go 2.1 miles, and then turn left onto fair dirt road Forest Road 2N13C, which climbs 2.5 miles to a parking area below the Butler Peak Fire Lookout. Note that 2N13C may be gated when the lookout is closed. It crosses a creek that, during high water, may be passable only in high-clearance vehicles.

Butler Peak (8,531') is one of a network of mountaintops in the San Bernardino National Forest hosting historic fire lookouts. Other lookouts include Keller Peak, Strawberry Peak, Morton Peak, Red Mountain, Black Mountain, and Tahquitz Peak. The 360-degree views from Butler Peak are among the most impressive, encompassing Big Bear Lake to the east, San Gorgonio to the southeast, the Santa Ana River Canyon and Keller Peak to the south, Lake Arrowhead to the west, and Holcomb Creek and the desert slopes to the north. The hike to the summit is very short, but it's steep and rocky and not suited for those who are unsteady on their feet. The tower is open 9 a.m.–5 p.m. on weekends, holidays, and some weekdays from Memorial Day to Labor Day. However, the high summit may be snowbound until June in wet years.

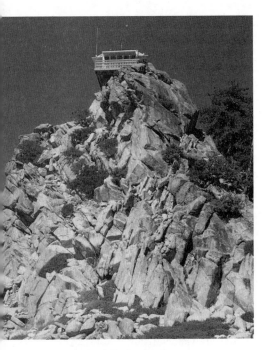

Butler Peak Fire Lookout

In September 2007, the Butler 2 Fire burned 14,000 acres northwest of Big Bear Lake, including Butler Peak itself. Vast sections of the forest in this area were incinerated. The Forest Service didn't reopen the access road until 2016. The groundcover has fully returned, but burnt tree trunks leave a stark reminder of the inferno.

From the parking area, follow the trail that switchbacks up to the fire lookout, which is precariously perched on the rocky summit outcrop. Climb two flights of steep stairs to the lookout.

The fire lookout was constructed in 1931 by the Civilian Conservation Corps (CCC) and was staffed for decades by the U.S. Forest Service. Today it's staffed by trained volunteers, who are also happy to show visitors the sights as well as explain how the structure works. If you're interested in becoming a volunteer, visit mountainsfoundation.org, or ask the volunteers at the lookout for more information.

trip 4.18   Granite Peaks

Distance	6 miles (out-and-back)
Hiking Time	5 hours
Elevation Gain	1,800'
Difficulty	Strenuous
Best Times	September–November, March–May
Agency	San Bernardino National Forest (Big Bear Discovery Center)
Required Map	USGS *Rattlesnake Canyon* 7.5'

see map on next page

DIRECTIONS A high-clearance vehicle is recommended. From Highway 18 just north of mile marker 18 SBD 61.00 (3.5 miles northeast of Baldwin Lake), turn east onto dirt Cactus Flat/Smarts Ranch Road (3N03). In 4.9 miles, park where the road crosses Arrastre Creek.

The Granite Peaks are the most interesting summits in the trailless and seldom-visited Bighorn Wilderness at the east end of the San Bernardino Mountains where the pine forests give way to the desert. This trip, although short in distance, involves rugged cross-country travel and challenging navigation. A GPS is very helpful, although expert application of map and compass is also sufficient. The Granite Peaks are a trio of boulder mounds atop a high ridge. The western summit, most visible from Lone Valley, is called Granite Peak (7,497'). The central summit is Granite Point (7,512'). The true high point and the destination of this trip is the eastern summit, East Peak (7,527'). The summit boulders offer splendid panoramic views. Long pants and gaiters are recommended to ward off the prickly desert vegetation.

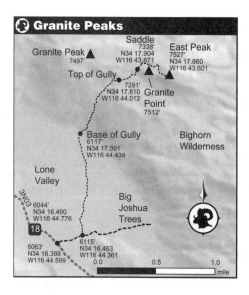

Granite Peaks

Granite Peak 7497'

Saddle 7338'
N34 17.904
W116 43.871

East Peak 7527'
N34 17.860
W116 43.601

Top of Gully 7291'
N34 17.810
W116 44.012

Granite Point 7512'

Base of Gully 6117'
N34 17.391
W116 44.439

Bighorn Wilderness

Lone Valley

3N03

6044'
N34 16.490
W116 44.776

18

6063'
N34 16.388
W116 44.599

6115'
N34 16.463
W116 44.361
0.0

Big Joshua Trees

0.5

1.0
mile

During deer season (October–November), hunters frequent this area.

Continue up Forest Road 3N03 for 0.2 mile to a closed road on the left. (Unless Arrastre Creek is high, you may be able to drive this stretch.) Walk 0.3 mile east on the closed road to the old parking area. Looking due north, pick out the high point at the north end of the ridge; this is Granite Peak. Then look for the first reasonably prominent gully to the right of the peak (a creek is shown in this gully on the USGS topo map). Your first goal is to hike 1.1 miles across Lone Valley to the base of this gully. East Peak is hidden behind the ridge. Lone Valley is one of the most starkly beautiful in the San Bernardino Mountains, dotted with huge Joshua trees, junipers, pinyon pines, cacti, Mormon tea, and other drought-resistant scrub. Watch out for and try to avoid cryptobiotic soil; these dark hummocks are composed of cyanobacteria and cyanolichens that hold the sandy soil together, retain moisture, and greatly improve the fertility of the desert. When disturbed, the soil takes decades to recover.

Granite Peak ascent route

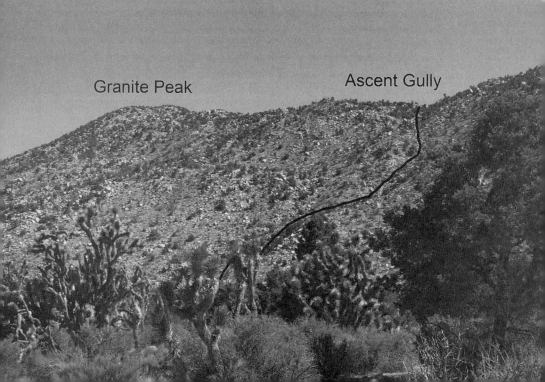

Granite Peak   Ascent Gully

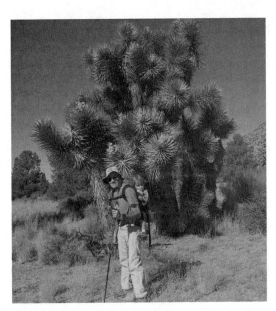

Joshua Tree in Lone Valley

Pick your way up the long, steep gully, veering to one side or the other as you see fit to find the easiest course. Watch for Mojave yuccas, nolinas, Mojave mound cactus, and pancake prickly pear. Near the top, keep in the gully as it veers left. You may start seeing ducks marking the path. After the gully levels out, continue up the sandy wash until you reach the top of the ridge.

This area is confusing, so note your landmarks carefully and be sure you'll be able to find your way back to this point. Looking straight ahead (east), pick out the two rocky peaks ahead. The one on the left is Granite Point, while the more distant one on the right is your goal, East Peak. The easiest way to reach East Peak is to circle around behind Granite Point. Aim for a low spot immediately left of Granite Point. To reach it, you'll cross a broad flat area, veer right down a wash about 100 feet, and then exit left and scramble up huge boulders to a saddle. You'll probably see ducks marking the route.

After crossing the saddle, curve around to the north and then east side of Granite Point. You'll soon encounter easy walking in a sandy, cactus-studded valley. After passing Granite Point, look for the rocky summit of East Peak to the east. The easiest way up follows the prominent pinyon-filled gully to the ridgeline; then it turns left and scales the final summit boulders to the peak. The bare summit of San Gorgonio is barely visible over the ridge to the left of Sugarloaf Mountain. Baldwin and Big Bear Lakes and the forests to the west stand in stark contrast to the desert where you stand. To the east, rugged slopes drop down to the Mojave Desert.

Retrace your steps carefully. Once you're back to Lone Valley, the gray rocks on a low ridge protruding into the south end of the valley make a helpful landmark for navigating back to the old parking area, or you may shortcut cross-country back to Arrastre Creek.

VARIATION

If time permits, explore a grove of enormous Joshua trees in Lone Valley 0.5 mile east of the old parking area. The largest known Joshua tree, almost 15 feet in circumference, was in this grove but was shot to death and toppled by hooligans before 2005. Hike east from the trailhead, looking for traces of an old jeep trail into the grove. The roads in this area were closed to prevent further vandalism.

chapter 5

San Bernardino Mountains: San Gorgonio Wilderness

The San Bernardino Mountains are part of California's unusual Transverse Ranges, running east to west rather than southeast to northwest. They've long attracted the attention of humans, at first for hunting, logging, and gold, but now most of all for recreation. The range is so large that trips for this area are divided into three chapters. This chapter explores the steep and rugged San Gorgonio Wilderness on the southeast side of the range, cut off from Big Bear by the deep trench of the Santa Ana River. Chapter 3 describes the western end, especially around Lake Arrowhead and the alluring creeks at the interface of forest and desert. Chapter 4 focuses on the eastern end, where richly forested hills circle the jewel-like Big Bear Lake.

San Gorgonio Wilderness, located in the southeast portion of the San Bernardino Mountains, is home to California's tallest mountains south of the Sierra Nevada. The biggest peaks are located along the 7-mile crest of the Great San Bernardino Divide stretching from San Gorgonio Mountain to San Bernardino Peak. This divide drops below 10,000 feet at only one point, Dollar Lake Saddle, and separates the Santa Ana River Canyon and Big Bear areas to the north from Mill Creek, the Yucaipa Ridge, and the eastern Los Angeles Basin to the south. This chapter also describes hikes on the nearby Yucaipa Ridge and Santa Ana River even though they're outside the wilderness area proper.

The San Gorgonio Wilderness is within the Sand to Snow National Monument, a 154,000-acre monument designed by President Barack Obama in 2016. The monument also encompasses the eastern slopes of the San Bernardino Mountains, providing a critical wildlife link between Joshua Tree National Park and the San Bernardinos necessary for the genetic diversity of large mammals. More than 60,000 acres along these slopes were privately acquired by The Wildlands Conservancy and others to protect them from development before they were transferred to the monument.

The San Bernardino Mountains were once of interest only to a handful of miners and loggers, but by the 1920s had become a center of Southern California recreation. Nearly 100,000 people visited the range each year and roads were cut across many of the slopes. Soon, winter-sport interests were calling for a ski resort on the north face of San Gorgonio Peak. Conflicts between developers and conservationists raged for decades. In 1964, the Wilderness Act was passed by Congress, setting aside untrammeled wild areas for the benefit of present and future generations. The 58,969-acre San Gorgonio Wilderness is one of these areas.

The peaks of San Gorgonio Wilderness hold distinguished roles in the history of Southern California. In 1852, Colonel Henry Washington established the first survey point in Southern California to begin surveying the newly admitted state. He selected San Bernardino Peak because it was prominently visible from much of the Los Angeles Basin. He led a crew of 12 sturdy men up the arduous, trailless, chaparral-clad north slope and established a 24-foot-tall survey marker half a mile west of the true summit. Measurements were distorted by the heat waves rising off the valley, so enormous fires were lit on the mountain and at various other points in the valley for nighttime surveying. Base Line Road in the Inland Empire still essentially follows the east–west line designated by the survey.

In 1872, Watson Goodyear of the California Geological Survey and Mark Thomas of San Bernardino claimed the first recorded ascent of San Gorgonio Mountain, known as Old Grayback at the time. There is some controversy about whether this party reached the correct summit, but numerous other parties climbed the mountain in the subsequent decade.

The most heavily used routes to the top of San Gorgonio Mountain are the steep Vivian Creek Trail from the south and the long South Fork Trail from the north. The long traverse across the ridge is a three-day rite of passage for many Boy Scouts, and successful trekkers proudly wear their "I Climbed the Nine Peaks" patch. Aspen Grove is also a great place to watch the leaves changing in the fall. However, there are many other lesser-traveled trails and cross-country routes on the mountain where the intrepid hiker can find solitude and beauty.

Access to the mountains in this area is a growing issue. The Falls Creek Trail from Mill Creek was built in 1898 by John Dobbs and was used by the public for a century, but it was closed because of complaints from a landowner, adding 3 miles each way to the climb to Dollar Lake Saddle. Also, the Banning Water Division and the Morongo Indians have closed southern access to the San Gorgonio Wilderness. When the Southern Pacific Railroad laid tracks through Banning Pass, it received every other section of land for several miles on both sides of the tracks as incentive to build. Southern Pacific sold much of the land to finance construction. Now, more than a century later, the Yucaipa Ridge is still a checkerboard of public and private land as a result of this grant. No fewer than three dirt

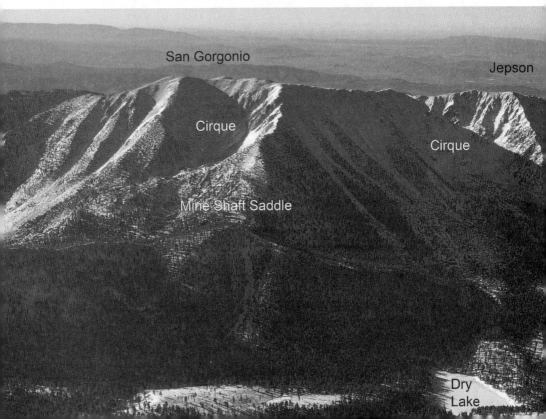

Winter aerial view of San Gorgonio from the north. Notice Dry Lake and the glacial cirques.

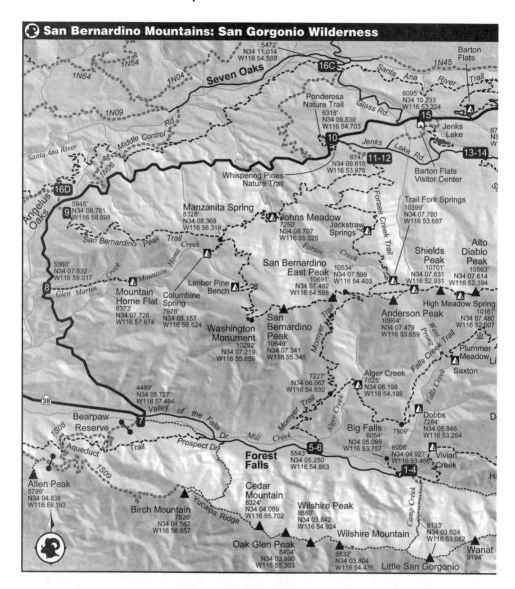

San Bernardino Mountains: San Gorgonio Wilderness

roads and three trails once served the ridge, but not a single one remains accessible now that private landowners have forbidden access to hikers.

A wilderness permit, which is required to camp overnight in San Gorgonio Wilderness, can be obtained at no charge from the Mill Creek Ranger Station (see Appendix B). Permits for some trails can be self-issued, permits for the most popular routes can be obtained at the station when it's open, and advance reservations can be made by mail or fax. The largest number of hikers and campers flock to the wilderness on summer weekends, and quotas for the popular trails fill up weeks in advance. If you find yourself unable to get a permit for Vivian Creek or South Fork, consider Fish Creek as a great alternative. The fall is a better time to seek seclusion. Hardy mountaineers equipped with skis, snowshoes, or crampons venture into the high country in the winter and spring. As of September 2017, day hikers

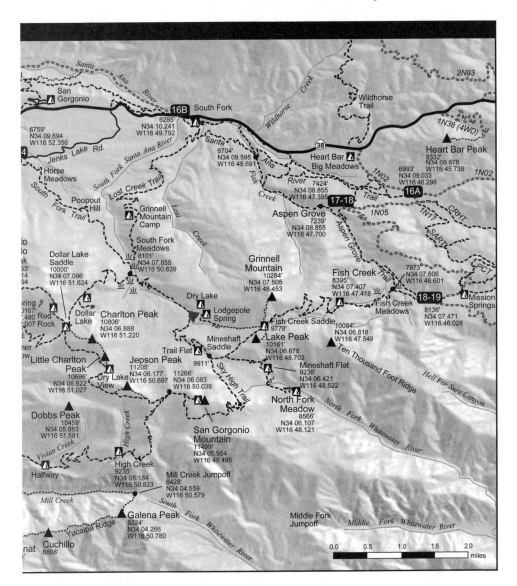

no longer need a wilderness permit but may file one voluntarily to notify rangers of where they will be traveling.

Summer also brings a pattern of afternoon thundershowers, especially in July and August. Moisture from the ocean is forced upward by the prevailing westerly breezes as it hits the wall of mountains. Heated by the afternoon sun, towering cumulus clouds build over the summit and dump their contents in violent storms. Hikers typically have advanced warning as the clouds gather and the sky darkens before the storm hits. On these days, it's best to be off the exposed ridges before noon to avoid lightning strikes. Hikers aiming for a single-day ascent of San Gorgonio in the summer should plan on a very early start.

Good campsites are labeled on the map above. Many of the higher sites are dry, so plan ahead and fill your water bottles at the last dependable source. Bears are active in some of these areas and have learned to steal food hanging from tree branches; bear canisters can be purchased or rented from the Mill Creek Ranger Station. Campfires are prohibited in the wilderness at any time.

San Gorgonio Wilderness is served by a large and active volunteer group called the San Gorgonio Wilderness Association (SGWA), which works with the grievously underfunded U.S. Forest Service to provide visitor information, patrol and maintain trails, and protect the wilderness. They have an information-packed website (including current trail conditions and water reports) at sgwa.org and also welcome new volunteers each year.

The northern half of the San Gorgonio Wilderness burned in the June 2015 Lake Fire. This 31,000-acre blaze swept through mature forest that had been weakened by the prolonged drought. The cause remains under investigation but arson is suspected.

For further reading about this area, see John W. Robinson's books *The San Bernardinos* and *San Gorgonio: A Wilderness Preserved.*

trip 5.1 San Gorgonio via Vivian Creek

see map on p. 102

Distance	17 miles (out-and-back)
Hiking Time	9 hours
Elevation Gain	5,500'
Difficulty	Strenuous
Trail Use	Dogs allowed, suitable for backpacking
Best Times	June–October
Agency	San Bernardino National Forest (Mill Creek Ranger Station)
Recommended Maps	Tom Harrison *San Gorgonio Wilderness* or USGS *Forest Falls* and *San Gorgonio Mountain* 7.5'
Permit	San Gorgonio Wilderness Permit required for overnight camping

DIRECTIONS From Redlands, drive east on Highway 38 to the huge hairpin turn at mile marker 038 SBD 15.00. Turn right onto Valley of the Falls Drive and proceed 4.5 miles to its end. Turn left and park at the Vivian Creek Trailhead.

At 11,499 feet, San Gorgonio Mountain is the tallest summit in Southern California and is an obligatory climb for serious local mountaineers. The Vivian Creek Trail was the original route to the summit of San Gorgonio. Albert Vivian of Yucaipa hewed the trail up the rugged mountainside for the enjoyment of patrons of the Forest Home resort in Mill Creek.

Now that there are numerous excellent trails on the mountain, many hikers still believe Vivian Creek is the best. It is steep and direct, offers fantastic views, and passes three fine trail camps en route. If you plan to hike this route on a summer weekend, request your permit long in advance because the quotas frequently fill two to four weeks ahead of time. Vivian Creek is also a good but demanding snow route in the spring; snowshoes, ice ax, and crampons may be required, depending on the conditions.

From the signed Vivian Creek Trailhead at the east end of the parking area, hike east along the trail, which is an old dirt road; ignore forks that lead to nearby cabins. In 0.5 mile, the Vivian Creek Trail turns north and crosses Mill Creek (occasionally hazardous when the water is high).

The trail then switchbacks steeply northward through the forest of oaks until, in 1 mile, it rounds a corner and enters a hanging valley carved by Vivian Creek. There is year-round water and scenic camping here beneath the incense cedars, white firs, and Jeffrey pines, though it's too low to be a practical campsite for summit-goers. Vivian Creek is lined with lush ferns and wildflowers. Lilies bloom in the spring, giving way to penstemon, Indian paintbrush, scarlet monkeyflower, and columbine by late summer.

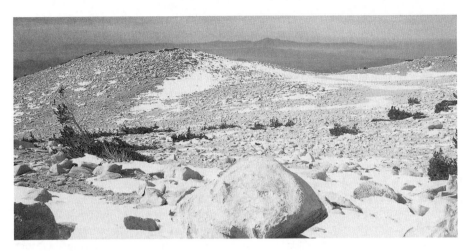

San Gorgonio summit

The trail turns east and follows Vivian Creek up the valley 1.3 miles to Halfway Camp (seasonal water) before making broad switchbacks up the next ridge and turning a corner in 2.3 miles to High Creek Camp, situated on High Creek, which tumbles year-round down the south wall of San Gorgonio. This site, at 9,400 feet amidst the hardy lodgepole pines, can be bitterly cold even on summer nights, but is most convenient for those backpacking the mountain.

Beyond High Creek Camp, the trail makes numerous gratuitously flat switchbacks as it climbs east to the next ridge at Bighorn Saddle, then turns north and follows the ridge up to treeline. If the mountain is covered in snow, you're better off going due east straight up to the ridge rather than attempting to follow the switchbacks. The lodgepole (two needles) and limber pines (five needles) have been beaten down by extreme winds and ice into a low-growing shrublike form called krummholz. San Gorgonio Mountain is one of Southern California's few summits above treeline, earning the nickname "Old Grayback" for the bare, sandy soil on the summit ridge. Reach a T-junction 2.4 miles from High Creek Camp. Turn right (east), proceed 0.2 mile to another junction with the Sky High Trail, stay left, and continue 0.4 mile to the windswept summit boulders.

Some backpackers spend a night on the summit. This site is fully exposed to the elements, but offers solitude and spectacular views. Return the way you came, or if you've arranged a shuttle, descend any of the other trails described in this chapter. The 21-mile loop via Dollar Lake Saddle and Falls Creek Trail is very enjoyable and requires only a 1.6-mile shuttle or walk or bike ride between trailheads.

trip 5.2 Little San Gorgonio Peak

see map on p. 102

Distance	5 miles (out-and-back)
Hiking Time	6 hours
Elevation Gain	3,100'
Difficulty	Strenuous
Best Times	March–November
Agency	San Bernardino National Forest (Mill Creek Ranger Station)
Required Map	Tom Harrison *San Gorgonio Wilderness* or USGS *Forest Falls* 7.5'

DIRECTIONS From Redlands, drive east on Highway 38 to the huge hairpin turn at mile marker 038 SBD 15.00. Turn right onto Valley of the Falls Drive and proceed 4.5 miles to its end. Turn left and park at the Vivian Creek Trailhead.

Little San Gorgonio Peak (9,133') is the second-highest point on the Yucaipa Ridge and the most difficult summit to reach. An insidiously direct cross-country route leads up Camp Creek, gaining 3,000 feet in 1.3 horizontal miles, for an astonishing average grade of 23 degrees. Despite the short distance, the trip is suited only to experienced cross-country climbers with strong route-finding skills. If in doubt, try the significantly easier Galena Peak first (see Trip 5.3). Camp Creek is also a natural avalanche chute, and accumulated snow in the north-facing gully can linger into early summer. This is an excellent snow climb in early spring when continuous well-consolidated snow covers the talus, waterfalls, and bushes. Be careful to assess the avalanche risk before you venture up. By late spring, the snow bridges over the creek have thinned, and present a falling hazard, but reveal delightful waterfalls. The creek dries up later in the season. An ice ax and crampons are necessary in early season and a helmet is prudent any time of year. Whenever you visit, your exertions are rewarded with solitude and stunning views of the peaks along the San Bernardino Divide and Yucaipa Ridge.

From the signed Vivian Creek Trailhead at the east end of the parking area, hike east along the trail, which is an old dirt road; ignore forks that lead to nearby cabins. In 0.2 mile, look for the narrow gravel wash of Camp Creek crossing the trail in a grove of incense cedars. It comes down from the first prominent canyon you pass along the hike. Turn right and ascend

Stairstep Falls, where the route exits Camp Creek and climbs southward

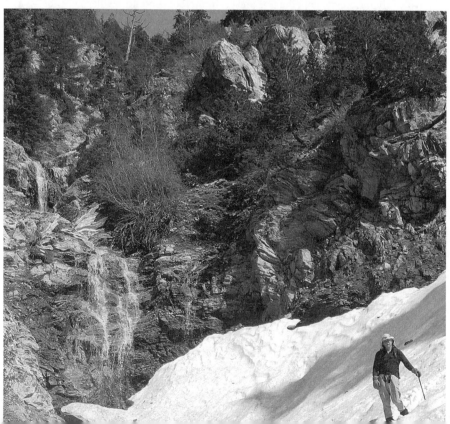

the creek (dry later in the season). In 0.1 mile, cross a dirt road. The forest opens, revealing views up the canyon. The shattered rock ridges on both sides are extremely unstable.

In 0.3 mile, the canyon narrows. In another 0.1 mile, stay left in the main canyon at a fork with a tributary. Beyond that, in another 0.1 mile, reach a waterfall that can be bypassed by climbing the slope to the west and then traversing back above.

In yet another 0.1 mile, the canyon veers left (southeast) and you reach the second waterfall—actually a series of falls stairstepping up the canyon. Although you can pick a path around the falls, the recommended route is to depart Camp Creek at this point and climb south directly to Yucaipa Ridge.

Hike up the steep slope until it's convenient to veer slightly left and gain a ridgeline. As you climb the relentless slopes, the ponderosa pines and incense cedars give way to lodgepole pines; white firs and sugar pines also keep you company nearly all the way to the ridge. Views across Mill Creek toward San Bernardino Peak and San Gorgonio steadily improve as you get higher. After 0.8 mile of strenuous climbing, reach the crest of Yucaipa Ridge about 0.2 mile east of an antenna site. Take a moment to identify where you are so you can find the same point for your descent later on.

The Oak Glen Divide Trail once ran along this ridge, and traces of it are still visible threading through the chinquapin. Turn left (east) and hike 0.5 mile to the summit of Little San Gorgonio Peak. Enjoy the dramatic views, and then return the way you came. For a very strenuous alternative, follow the ridge east or west to climb more peaks (see Trip 5.21).

---

trip 5.3   ## Galena Peak

Distance	8 miles (out-and-back)
Hiking Time	6 hours
Elevation Gain	3,400'
Difficulty	Strenuous
Trail Use	Suitable for backpacking
Best Times	May–November
Agency	San Bernardino National Forest (Mill Creek Ranger Station)
Recommended Maps	Tom Harrison *San Gorgonio Wilderness* or USGS *Forest Falls* and *San Gorgonio Mountain* 7.5'

see map on p. 102

DIRECTIONS From Redlands, drive east on Highway 38 to the huge hairpin turn at mile marker 038 SBD 15.00. Turn right onto Valley of the Falls Drive and proceed 4.5 miles to its end. Turn left and park at the Vivian Creek Trailhead.

At 9,324 feet, Galena Peak is the tallest and most dramatic summit on the long Yucaipa Ridge. Its north face has been carved into soaring buttresses and forbidding ravines. After a fresh coat of snow in the spring, Galena Peak looks like it could have been transported to Southern California from the Swiss Alps. Moreover, Galena Peak provides fantastic views of San Gorgonio Mountain. The steep and crumbling rock on the north face is too dangerous to climb directly, so the peak is best reached from the Mill Creek Jumpoff via the northeast ridge. Even so, this is a strenuous and challenging cross-country hike. It follows Mill Creek's channel for several miles, so the route is best avoided during times of high water.

From the signed Vivian Creek Trailhead at the east end of the parking area, hike east along the trail, which is an old dirt road; ignore forks that lead to nearby cabins. In 0.5 mile, the Vivian Creek Trail turns north and crosses Mill Creek, but our route continues east. In 0.1 mile, the trail disappears entirely and you must hike east up the creekbed. The best route may change as flash floods churn up the channel, but at this writing, staying in the bed near the south bank avoided the worst of the boulder-hopping.

After about 2 miles, the channel narrows and you come to two waterfalls. Adept rock scramblers can pass the waterfalls on the slabs and steep dirt immediately to the right, but an easier way is to climb out of the riverbed on the right and follow a use trail 0.1 mile past the falls and back down into Mill Creek.

Beyond, the canyon steepens, and then abruptly rises to the infamous and phenomenally loose Mill Creek Jumpoff. The face is continually eroding; a big storm in 2013 shaved off about 10 feet of the shelf on the top. You'll have to assess the least bad route under current conditions. Rockfall is almost inevitable, so large groups should take special care here; helmets would be prudent. The top of the jumpoff is 3.2 miles from the trailhead.

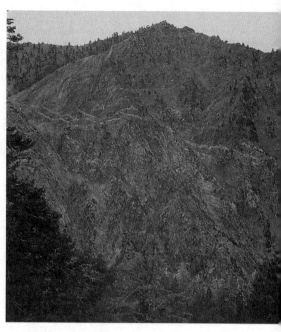

North face of Galena Peak

From Mill Creek Jumpoff, you can see the east summit of Galena Peak to the south. Follow a use trail up the ridge, enjoying stunning views into the abyss of Galena's northwest face. The trail used to be easy to follow and bypassed all nasty brush, but parts have been eroded in a 2007 thunderstorm, and some of the lower trail along the lip was swept away by the 2013 storm. The distance is only 0.5 mile, but the climbing is steep and strenuous.

Galena has east and west summits. The east summit where the trail ends is the official peak and is where the climbing register can be found. If you have time and energy remaining, consider taking the 10-minute walk along the ridge to the west summit, which is 15 feet taller. The west summit also offers breathtaking views along the jagged Yucaipa Ridge toward Little San Gorgonio Peak.

Return the way you came. Do not be lured down the loose and dangerous cliffs of the north face.

---

trip 5.4   Big Falls

Distance	0.6 mile (out-and-back)
Hiking Time	30 minutes
Elevation Gain	100'
Difficulty	Easy
Trail Use	Dogs allowed, good for kids
Best Times	All year
Agency	San Bernardino National Forest (Mill Creek Ranger Station)
Optional Map	Tom Harrison *San Gorgonio Wilderness* or USGS *Forest Falls* 7.5'

see map on p. 102

DIRECTIONS From Redlands, drive east on Highway 38 to the huge hairpin turn at mile marker 038 SBD 15.00. Turn right onto Valley of the Falls Drive and proceed 4.3 miles to the Big Falls parking area on the left. If you reach the Vivian Creek Trailhead, you've gone 0.2 mile too far.

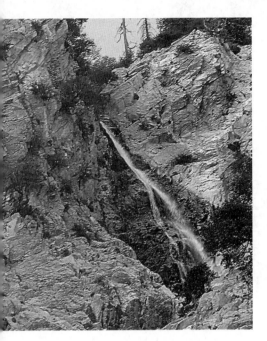

Big Falls

Mill Creek cuts a deep swath through the loose rocks south of San Gorgonio Mountain. Numerous waterfalls along the lateral streams pour down the steep faces into Mill Creek. Falls Creek has the most impressive waterfall, uncreatively named Big Falls. It's hidden behind the mouth of the canyon but can be viewed from this short hike.

Bring sandals and a swimsuit. The creek and pools along the way are popular for water play on a warm day. However, be careful in the spring or during other times of high water when Mill Creek can be hazardous to cross.

From the north edge of the Big Falls Trailhead parking lot, look for a trail marker and follow the trail west along the bank of Mill Creek. Falls Creek Canyon is the first canyon on the north to the west of the parking area. As you approach, cross Mill Creek (the trail is washed out here every spring), and follow the Big Falls Trail into the mouth of Falls Creek Canyon and up the slope to a viewing platform with a metal railing.

Do not be tempted to climb the slick and unstable rocks adjacent to Big Falls. The Valley of the Falls Search and Rescue Team was established here in 1958 after a particularly gruesome accident, and rescuers continue to respond many times a year. One of the boulders at the base is known as Blood Rock in memory of the victims who have fallen here.

trip 5.5   Alger Creek or Dobbs Trail Camp

see map on p. 102

Distance	7–11 miles (out-and-back)
Hiking Time	4–6 hours
Elevation Gain	2,100'/2,800'
Difficulty	Moderate
Trail Use	Dogs allowed, suitable for backpacking
Best Times	June–November
Agency	San Bernardino National Forest (Mill Creek Ranger Station)
Recommended Maps	Tom Harrison *San Gorgonio Wilderness* or USGS *Forest Falls* and *San Gorgonio Mountain* 7.5'
Permit	San Gorgonio Wilderness Permit required for overnight camping

DIRECTIONS From Redlands, drive east on Highway 38 to the huge hairpin turn at mile marker 038 SBD 15.00. Turn right onto Valley of the Falls Drive and proceed 2.9 miles to the Momyer Trailhead, on the left. If you reach the fire station, you've gone about 100 yards too far.

The southern face of the San Bernardino Divide is lightly visited. Tucked away halfway up the slopes are two splendid trail camps, located alongside rushing creeks and shaded beneath towering incense cedars. Backpackers looking for solitude can find it here. In the summer when popular trails are reserved weeks in advance, these camps are usually available.

The Momyer Creek Trail, named for Joe Momyer, who was instrumental to the protection of San Gorgonio Wilderness, departs the northwest corner of the parking area. It crosses the boulder-strewn bed of Mill Creek to reach a sign on the north side. Beyond the sign, turn right and follow the trail parallel to the creek through the forest before you turn back north. Climb out of the forest and begin switchbacking through the sunbaked chaparral with great views of the steep Yucaipa Ridge to the south across the valley. At the first major switchback, you may see traces of an abandoned trail coming up from Torrey Pines Road. Soon, you climb back into the oak forest, where squirrels busily scamper about, stocking up their winter supply of acorns. At 2.5 miles, cross the wilderness boundary, and 0.15 mile farther, come to a signed junction.

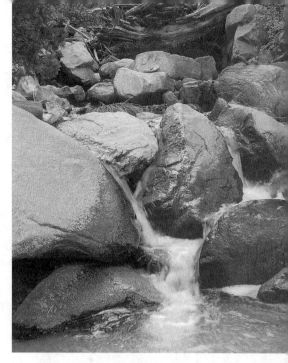

Falls Creek below Dobbs Trail Camp

The Momyer Creek Trail climbs to the left, but we turn right (east) and contour along the slope 0.8 mile, passing a spring and then switchbacking steeply down into the canyon cut by Alger Creek. On the west bank is the Alger Creek Trail Camp with year-round water.

VARIATION

For those seeking a taste of history and an even more remarkable camp, cross Alger Creek and continue southeast 1.5 miles to a junction at the south end of a long ridge. Follow the trail that descends northeast, switchbacking down 0.5 mile to the confluence of two forks of Falls Creek. At the end of the 19th century, the mountain man John Dobbs built his cabin immediately above the two streams on a flat clearing beneath the mighty cedars. Now, scarcely a trace of the dwelling remains, but the Dobbs Trail Camp is one of the most scenic in all of Southern California. Water is reliable year-round.

Return the way you came. The Falls Creek Trail, built by John Dobbs in 1898 and used by the public for a century, once cut off 3 miles each way of the hike to Dobbs Trail Camp, but now it has been closed by the Forest Service because of complaints by a private landowner.

trip 5.6 Momyer to Falls Creek Loop

Distance	20 miles (loop)
Hiking Time	10 hours
Elevation Gain	5,900'
Difficulty	Strenuous
Trail Use	Dogs allowed, suitable for backpacking
Best Times	June–October
Agency	San Bernardino National Forest (Mill Creek Ranger Station)
Recommended Maps	Tom Harrison *San Gorgonio Wilderness* or USGS *Forest Falls, Big Bear Lake, Moonridge,* and *San Gorgonio Mountain* 7.5'
Permit	San Gorgonio Wilderness Permit required for overnight camping

see map on p. 102

DIRECTIONS From Redlands, drive east on Highway 38 to the huge hairpin turn at mile marker 038 SBD 15.00. Turn right onto Valley of the Falls Drive and proceed 2.9 miles to the Momyer Trailhead, on the left. If you reach the fire station, you've gone about 100 yards too far.

Few hikers venture up the unrelenting switchbacks on the enormous southern wall of the San Bernardino Divide. But those who do are rewarded with solitude, a unique perspective on the mountain, and a first-rate workout. This trip climbs the Momyer Creek Trail, which is the shortest and steepest route to the crest. It follows the flat ridgetop east to Dollar Lake Saddle, and then descends the Falls Creek Trail to form a great loop. This route is handy when the more popular trailheads book up in the summer or as a speedy way to the ridgeline for avid peak baggers. It also tours a diverse forest featuring many species of pines (Jeffrey, ponderosa, limber, lodgepole, sugar, and Coulter) and oaks (black, canyon live, and scrub), white firs, bigcone Douglas-fir, incense cedars, and, of course, endless chaparral. The upper Momyer Creek Trail is seldom maintained and long pants are helpful, but the worst of the brush is still cut back from the trail.

The Momyer Creek Trail departs the northwest corner of the parking area and crosses the boulder-strewn bed of Mill Creek to reach a sign on the north side. Beyond the sign, turn right and follow the trail parallel to the creek through the forest before you turn back north. Climb out of the forest and begin switchbacking through the sunbaked chaparral with great views of the steep Yucaipa Ridge to the south across the valley. At the first major switchback, you may see traces of the old trail coming up from Torrey Pines Road. Soon, you climb back into the oak forest, where squirrels busily scamper about. At 2.5 miles, cross the wilderness boundary, and 0.15 mile farther, come to a signed junction. Stay left up the Momyer Creek Trail toward San Bernardino Peak; you'll later return to this point on the

Falls Creek Canyon

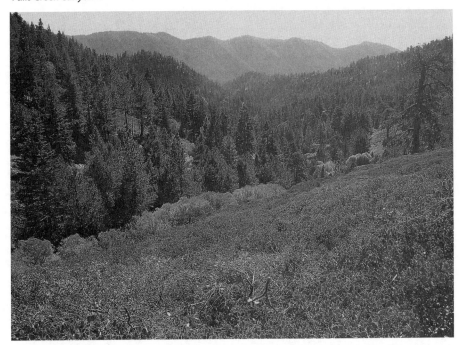

Falls Creek Trail from Dollar Lake Saddle and Alger Creek. The 2011 Momyer Fire burned 150 acres near the trail junction.

The Momyer Creek Trail climbs through a zone where the trees have been devastated by bark beetles and the path can be hard to follow at times when it's covered with debris of downed firs and pines. At about 8,500 feet, the forest yields to a vast field of manzanita, buckthorn, chinquapin, and other chaparral. On a clear day, you can see over the Yucaipa Ridge to Lake Perris (with a distinctive island), saddle-backed Santiago Peak, and even the Pacific Ocean. At 10,000 feet, the trail crosses the south ridge of San Bernardino East Peak and gradually climbs to the east; it then switches back to meet the crest at a signed junction east of the peak, 6.8 miles and 4,800 feet up from the trailhead.

Turn right and follow the trail east through the fine lodgepole forest atop the San Bernardino Divide. Stay on the main trail; don't be lured down the Forsee Creek Trail. Along the way, pass Anderson Peak, Shields Peak, and the formidable Alto Diablo Peak. Enjoy the views north across the Santa Ana River Canyon to Big Bear Lake, which looks like a sapphire floating in the sky. Northwest of Alto Diablo is a cirque littered with avalanche debris, which has two terminal moraines left over from the last ice age when a glacier hung on the north face of the ridge. Also, pass trail camps at Anderson Flat, Shields Flat, High Meadow Springs, and Red Rock Flat. High Meadow Springs (reliable year-round) is 250 feet below the trail and requires cross-country travel; a GPS or good navigation skills are recommended. After 3.6 miles, arrive at the four-way junction of Dollar Lake Saddle at 10,000-foot elevation.

Turn right (southwest) and descend toward Plummer Meadows. This is one of the best trails to observe conifers as you drop through many climate zones. The tall lodgepole pines have two needles, thin flaky bark, and golf ball–sized cones. The limber pines might be difficult to distinguish from a distance but have five needles and skinny cones to 4 inches. After crossing the main fork of Falls Creek at 9,000 feet in 1.4 miles (reliable water and wildflowers), enter stands of Jeffrey pines (with three needles and shapely 6-inch cones) and white fir (needles in rows rather than bundles, green cones growing upright near the treetops and disintegrating before falling to the ground).

In another mile, watch for the signed Saxton Trail Camp just off the trail, where a large group could stay. Water is reliable at the West Prong of Falls Creek in another 0.3 mile. By the time you drop to 8,200 feet, occasional sugar pines (five needles and very long, skinny cones) join the mix, soon followed by canyon live oak and incense cedar. Follow the east side of a long ridge to a trail junction, 4.1 miles down from the saddle. Consider a brief tour east to Dobbs Trail Camp (see Trip 5.5), but the main trail turns west.

At a prominent bend in the trail is the obscured junction with the old Falls Creek Trail, built by John Dobbs in 1898 and used by the public for a century as the most popular route into San Gorgonio Wilderness high country. The trail is now closed because of complaints by a private landowner. Instead, veer north, cross a small creek, and then descend into the deep canyon carved by Alger Creek. On the west side is a fine trail camp shaded beneath the cedars, 1.5 miles from the Dobbs turnoff. Switchback up to the north; then contour southwest 0.8 mile back to the junction with the Momyer Creek Trail. During the descent, the Jeffrey pines give way to ponderosa pines, which also have three needles and a similar appearance but smaller cones, usually less than 4 inches. Watch for Coulter pines with three needles and huge "widow-maker" cones, and bigcone Douglas-fir (needles growing on all sides of the branches individually rather than in bundles, and skinny cones of 4–7 inches that are big compared only with those of ordinary Douglas-fir). Turn left and descend to the trailhead.

see
map on
p. 102

trip 5.7 Aqueduct Trail

Distance	4.5 miles (loop)
Hiking Time	3 hours
Elevation Gain	700'
Difficulty	Moderate
Trail Use	Dogs allowed
Best Times	All year
Agency	The Wildlands Conservancy Bearpaw Reserve
Required Map	USGS *Forest Falls* 7.5'
Permit	Bearpaw Reserve Permit required

DIRECTIONS From Redlands, drive east on Highway 38 to the huge hairpin turn at mile marker 038 SBD 15.00. Turn right onto Valley of the Falls Drive and then immediately right again onto the Bearpaw Reserve road crossing Mill Creek. Park in a dirt turnout on the far side of the creek.

This is an obscure hike on a lightly maintained but passable trail that follows an aqueduct of historic interest. Mill Creek's hydropower was harnessed in 1893 to drive the first commercial three-phase power plant in America. The 250-kilowatt generator supplied electricity to the citrus industry in Redlands for lighting and ice making. Three-phase power proved superior to direct current and one-phase alternating current and has been used ever since. In 1903, Edison added the Mill Creek No. 2 and No. 3 Powerhouse,

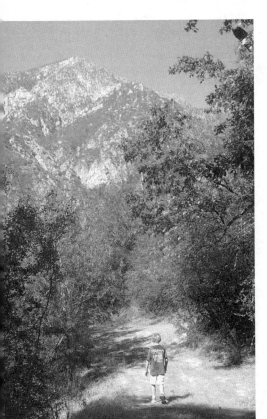

located along Highway 138 just north of the Mill Creek Ranger Station. A long pipe carries the water from the 5,000-foot contour on Mill Creek in Forest Falls down to the powerhouse at 2,924 feet, providing the water pressure to spin the turbines. This trip follows a service trail on top of the aqueduct from Bearpaw Reserve to Forest Falls, then returns along the Mill Creek wash.

The hike passes through The Wildlands Conservancy's Bearpaw Reserve. **Note:** You must obtain a free permit to hike through the preserve. Email mountainpreserves@twc-ca.org for a permit application.

From the turnout, walk 0.2 mile to a gate. Enter the code provided with your permit and continue along the main road 0.5 mile to the road-end at the Bearpaw Reserve. Across a field to the left, look for a kiosk where you sign in and join a trail. This trail climbs steeply 0.1 mile to meet Forest Road 1S08 (Bearpaw Ridge Road). If you're there in the wet season, it's worth turning right on the road and taking a 0.1-mile detour to the tall but seasonal Columbine Falls. However, this

San Bernardino Peak towers above the Aqueduct Trail.

trip turns left and in 0.1 mile reaches a signed service road that heads up to the Aqueduct Trail. After a stiff 0.6-mile climb, the road ends at the trail over the buried aqueduct.

The easily overlooked Aqueduct Trail on the left leads east, clinging to the steep hillside through canyon live oaks and bigcone Douglas-fir. Oaks at this elevation harbor obnoxious gnats that swarm hikers' faces. The narrow trail is washed out in places and receives little maintenance, but is readily followed by adventurous hikers. You eventually pass a tributary pipe and evidence of an old mine shaft.

In 1.9 miles, the trail ends at Oak Creek, yards short of the cabins on Prospect Drive in Forest Falls. (Finding the trail from the road would be difficult in the jumbled terrain if you weren't already familiar with it.) To make a loop, descend Oak Creek 0.2 mile to reach the wide rocky wash of Mill Creek. Turn left and pick a path westward along the wash for 0.7 mile to return to your starting point.

trip 5.8 Mountain Home Flats

Distance	3.5 miles (out-and-back)
Hiking Time	2.5 hours
Elevation Gain	1,100'
Difficulty	Moderate
Trail Use	Dogs allowed, suitable for backpacking
Best Times	April–November
Agency	San Bernardino National Forest (Mill Creek Ranger Station)
Required Map	Tom Harrison *San Gorgonio Wilderness* or USGS *Big Bear Lake* 7.5'

see map on p. 102

DIRECTIONS From Redlands, drive east on Highway 38. Take the huge hairpin turn at the mouth of Mill Creek Canyon, and then continue 3.4 miles to a bridge over Glen Martin Creek at mile marker 038 SBD 18.44. There is very limited parking just south of the bridge, and more at a turnout 0.25 mile north. Do not mix up this trailhead with Mountain Home Creek, which is 1.5 miles farther south.

Mountain Home Flats Trail Camp

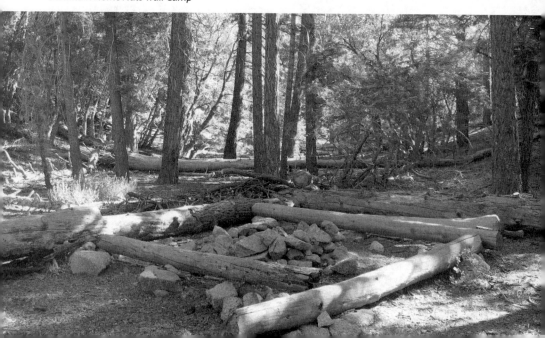

Nestled among the firs, pines, and cedars in a sheer canyon beneath San Bernardino Peak is a trail camp perched on a small flat. Though it's less than 2 miles from the highway, few visitors make the steep and wild climb and you're likely to have the spot to yourself. This is an enjoyable destination for a picnic or short backpacking trip.

A narrow trail starting at the south end of the bridge leads east into Glen Martin Canyon beneath the shady oaks. It soon drops down to the floor of the creek and briefly crosses to the north side. The creek soon divides and the trail follows the south fork. This part of the forest is home to many Coulter pines, with their enormous "widow maker" pinecones, which are uncommon higher up in the San Bernardino Mountains.

The trail soon veers right and switchbacks up to the south ridge of the canyon. Several poor use trails split off where hikers missed a switchback; take care to stay on the main trail because it's the easiest. In 1.0 mile, cross the ridge into the forested upper reaches of Mountain Home Creek. The trail claims your attention as it clings to the edge of a decomposing cliff; then it descends to the creek, crossing just above a series of pools connected by a small waterfall. The trail switchbacks steeply up again before leveling out in another 0.7 mile near the trail camp at Mountain Home Flats.

Several good tent sites can be found under the stately trees. You can make a short but steep descent to seasonal Mountain Home Creek directly north of camp to fetch water. Return the way you came.

trip 5.9 San Bernardino Peak

see maps on pgs. 102 & 126

Distance	16 miles (out-and-back)
Hiking Time	8 hours
Elevation Gain	4,700'
Difficulty	Strenuous
Trail Use	Dogs allowed, suitable for backpacking
Best Times	June–October
Agency	San Bernardino National Forest (Mill Creek Ranger Station)
Recommended Maps	Tom Harrison *San Gorgonio Wilderness* or USGS *Big Bear Lake* and *Forest Falls* 7.5'
Permit	San Gorgonio Wilderness Permit required for overnight camping

DIRECTIONS From Redlands, drive east on Highway 38 to Angelus Oaks. Follow the signs for the San Bernardino Peak Trail (1W07): First, turn right off Highway 38 onto Manzanita Avenue toward the fire station at mile marker 038 SBD 20.00. Then make an immediate left and drive 0.1 mile, passing the station. Make a right onto a fair dirt road past the station at a brown sign indicating SAN BERNARDINO PEAK TRAIL 1W07. Stay right at two forks, and go 0.3 mile to a large dirt parking area with the signed San Bernardino Peak Trailhead.

San Bernardino Peak anchors the west end of the great San Bernardino Ridge. The rolling ridge continues east to San Gorgonio Mountain and beyond, generally maintaining an altitude in excess of 10,000 feet until abruptly plummeting into Hell for Sure Canyon. From the western parts of the Inland Empire, San Bernardino Peak is the most prominent portion of the ridge. On a clear winter day, its white summit towers proudly above the valley cities. San Bernardino Peak is also noteworthy because Southern California was first surveyed from a vista near the summit. This strenuous hike from the hamlet of Angelus Oaks to the summit of San Bernardino Peak offers ever-expanding views and a tour of many of the vegetation zones of San Gorgonio Wilderness.

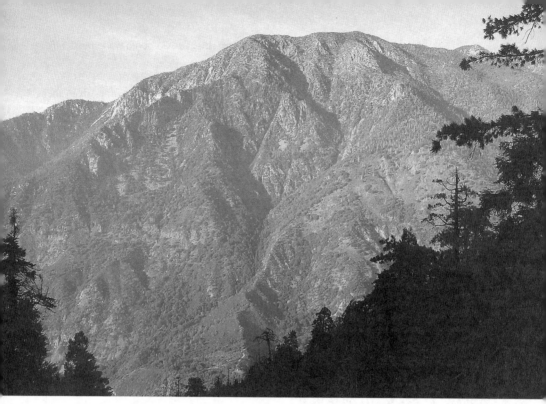

San Bernardino Peak from the south

The San Bernardino Peak Trail begins steadily switchbacking up the ridge through a forest of pines, oaks, and white firs. After 2 miles and nearly 1,600 feet of elevation gain, you pass a sign marking the San Gorgonio Wilderness boundary. Soon after, the grade abruptly eases as you reach a long bench covered in chaparral. Near the east end of the bench, in another 2.3 miles, a side trail to the right leads down to Manzanita Springs and then on to Columbine Spring Trail Camp; water is available in early summer at the first spring and sometimes through midsummer at the second.

The main trail begins climbing again. In 1.4 miles and 1,000 feet of gain, reach Limber Pine Bench Trail Camp. This is a large and popular site for those backpacking the mountain, and water is usually available from Limber Pine Springs near the next major switchback on the trail. On a clear night, there are breathtaking views of the city lights laid out below.

The trail continues through an open forest of lodgepole pine, switchbacking up to gain the west ridge of San Bernardino Peak in 1.5 miles. Once you reach the ridge, keep your eyes open for a side trail marked by a plaque leading to Washington Monument, 50 feet off the main trail. This large rock pile marks the site from which Col. Henry Washington established the initial point for surveying Southern California in 1852. Heat waves distorted the measurements, so bonfires were built at each triangulation point and the surveys were completed at night. Base Line Road still follows the east–west line established in the survey.

The main trail continues up the ridge. In another 0.7 mile, it passes along the north side of San Bernardino Peak. A side trail climbs the short distance to the 10,649-foot summit, where you can enjoy views of the San Bernardino Ridge, Mill Creek, the Yucaipa Ridge, San Jacinto, Baldy, and beyond.

Return the way you came. Or, with a shuttle, descend the Momyer Creek Trail (see Trip 5.6), the Forsee Creek Trail (Trip 5.12), or any of the other fine trails farther along the ridge.

| trip 5.10 | **Whispering Pines and Ponderosa Vista Nature Trails** |

Distance	0.7 mile each (loops)
Hiking Time	30 minutes
Elevation Gain	200', 150'
Difficulty	Easy
Trail Use	Dogs allowed, good for kids
Best Times	April–November
Agency	San Bernardino National Forest (Mill Creek Ranger Station)
Optional Map	USGS *Big Bear Lake* 7.5'

see map on p. 102

DIRECTIONS From Redlands, drive east on Highway 38. Just before mile marker 038 SBD 25.51 and Jenks Lake Road, pull off on either side of the road. The Ponderosa Vista Trailhead is on the north side and the Whispering Pines Trailhead on the south.

These two nature trails are conveniently located for families camping in the Barton Flats Area or driving the back way to Big Bear.

The Whispering Pines Trail (1E33) was constructed in 1969 for an episode of the TV show *Lassie,* in which a blind girl followed the dog Lassie and a ranger around the trail to learn about the forest. The trail winds counterclockwise through the oaks and pines up a gradual hill. In the late spring, this can be a good place to see wildflowers. Woodpeckers have perforated the tall trees atop the hill. There are 10 signs along the path, and a booklet describing the sights at each sign is usually available at the trailhead for a fee.

The Ponderosa Vista Nature Trail (1E19) makes a counterclockwise loop to a scenic overlook with views across the Santa Ana River Canyon to the dramatic face of Slide Peak and beyond to the San Gabriel Mountains. Signs explain some of the sights along the way. There was once a 0.3-mile short loop that returned directly from the overlook, but it has been obliterated by downed trees and lack of use; the longer 0.7-mile loop is presently the only option.

Examining tree rings on the Ponderosa Trail

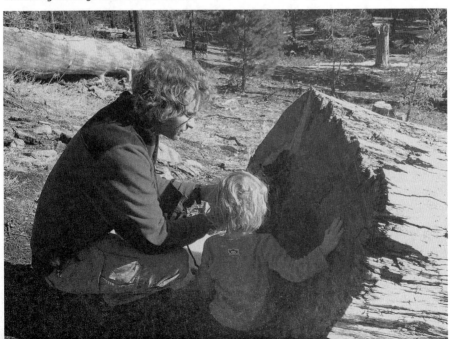

trip 5.11 **Johns Meadow**

Distance	6 miles (out-and-back)
Hiking Time	3 hours
Elevation Gain	800'
Difficulty	Moderate
Trail Use	Dogs allowed, suitable for backpacking
Best Times	May–November
Agency	San Bernardino National Forest (Mill Creek Ranger Station)
Recommended Map	Tom Harrison *San Gorgonio Wilderness* or USGS *Big Bear Lake* 7.5'
Permit	San Gorgonio Wilderness Permit required for overnight camping

see map on p. 102

DIRECTIONS From Redlands, drive east on Highway 38 to Jenks Lake Road, just before mile marker 038 SBD 25.51. Turn right (southeast). After 0.3 mile, bear right again onto a fair dirt road where a sign reads FORSEE CREEK TRAIL. Drive 0.5 mile to the large parking area at the trailhead, on the right (south) side of the road.

Unlike most of the long and steep trails climbing into the San Gorgonio Wilderness, the Johns Meadow Trail offers a moderate hike, which samples the pleasures of the woods and creeks. Though there is scarcely any meadow any longer, the trail ends at a pleasant camp shaded beneath the white fir on a bench above Forsee Creek. The trail was built by hardy San Bernardino Boy Scouts starting in 1969. The meadow was named in honor of John Surr of San Bernardino, a charter member of Defenders of the San Gorgonio Wilderness, who died in 1971 while hiking on San Bernardino Peak. This is a popular destination for a picnic or easy backpacking trip and often attracts Boy Scout groups. Quiet hikers will likely hear birds calling to one another and scolding interlopers; squirrels and lizards are also common and the forest's larger denizens are sometimes sighted. In the summer, the wild berries and flowers along the creeks add to the trip's delights.

The first part of the trail is one of the steepest, climbing the slopes beneath white firs, ponderosa pines, incense cedars, and black oaks. In 0.3 mile, pass the San Gorgonio Wilderness Boundary sign; then in another 0.1 mile, reach a fork. The Forsee Creek Trail continues straight toward the San Bernardino Divide, but this trip turns right toward Johns Meadow.

The trail becomes fairly level as it contours along the slope. Majestic sugar pines shade parts of the trail, and you may see their long cones heavily loading the branches or fallen on the ground below. The trail crosses a seasonal creek, rounds a hill, and descends to another seasonal creek before climbing to a small saddle overlooking Forsee Creek. It's worth making the very short scramble up the nearly bald hill northwest of the saddle for some of the best views of the trip into the Santa Ana River Canyon and to the surrounding mountains.

Descend from the saddle and cross Forsee Creek (water available year-round). A mammoth avalanche swept down the creek in 2005 and you can still see the shards of trees

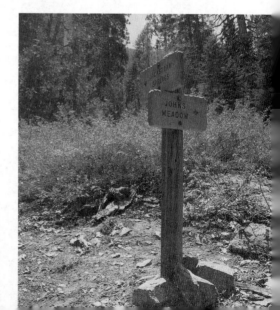

Johns Meadow trail junction

scattered about like broken matchsticks. Up the hill on the far side, reach the spacious campsites in the soft duff, 3 miles from the trailhead.

<hr>

VARIATION

For a longer jaunt, continue on an unmaintained trail up to Manzanita Springs. The trail picks up on the far (southwest) side of the campsites and crosses a tributary creek. Beyond the creek, it immediately forks; both branches have faint sections, and both rejoin in 0.3 mile at a switchback. The trail then climbs the hill and is in remarkably good condition for the remainder of the way. Pass stands of manzanitas and buckthorns, and then reach lodgepole pines just before you arrive in 1.9 miles at the San Bernardino Peak Trail. This option adds another 1,000 feet of elevation gain. Beyond the Manzanita Springs trail junction, you can continue south 0.5 mile, dropping 300 feet to the seasonal Columbine Spring, where there is another trail camp.

<hr>

trip 5.12   San Bernardino Peak via Forsee Creek

see map on p. 102

Distance	17 miles (loop)
Hiking Time	10 hours
Elevation Gain	4,000'
Difficulty	Strenuous
Trail Use	Dogs allowed, suitable for backpacking
Best Times	June–October
Agency	San Bernardino National Forest (Mill Creek Ranger Station)
Required Maps	Tom Harrison *San Gorgonio Wilderness* or USGS *Big Bear Lake* and *Forest Falls* 7.5' (not all of trail shown on map)
Permit	San Gorgonio Wilderness Permit required for overnight camping

DIRECTIONS From Redlands, drive east on Highway 38 to Jenks Lake Road, just before mile marker 038 SBD 25.51. Turn right (southeast). After 0.3 mile, bear right again onto a fair dirt road where a sign reads FORSEE CREEK TRAIL. Drive 0.5 mile to the large parking area at the trailhead, on the right (south) side of the road.

The Forsee Creek Trail scales the precipitous northern face of the San Bernardino Divide. In combination with the San Bernardino Peak Divide and Johns Meadow Trails, it offers a scenic and varied loop hike scaling San Bernardino Peak. The Forsee Creek Trail receives fewer visitors than the traditional western approach of Trip 5.9, and permits may be easier to come by. It also has more shade and is cooler on the ascent. Forsee Creek is named for Peter Forsee, the first known resident of Mill Creek Canyon, who grew apples and guided visitors through the mountains from around 1868 to 1888.

The trail leads south beneath white firs, ponderosa pines, incense cedars, and black oaks. In 0.3 mile, pass the San Gorgonio Wilderness Boundary sign; then in another 0.1 mile, reach a fork. The right branch leads to Johns Meadow (see Trip 5.11), but our route continues straight up the Forsee Creek Trail. The trail diagonally crosses the steep slope before making numerous switchbacks. When trees aren't in the way, the trail has fine views of the Santa Ana River Canyon. Around 8,600 feet, the forest abruptly transitions to pure stands of lodgepole pines. The trail then gains a gentler bench, turns west, and then turns south again, 4.2 miles from the trailhead. Immediately after this turn, look for a side trail on the right leading to Jackstraw Springs Trail Camp. The sign is high up on a lodgepole and easy to miss. The fine camping spots beneath the tall lodgepoles lie 0.2 mile west of the main trail. Water is available in early season from two small brooks that you cross just before you reach the camp.

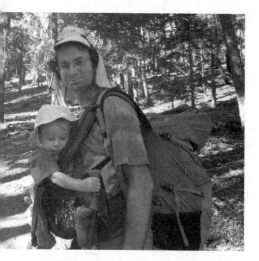

Double load on the Forsee Creek Trail

The main trail continues up the narrowing ridge between Forsee Creek on the right and Barton Creek on the left. Panoramic views to the north over Big Bear Lake continue to improve. The rocky debris near the head of Forsee Creek was deposited by a glacier during the ice age. In 1.8 miles, reach a trail junction. Adjacent to this junction is a heavily vegetated area where water can often be found at Trail Fork Springs. At the first switchback immediately below the junction, an obscure trail climbs the slope to Trail Fork Springs Camp, an outstanding spot to watch the sunset.

From the junction, the trail to the left leads toward Dollar Lake Saddle and on to San Gorgonio. This trip, however, takes the right (west) fork. In 0.5 mile, it joins the main San Bernardino Peak Trail atop the divide.

Continue west past the Momyer Creek Trail junction and the summit of San Bernardino East Peak. In 1.8 miles, reach a short side trail to the summit of San Bernardino Peak.

Descend the San Bernardino Peak Trail to the west (see Trip 5.9). In 0.7 mile, pass the signed turnoff for the Washington Monument. In 1.2 miles, reach Limber Pine Springs (which often flows all summer); then, in another 0.3 mile, pass Limber Pine Bench Trail Camp. In 1.4 miles, reach a flat area with a signed junction for Manzanita Springs to the left (south, early-season water). An unmarked and unmaintained but surprisingly good trail leads to the right from this point 1.9 miles to Johns Meadow (see Trip 5.11). Shortly before the meadow, the trail forks, but both branches rejoin. Water is available from the reliable Forsee Creek at the meadow. Follow the Johns Meadow Trail 2.6 miles east back to its junction with the Forsee Creek Trail; then turn left and descend the last 0.4 mile to the trailhead.

VARIATION

With a car shuttle, it's slightly shorter to continue 4.3 miles west from Manzanita Springs down to the San Bernardino Peak Trailhead (see Trip 5.9).

---

trip 5.13 South Fork Meadows

Distance	8 miles (out-and-back)
Hiking Time	4 hours
Elevation Gain	1,400'
Difficulty	Moderate
Trail Use	Dogs allowed
Best Times	May–November
Agency	San Bernardino National Forest (Mill Creek Ranger Station)
Recommended Map	Tom Harrison *San Gorgonio Wilderness* or USGS *Moonridge* 7.5'
Permit	San Gorgonio Wilderness Permit required for overnight camping

see map on p. 102

DIRECTIONS From Redlands, drive east on Highway 38 to Jenks Lake Road, 50 yards before mile marker 038 SBD 25.51. Turn right (southeast) and follow Jenks Lake Road 2.5 miles to the vast South Fork Trailhead parking area, on your left.

outh Fork Meadows is tucked away on the north side of San Gorgonio Wilderness in a forested valley beneath the tall peaks. It's one of the few places where hikers can venture into the wilderness without grueling climbs up the steep slopes. In the summer, the trail is dotted with wildflowers and a quiet brook bubbles through the ferns in the meadow. There are so many springs bursting forth that the meadow was once known as Valley of the Thousand Springs. In the winter, backcountry skiers test their mettle on the trail and sometimes on the open slopes above. (A hardy group of Pomona College students made the first ski ascent of San Gorgonio on February 3, 1931.) The meadow was once a popular campsite, but has suffered from overuse and is now closed; Dry Lake, 1.8 miles farther up the trail, is a reasonable alternative.

The South Fork Trail (1E04) leads south from the trailhead through a stately forest of Jeffrey pines and white firs. In 1.3 miles, it passes through Horse Meadows; 0.8 mile beyond, it reaches the wilderness boundary, 1,000 feet up from the start. Look for a sign pointing out a short trail to the east leading up Poopout Hill to a vista of San Gorgonio framed by the trees. (Poopout Hill got its name in the 1930s, when youth groups coming up from camps near Barton Flats would turn around here.)

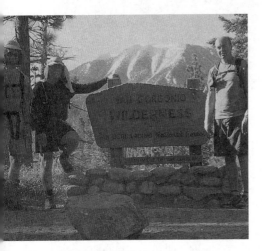

San Gorgonio Wilderness Boundary

Return to the main trail and continue southeast. In 1.4 miles, pass a junction with the Lost Creek Trail coming in from the north via Grinnell Ridge. Just 0.3 mile beyond, arrive at the lush South Fork Meadows, where you can enjoy a picnic and admire some of the most spectacular wildflowers in the San Bernardino Mountains. The trail forks here, with one branch leading to Dollar Lake and the other to Dry Lake (see Trip 5.14), but this trip ends here and returns the way you came.

trip 5.14   San Gorgonio via Dollar and Dry Lakes

see map on p. 102

Distance	21 miles (loop)
Hiking Time	11 hours
Elevation Gain	4,700'
Difficulty	Strenuous
Trail Use	Dogs allowed, suitable for backpacking
Best Times	June–October
Agency	San Bernardino National Forest (Mill Creek Ranger Station)
Recommended Maps	Tom Harrison *San Gorgonio Wilderness* or USGS *Moonridge* and *San Gorgonio Mountain* 7.5'
Permit	San Gorgonio Wilderness Permit required for overnight camping

DIRECTIONS From Redlands, drive east on Highway 38 to Jenks Lake Road, 50 yards before mile marker 038 SBD 25.51. Turn right (southeast) and follow Jenks Lake Road 2.5 miles to the vast South Fork Trailhead parking area, on your left.

his loop up and over San Gorgonio from the north is longer than the Vivian Creek approach, but is arguably even more scenic. It features a fine forest, verdant meadows

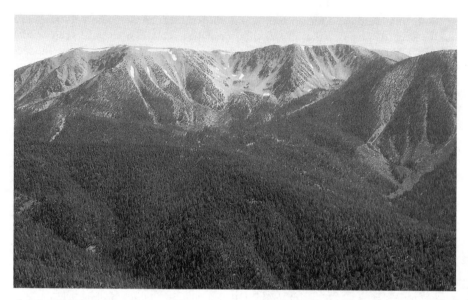

San Gorgonio from the north

with wildflowers, an extended traverse at and above treeline, and visits to both of the tiny lakes in San Gorgonio Wilderness. This trip can be done as a long day hike or as a two- to three-day backpacking trip. If you're backpacking, check sgwa.org for the latest information on availability of water. This side of the mountain can hold its snowpack into the early summer, so check conditions and bring appropriate gear.

The South Fork Trail (1E04) leads south, climbing gradually but steadily through the forest of Jeffrey pines and white firs. In a good summer, it passes fields of wildflowers. In 1.5 miles, pass Horse Meadows. In another 1.0 mile, reach the wilderness boundary. Take a short side trail to the left (east) to a worthwhile viewpoint on Poopout Hill where San Gorgonio Mountain is framed between the trees; then return to the main trail.

Continue 2.1 miles to South Fork Meadows, where several springs and creeks converge to support a lush fern-filled bog. In the later summer and fall, this may be the last convenient reliable source of water. The trail forks, with one branch to Dry Lake and the other to Dollar Lake. Take the left (southeast) fork toward Dry Lake. As you climb, the diverse forest gives way to pure stands of lodgepole pines. In 1.8 miles, reach the outlet of Dry Lake, where you can enjoy another fine view of the mountain ahead. By midsummer, the lake is usually a boggy meadow. Deer can frequently be seen here, grazing and drinking. The Dry Lake and Lodgepole Spring campsites are located along the east side of the lake, but the main trail leads south along the west side, then switchbacks up, passing the small Trail Flat campsite at a switchback at 9,600 feet before arriving at 9,936-foot Mineshaft Saddle in 2.2 miles, where the Fish Creek Trail comes in from the east.

Continue on to the right and up Sky High Trail as it spirals around the mountain to gain the last 1,500 feet of elevation on a gradual slope. The trail passes limber and lodgepole pines, which become shorter and more weather-beaten until being reduced to stunted krummholz at treeline. It initially leads southeast, offering views across the north fork of the Whitewater River to the Ten Thousand Foot Ridge, which drops down into Hell for Sure Canyon. Pass the wreckage of a C-47 transport plane that splattered against the mountainside in 1952 en route from Tucson to March Air Force Base during a December blizzard. Then climb eight switchbacks and traverse around to a junction west of the summit in 3.8 miles. Finally, turn right and hike the last 0.4 mile to the top of San Gorgonio Mountain. Hardy backpackers may pitch their tents on the windswept summit for a magical night beneath the stars.

To complete the loop, return to the junction west of the summit and continue west. In 0.2 mile, pass another junction where the Vivian Creek Trail comes up from the south. Continue west for 3.2 miles around Jepson, Little Charlton, and Charlton Peaks to a four-way junction at Dollar Lake Saddle, where you dip below 10,000 feet for the first time since Mineshaft Saddle. Descend the Dollar Lake Trail 0.5 mile to a turnoff for tiny Dollar Lake, which was formed when a terminal moraine dammed a small valley as the last glaciers retreated from San Gorgonio's north face. Another trail camp is located near the lake, though water may not be reliable after early season. Continue down the main trail 1.8 miles to South Fork Meadows, go left on the South Fork Trail and finally grind out the last 4.6 miles back to the trailhead.

---

trip 5.15   **Jenks Lake**

see map on p. 102

Distance	3 miles (semiloop)
Hiking Time	2 hours
Elevation Gain	600'
Difficulty	Easy
Trail Use	Dogs allowed, good for kids, suitable for mountain biking, suitable for equestrians
Best Times	May–October
Agency	San Bernardino National Forest (Mill Creek Ranger Station)
Required Map	Tom Harrison *San Gorgonio Wilderness* or USGS *Big Bear Lake* 7.5'

DIRECTIONS From Redlands, drive east on Highway 38 to the Barton Flats Visitor Center, at mile marker 038 SBD 26.84. Park in the visitor center lot or in the wide turnout alongside the highway. Note that the visitor center closes at 4:30 p.m., so park outside if you don't think you'll be back in time.

Captain Lorin Shaw Jenks built a trout pond in the 1870s, using a small dam and diverting water from the South Fork of the Santa Ana River along a 1.5-mile ditch. He raised fish and sold them in San Bernardino. Captain Jenks also founded a resort by the lake and was renowned for regaling his guests with tall tales, but the business failed because the three-day burro ride from town was too long for most visitors. His lake, nestled beneath the tall mountains and surrounded by splendid forest, is now a popular destination for anglers, youth groups, and families. It's stocked with bluegill, sunfish, largemouth bass, and rainbow trout. Unfortunately, the water is now closed to swimming. While the lake can be reached from the paved Jenks Lake Road, it's more enjoyable to take the short hike up from Barton Flats Visitor Center, and then saunter around the lake before returning the way you came.

The Barton Flats Visitor Center is normally open 7:30 a.m.–4:30 p.m., Thursday–Sunday from May through October. It was closed in the 1970s by the understaffed U.S. Forest Service, but it reopened in 1986 and has been operated ever since by volunteers from the San Gorgonio Wilderness Association. If you're camping nearby, inquire here about nature walks and interpretive programs. The flats got their name from Dr. Ben Barton, who raised sheep in Redlands in the 1860s and drove them each summer to graze in the mountain meadows. Barton Flats is now the site of 25 youth camps, the densest collection of camps in any National Forest. More than 30,000 children a year spend time at these camps.

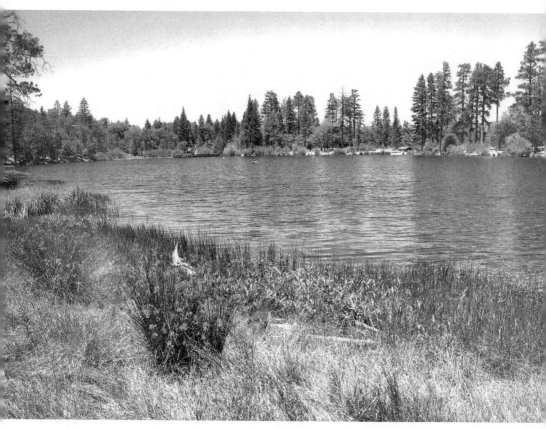

Jenks Lake

The trail, marked with a sign reading RIO MONTE PANORAMA, starts next to the gate at the east end of the Barton Flats Visitor Center. It leads east between Highway 38 and Frog Creek through a forest of incense cedars, black oaks, ponderosa pines, and white firs. In 0.2 mile, reach a signed Jenks Lake Trail marker. The entrance to Camp Arbolado is across the highway and this is an alternative starting point. Just beyond the marker, the trail turns right onto a dirt Forest Service road. Immediately after this turn, stay on the dirt road and pass another spur road leading along some power lines. In another 0.2 mile, cross Frog Creek at a lovely spot shaded beneath incense cedars. Then, in another 0.2 mile, turn left onto another dirt road at a trail marker; the main road continues up to private cabins. The trail makes two more switchbacks before arriving at Jenks Lake near the outlet and a wooden pier.

Turn left and make a clockwise loop around the lake. You're likely to see ducks, squirrels, and butterflies along the way. The first part of the trail is paved and passes a picnic ground and outhouse. At the end, continue around the lake on a dirt access road to reach the southeast corner, where you may meet youth groups launching boats. A narrow dirt footpath continues along the south side of the lake. Hikers unsure of their footing will want a walking stick or helping hand along this stretch. Unfortunately, inconsiderate visitors leave quite a bit of litter along this beach; if you bring a trash bag and carry some out, you'll make the lake more enjoyable for everyone. Reach the parking area at the west end of the lake, and circle back to the trail you came up.

trip 5.16　Santa Ana River Trail

Distance	38 miles (one-way)
Hiking Time	2–5 days
Elevation Gain/Loss	2,800'/7,800'
Difficulty	Moderate–strenuous backpack
Trail Use	Dogs allowed, suitable for backpacking, suitable for mountain biking, suitable for equestrians
Best Times	March–November
Agency	San Bernardino National Forest (Mill Creek Ranger Station)
Required Maps	USGS *Moonridge, Big Bear Lake, Keller Peak,* and *Yucaipa* 7.5' (trail not depicted fully)

DIRECTIONS This lengthy hike is divided into six segments. The driving directions for each trailhead follow, starting at Highway 38 east of Redlands:

(A) Big Meadows Drive to the Heart Bar Campground turnoff, just past the 038 SBD 33.48 mile marker. Turn right (south) and follow Forest Road 1N02 for 1.3 miles to a junction with 1N05. Park in a dirt clearing next to this junction.

(B) South Fork Campground Drive to a paved trailhead parking area on your left (north), just past mile marker 038 SBD 30.74 and 100 feet before the South Fork Campground turnoff to the right.

(C) Glass Road Drive to Glass Road between Jenks Lake Road and Barton Flats near mile marker 038 SBD 26.54. Turn left (north) onto Glass Road and descend 2.1 miles to the signed Santa Ana River Trailhead. If you reach an intersection on the canyon bottom, you've gone 0.1 mile too far.

(D) Angelus Oaks Drive to Angelus Oaks and, just past mile marker 20.00, turn left (west) into the parking area for The Oaks Restaurant. Stay right through the parking area and pass the post office; then turn left onto dirt Forest Road 1N12. Immediately stay right at a sign reading THOMAS HUNTING GROUNDS, and pass through a gate. In 0.2 mile, park at the signed trailhead.

(E) Thomas Hunting Grounds Drive to Angelus Oaks and, just past mile marker 20.00, turn left (west) into the parking area for The Oaks Restaurant. Stay right through the parking area and pass the post office; then turn left onto dirt Forest Road 1N12. Immediately stay right at a sign reading THOMAS HUNTING GROUNDS, and pass through a gate. Follow the road 3.5 miles to a junction where the Santa Ana River Trail crosses the road, marked by a small sign. Many fine yellow-post campsites are scattered about this area.

(F) Morton Peak Fire Lookout　Note: A high-clearance vehicle is recommended. From Highway 38, 0.1 mile east of mile marker 038 SBD 10.50, turn left (north) onto fair dirt Forest Road 1N12. Drive 1.2 miles up the road to a junction. A gated road turns left up to the Morton Peak Fire Lookout. If the gate is open, turn left and drive 1.4 miles to the lookout. Otherwise, leave your vehicle at the junction.

(G) Seven Oaks Dam In Mentone, 0.4 mile east of mile marker 038 SBD 05.00, turn left (north) onto Garnet Street, which crosses Mill Creek on a narrow bridge, makes two sharp turns, and becomes Greenspot Road. Drive 2.5 miles to the unmarked Front Line fire road, on your right (east). Park here outside the locked gate—please don't block the gate. If you reach a second bridge over the Santa Ana River near the Seven Oaks Dam, you've gone 0.3 mile too far.

The Santa Ana River is fed by snowmelt and alpine springs flowing down from the north face of San Gorgonio and from Big Bear Lake. As the river gathers strength, it carves a deep canyon between San Gorgonio and Big Bear, plunging down to the Seven Oaks Dam before joining with Mill Creek and flowing past Redlands and San Bernardino en route to the sea. The Santa Ana River Trail (2E03) follows the wild upper portion of the river to the point where the river is tamed by the dam. This trail is part of a 110-mile planned trail

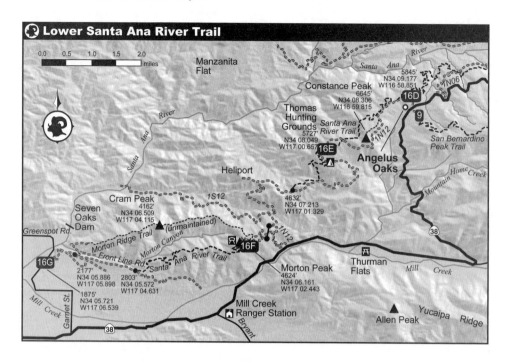

Lower Santa Ana River Trail

system that has been under sporadic construction since the 1960s. A paved bikeway will follow the river from Seven Oaks Dam to the sea.

It's hard to say whether the Santa Ana River Trail is an underused gem-in-the-rough or a sad mistake in trail planning. The river is rarely in sight of the trail, and comes in direct contact with the trail only at South Fork Campground. Some portions are poorly marked. Several miles of the route above Morton Peak follow a dirt road rather than trail. On the other hand, the trail offers good views as it traverses conifer and oak forests, riparian zones, a meadow, and chaparral-clad hillsides. Its length is exceeded in the Inland Empire only by that of the Pacific Crest Trail (PCT). And traveling the full distance gives a unique perspective into one of the region's major watersheds.

The top segment from Big Meadows to South Fork Campground is most popular among hikers and equestrians because it's conveniently located near many campgrounds and offers a loop option. The next two segments from South Fork Campground to Angelus Oaks are heavily used by serious mountain bikers. The trail is exposed, narrow, and uneven. Some cyclists consider this to be one of the best rides in Southern California. The lower segments receive sparse use and offer solitude and sweeping views. The long trail has strong promise for backpacking or extreme trail running, and the periodic road crossings make caching water or food easy.

Note that Forest Road 1N17 between Big Meadows and the PCT is officially designated as part of the Santa Ana River Trail as well. This rugged jeep road begins 0.2 mile south of Segment A on 1N05 and leads 2.7 miles up to the PCT. Stay right at forks near the start and in the middle. To make a 5.7-mile loop with 1,100 feet of elevation gain, turn left onto the PCT and go 0.7 mile; then turn left again and descend a little-used and easily overlooked segment of the California Riding and Hiking Trail along Heart Bar Creek.

trip 5.16 **SEGMENT A: Big Meadows to South Fork Campground**

Distance	5.5 miles (one-way), 11 miles (out-and-back or loop)
Hiking Time	3 hours (one-way)
Elevation Gain/Loss	200'/800' (one-way)
Required Map	Tom Harrison *San Gorgonio Wilderness* or
	USGS *Moonridge* 7.5' (trail not depicted accurately on either map)

see map on p. 103

This segment can be done as a one-way hike with a car or bicycle shuttle, as an out-and-back hike, or as a loop returning along a poorly marked parallel trail. It has a number of unmarked side trails that can be confusing.

The trail starts at a large SANTA ANA RIVER TRAIL sign on the west side of the road, opposite the parking area at the junction of 1N02 and 1N05. In 0.3 mile, pass a junction on the right leading back to 1N02 near the Wild Horse Equestrian Campground. In another 0.6 mile, pass a junction on the left, marked ASPEN GROVE/FISH CREEK, which climbs steeply up to the Aspen Grove Trailhead. Pass above the aptly named Big Meadows. Although it's hard to see, another trail runs parallel at the edge of the meadow and several side trails drop down to it. In 1.2 miles, pass an unmarked trail on the left, which climbs to Fish Creek below Aspen Grove. In 0.3 mile, pass the top of a closed jeep road.

The trail continues contouring through the forest and then descends into the Fish Creek drainage. In 0.7 mile, reach a hairpin turn. An unmarked trail at this turn also leads left up Fish Creek to Aspen Grove (see Trip 5.17). But our trail heads downstream 0.1 mile and then turns left. The right fork leads down to a defunct camp. The trail has been rerouted around here and isn't indicated properly on current maps. Look for signs reading 2E03 that mark the correct route.

The Santa Ana River Trail generally contours along the mountainside, winding in and out of various drainages. The forest is characteristic of the northern San Gorgonio region, including a mixture of ponderosa and Jeffrey pines, white firs, and black oaks. In 1.5 miles, reach a junction with the Lost Creek Trail (1E09) on the left, which makes a long climb to South Fork Meadows, but our trail turns right and descends.

Near Big Meadow after a summer thunderstorm

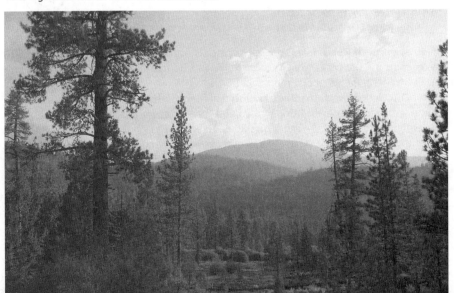

In 0.6 mile, reach the paved entrance to South Fork Campground. This is a good turn-around point for a loop trip. If you're making a one-way trip, the lower trailhead parking is located directly across Highway 38. However, a more pleasant alternative to braving the busy road is to cross the campground entrance road to a trail sign, and then veer left under a highway bridge alongside the Santa Ana River. Then follow the edge of the river beneath beautiful incense cedars. In the summer, expect to see red-tipped Indian paintbrush and other wildflowers. Reach the trailhead parking at another large sign.

ALTERNATIVE FINISH ───────────────────────────────

If you don't have a vehicle waiting, the least confusing option is to return the way you came. If you feel adventurous, return to the trail sign at the entrance of South Fork Campground. Follow an intermittent trail east between the river and the edge of the campground. After passing the end of the campground, the trail continues along the river. In 0.6 mile, reach a fuel tank beside the trail. The trail soon vanishes at a defunct camp, so a better choice is to ford the river and pick up another path leading east between the river and the highway. Pass the gated access road at the mouth of the camp and continue close to Highway 38. Immediately before you reach another paved road leading southeast from the highway, turn right and follow the trail back across the river. The trail then leads southeast and soon follows the edge of Big Meadows. Various spurs lead south back up to the main Santa Ana River Trail. This area is a maze of equestrian trails and requires good navigational skills.

VARIATION ───────────────────────────────

You can make a fine long loop by following the Lost Creek Trail to South Fork Meadows and then continuing up to Dry Lake and taking a faint path up to Fish Creek Saddle. Descend the Fish Creek Trail to Fish Creek Meadows. Follow the Aspen Grove Trail down, and then take the Santa Ana River Trail back to the trailhead. This route requires a San Gorgonio Wilderness Permit. This route is approximately 20 miles, depending on the exact path selected. **Note:** Lost Creek was affected by the 2015 Lake Fire and remained closed at press time.

---

trip 5.16   **SEGMENT B: South Fork Campground to Glass Road**

Distance	6 miles (one-way)
Hiking Time	3 hours
Elevation Gain/Loss	300'/1,100'
Required Map	USGS *Big Bear Lake* 7.5'.

see map on p. 103

This segment descends along the upper reaches of the Santa Ana River Canyon. This segment and the next traverse a steep hillside with infrequent opportunities for camping. The trail is popular among mountain bikers.

From the signed Santa Ana River Trailhead parking northwest of the South Fork Campground entrance, walk west through a conifer forest along a Forest Service road, which crosses the South Fork of the Santa Ana River. In 0.1 mile, a signed trail begins on the left side of the road. The slope starts to drop away as you contour above the head of the river canyon. Sugarloaf Mountain looms to the north, forming the opposite wall of the canyon. In 0.6 mile, reach a signed spur trail on the left leading up to Highway 38 across from Jenks Lake Road East. Dispersed camping is allowed along this spur trail in the East Flat area north of the highway. The plant communities change as the slope becomes steep and sunbaked, giving way to live oaks, manzanitas, even prickly pear cacti. In another 2.4 miles, reach a signed four-way junction. The left fork climbs 1 mile up to Barton Flats and San Gorgonio Campgrounds. The right fork once led down to the river and Forest Road 1N45,

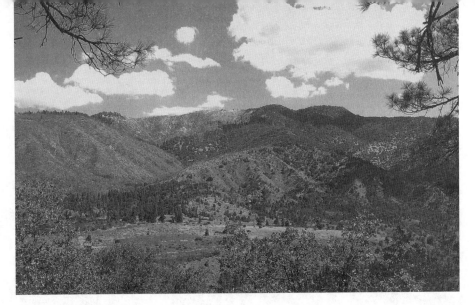

Santa Ana River Canyon

but it hasn't been maintained recently and is blocked with fallen trees and washouts. The main trail continues west, gradually descending into the river canyon, and reaches a signed junction with Glass Road in another 3 miles.

trip 5.16 SEGMENT C: Glass Road to Angelus Oaks

see map on p. 102

Distance	8 miles (one-way)
Hiking Time	5 hours
Elevation Gain/Loss	1,200'/800'
Required Map	USGS *Big Bear Lake* 7.5'

This segment follows the edge of the Santa Ana River Canyon past the resort community of Seven Oaks before climbing back up to cross Middle Control Road and travel on to Angelus Oaks. The undulating trail curves in and out to cross numerous tributary creeks, where wildflowers, firs, oaks, and a variety of pines can be found. Camping opportunities are limited. Mountain bikers use this trail heavily, but a fall on some of the steep slopes could be serious.

Starting from the trailhead at Glass Road, head west along the Santa Ana River Trail (2E03). In 0.5 mile, cross Barton Creek. In another 0.8 mile, an unmarked trail drops down toward the resorts. In 1.2 miles, reach an overlook where you can gaze west over the river canyon to the dramatic slope of Slide Peak. Keller Peak Fire Lookout stands on the high point just above Slide Peak. In 0.4 mile, cross Forsee Creek, where tasty blackberries ripen in late summer.

In 0.3 mile, reach a rutted dirt road. Follow the road downhill; it soon narrows back down to a trail following the path of the old road cut. In 0.9 mile, reach a junction. The right fork ends in 0.25 mile at Middle Control Road at a 2E03 sign. But this trip takes the left fork to stay on the main trail. Cross Schneider Creek; then, in 0.9 mile, cross Kilpecker Creek to arrive at Middle Control Road (1N06) at another 2E03 sign. (This junction is 2.0 miles down Middle Control Road from Highway 38.)

The trail resumes on the west (right) side of the road and follows another old road cut. In 1.1 miles, cross the jumbled granite blocks of Cold Creek Canyon. In another 0.5 mile, the trail begins switchbacking upward in earnest. Stay on the main trail, passing a faint side path

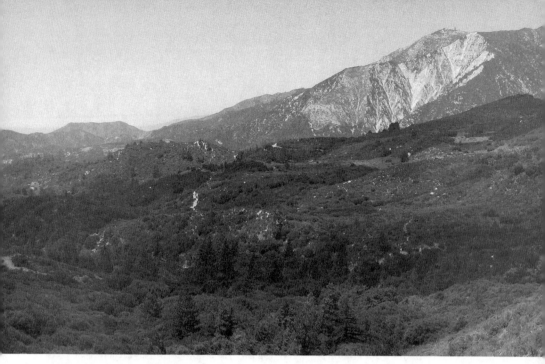

Slide Peak from Santa Ana River Trail

leading right at the first switchback. In another 1.7 miles, reach the end of a logging road. A side trail to the left leads 0.2 mile up to the Santa Ana River Trailhead at Angelus Oaks, while the main trail continues southwest. Dispersed dry camping is feasible in this area.

trip 5.16   SEGMENT D: Angelus Oaks to Thomas Hunting Grounds

Distance	4 miles (one-way)
Hiking Time	2 hours
Elevation Gain/Loss	400'/500'
Required Maps	USGS *Big Bear Lake* and *Keller Peak* 7.5'

see map on p. 126

This short segment winds along the west shoulder of Constance Peak, with dramatic views into the deep Santa Ana River Canyon and to the mountains beyond.

If you're starting at the Angelus Oaks Trailhead described in the driving directions, hike 0.2 mile down to meet the main trail at a logging road. Turn left and hike southwest on the trail. In 1.3 miles, cross another logging road. Hike through a forest of pines, firs, and oaks. Enjoy the expansive views over the Santa Ana River up Bear Creek, over Manzanita Flat, and out to Slide Peak. From here, you can see the fire lookouts atop both Butler and Keller Peaks.

The forest gives way to chaparral as it crosses the west side of Constance Peak. In 1.9 miles, cross Forest Road 1N12 at an unsigned point west of the peak. Follow a spur road, which soon ends at a signed clearing where the trail resumes. In 0.7 mile, reach 1N12 again, where this segment terminates. This beautiful area is called Thomas Hunting Grounds, and several fine yellow-post campsites can be found in the open woodland. The origin of the place name is uncertain, but John Robinson speculates that it was named for Mark Thomas of San Bernardino, who guided W. A. Goodyear of the California Geological Survey on the first claimed ascent of San Gorgonio in 1872.

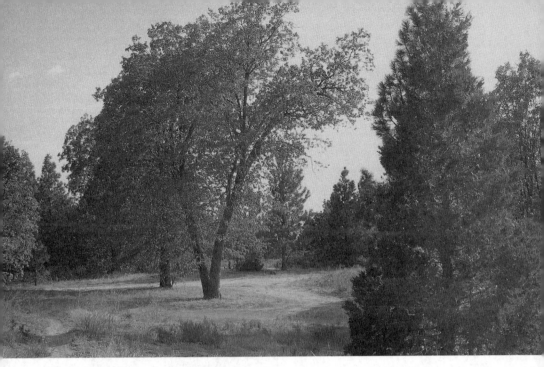

Approaching Thomas Hunting Grounds

trip 5.16 **SEGMENT E: Thomas Hunting Grounds to Morton Peak Fire Lookout**

see map on p. 126

Distance	7.5 miles (one-way)
Hiking Time	4 hours
Elevation Gain/Loss	700'/1,800'
Required Maps	USGS *Keller Peak* and *Yucaipa* 7.5'

This segment follows a short stretch of trail and then joins a dirt road. The trail is exposed to the merciless sun and can be unpleasantly hot on a summer afternoon; bring plenty of water. During the fall hunting season, wear bright colors and be particularly alert for the first half mile.

From Thomas Hunting Grounds, find the small sign at the trailhead on Forest Road 1N12 and hike west on the Santa Ana River Trail. In 0.2 mile, reach an unmarked junction with a dirt road. The trail follows the road 50 yards and then splits off to the left at a sign reading NO MOTOR VEHICLES. Pass above some yellow-post campsites and near another dirt road before switchbacking down a steep slope. In 1.5 miles, reach a notch in the ridge where the trail meets 1N12 again. Instead of crossing the road, take the trail that continues west on the north side of the ridge. In 0.8 mile, the trail terminates at the road.

Turn right and descend 1N12. A mountain bike ride is particularly appealing for travel on this segment. Pass a spur road on the right at a switchback in 1.1 miles, and then a second spur on the right in another 1.9 miles. In another 0.6 mile, reach a junction with a road on the right, labeled 2E03, leading up to the Morton Peak Fire Lookout. The gate is locked when the lookout is closed.

If you're not planning to visit the lookout, you can meet a vehicle here or descend 1N12 another 1.2 miles to Highway 38. To reach the lookout, hike west up the road 1.2 miles to a junction. A signpost beside a trail on the left, reading PLEASE STAY ON EXISTING ROADS

AND TRAILS, marks the continuation of the Santa Ana River Trail. However, it's worth continuing up the road 0.2 mile to the lookout on Morton Peak, where you can enjoy spectacular views in all directions. The lookout is normally staffed by volunteer fire-lookout hosts from May through October; these volunteers enjoy sharing their wealth of knowledge with visitors.

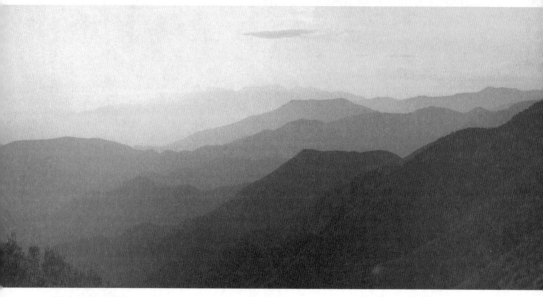

Sunset over the San Bernardino and San Gabriel Mountains

trip 5.16 SEGMENT F: Morton Peak Fire Lookout to Seven Oaks Dam

see map on p. 126

Distance	6.5 miles (one-way)
Hiking Time	3.5 hours
Elevation Loss	2,800'
Required Map	USGS *Yucaipa* 7.5'

The final segment of the Santa Ana River Trail descends a ridge overlooking Morton Canyon. It then follows the dirt Front Line Road down to paved Greenspot Road beneath Seven Oaks Dam. This is the lowest and hottest section of the trail and isn't recommended in the summer. The south side of the ridge was incinerated in the August 2006 Emerald Fire, which was started by illegal and negligent target shooting. The chaparral has mostly recovered.

From the top of Morton Peak, descend the access road east 0.2 mile. Look for an old road cut on the left. This was once the Morton Ridge Trail that led to Cram Peak and down to Seven Oaks Dam, but it hasn't been maintained in years and is badly overgrown with chaparral; the route isn't particularly enjoyable today.

About 20 feet beyond the road cut, a trail on the right side is marked with a sign reading PLEASE STAY ON EXISTING ROADS AND TRAILS. This is the continuation of the Santa Ana River Trail, although the signage currently gives no clue of this fact. The good trail descends

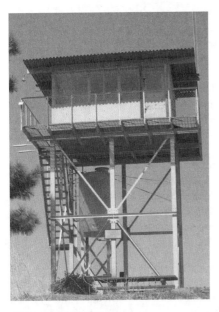

Morton Peak Fire Lookout

switchbacks to the south before following the ridge west. An excessive number of trail markers warn mountain bikers to stay in control. At a point south of Cram Peak, the trail makes several more switchbacks to drop off the toe of the ridge and join Front Line Road (1S14) at a gap in the fence, 4.4 miles down. This junction is marked with another PLEASE STAY ON EXISTING ROADS AND TRAILS sign, but no Santa Ana River Trail marker.

Turn right and follow Front Line Road west along a low ridge. In 1.2 miles, pass a road coming in sharply from the left above old orchards. Just after, another road descends right into Morton Canyon. (This road meets the Morton Ridge Trail on the north side of the canyon.)

Beyond this point, the USGS topographic map is no longer accurate, and the maze of dirt roads can be confusing. Your goal is to get down to paved Greenspot Road to the west. In 0.2 mile, turn left (south) and descend to another dirt road. Turn right and follow the road northwest above more orchards. In 0.1 mile, turn left. In another 0.3 mile, pass a junction on the left leading east into the orchards, but stay on the main road, which leads another 0.2 mile west to the unsigned terminus of the Santa Ana River Trail at Greenspot Road.

trip 5.17 Aspen Grove

see map on p. 103

Distance	1.8 miles (out-and-back)
Hiking Time	1 hour
Elevation Gain	350'
Difficulty	Easy
Trail Use	Dogs allowed, good for kids
Best Times	October
Agency	San Bernardino National Forest (Mill Creek Ranger Station)
Recommended Map	Tom Harrison *San Gorgonio Wilderness* or USGS *Moonridge* 7.5'

DIRECTIONS From Redlands, drive east on Highway 38 to the Heart Bar Campground turnoff, just past the 038 SBD 33.48 mile marker. Turn right and follow Forest Road 1N02 for 1.3 miles, passing the campground entrance. At a junction, turn right onto 1N05, a fair dirt road, and proceed 1.6 miles to the signed Aspen Grove Trailhead at a hairpin turn in the road.

Note: *This area was affected by the 2015 Lake Fire and remained closed at press time.*

In October each year, the leaves of quaking aspens (*Populus tremuloides*) turn bright yellow for a few short weeks, and then drop from the trees. Aspen Grove is one of only two places in California outside the Sierra Nevada where the splendid trees can still be seen. This hike follows Fish Creek through four groves of aspens. The willows in the creek also change colors, adding to the festive display beneath the evergreen firs and pines. Call the Mill Creek Ranger Station for current foliage information. Neither of the recommended maps is quite accurate at depicting the maze of trails around Big Meadows, but the main trail from the Aspen Grove Trailhead is clearly marked.

From the trailhead, walk south 0.3 mile down to Fish Creek. Cross the creek and immediately reach a trail junction in a dense grove of aspen. It can be hard to get a perspective on the trees because you're right beneath them. Trails lead north and south from this junction along the west side of Fish Creek, which the trail crosses several times.

The naming of the trails is somewhat confusing. The Aspen Grove Trail leads south to join the Fish Creek Trail beyond Lower Fish Creek Meadow (see Trip 5.18). An unnamed trail leads north to join the Santa Ana River Trail. The best groves of aspen are actually found to the north.

Turn right (north) and follow the trail downstream along the creek. The forest is unusual because it consists predominantly of white firs, though Jeffrey pines are also plentiful. In 0.25 mile, pass a second grove of aspens mixed with willows and cross back to the east side of the creek. In another 0.15 mile, look for a stately grove of aspens lined up on the far side of the creek. In another 0.2 mile, cross Fish Creek three more times and reach a fourth grove of aspens. Return the way you came.

VARIATION

For a 4.5-mile walk, consider continuing down Fish Creek to the junction with the Santa Ana River Trail (see Trip 5.16) and then heading east along the river trail to an unmarked junction where you can climb back up. This is recommended only if you're familiar with the area and comfortable navigating; the trails aren't properly indicated on the recommended maps.

Aspen Grove

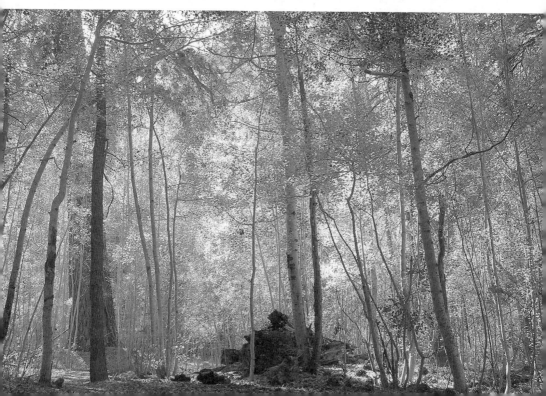

see map on p. 103

trip 5.18   **Fish Creek Meadows**

Distance	4 miles (out-and-back)
Hiking Time	2 hours
Elevation Gain	650'
Difficulty	Easy
Trail Use	Dogs allowed
Best Times	May–November
Agency	San Bernardino National Forest (Mill Creek Ranger Station)
Recommended Map	Tom Harrison *San Gorgonio Wilderness* or USGS *Moonridge* 7.5'

DIRECTIONS From Redlands, drive east on Highway 38 to the Heart Bar Campground turnoff, just past the 038 SBD 33.48 mile marker. Turn right and follow Forest Road 1N02 for 1.3 miles, passing the campground entrance. At a junction, turn right onto 1N05, a fair dirt road, and proceed 1.6 miles to the signed Aspen Grove Trailhead at a hairpin turn in the road.

If you plan to do a one-way hike, leave another vehicle 4.7 miles farther up 1N05 at the Fish Creek Trailhead. Along the way, stay right at three forks, not all of which are marked.

Note: *This area was affected by the 2015 Lake Fire and remained closed at press time.*

Fish Creek defines the northeastern boundary of the San Gorgonio Wilderness. This pleasant hike up the valley leads to a small meadow. A short detour to the north leads to several stately groves of aspens.

From the Aspen Grove Trailhead, walk south 0.3 mile and cross Fish Creek to reach a fork. The trail to the right leads down to Aspen Grove (see Trip 5.17), but this trip turns

Lower Fish Creek Meadow

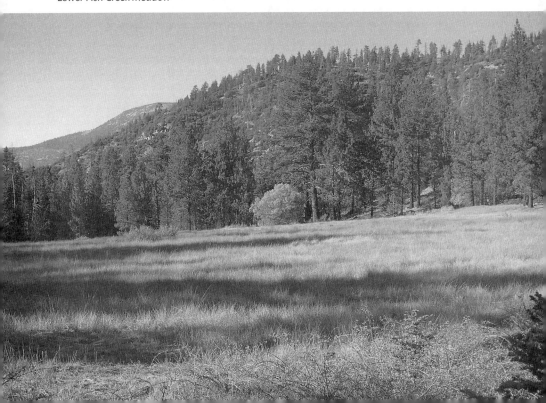

left. Hike south along the west bank of the creek through a forest of tall white firs. In 1.2 miles, cross to the east side of the creek and stay right at an unmarked fork. (The left fork passes along the east edge of Lower Fish Creek Meadow and leads to the Fish Creek Trailhead in 1.1 miles.) Shortly beyond, Lower Fish Creek Meadow comes into view beside the trail and, in 0.6 mile, you'll reach a signed trail junction with the Fish Creek Trail. At this point, you can retrace your steps to the trailhead.

VARIATION

To visit more of Fish Creek Meadows, turn right (west) at the junction and proceed 0.5 mile to Upper Fish Creek Meadow, where you may find columbine, Indian paintbrush, and corn lilies.

ALTERNATIVE FINISH

Alternatively, for a one-way hike, turn left (east) and go 0.6 mile to the Fish Creek Trailhead at the end of 1N05. This requires a 4.7-mile car or bicycle shuttle; mountain bikers should beware that there is uphill travel in both directions.

---

trip 5.19 San Gorgonio via Fish Creek

Distance	19 miles (out-and-back)
Hiking Time	10 hours
Elevation Gain	3,600'
Difficulty	Strenuous
Trail Use	Dogs allowed, suitable for backpacking
Best Times	June–October
Agency	San Bernardino National Forest (Mill Creek Ranger Station)
Recommended Maps	Tom Harrison *San Gorgonio Wilderness* or USGS *Moonridge* and *San Gorgonio Mountain* 7.5'
Permit	San Gorgonio Wilderness Permit required for overnight camping

DIRECTIONS From Redlands, drive east on Highway 38 to the Heart Bar Campground turnoff, just past the 038 SBD 33.48 mile marker. Turn right and follow Forest Road 1N02 for 1.3 miles, passing the campground entrance. At a junction, turn right onto 1N05, a fair dirt road, and proceed 6.3 miles, staying right (on the main road) at three forks, to the signed Fish Creek Trailhead at the end of the road.

Note: *This area was affected by the 2015 Lake Fire and remained closed at press time.*

Fish Creek drops down the northeast slopes of San Gorgonio Mountain. A long dirt road leads high up into its headwaters. The Fish Creek Trail, completed in 1971, is the easiest route to the summit, and is also one of the most lightly used, so you're likely to be able to get a permit when the more popular Vivian Creek and South Fork Trails have reached their quotas. The forests, meadows, and wide-ranging views are magnificent and this route would likely see as much travel as the others if the trailhead were closer to the highway. Fish Creek also provides backpackers access to excellent camping at Mineshaft Flat.

The Fish Creek Trail (1W07) leads west from the southern end of the parking area into a forest of Jeffrey pines and white firs. In 0.6 mile, come to a junction near Lower Fish Creek Meadow. The right fork leads to Aspen Grove (see Trips 5.17 and 5.18), while the Fish Creek Trail continues straight. Stay on the Fish Creek Trail, cross two trickling forks of Fish Creek, and hike alongside the bushy Upper Fish Creek Meadow.

In 1.2 miles, reach Fish Creek Trail Camp at the bottom of a draw, with tent sites cleared beneath the towering firs. Great forested slopes rise on three sides, with Ten Thousand Foot Ridge to the south and Grinnell Mountain to the west. Water might be available from the draw just up the trail; check conditions in advance before depending on it.

The trail follows the draw, then soon crosses it and begins long switchbacks up the east slope of Grinnell Mountain. The mountain was named for Joseph Grinnell, a zoologist from the University of California who made the classic study of animals in the eastern San Bernardino Mountains from 1905 to 1907. Lodgepole pines begin appearing, with their distinctive flaky bark and small cones, and soon crowd out all the other trees. After 3 miles of steady climbing, reach Fish Creek Saddle and yet more dry camping. (A faint, unmaintained trail leads west down the draw to Lodgepole Spring, just above Dry Lake, where you may find water.) Continue southwest 0.8 mile, through a ghost forest of dead lodgepoles on the north slopes of Lake Peak, to a saddle with a trail junction leading 1.2 miles down to Mineshaft Flat overlooking the Whitewater River's North Fork.

VARIATION

Mineshaft Flat is a great destination for a backpacking trip if you don't care to hike all the way to San Gorgonio. This round-trip is 14 miles with 3,000 feet of elevation gain. You'll beat the crowds and find plenty of camping on soft ground beneath the lodgepoles under Gorgonio's steep slopes. Tremendous avalanches sweep down these slopes in the winter every few decades, laying waste to all trees in their path. Watchful and lucky hikers may see the herd of desert bighorn sheep that roam the ridges and canyons where humans rarely visit. Mineshaft Flat was the site of an unsuccessful mining operation early in the 20th century. Water is usually available from a spring below the trail 0.4 mile below the flat where the trail crosses the Whitewater River. You might choose to continue another 0.8 mile down the canyon to North Fork Meadows where there was once camping beside Big Tree. The flat sites are now overgrown, but it's a quiet destination for lunch and peaceful contemplation.

From Fish Creek Saddle, pass along the south side of a hill, locally known as Zahniser Peak, for 0.2 mile to a second junction at Mineshaft Saddle. Take the Sky High Trail to the left (south), which spirals around the mountain to gain the last 1,500 feet of elevation on a gradual slope. It passes limber and lodgepole pines, which become shorter and more weatherbeaten until they're reduced to isolated shrubs at treeline. At about 10,400 feet, pass the wreckage of a C-47 transport plane that splattered against the mountainside on a stormy night in 1952. Then climb eight switchbacks and traverse around to a junction west of the summit in 3.8 miles. Finally, turn right and hike the last 0.4 mile to the top of San Gorgonio Mountain. Hardy backpackers may pitch their tents on the windswept summit for a magical night beneath the stars.

VARIATION

Dedicated peak baggers might choose to hike Lake Peak and/or Grinnell Mountain from Fish Creek Saddle on the return. To reach Lake Peak, hike south up to the ridge; then turn right and follow the ridge to the boulder pile that forms the summit. This adds 400 feet of gain and 0.3 mile each way.

Upper Fish Creek Meadow (on the right) after the Lake Fire

VARIATION ——

To reach Grinnell Mountain, hike north along the ridge, bypassing some obstacles on the left. You may find traces of a use trail along the way. The summit is broad, flat, and forested, but the true high point is marked by a cairn near the east side. This adds 500 feet of gain and 0.6 mile each way.

---

trip 5.20   San Gorgonio Nine Peaks Challenge

Distance	25 miles (one-way)
Hiking Time	14 hours
Elevation Gain	8,000'
Difficulty	Very strenuous
Trail Use	Dogs allowed, suitable for backpacking
Best Times	June–October
Agency	San Bernardino National Forest (Mill Creek Ranger Station)
Required Maps	Tom Harrison *San Gorgonio Wilderness* or USGS *Forest Falls, San Gorgonio Mountain, Moonridge,* and *Big Bear Lake* 7.5'
Permit	San Gorgonio Wilderness Permit required for overnight camping

DIRECTIONS Hikers have many choices for where to start and end this trip. This version assumes you start at the Vivian Creek Trailhead and end at the San Bernardino Peak Trailhead, arranging a half-hour car shuttle.

To drop a vehicle at the San Bernardino Peak Trailhead, drive east on Highway 38 from Redlands to Angelus Oaks. Follow the signs for the San Bernardino Peak Trail (1W07): First, turn right off Highway 38 onto Manzanita Avenue toward the fire station at mile marker 038 SBD 20.00. Then make an immediate left and drive 0.1 mile, passing the station. Make a right onto a fair dirt road past the station at a brown sign indicating SAN BERNARDINO PEAK TRAIL 1W07. Stay right at two forks, and go 0.3 mile to a large dirt parking area with the signed San Bernardino Peak Trailhead.

To reach the Vivian Creek Trailhead, descend Highway 38 and head southwest to the huge hairpin turn at mile marker 038 SBD 15.00. Turn left (east) onto Valley of the Falls Drive and proceed 4.5 miles to its end. Turn left and park at the Vivian Creek Trailhead.

The great San Bernardino Divide forms the backbone of the San Gorgonio Wilderness and is the highest ridge in California south of the Sierra Nevada. The west end is anchored by San Bernardino Peak, while the east end culminates above treeline on the towering summit of San Gorgonio Mountain. A well-built trail, constructed by the Forest Service in 1938, runs the length of the gently undulating crest, passing seven other minor peaks along the way. A worthwhile challenge is to climb all nine of these summits; the undertaking has become so popular that the San Gorgonio Wilderness Association sells an "I Climbed the Nine Peaks" arm patch to commemorate the deed. Boy Scout troops do the hike as a three-day backpacking trip. Experienced mountaineers can do it in one long day. This trip is recommended for those who already know the area well because it usually involves some hiking before dawn and/or after dark. Good navigation skills are required to locate the minor peaks on the ridge. Although this is a very strenuous route, it's easier than the other Nine Peaks challenges around Mount Baldy and the Desert Divide.

Carefully study the map and choose the route you want to take. This description assumes a start up the Vivian Creek Trail to San Gorgonio Mountain followed by an east–west traverse ending at Angelus Oaks. It has the advantage of giving you the hardest climb in the morning while you're fresh and being mostly downhill thereafter. Another alternative is to start up the Fish Creek Trail; this route has less elevation gain but a much longer car shuttle. If only one vehicle is available, you can ascend Vivian Creek, descend the Momyer Creek

Trail, and then hike or cycle Valley of the Falls Drive 2 miles back to the Vivian Creek Trailhead. If you plan to backpack the route, study the map for campsites and springs.

Many of the peaks along the ridge were named by a young surveyor named Donald McLain in 1920 as he spent the summer roaming and mapping the high country. Those honored by place names include Willis Jepson, the University of California botanist who wrote *A Manual of the Flowering Plants of California;* Rushton Charlton, McLain's boss and the supervisor of Angeles National Forest, who ironically opposed wilderness protection for San Gorgonio; Leila Shields, manager of Camp Radford on the Santa Ana River; and Lou Anderson, the Barton Flats ranger.

Backpackers must plan their trip around the availability of water. Water is usually available at Vivian Creek and High Creek. High Meadow Springs is reliable but off the trail and takes some effort to locate. Trail Fork and Limber Pine Springs may run into the summer but could dry up sooner in a drought year. Manzanita and Columbine Springs run only in early season. Contact the ranger about current conditions before your trip.

Climb the Vivian Creek Trail (see Trip 5.1) 8 miles to the trail junction on the crest. Just above this junction is a vista point with a fine view west along the entire San Bernardino Divide. Turn right (east) and proceed 0.6 mile to the summit of San Gorgonio. At this point, you've completed two-thirds of the elevation gain but only one-third of the distance. Return to the junction and hike west past the junction of the Vivian Creek Trail. As the trail descends near Jepson Peak, hike cross-country to the summit; then descend to rejoin the trail. Follow the trail around Jepson Peak to a bend north of the peak. Hike cross-country from here up Little Charlton and Charlton Peaks, and then descend to Dollar Lake Saddle.

Follow the trail northwest as it passes the insignificant rock pile which has been informally dubbed Alto Diablo Peak, and scramble to the top. The crux of this climb is to identify the summit, which is marked on the Tom Harrison map but not on the USGS topo. It's the first high point reached after the climb from Dollar Lake Saddle—if you begin switchbacking down toward Shields Flat, you've just missed it.

The trail then follows the north side of the ridge. The tall lodgepole pines and fine views more than compensate for your fatigue. Make similar short excursions to the summits of Shields Peak, Anderson Peak, San Bernardino East Peak, and finally San Bernardino Peak, 9 miles from San Gorgonio. Then descend the last weary 8 miles to Angelus Oaks (see Trip 5.9).

San Bernardino Divide

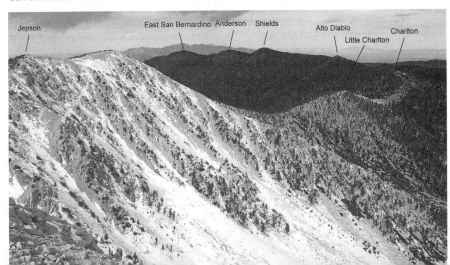

VARIATION ———————————————————————————————

Extraordinarily ambitious peak-baggers can scale even more summits in this beautiful high country. For example, at least two mountaineers have day-hiked all 17 named peaks: Grinnell, Ten Thousand Foot Ridge, Lake, Zahniser, Bighorn, Dragon's Head, San Gorgonio, Jepson, East Dobbs, Dobbs, Little Charlton, Charlton, Alto Diablo, Shields, Anderson, San Bernardino East, and San Bernardino. This 38-mile loop with 12,000 feet of elevation gain can be done without a car shuttle by starting at the South Fork Trailhead and descending the Forsee Creek Trail.

---

trip 5.21   Ten Peaks of the Yucaipa Ridge

Distance	19 miles (one-way)
Hiking Time	15 hours
Elevation Gain	6,700'
Difficulty	Very strenuous
Best Times	May–November
Agency	San Bernardino National Forest (Mill Creek Ranger Station)
Required Maps	Tom Harrison *San Gorgonio Wilderness* or USGS *Forest Falls* and *San Gorgonio Mountain* 7.5'
Permit	Bearpaw Reserve Permit required

see map on pgs. 102 & 103

DIRECTIONS The hike requires a 5-mile shuttle between trailheads. From Redlands, drive east on Highway 38 to the huge hairpin turn at mile marker 038 SBD 15.00. Turn right onto Valley of the Falls Drive and then immediately right again onto the Bearpaw Reserve road, crossing Mill Creek. In 0.3 mile, reach a gate where you'll enter the code provided with your Bearpaw Reserve permit. In 0.2 mile, pass the Audubon parking area on the left. In another 0.3 mile, the road ends at the Bearpaw Reserve Trailhead. Leave a vehicle here.

Return to Valley of the Falls Drive and continue east 4.5 miles to its end. Turn left and park at the Vivian Creek Trailhead.

The Oak Glen Divide or Yucaipa Ridge, running parallel to and south of the San Bernardino Divide, separates Mill Creek Canyon from Oak Glen and Yucaipa. The ridge tapers from a jagged knife-edge at the east end to a rounded series of humps on the lower west end. This trip follows the crest all the way from Galena Peak to Allen Peak, visiting Wanat, Cuchillo, Little San Gorgonio Peak, Wilshire Mountain, Wilshire Peak, Oak Glen Peak, Cedar Mountain, and Birch Mountain along the way. It involves cross-country travel most of the way, and has some extremely steep and loose sections; the trip is suitable only for highly experienced navigators who are comfortable moving quickly on difficult terrain.

The USGS topographic maps are strongly advisable because they provide far more detail than can be shown on a larger-scale map. In 2014, the USGS officially named Peak 9,164' Wanat (a Serrano Indian word for "mountain lions," which frequent this remote country) and Peak 8,868' Cuchillo (Spanish for "knife," due to the knife-edge ridge).

The hike exits through The Wildlands Conservancy's Bearpaw Reserve. You must obtain a free permit and gate code to enter the preserve; the permit will also allow you to park at the preserve. E-mail mountainpreserves@twc-ca.org for a permit application. You could descend to Forest Falls from the Cedar–Birch Saddle and avoid Bearpaw, but this involves tedious travel over steep rock.

The trip's difficulty can be reduced somewhat by doing only the section from Galena Peak to Little San Gorgonio Peak, or from Little San Gorgonio Peak to Allen Peak, but both of these options are still serious undertakings. Long pants and gaiters are strongly

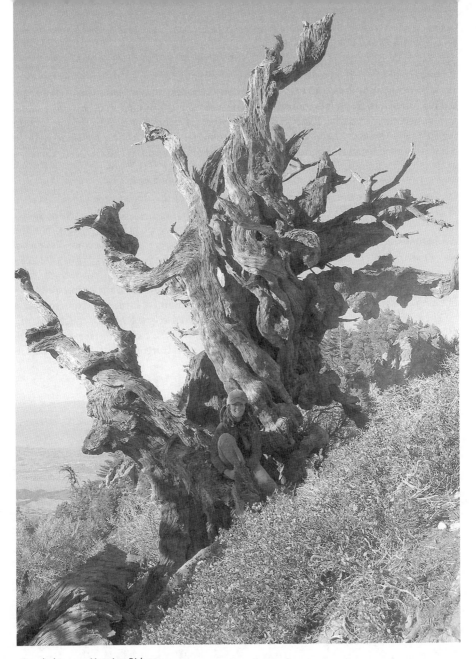

Gnarled tree on Yucaipa Ridge

recommended because some patches of brush are inevitable. A hiking pole or work gloves are also handy on the unstable terrain. Large parties may want helmets because rockfall is almost certain. USGS 7.5' maps are indispensable for cross-country navigation. They show the Oak Glen Divide Trail along the top of the Yucaipa Ridge, but it hasn't been maintained in years and is scarcely visible. Access to the ridge from all directions has also been severely curtailed by private-property owners.

The hike begins at the Vivian Creek Trailhead and ends on Prospect Drive in Forest Falls. Start by climbing Galena Peak by way of Mill Creek Canyon and the Mill Creek

Jumpoff (see Trip 5.3). Hike over to the west summit and inspect the route to the west. Little San Gorgonio Peak, the high point visible 2.3 miles away, is lower than Galena, but the next stretch to reach it is more demanding and time-consuming than the entire climb to Galena Peak. A gnarly ˙hiker named Rick Kent describes the traverse in the summit register as "a wickedly diabolical route!" The route follows the knife-edge ridge studded with rocky gendarmes and dotted with brush. Most of the terrain is class two, but there are a few third-class moves involved. Along the way, savor some of the finest viewpoints of the four Saints: San Gorgonio, San Bernardino, San Jacinto, and San Antonio.

The crux of the traverse is to descend the first part of the ridge to the saddle between Wanat and Cuchillo. The easiest path tends to follow the crest, or just below on the south, but occasionally has to dip farther down on the south to escape brush or to veer onto the crumbling north face to bypass obstacles. Beyond the saddle, the ridge becomes less steep and a use trail can occasionally be found. There are many large patches of brush that can be circumvented with careful route-finding. Climb over Cuchillo, then down to the next saddle, then up over the rocky top of Peak 9,040', and then down into the saddle at the top of Camp Creek. Finally, hike up the open slopes to the summit of Little San Gorgonio Peak.

The remainder of the Yucaipa Ridge loses its knife-edge character and is much easier to follow. Moreover, the Oak Glen Divide Trail once followed the crest and traces of it are still visible, guiding you past patches of brush. From Little San Gorgonio Peak, descend west to

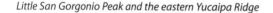

Little San Gorgonio Peak and the eastern Yucaipa Ridge

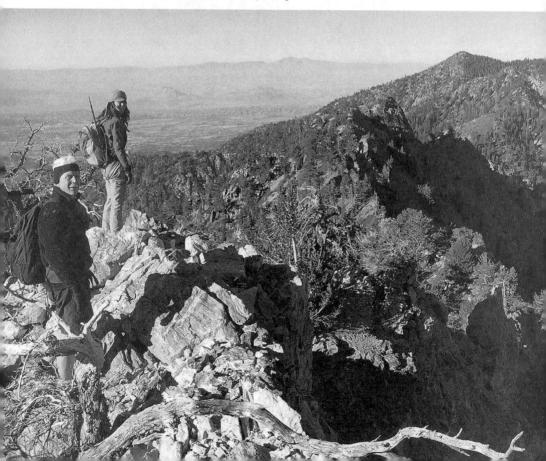

a saddle and then climb to a hill with a communications tower. If you need to escape the ridge because of a shortage of time or energy, the best way down begins about 0.2 mile east of the tower and descends northward onto a ridge that drops into Camp Creek (see Trip 5.2). Otherwise, follow the dirt service road west down and then gently up to Peak 8,832′, which is called Wilshire Mountain by the Sierra Club. When the service road turns left (south) and begins to descend, leave it and hike to the nearby flat wooded summit.

Descend northwest and then hike back up southwest to Wilshire Peak (not to be confused with Wilshire Mountain). Wilshire Peak is named for Joe Wilshire, a pioneer apple grower in Oak Glen. The old trail is marked by single rock cairns in places and tends to follow the crest. It's convenient when you can locate it, but it's not worth too much effort to precisely follow because it has been completely obliterated in places. Descend the steep northwest ridge of Wilshire Peak; then take the easy hike over nearby Oak Glen Peak to Cedar Mountain. Sadly, no cedars are to be found on the summit.

Just 0.1 mile west of the summit is a sign marking the junction of the 1W08 Oak Glen Divide Trail and the 1E10 Wilshire Peak Trail leading up from Oak Glen, though both trails are scarcely visible any longer. Unfortunately, the Wilshire Peak Trail also has private-property issues.

Hike northwest, passing on the south side of two bumps on the ridge, to the Birch–Cedar Saddle. The Oak Glen Divide Trail may be found contouring around the north slope of Birch Mountain, but it's easier to hike directly up the ridge to the summit of Birch Mountain. The complete traverse from Little San Gorgonio Peak involves 4.8 miles and 1,100 feet of elevation gain. Again, there are no birches on the summit. Birch Mountain was apparently named for Birch Creek, which itself was named for misidentified trees.

Return to the Birch–Cedar Saddle and make a long westward descent on the Oak Glen Divide Trail, which eventually becomes the Yucaipa Ridge Road. In 4 miles, reach the deep Allen–Birch Saddle. A road leads north from here down through Bearpaw Reserve, but intrepid peak baggers have one last piece of business.

Allen Peak's sheer east face looms large above the saddle. Follow the Yucaipa Ridge Road west, immediately passing a gate to exit Bearpaw Reserve. In 0.3 mile, look for a faint climber's trail at a berm on the left at your first opportunity to gain the north ridge of Allen Peak. Follow this path southwest onto the ridge and then south up to the summit. The trail nicely avoids the manzanita and mountain mahogany on the ridge; if you find yourself bushwhacking, you've gone off-route.

Return to the Birch–Allen Saddle and turn left to descend the easy fire road through Bearpaw Reserve. In 1.0 mile, shortly after a pair of switchbacks, you may notice a grassy path on the right up to a hatch serving an aqueduct. This is a way to join the Aqueduct Trail, a narrow grassy path that clings to the edge of the steep hillside to follow a buried pipeline carrying water from Mill Creek to the Edison Mill Creek Hydroelectric Projects 2 and 3.

You can follow the trail and then drop down a service road to the Bearpaw Reserve Trailhead or continue to Mill Creek (Trip 5.7). But if you've done this complete trip, the hour is likely to be late, so the easiest choice is to continue down the road another 1.3 miles. A signed spur on the left leads 0.1 mile to the seasonal mossy 100-foot Columbine Falls. Stay on the road for another 0.1 mile to a second signed junction, where a trail on the left drops 0.1 mile to the Bearpaw Reserve Trailhead and your getaway vehicle.

VARIATIONS

Hikers have several alternatives to choose from for this trip. Local mountaineers have discovered a number of steep and devious routes from Forest Falls to the Yucaipa Ridge. You can climb to a point 0.5 mile west of Little San Gorgonio Peak from the Vivian Creek Trailhead by way of Camp Creek (see Trip 5.2). From here, you can make a shorter loop east to Galena Peak or west to Allen Peak.

You can also escape off the ridge into Forest Falls from the Birch–Cedar Saddle; this route is much shorter than descending through Bearpaw but isn't much faster. From the east end of the saddle, hike east into the canyon between Oak Creek and Bridal Veil Creek. It's convenient to aim for the ridge east of the canyon where the walking is unobstructed, but rock ribs separating upper forks of the canyon make the traverse very tedious. The ridge has been partially logged at about 6,600 feet. The route ends behind the houses on Prospect Drive.

The ultimate Yucaipa Ridge traverse continues 3 miles west on the Yucaipa Ridge Road, visiting Mill Peak. When the road turns left and drops down a spur ridge through private property, leave the road and hike west straight down the Aqueduct Trail to the Mill Creek Hydroelectric Plant.

Aerial view of western Yucaipa Ridge, separated from San Bernardino Ridge by the deep fault trench of Mill Creek Canyon

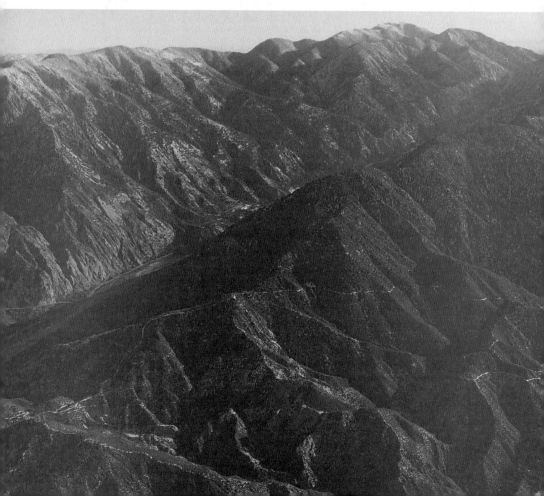

chapter 6

High Desert

The High Desert encompasses the Mojave Desert in San Bernardino County. It generally sits at elevations of 2,000–4,000 feet, in contrast to the Low (Colorado) Desert around the Coachella Valley, which is near or below sea level. The High Desert is thus cooler and moister than its lower counterpart. Creosote bush and Joshua tree are two of the characteristic plants. This chapter covers hikes in the vicinity of Victorville and Barstow, the High Desert's major communities. Chapters 15–20 cover other regions of the Mojave Desert.

The High Desert is a gigantic plateau that began pushing up about 140 million years ago as the Pacific and North American Plates crashed together. More recently, the same forces pushed up some of the minor desert mountain ranges and volcanoes. Until recently, geologically speaking, the region received regular rainfall and was the site of enormous lakes. Large land animals once roamed the area. About 10,000 years ago, at the end of the last ice age, the Mojave fell into the rain shadow of the rising Transverse and Peninsular Ranges (the San Gabriels, San Bernardinos, and San Jacintos), which were pushed up by

Upper Owl Canyon (see Trip 6.3)

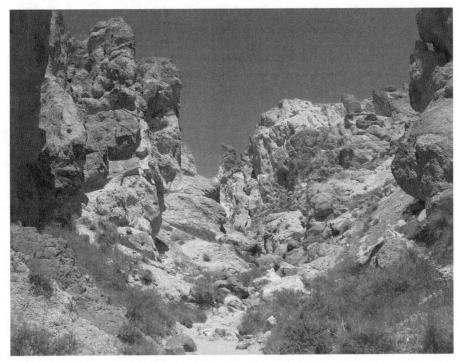

the infamous San Andreas Fault. Moisture from the ocean seldom crosses these formidable barriers, so the lakes dried up and the land changed dramatically.

The Mojave River is one of the few major water sources in this desert. Its waters flow briskly off the north slopes of the San Bernardino Mountains, but soon sink into the sands near Hesperia. The river mostly flows underground, but occasionally emerges to the surface at bottlenecks such as Afton Canyon, or when intense thunderstorms send flash floods down the riverbed. Flash floods can radically change the terrain in canyons and washes, so be prepared for conditions to differ from these route descriptions.

Although many people think of the desert as lifeless, a wide variety of animals scratch out a living in these harsh conditions. Dawn and dusk are great times to watch for wildlife, but observant hikers will see tracks and scat any time of day.

The best time to visit the High Desert is between late fall and early spring. Summer temperatures routinely exceed 100°F in the shade. However, subfreezing temperatures are not uncommon in the winter. The desert is especially beautiful after the occasional snowstorm. Temperatures can fluctuate dramatically between day and nighttime, so come prepared.

trip 6.1 Mormon Rocks Nature Loop

Distance	1 mile (loop)
Hiking Time	30 minutes
Elevation Gain	200'
Difficulty	Easy
Trail Use	Dogs allowed, good for kids
Best Times	October–April
Agency	Angeles National Forest (Lytle Creek Ranger Station)
Optional Maps	USGS *Telegraph Peak* and *Cajon* 7.5'

DIRECTIONS From the 15 Freeway (I-15) south of Cajon Pass, take Exit 131 west on Highway 138. Proceed 1.6 miles and turn left into the Mormon Rocks Forest Service Fire Station.

At the junction of the 15 Freeway and Highway 138, oddly tilted sedimentary rock formations stand sentinel below Cajon Pass. Officially named Rock Candy Mountains but locally known as the Mormon Rocks, the formations have been riddled with holes by strong winds and weather. Lizards, owls, and pack rats make their homes in these small caves. The wild contortions of the San Andreas Fault have thrust these cemented sandstone beds upward toward the sky. Although the Mormon Rocks appear to be weather-worn and crumbly, they remain standing because they erode more slowly than the sand and silt of the alluvial flats of the Cajon Canyon wash. This area burned in the 2016 Blue Cut Fire.

Behind the pine-shaded Mormon Rocks Fire Station and across a picturesque footbridge is a well-marked 1-mile nature trail. The trail was built by the Forest Service in 1975 to provide hikers with panoramic views of the Mormon Rocks and the Cajon Pass. The

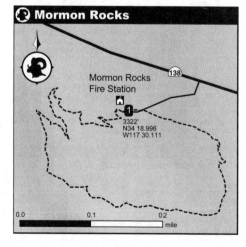

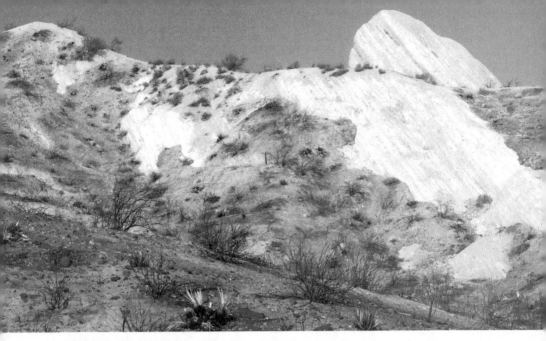

Mormon Rocks after the Blue Cut Fire

trail's numbered interpretive markers provide history and geological information about the surrounding area. Be sure to pick up the informative brochure at the beginning of the trail.

The trail switchbacks through areas of creosote and sage bushes, manzanitas, and yuccas. Note that this trail does not weave its way through the rocks themselves but is across the highway, providing expansive views of the formations. To explore the rock formations more closely, simply cross Highway 138 and wander to your heart's content.

trip 6.2   East Ord Mountain

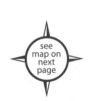

see map on next page

Distance	2.5 miles (out-and-back or semiloop)
Hiking Time	3–4 hours
Elevation Gain	2,000'
Difficulty	Moderate
Trail Use	Dogs allowed
Best Times	October–April
Agency	BLM Barstow Field Office
Required Maps	USGS *Fry Mountains, Camp Rock Mine,* and *Ord Mountain* 7.5'

DIRECTIONS A high-clearance vehicle is helpful to reach the trailhead. From Exit 153A or 153B off the 15 Freeway in Victorville, turn east on Highway 18 and proceed 25 miles to Lucerne Valley. At a stop sign, continue straight (east) to join Highway 247 and go 5.1 miles. At an intersection 0.4 mile east of mile marker 247 SBD 40.00, turn left (north) onto Camp Rock Road. In 4.0 miles, bear right to remain on Camp Rock Road. In another 2.3 miles, the road turns to excellent dirt. Continue 7.6 miles to a junction beneath the huge transmission lines; turn left onto fair dirt BLM Road OM 6657. Go 0.9 mile to a junction, and turn right onto OM 6659 and continue 0.7 mile up a rocky dirt road to a turnout beside the ruins of a corrugated metal water tank. If your vehicle and road conditions allow, you can continue 0.3 mile farther up the road to park at a second turnout where the road passes near the wash to the north.

East Ord Mountain is a volcanic desert peak overlooking the Lucerne Valley between Victorville and Joshua Tree. It's slightly shorter than its neighbor, Ord Mountain, but is

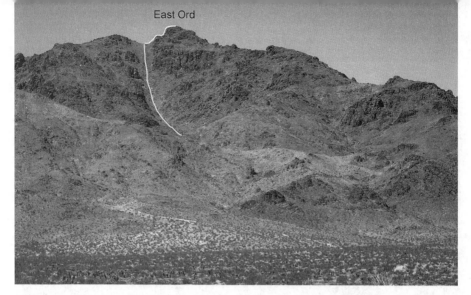

East Ord

Follow the gully to the saddle left of the peak.

nevertheless the most prominent mountain in the range. The Ord Mountains were named for Major General E. O. C. Ord, who led the first official survey of Los Angeles. Finding the remote trailhead is half the fun of this short but steep cross-country jaunt. Despite its short length, the trip isn't recommended for inexperienced desert travelers. The summit offers outstanding 360-degree views of snowcapped ranges and desert basins on a clear winter day, from San Gorgonio in the south to the Panamint Mountains to the north.

The mountain overlooks the Johnson Valley Off-Highway Vehicle Recreation Area; the incessant whine of dirt bikes and ATVs can detract from the wilderness experience.

From the lower parking area, hike west up the rough and rocky mining road 0.3 mile. After passing around a ridge coming down from the north, the road runs adjacent to a boulder-strewn dry wash before climbing steeply up a hill. 4WD vehicles can park here, just before the hill and a white cable fence. From this upper parking area, study the view of the peak to the north-northwest and pick out your route. The summit is identifiable by the brown line of cliffs underneath and the dirt saddle immediately to the left (west). This trip climbs the mountain by way of the saddle.

Leave the road at the 4WD parking area and hike up the wash 0.2 mile to the first place you can easily exit on the right (north). Follow a smaller gully system that leads up to the saddle left of the peak. This is steep hiking, climbing 1,500 feet in 1 mile and involves plenty of boulder-hopping, but no difficult climbing. The region is home to creosote bushes and hedgehog cacti, yielding to barrel

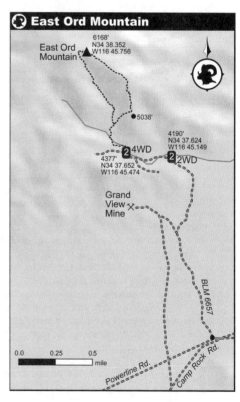

and Mojave mound cacti at higher elevations. Upon reaching the saddle, turn right (east) and climb 150 feet more to the summit. If you pick a careful path that loops around the north side, you can avoid scrambling up large rocks. Descend the way you came.

ALTERNATIVE FINISH

Climb or descend the southeast ridge to make a semiloop trip. The ridge is most easily accessed from a saddle next to Point 5,038'. The ridge route is of comparable difficulty to the gully route, involving mostly straightforward walking with one band of rock to navigate through.

---

trip 6.3 **Owl Canyon**

Distance	4 miles (out-and-back)
Hiking Time	3 hours
Elevation Gain	1,000'
Difficulty	Moderate
Trail Use	Dogs allowed, good for kids
Best Times	October–April
Agency	BLM Barstow Field Office
Recommended Map	USGS *Mud Hills* 7.5'

DIRECTIONS From the 15 Freeway in Barstow, take Exit 183 north onto Barstow Road. Go 1 mile to a T-junction at Main Street and turn left (west). In 0.2 mile, turn right (north) onto First Street, which crosses the rail yard and Mojave River. Train buffs won't want to miss a stop at the Western American Railroad Museum. In 0.9 mile, turn left onto Irwin Road. In another 5.9 miles, turn left onto good dirt Fossil Bed Road. In 2.9 miles, turn right (north) at a signed turnoff for Rainbow Basin Scenic Drive and Owl Canyon Campground. In 0.4 mile, come to a signed junction with a road leading right to Owl Canyon Campground.

The trailhead starts at the Owl Canyon Campground. Before you go there, however, it's worth taking a driving tour through Rainbow Basin. Continue straight (north) on the 3.7-mile, one-way loop through the spectacular multihued canyon, which is too narrow for motor homes or cars pulling trailers. Watch for the famous bent-rock bands of the Barstow Syncline.

When you get back to the main Fossil Bed Road, turn left and return 0.7 mile to the junction you'd originally reached leading to Rainbow Basin and Owl Canyon Campground. Drive 0.4 mile to the Owl Canyon turnoff and then 1.4 miles to the campground. Park at the far north end at the signed Owl Canyon Hiking Trail.

During the Barstovian Land Mammal Age, 12–16 million years ago, the Mojave Desert received much more rainfall and resembled the savannas of Africa. Large animals, including mastodons, camels, and dog-bears, roamed the grasslands. Their fossils can be found today in the green, brown, and white sedimentary rock around Rainbow Basin. The basin also contains a complex mix of older granite rock and recent volcanic rock, all of which has been bent and twisted by fault action into an exotic badland. Because of its unique paleontological and geological value, the area has been designated a National Natural Landmark and an Area of Critical Environmental Concern. Collecting fossils without a permit is illegal. Bring a flashlight to explore an unusual natural tunnel along the way.

Owl Canyon is one of the best places to see the geological splendors of this area for yourself. As interesting as the Rainbow Basin drive may be, navigating the rock formations up close as you hike and scramble through the narrows is far better. The well-situated Owl Canyon Campground has picnic tables, outhouses, and a playground, and sometimes tap water.

The signed "trail" leads down from the parking area into the wash and promptly vanishes. Follow the wash north; the majority of the hike is easy walking, but there is some rock-hopping and an occasional 6-foot dry waterfall to scramble up, so young children will need a boost. The geologic formations at the start are interesting and become even more dramatic as you ascend.

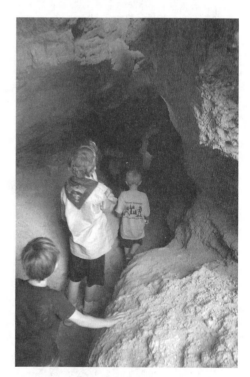

In 0.7 mile, reach a remarkable tunnel on the right side of the canyon. This rare feature penetrates about 100 feet through the sedimentary wall to reach the mouth of a tributary wash. The middle portion is completely dark. After exploring, return to the main canyon.

In another 0.1 mile, enter a section of spectacular narrows. In another 0.4 mile, the canyon opens up into an amphitheater splashed with swathes of green, orange, purple, and gray rock. At the north end, pass through a final section of narrows before you emerge in a valley below some hills.

The wash divides—take the right fork, which soon becomes a trail leading toward a huge purple rock formation. The hills here are chopped up with a maze of ATV trails. Climb a quarter mile for good views back over the valley before you return the way you came.

Cub Scouts explore a mud tunnel in Owl Canyon.

chapter 7

Urban Parks

This chapter covers a potpourri of trails scattered through urban areas in the Inland Empire. It would take a much larger book to describe every trail in every city, so these trips were selected because they're popular, noteworthy, and close to large numbers of people. Few people travel long distances to visit these parks. But, for those who live nearby, it's a great pleasure to take a stroll or jog in these hills at the start or end of a busy day. By watching the seasons pass and the plants and birds going through their cycles of life, you strengthen your connection to the land and enrich your own life.

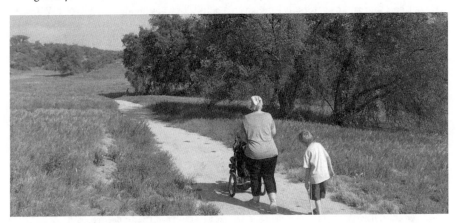

Family-friendly stroll in Oakmont Park (see Trip 7.12)

trip 7.1 Pacific Electric Trail

see map on next page

Distance	Up to 20 miles (one-way)
Hiking Time	Varies
Elevation Gain	Up to 300'
Difficulty	Variable
Trail Use	Dogs allowed, suitable for biking, suitable for equestrians
Best Times	All year
Agency	Cities along the route
Optional Maps	See cityofrc.us/cityhall/cs/parks/trails

DIRECTIONS See next page for the various access points along the trail.

The Pacific Electric Trail is Southern California's longest Rails-to-Trails effort, spanning 20 miles from Claremont to Rialto along the right-of-way of the former Pacific Electric

Pacific Electric Trail

Railway. The paved path is paralleled by a wide decomposed granite trail for part of the way, especially in Rancho Cucamonga. Walkers, joggers, cyclists, and equestrians use the trail for exercise or even commuting. The trail is rarely scenic, and it becomes tedious as it repeatedly detours to cross roads at traffic lights, but it's notable historically and is easily accessible to hundreds of thousands of Inland Empire residents.

Railroad baron Henry Huntington established the Pacific Electric Railway in 1901. The railroad soon reached from the Pacific to Redlands and more than 10,000 electric trains a day carried Californians across its extensive web. Its glory days ended after World War II as freeways replaced rail travel, and the tracks were largely abandoned. In 1991, San Bernardino County purchased the right-of-way to build a trail, and the route from the Los Angeles County line in Claremont to Cactus Avenue in Rialto was completed in 2015. In the future, the trail might be extended west to San Dimas. The trail is landscaped with drought-tolerant plants, including the desert willow, which produces striking pink blossoms in the summer.

For hundreds of thousands of Southern California residents, this is the closest trail to their home. Many health or budget-conscious residents are now using it to walk or ride to school or work.

Various access points from west to east are as follows:

MILE	LANDMARK	LOCATION
0.0	Claremont Terminus	Huntington Drive & Claremont Blvd., Claremont
5.1	Route 66 Trailhead	8500 Foothill Blvd., Rancho Cucamonga
6.8	Amethyst Trailhead	Amethyst Ave. north of Base Line Road, Rancho Cucamonga
9.1	Central Park	11200 Base Line Road, Rancho Cucamonga (*near north edge of park*)
9.7	Ellena Park	7139 Kenyon Way, Rancho Cucamonga
11.4	Etiwanda Depot	Etiwanda Ave. north of Base Line Road, Rancho Cucamonga
16.6	Seville Park	Juniper Ave. between Foothill Blvd. & Arrow Rte., Fontana
17.2	Fontana Civic Center	8353 Sierra Ave., Fontana
20.2	Rialto Terminus	Cactus Ave. between Foothill Blvd. & Rialto Ave., Rialto

The best 4-mile stretch of trail is from Route 66 to Central Park through Rancho Cucamonga. This section has few road crossings, is more scenic than most, and has good trailhead facilities at both ends.

You can jog or ride the entire trail, starting at the Claremont Metrolink station and ending at the Rialto Metrolink station, and take the train back. Cyclists should note that prevailing winds from the west favor an eastbound ride. Metrolink trains are infrequent on the weekends, so plan your trip accordingly.

trip 7.2 **Prado Lake**

Distance	2.5 miles (loop)
Hiking Time	2 hours
Elevation Gain	50'
Difficulty	Easy
Trail Use	Dogs allowed, good for kids, suitable for mountain biking, suitable for equestrians
Best Times	September–June
Agency	San Bernardino County Regional Parks District
Optional Map	*Prado Regional Park* (available at entrance station)
Permit	Day-use fee required ($8 weekdays, $10 weekends and holidays)

DIRECTIONS From the 10 (I-10) or 60 (SR 60) Freeway in Ontario, take Exit 51 or 35, respectively, south onto Euclid Avenue. Go 5.6 miles south of the 60 Freeway, and then turn left onto McCombs Way, the entrance road into Prado Regional Park. Pay the hefty entry fee at the gate and pick up a copy of the park map. Make a right at the first intersection and follow a short road to Parking Area 1.

Prado Regional Park is a popular destination for families and anglers. Located on 2,200 acres leased by San Bernardino County from the Army Corps of Engineers, it features a 60-acre lake, sports fields, an enormous playground, camping, picnicking, and, of course, a walking trail. It's located close to Chino Airport, which is home to excellent aircraft museums; you may see vintage bombers and fighter planes circling overhead. The Prado Flood Control Basin to the south attracts copious wildlife because it's one of the few remaining undeveloped areas in the region. The park is open year-round, though it can be very hot during summer days. For current hours and information, contact the park at 909-597-4260.

From the parking lot, a 2.5-mile trail leads around the many tentacles of this oddly shaped lake. Start walking west, then south around the small dam at the west end of the lake, and follow a series of trails counterclockwise around the lake. Native vegetation and plentiful wildlife are found on the south side of the lake, while the north side has grass, picnic areas, and playgrounds. In 0.8 mile, pass the outlet on the south end of the lake. Pass the campground and picnic area at the east end of the lake; then come to a huge playground and water play park. Rowboats and pedal boats can be rented at the nearby ramp. Continue north around the last tentacle of the lake past athletic fields, and return to your vehicle.

Turkey vultures in a tree by Prado Lake

trip 7.3   Mount Rubidoux

Distance	3.0 miles (loop)
Hiking Time	1.5 hours
Elevation Gain	450'
Difficulty	Easy
Trail Use	Dogs allowed, suitable for mountain biking
Best Time	All year, but hot in summer
Agency	City of Riverside Parks & Recreation
Optional Map	USGS *Riverside West* 7.5'

DIRECTIONS From the 60 Freeway, take Exit 50 south onto Rubidoux Boulevard in Riverside. In 0.3 mile, turn left (east) onto Mission Boulevard. Follow it 1.5 miles across the Santa Ana River to where the name changes to Mission Inn Avenue; then turn right onto Redwood Drive. In 0.5 mile, the name changes to Palm Avenue. In 0.2 mile, veer right onto Tequesquite Avenue, and continue 0.3 mile. Trailhead parking has been relocated to Ryan Bonaminio Park at 5000 Tequesquite Ave., solving a long-standing problem of parking in residential neighborhoods.

Mount Rubidoux is a prominent granite hill located west of downtown Riverside and south of the Santa Ana River. The mountain is named for Louis Rubidoux, who settled the area in the mid-1800s, but it was Frank Miller, one of Riverside's early promoters and the builder of the historic Mission Inn, who transformed Mount Rubidoux from an anonymous bump to a much-loved and inspirational park. Miller originally intended to develop the mountain for expensive homes, but his plans failed. Instead, Miller graded a road circling up the mountain; it's this road that hikers, cyclists, joggers, and strollers enjoy today.

Miller's estate donated Mount Rubidoux to the people of Riverside in 1955, and it's now a favorite city park attracting throngs of walkers, joggers, baby strollers, and boulderers on a pleasant day. The long list of restrictions at the entrance gate forbids alcohol, smoking, fires, gambling, weapons, unleashed dogs, off-trail travel, skateboards, horses, camping, motorized vehicles, fireworks, cutting plants, and, last but not least, soliciting. The park is open year-round from a half hour before sunrise to a half hour after sunset.

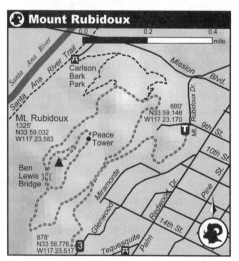

Two paved trails wind up the mountain like intertwined corkscrews. The gentle route is 2 miles long and loops the mountain twice, while the steeper route is also shorter, at 1 mile, and loops the mountain only once. The two trails intersect twice.

From Bonaminio Park, walk northeast on San Andreas Avenue. In 0.2 mile, enter Frank Miller Mount Rubidoux Memorial Park on your left and take the road climbing onto the hillside. In 0.3 mile, reach a signed four-way junction and stay straight to take the longer trail. Gnarly prickly pear cactus intermingle with brittlebush and invasive mustard and drift downward into the backyard gardens of homes at the base of the mountain. The yuccas, aloes, agaves, and cacti were planted by Miller. As you climb there are views of downtown Riverside, Evergreen Memorial Historic Cemetery, the Santa Ana River, and Flabob Airport. Flabob is one of the older airports in America and

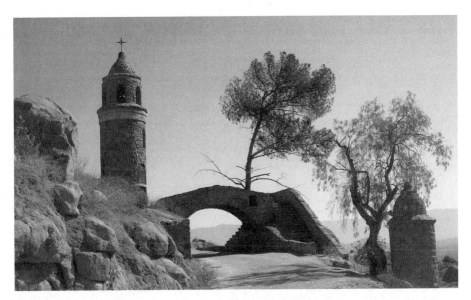

Peace Tower

is a famous base for antique and home-built aircraft. Keep your eyes out for unusual planes on approach into the field.

Pass the short trail a second time as you cross under the Ben Lewis Bridge; then reach the Peace Tower, built by "friends of Frank Augustus Miller in recognition of his constant labor in the promotion of civic beauty, community righteousness, and world peace." Once you reach the top of the mountain, explore the amphitheater, the plaque honoring Father Junipero Serra, the flagpole, and the large cross. On a clear day there are spectacular views south over Riverside.

Return via the steeper trail, which leads west along the north side of the mountain and over the Ben Lewis Bridge. When you reach the junction on the southeast side, turn hard right and take your original route back to the trailhead.

VARIATION

Mount Rubidoux can also be reached on a steeper trail from the Carlson Bark Park, on Mission Boulevard just north of the mountain.

---

trip 7.4   Box Springs: Two Trees Trail

see map on next page

Distance	2.6 miles (out-and-back)
Hiking Time	2 hours
Elevation Gain	1,000'
Difficulty	Moderate
Trail Use	Dogs allowed, suitable for mountain biking, suitable for equestrians
Best Times	September–June
Agency	Riverside County Regional Park and Open-Space District
Optional Maps	USGS *Riverside East* and *San Bernardino South* 7.5'

DIRECTIONS From the 215 Freeway (I-215) in Riverside, take Exit 33 onto Blaine Street and drive east 1.8 miles. Turn left onto Belvedere Drive; then, in 0.2 mile, turn right onto Two Trees Road and follow it 0.2 mile to the trailhead parking area, where the road turns to dirt.

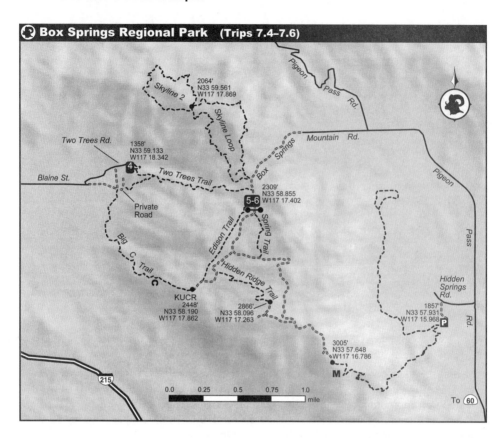

Box Springs Regional Park   (Trips 7.4–7.6)

2064'
N33 59.561
W117 17.869

Skyline 2

Skyline Loop

Pigeon Pass Rd.

Mountain Rd.

Two Trees Rd.

1358'
N33 59.133
W117 18.342

4

Two Trees Trail

Box Springs

Blaine St.

Private
Road

2309'
N33 58.855
W117 17.402

5-6

Spring Trail

Edison Trail

Big C Trail

Pigeon

Pass

Hidden Ridge Trail

Hidden
Springs
Rd.

KUCR
2448'
N33 58.190
W117 17.862

2866'
N33 58.096
W117 17.263

1857'
N33 57.931
W117 15.968

Pass Rd.

P

3005'
N33 57.648
W117 16.786

M

215

0.0   0.25   0.5   0.75   1.0
mile

To 60

The Two Trees Trail offers a short and steep workout with convenient access from Riverside. It follows a canyon from the edge of town to the trailhead on the ridge. From there, you can make a longer hike by linking up with the Skyline Trail or Towers Loop (see Trips 7.5 and 7.6).

This trip and the next two are in Box Springs Mountain Reserve Park, which encompasses 1,155 acres overlooking the University of California, Riverside. The boulder-studded hills are laced with numerous trails popular among hikers, equestrians, and mountain bikers. The park is located in a transitional zone between coastal sage scrub and chamise chaparral. The park provides habitat for many species of reptiles, mammals, and birds that are under pressure because of the unrelenting urban growth in the Inland Empire. The park is open daily, 8 a.m.–sunset.

From the parking area, walk 50 yards up the dirt road to the signed Two Trees Trailhead next to a gate. Cross a small bridge and

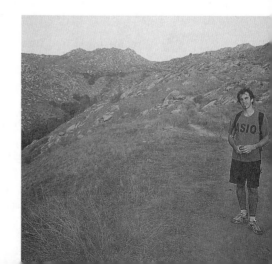

Box Springs: Two Trees Trail

pass a sycamore-filled canyon; then hike up to a ridge where you may see another equestrian trail coming up from the houses at the end of Blaine Street. Continue east up to the trail's end on Box Springs Mountain Road, 1.3 miles from the start. The upper trailhead parking area is located to the right (south) beyond a private residence. Please respect the homeowner's privacy.

| trip 7.5 | **Box Springs: Skyline Trail** |

Distance	3 or 4.5 miles (loop)
Hiking Time	2 hours
Elevation Gain	600' or 1,300'
Difficulty	Moderate
Trail Use	Dogs, cyclists, equestrians
Best Times	September–June
Agency	Riverside County Regional Park and Open-Space District
Optional Maps	USGS *Riverside East* and *San Bernardino South* 7.5'

DIRECTIONS From the 60 Freeway in Moreno Valley, take Exit 60 onto Pigeon Pass Road, following it north and then west 4.6 miles to where the road turns right (north) in the pass. Stay straight (west) on Box Springs Mountain Road, which soon turns to dirt. In 1.2 miles, reach the trailhead parking area on the right, beside a gate and a private residence.

The Skyline Trail makes a loop on the northern end of the Box Springs Mountain ridge. On a clear day, it has terrific views of the Inland Empire's major peaks towering over the endless suburban sprawl.

From the parking area, walk north back down Box Springs Mountain Road 0.2 mile, passing the top of the Two Trees Trail. Look on the left side of the road for the start of the Skyline Trail at the foot of a small hill. The Skyline Trail promptly forks. It makes a 2.5-mile loop around the ridge, with fine views along the way. Consider scrambling up one of the hills near the start of the trail for even better vistas.

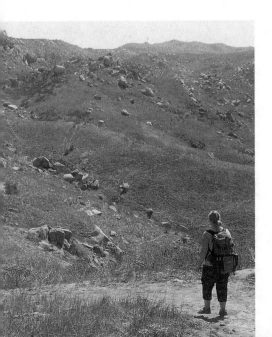

VARIATION

At the northwest end where the Skyline Trail crosses a saddle on the ridge, less-maintained Skyline 2 Trail continues northwest around the next part of the ridge. If you choose to take the second loop, you can add 1.5 miles and 700 feet of elevation gain and loss on numerous steep ups and downs. The park map shows a third loop farther west, but it was not yet established at this writing.

Box Springs: Skyline Trail

see
map on
p. 156

trip 7.6 Box Springs: Towers Loop

Distance	3.5 miles (loop, with many possible variations)
Hiking Time	2 hours
Elevation Gain	800'
Difficulty	Moderate
Trail Use	Dogs allowed, suitable for mountain biking, suitable for equestrians
Best Times	September–June
Agency	Riverside County Regional Park and Open-Space District
Optional Maps	USGS *Riverside East* and *San Bernardino South* 7.5'

DIRECTIONS From the 60 Freeway in Moreno Valley, take Exit 60 onto Pigeon Pass Road, following it north and then west 4.6 miles to where the road turns right (north) in the pass. Stay straight (west) on Box Springs Mountain Road, which soon turns to dirt. In 1.2 miles, reach the trailhead parking area on the right, beside a gate and a private residence.

The Towers Loop climbs to the antennas on the tallest hills of Box Springs Mountain. On a clear winter day, it offers stunning views over Riverside and Moreno Valley. You can choose your route, staying mostly on dirt service roads or exploring the trails that parallel the road.

The Towers Loop begins at the service road leading south past the gate from the parking area. In 0.1 mile, it reaches the Spring Trail sign warning DANGER: NO HORSES. You can follow this past Cassina Springs 0.4 mile to where it rejoins the service road. Alternatively, continue on the service road 0.6 mile, staying left at a fork, to where it meets the southern terminus of the Spring Trail.

The service road climbs the hill toward the antenna farm. In 1.0 mile, it branches again at a cluster of antennas. The left fork leads down to an overlook above Moreno Valley's Big

The University of California, Riverside, from Box Springs Mountain

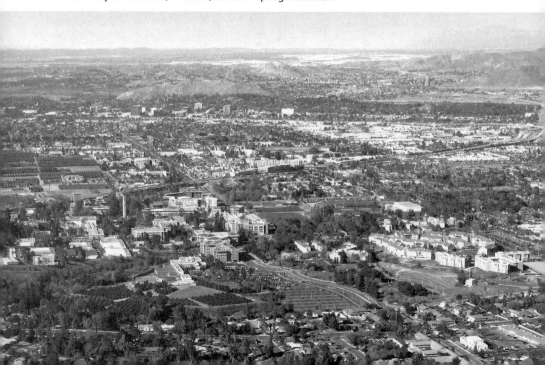

M sign, while the right fork continues past more antennas on the ridge. Take the right fork; then stay right again at a second junction to reach the road's end, in 0.4 mile at a rectangular tower with white horns.

From this tower, the enjoyable Hidden Ridge Trail descends 0.7 mile northwest toward the lone KUCR antenna. The trail ends at another service road. Turn right at the service road junction and go 0.3 mile back to the main service road, which leads north back to the trailhead.

ALTERNATIVE FINISHES —————————————————————

From the bottom of Hidden Ridge Trail, you can turn left and follow the service road southwest. In 0.2 mile, reach the Edison Trail, which leads north-northeast 0.8 mile under the power lines to the trailhead.

Yet another option is to continue 0.1 mile farther on the service road to the solitary antenna. From here, you can descend to UC Riverside's Big C sign; a steep and loose trail continues down from the C to the railroad tracks, then turns north toward Blaine Street, where you could loop back on the Two Trees Trail (see Trip 7.4).

---

trip 7.7	**Sycamore Canyon Wilderness Park**

Distance	2–10 miles (many options)
Hiking Time	Varies
Elevation Gain	Modest
Difficulty	Easy–moderate
Trail Use	Dogs allowed, good for kids, suitable for mountain biking
Best Times	October–April
Agency	City of Riverside Parks & Recreation
Optional Map	USGS *Riverside East* 7.5'

Sycamore Canyon Wilderness Park is laced with miles of trails.

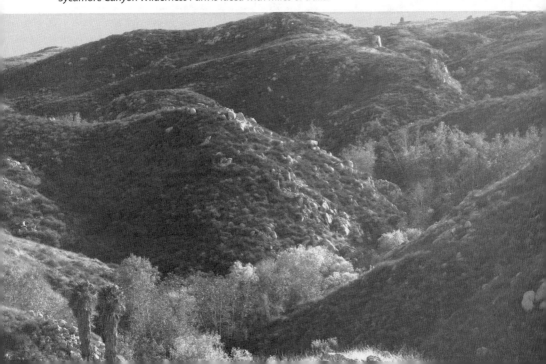

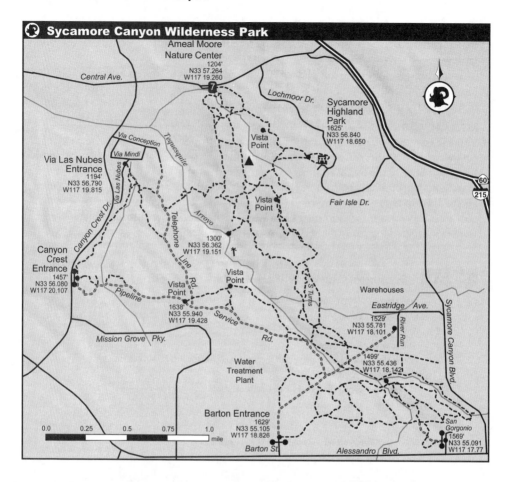

Sycamore Canyon Wilderness Park

Ameal Moore Nature Center
1204'
N33 57.264
W117 19.260

Central Ave.

Lochmoor Dr.

Sycamore Highland Park
1625'
N33 56.840
W117 18.650

Via Conception

Vista Point

Via Las Nubes Entrance
1194'
N33 56.790
W117 19.815

Via Mindi

Tequesquite

Canyon Crest Dr.

Via Las Nubes

Telephone Line Rd.

Arroyo

Vista Point

Fair Isle Dr.

1300'
N33 56.362
W117 19.151

Canyon Crest Entrance
1457'
N33 56.080
W117 20.107

Pipeline

Vista Point

Vista Point

S. Turns

Warehouses

Eastridge Ave.

1529'
N33 55.781
W117 18.101

River Run

Sycamore Canyon Blvd.

1638'
N33 55.940
W117 19.428

Service

Rd.

1499'
N33 55.436
W117 18.142

Mission Grove Pky.

Water Treatment Plant

Barton Entrance
1629'
N33 55.105
W117 18.826

San Gorgonio
1569'
N33 55.091
W117 17.77

0.0   0.25   0.5   0.75   1.0   mile

Barton St.

Alessandro Blvd.

DIRECTIONS The City of Riverside recommends that visitors use the Central Entrance, on the south side of Central Avenue, 1 mile west of Exit 30B off the 60/215 Freeway. This entrance has a large parking area and a drinking fountain beside the Ameal Moore Nature Center. Street parking is also available at entrances on Barton Street, Via Las Nubes, and Sycamore Highlands Park. Regular visitors will discover numerous other unofficial access points, although parking at these other entrances may be problematic.

Riverside, founded in 1870, is one of the oldest cities in the Inland Empire. It's the birthplace of the Southern California citrus industry and the home of many treasures, not the least of which is the Sycamore Canyon Wilderness Park. The park, owned by the City of Riverside and the California Department of Fish and Wildlife, protects nearly 1,500 acres of habitat and watershed and offers an important wildlife corridor. It is a core reserve for the endangered Stephens' kangaroo rat.

The Nature Center facilitates a popular citizen science program in which visitors help build an inventory of the park's flora and fauna. See mysycamorecanyon.com to download the Riverside Nature Spotter app and to find a calendar of events.

The wilderness park is laced with countless trails tempting the hiker to explore. It's extremely popular among mountain bikers, who consider it a prime riding location in the Inland Empire. Although the park can be enjoyed year-round, it gets very hot in the summer. Springtime is a particularly enjoyable time to visit and enjoy the abundant wildflowers. The park is open from a half hour before sunrise to a half hour after sunset.

At present, the wilderness park has almost no trail markers. A first-time visitor would need extraordinary navigational skills to follow a particular route. Nevertheless, anyone with a reasonable sense of direction will be able to wander the trails and find the way back to the trailhead as long as he or she keeps an eye on the landmarks. Thus, instead of recommending a specific loop through the park, this trip simply describes some of the major features and encourages you to roam as far as you care to explore. You can readily choose 3- to 5-mile loops from any of the trailheads or aim for an 8- to 10-mile loop encompassing the entire wilderness park. For example, from the Nature Center, consider taking the lefthand trail and work your way up to Sycamore Highlands Park; then circle back on another of the trails.

Overall, the east end of the park is the flattest, while Sycamore Canyon becomes quite deep to the northwest. The canyon presents a significant barrier to travel and is crossed by trails in only a limited number of locations. Plan your loop accordingly. Keep your eyes out for the abundant wildlife in the park. Snakes are not uncommon, so pay attention to where you place your feet. Wear shoes with good traction, because some trails can be steep and slippery.

While the author has made a substantial effort to walk each trail (more than 20 miles) and depict the trails accurately on the map, the trail system presently lacks vigorous management, and thoughtless users are steadily creating new unplanned trails. *Please stay on established paths.*

trip 7.8   Olive Mountain

Distance	2.4 miles (out-and-back)
Hiking Time	1.5 hours
Elevation Gain	900'
Difficulty	Moderate
Trail Use	Dogs allowed, suitable for mountain biking
Best Times	October–June
Agency	City of Moreno Valley Parks and Community Services
Optional Map	USGS *Sunnymead* 7.5'

see map on next page

DIRECTIONS From the 60 Freeway in Moreno Valley, take Exit 62 north onto Perris Boulevard. In 1.2 miles, turn right onto Kalmia Avenue; then, in 0.5 mile, turn left onto Kitching Street and park at the end of the road in 0.3 mile.

Bouldery Olive Mountain from Reche Mountain

The many granite-bouldered hills in the Moreno Valley area are alluring destinations for a walk. Olive Mountain is a relatively short climb but provides a vigorous workout and terrific views.

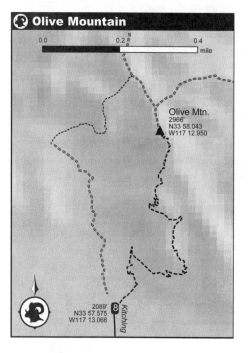

A confusing network of unsigned paths radiates out from the end of the road. Walk northeast across a field toward a triangular rock in the field. Pass the rock and continue up a broad path in the same direction toward the mountain. At the base of the mountain, the path narrows and turns sharply left, becoming a distinct trail. Switchback up the brittlebush-clad slopes past rocks that are unfortunately scarred by graffiti. The trail eventually reaches the ridge and follows it up to the summit.

From the top of Olive Mountain, you have great views of three county high points: San Gorgonio, San Jacinto, and Santiago Peaks. San Antonio is just obscured by the tall ridge of Ontario Peak. The San Timoteo Badlands to the east contrast with the subdivisions that stretch for miles across the valleys.

A rough fire road leads north from the summit. The myriad use trails in the area suggest that some hikers continue north and then loop back via one of the other paths.

---

trip 7.9   Terri Peak

Distance	4 miles (out-and-back)
Hiking Time	2 hours
Elevation Gain	800'
Difficulty	Moderate
Trail Use	Suitable for mountain biking, suitable for equestrians
Best Times	October–May
Agency	Lake Perris State Recreation Area
Optional Maps	USGS *Perris* and *Sunnymead* 7.5'
Permit	$10 day-use fee required

DIRECTIONS From the 60 Freeway in Moreno Valley, 6 miles east of the 215 Freeway, take Exit 65 south onto Moreno Beach Drive. Follow Moreno Beach Drive 3.4 miles, and turn left onto Via Del Lago.

This hike can begin inside or outside Lake Perris State Recreation Area. To begin outside, pull off the right side of Via Del Lago in 0.4 mile at the south end of a gated development near the beginning of a white-fenced walking trail. To begin inside, continue another 0.8 mile to the entry station and pay your admission fee. Turn right onto a paved road 0.1 mile beyond the entry station. Go 0.4 mile; then, immediately beyond the Campfire Center, turn right onto a good dirt road to the Horse Group Camp. Follow it 0.4 mile, staying left at a junction with a service road, and park near a corral, taking care not to block anyone camping there.

Lake Perris was built in 1973 as a reservoir at the southern end of the 444-mile California Aqueduct. Each year nearly 100 billion gallons of water flow through the lake and on to Riverside and San Diego Counties. The land around Lake Perris has been set aside as a California State Recreation Area. It primarily draws boaters, picnickers, and anglers, but the hills surrounding the lake are of interest to hikers and rock climbers. Terri Peak overlooks the facilities on the northwest side of the lake and offers a moderate climb with fine views of the lake and nearby communities. It's especially worth visiting in March and April, when the wildflowers are in bloom.

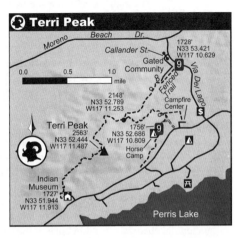

The hike can begin inside or outside the State Recreation Area and can involve a simple jaunt to the peak and back or a longer loop. Starting inside involves paying a substantial admission fee and the trailhead lacks good parking and signage, so the outside start is recommended unless you want to visit the Ya'i Heki' Regional Indian Museum and picnic by the lake.

If you start on the north side outside the park, follow the fenced walking path along the southeast boundary of the gated community. Young children may be frightened by aggressively barking dogs roaming the backyards. In 0.4 mile, reach a water tank and flood-control basin. Turn left, pass a gate, and follow a paved road up toward another water tank. In 0.1 mile, just before you reach the second tank, turn left again, pass another gate, and hike up a dirt road that's now closed to vehicles. The road leads past brittlebushes and other coastal sage scrub for 0.6 mile to a T-junction with the trail from Horse Group Camp. Turn right and continue 0.9 mile to the summit.

If you start at the Horse Group Camp, walk back up the road 0.1 mile, and turn left onto an unmarked trail that shortcuts to the service road that you passed on the way in. Follow the road up another 0.1 mile to a water tank in a grove of trees. On the north side of the road, look for two trails. One leads east down to the campfire circle, but our trail goes northwest up the mountain. It gradually climbs 0.7 mile to reach the junction with the trail from the north side of the mountain. Continue up another 0.9 mile to the summit. Retrace your steps to your vehicle.

ALTERNATIVE FINISH

If you started in the park, consider making a longer loop down to the Ya'i Heki' Regional Indian Museum and back along the lakeshore. A faint 1.2-mile trail continues west from Terri Peak and descends the southwest ridge before turning south and arriving at a marker at the west end of the parking area for the Indian museum. Unfortunately, the path is rarely maintained and can be overgrown with scratchy brush, which detracts from this otherwise appealing route. Long pants are highly recommended. At this writing, the museum was open 10 a.m.–4 p.m. on weekends and 10 a.m.–2 p.m. on Fridays.

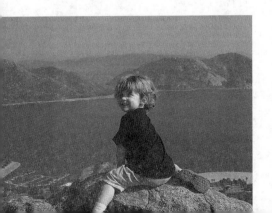

Lake Perris from Terri Peak

trip 7.10   South Hills Preserve: Jedi Trail

Distance	5 miles (out-and-back)
Hiking Time	2.5 hours
Elevation Gain	800'
Difficulty	Moderate
Trail Use	Suitable for mountain biking, suitable for equestrians
Best Times	October–April
Agency	Loma Linda Public Works Department
Optional Map	USGS *Redlands* 7.5'

DIRECTIONS From the 10 Freeway, take Exit 75 for Mountain View Avenue and drive south through Loma Linda 2 miles. At the entrance of Hulda Crooks Park, veer left and park on the east side of the basketball and tennis courts. The trail starts at the south end of the parking lot. On the opposite side of the courts is an attractive playground with picnic benches and a restroom.

The hills on the south side of Loma Linda represent the last gasp of the Peninsular Ranges, which extend from San Jacinto south into Baja California. Thrust up from an ancient lakebed by the confluence of the San Jacinto, Banning, and Loma Linda Faults, the sedimentary hills are now laced with an intricate web of trails and dirt roads. Tremendously popular with mountain bikers, they also draw large numbers of hikers. The most popular route ascends Scott Canyon to the narrow, winding Jedi Trail. The ridge at the end of the trail offers spectacular views in all directions. My favorite time is winter, when the grass grows green and the snowcapped peaks ringing the basin stand out in the crisp air. Hulda Crooks Park is named in honor of an American mountaineer and longtime Loma Linda

Snowy San Bernardino Peak towers beyond South Hills Preserve.

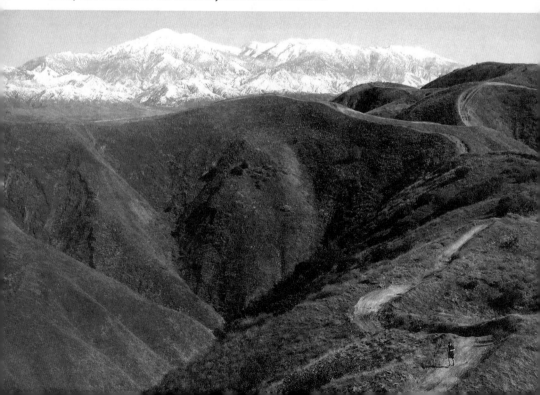

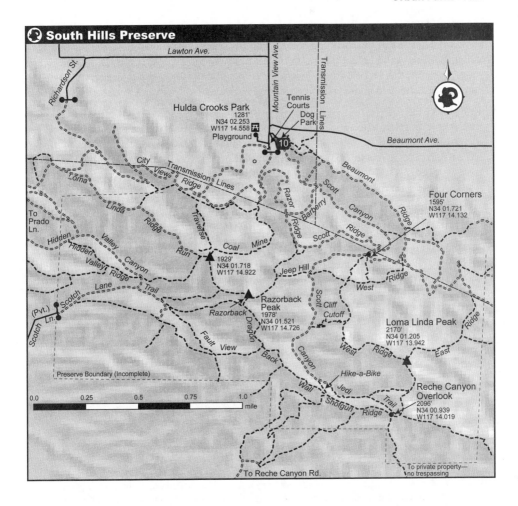

South Hills Preserve

Lawton Ave.

Richardson St.

Mountain View Ave.

Transmission Lines

Hulda Crooks Park
1281'
N34 02.253
W117 14.558
Playground

Tennis
Courts
Dog
Park

10

Beaumont Ave.

City
View

Transmission Lines

Loma

Linda

Ridge

Traverse

Beaumont

Scott

Razor Ridge

Barberry

Canyon

Scott
Ridge

Four Corners
1595'
N34 01.721
W117 14.132

Ridge

To
Prado
Ln.

Hidden

Hidden
Valley

Valley

Ridge

Canyon

Run

Coal   Mine
1929'
N34 01.718
W117 14.922

Jeep Hill

Ridge

West

Lane

Trail

Scotch

Scott

Cliff
Cutoff

(Pvt.)

Scotch Ln.

Razorback

Dragon

Razorback
Peak
1978'
N34 01.521
W117 14.726

Loma Linda Peak
2170'
N34 01.205
W117 13.942

Ridge

Fault
View

Back

Canyon

West   Ridge

East

Preserve Boundary (Incomplete)

Wall

Hike-a-Bike

Jedi

Reche Canyon
Overlook
2096'
N34 00.939
W117 14.019

0.0   0.25   0.5   0.75   1.0
mile

Shotgun   Ridge

Trail

To Reche Canyon Rd.

To private property—
no trespassing

resident. Known as "Grandma Whitney," Crooks scaled California's tallest peak 23 times between the ages of 65 and 91.

The City of Loma Linda established the South Hills Preserve in 2008. It's presently the Wild West of city wilderness parks: the trailheads are unmarked, and one key entry point is still posted with a defunct NO TRESPASSING sign. Some of the trails are extremely steep with dramatic drop-offs or severe erosion. Teams of daredevil cyclists, acting on their own authority, are often seen building new jumps and obstacles. Although the park is legally closed to motorized vehicles, the closure isn't yet posted and the southern portion of the preserve commonly buzzes with the whining of motorbikes that are tearing up ridges and causing erosion. The boundaries of the city land are unmarked, and many trails lead out of the preserve onto private land, but all of the trails have had a long tradition of use by hikers and cyclists dating back before the city acquired the land. The hills are a vital wildlife corridor and are home to coyotes and rattlesnakes as well as deer, redtail hawks, and an occasional cougar. As you would anywhere, watch your step and travel in a group for safety.

From the far (south) end of the parking area, walk south toward a concrete dam and debris basin on a wide dirt road. Skirt the left edge of the basin and follow the dirt road up Scott Canyon. Numerous side trails tempt the curious, but this trip stays on the main road along the canyon bottom. In 1.1 miles, reach Four Corners where the Scott Ridge and Beaumont Ridge Roads meet the canyon. Continue up Scott Canyon. In another mile, the road deteriorates to a winding rutted trail that mountain bikers find challenging and delightful. Stay on the main path as you pass trails entering side canyons. In another 0.5 mile, emerge at the Reche Canyon Overlook Trail junction atop Shotgun Ridge, where you can catch your breath and admire the views.

VARIATIONS

The simplest option is to return the way you came. However, the adventurous hiker will investigate one of the countless more interesting alternatives. One popular route is to turn left and climb to Loma Linda Peak, the high point of the preserve. Veer left down the narrow West Ridge Trail. When the West Ridge Trail ends at a power line service road, continue straight onto the Beaumont Ridge Road, which leads north and then northwest back to the trailhead. This option has great views and is scarcely longer.

Another great route is to turn right and follow Shotgun Ridge, named for a former landowner known for aggressively dissuading trespassers. Climb the aptly named Wall and continue along Dragon Back to the short but dramatic Razor Back that leads to Razorback Peak. Turn left and follow the Loma Linda Ridge Run to a second hilltop; then turn right and drop down the Coal Mine Trail on the way back to the trailhead. This option is also scarcely longer, although it crosses some wild and poorly signed portions of the preserve.

---

trip 7.11   San Timoteo Nature Sanctuary

Distance	3.4 miles (loop)
Hiking Time	2 hours
Elevation Gain	200'
Difficulty	Easy
Trail Use	Dogs allowed, suitable for mountain biking, suitable for equestrians
Best Times	October–June
Agency	Redlands Conservancy
Optional Map	USGS *Redlands* 7.5'

DIRECTIONS From the 10 Freeway in Redlands, take Exit 76 south for California Street. In 1.3 miles, turn left onto Barton Road. In 0.5 mile, turn right onto San Timoteo Canyon Road. In 3.6 miles, turn left onto Alessandro Road. In 0.4 mile, park in the dirt on the left side of the road, by the signed entrance to the nature sanctuary.

San Timoteo Nature Sanctuary is a 166-acre preserve alongside San Timoteo Creek owned by the City of Redlands and managed by the Redlands Conservancy. It serves as a wildlife corridor connecting open space in the region, and as riparian habitat. This trip follows a historic carriage road through the canyon and up to a vista point. Keep your eyes open for wildlife. Native Americans have used this canyon as a trade route for centuries. More recently, it has served as a stagecoach route and the Southern Pacific Railroad route; it also was considered as a possible route for the 10 Freeway.

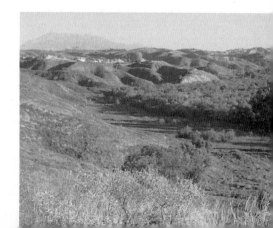

Citrus orchards and South Hills beyond San Timoteo Creek

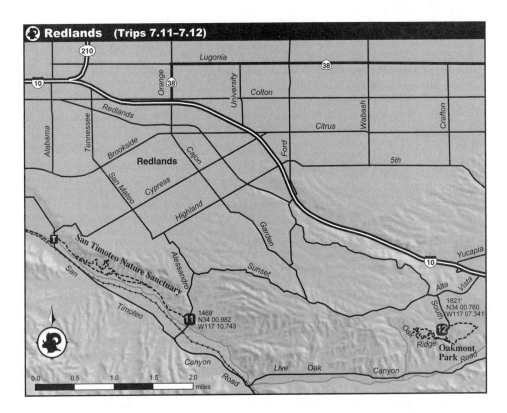

Enter through the gate and sign in at the register. Follow Carriage Road, a trail originally constructed in the late 1800s by the Smiley brothers, two of Redlands' founding fathers. Visitors used the path to reach Canyon Crest Park, a 200-acre botanical garden on the Smileys' resort. After repeated wildfires, dryland farming, and sheep grazing, the native sage scrub has been supplanted by invasive tumbleweeds. Restoration will be a major undertaking.

The trail passes the Bobcat Bowl assembly area, and then the canyon narrows and becomes more scenic. Squeeze between the willow-lined creek and the sheer canyon wall. At 0.7 mile, come to a fork. Stay right on the Carriage Trail, which, in another 0.7 mile, enters a side canyon with a eucalyptus grove planted by the Smileys.

Take a spur on the right that climbs to the Canyon Lookout on the hill. From here, you can take in views of the South Hills Preserve over the citrus orchards. San Jacinto and Cucamonga Peaks are visible on opposite skylines. Ridgetop mansions stand just above you, and the San Timoteo Landfill is cut into the South Hills. The Union Pacific tracks run through the canyon and you'll likely see or hear a train roll through during your hike. Brittlebush is the dominant scrub, appearing dead in the summer and fall but turning green and sprouting a beautiful yellow flower after the winter rains.

Return to the main trail and continue out of the side canyon to a connector trail on the left that descends to the Cocomaricopa Trail paralleling the creek. Turn left again and return to the parking area.

VARIATION

Continue on the Carriage Trail to meet San Timoteo Canyon Road at the northwest end of the sanctuary. Going out and back on this segment adds 1.9 miles to the trip.

trip 7.12 **Oakmont Park**

Distance	3.4 miles (loop)
Hiking Time	2 hours
Elevation Gain	400'
Difficulty	Easy
Trail Use	Dogs allowed, good for kids, suitable for mountain biking, suitable for equestrians
Best Times	October–June
Agency	Redlands Conservancy
Optional Maps	USGS *Yucaipa* and *Redlands* 7.5'

see map on previous page

DIRECTIONS From the 10 Freeway, take Exit 83 south for Yucaipa Boulevard. In 0.1 mile, turn left onto the frontage road. In 0.3 mile, turn right onto Alta Vista Drive. In 0.7 mile, turn left onto South Lane. In 0.6 mile, turn left into unsigned Oakmont Park.

Oakmont Park is a great place for a ramble about the oaks, wildflower-strewn meadows, and viewful ridges. The park features two loop trails: the Oakmont Trail to the east (with more trees and meadows) and the Oak Ridge Trail to the west (steeper, with more views). This trip takes you on both.

From the parking area, walk back to the park entrance and turn right onto unsigned Oakmont Trail, following the fenceline along South Lane. The trail soon veers right away from the road and climbs a hill, reaching a junction in 0.3 mile. Go left, cross the meadow, and make an immediate right on the far side. In 0.1 mile, continue straight onto a fire road.

Take the fire road down into the oak-studded canyon, where you reach another junction by a large coast live oak in 0.3 mile. Turn hard right and continue down the canyon, crossing some social trails. In 0.4 mile, turn right to leave the canyon and return to a kiosk at the bottom of Oakmont Park.

To make the Oak Ridge Loop, turn left at the kiosk onto a trail signed TRAIL NO. 1, and climb the switchbacks 0.4 mile to a junction on the ridge. From here, you have fine views of the San Bernardino Mountains over the park. Turn right to make a counterclockwise loop. In another 0.4 mile, reach paved Silverleaf Court. Cross the road and pass through a gate onto a paved service road, which you descend 0.1 mile to where the trail resumes on the left. This unusual trail weaves in and out of each canyon before returning to the ridgetop junction to complete the loop.

Descend to the kiosk, and then turn left to walk through the live oaks and return to your vehicle.

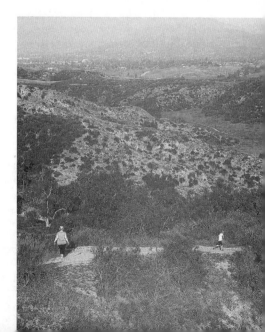

Descending the ridge to Oakmont Park

see map on next page

trip 7.13 **Wildwood Canyon State Park**

Distance	2.6 miles (loop)
Hiking Time	1.5 hours
Elevation Gain	500'
Difficulty	Easy
Trail Use	Good for kids, suitable for mountain biking, suitable for equestrians
Best Times	All year, but hot in summer (day use only)
Agency	California State Parks (in development)
Optional Map	USGS *Forest Falls* 7.5' (trails not marked)

DIRECTIONS From the 10 Freeway, take Exit 83 east for Yucaipa Boulevard and go 5 miles to Bryant Street. Turn right (south) and go 1.2 miles to Wildwood Canyon Road. Turn left (east) and go 1.8 miles to narrow Canyon Drive, the first left turn past Mesa Grande Drive. Go 0.1 mile and park in the large dirt equestrian staging area on the right side of Canyon Drive.

Wildwood Canyon, scarcely a stone's throw from Yucaipa's bustling center, invites you to hike along shady trails past historic ranches. It's enormously popular with local equestrians but was until recently a well-kept secret outside of Yucaipa. A developer purchased the canyon in the 1980s and planned to build thousands of homes, but a fortuitous accidental fire and subsequent flooding delayed construction and ultimately the developer sold the land to the Yucaipa Valley Conservancy. The State of California purchased the 850-acre parcel to establish a new state park, dedicated in 2003. Unfortunately, California State Parks has been inadequately funded, and the park has seen very little development.

Wildwood Canyon is laced with trails on seemingly every ridge and canyon. Fast-growing brush periodically overtakes some of the trails until dedicated volunteers cut them clear. When the state park opens, it's possible that some trails will change. By the time you visit, the map and trail description may no longer exactly match the situation. Take a careful look at the landmarks and remember that traveling downhill or southwest will generally lead you back toward the trailhead should you become disoriented. This trip describes a

Oaks in Wildwood Canyon

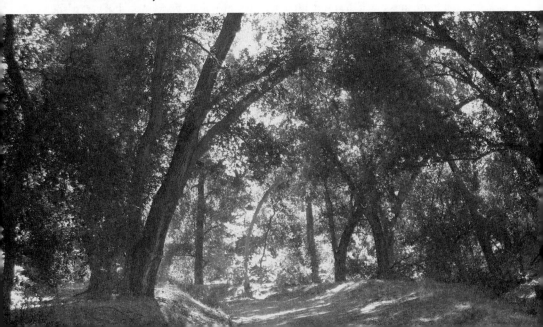

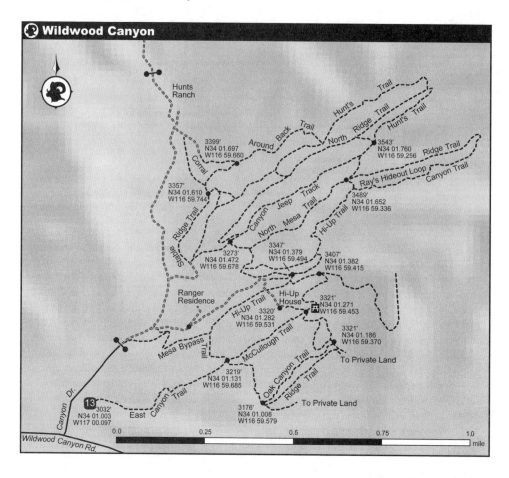

Wildwood Canyon

Hunts Ranch

Hunt's Trail

Trail

North Ridge Trail

Hunt's Trail

3399'
N34 01.697
W116 59.660

Around Back Trail

Ridge Trail

3543'
N34 01.760
W116 59.256

Corral

3357'
N34 01.610
W116 59.744

Ridge Trail

Ray's Hideout Loop

Canyon Trail

Canyon Jeep Track

3489'
N34 01.652
W116 59.336

North Mesa Trail

Hi-Up Trail

Stable

3273'
N34 01.472
W116 59.678

3347'
N34 01.379
W116 59.494

3407'
N34 01.382
W116 59.415

Ranger Residence

Hi-Up Trail

Hi-Up House

3321'
N34 01.271
W116 59.453

Hi-Up Trail

3320'
N34 01.282
W116 59.531

McCullough Trail

3321'
N34 01.186
W116 59.370

Mesa Bypass Trail

Oak Canyon Trail

To Private Land

3219'
N34 01.131
W116 59.685

Ridge Trail

To Private Land

Canyon Dr.

East Canyon Trail

13
3032'
N34 01.003
W117 00.097

3176'
N34 01.008
W116 59.579

0.0   0.25   0.5   0.75   1.0

mile

Wildwood Canyon Rd.

short loop through some of the most attractive parts of Wildwood Canyon, but part of the fun of the park is to roam the twisting maze and explore the rich trail network.

The Cahuilla and Serrano Indians used to come to Wildwood Canyon to gather acorns before continuing up to Yucaipa Ridge in search of pine nuts. Canyon Road follows one of their ancient trails, and shards of pottery can still be found. More recently, miners and ranchers have occupied the canyon, which was long known as Hog Canyon until a developer decided that "Wildwood" was more marketable. Feral pigs roamed the canyon into the 1990s. Animals and birds now visit the canyon in search of water and food. If you're fortunate, you may see deer, bears, or even shy mountain lions.

The East Canyon Trail starts beside the ruins of a 1920s lodge and leads east into the mysterious oak groves. Water once ran year-round in the creek, but Southern California's insatiable demand for water has lowered the water table and dried up the creek. In 0.5 mile, come to a four-way junction. Turn right and hike 0.2 mile to another junction in a ravine. Turn left here onto the Oak Canyon Trail and follow the cool canyon, which lights up with wildflowers in the spring. Watch out for poison oak and look for the spiny and inedible wild cucumber growing on vines.

In 0.3 mile, come to a T-junction on a ridge. Turn left and promptly reach another junction. An unmaintained old wagon road veers right, but this trip curves left on the trail that cuts through the chamise. Enjoy the views; to the south is Black Mountain and the Hidden Meadows subdivision, and to the southwest is Santiago Peak, the high point of Orange County. Pass the wagon road again on your right before you reach another four-way junction. The trail straight ahead leads to the Hi-Up House, and the Hi-Up Trail to the left returns to the trailhead, but this trip turns right toward a picnic bench and tie rail.

The trail curves around and reaches a T-junction with a wagon road in 0.2 mile. The McCullough family cut this road decades ago to climb onto the hill to the right where they could watch glorious sunsets. This trip turns left down the road and passes fields of buckwheat. Veer right where the road becomes overgrown, and pass a trail on the left leading down toward the house. Shortly after, reach another T-junction. The right path leads to the former site of Huebner's Ranch, but we turn left (west) and reach a graded dirt road.

Consider making a short excursion to the left (south) on the dirt road to see the Hi-Up House, well situated to command an excellent view. The resourceful McCollough family built the house during the Great Depression using mostly recycled materials. The blocks are from an icehouse that burned down in Yucaipa. Surplus wood came from a job site at March Air Force Base. Boulders were collected from Mill Creek.

Return along the dirt road, which turns west. Follow it down through a lovely grove of oaks that arch gracefully over the road. When you reach a T-junction with the main road, turn left and follow it down past a gate to the trailhead.

VARIATION

If you haven't had enough, you can explore more of the intricate web of trails that follow almost every ridge and valley in Wildwood Canyon. Beware that trail conditions are highly variable, but the fun is in the discovery. The chaparral provides shelter and food for numerous birds, lizards, and other small animals. It's not uncommon to hear the piercing cry of a hawk circling overhead in search of prey. Be particularly alert on these trails for poison oak bushes in the canyons and rattlesnakes prowling the tall grass looking for rodents.

---

trip 7.14   Crafton Hills: Park-to-Peak Loop

Distance	5 miles (loop)
Hiking Time	2.5 hours
Elevation Gain	1,100'
Difficulty	Moderate
Trail Use	Dogs allowed, suitable for mountain biking
Best Times	October–April
Agency	Crafton Hills Open Space Conservancy, Yucaipa Regional Park
Optional Map	USGS *Yucaipa* 7.5'

see map on next page

Crafton Hills

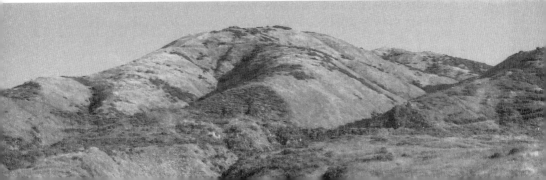

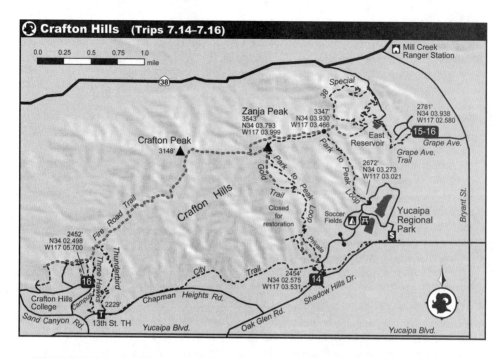

Crafton Hills (Trips 7.14–7.16)

DIRECTIONS From the 10 Freeway, take Exit 83 north/east for Yucaipa Boulevard. Proceed 2.9 miles, and then veer left onto Oak Glen Road. In 1.0 mile, turn left into the Oak Glen Road Trailhead parking area, opposite Shadow Hills Drive.

This loop is the shortest way to reach Zanja Peak and offers the greatest diversity of scenery. The steep climb provides a great workout. Gold Gulch, just west of the trail, was the site of California's first gold-mining operations from 1820 to 1840. Dozens of adits (horizontal mine shafts), most tight enough to require crawling, were chopped into the hillside in search of the precious metal. The shafts are now unsafe for entry. The trip ends with a walk through Yucaipa Regional Park. Tent and RV camping is available at the regional park.

Starting from the message board/trail map, hike northeast up the paved road beyond a gate. In 0.2 mile, take a dirt road to the left. In 60 yards, a trail forks right and a dirt road forks left, but stay straight on the main path. In another 300 yards, the road comes to an end in the canyon, and you take the marked trail on the left that switchbacks onto a ridge.

In 0.4 mile, come to an unsigned fork at an old road cut. The path to the left joins an old firebreak that climbs extremely steeply up the ridge (and is closed for restoration), but the Zanja Peak Trail stays right and follows a good trail that soon climbs along the west wall of a scenic canyon. About two-thirds of the way up, come to a fork with the Gold Trail on the left that climbs to join the upper part of the firebreak; both paths run parallel, so you can take either one and rejoin just below Zanja Peak. Continue up to the high point of the Crafton Hills.

After enjoying the summit views, follow a trail to the right that leads northeast along the crest of the Crafton Hills. In 0.6 mile, the trail passes alongside a fire road that also runs along the crest. But stay right on the trail and descend 1.1 miles through another canyon to reach the paved road at a trailhead marker in Yucaipa Regional Park.

Families with young children may enjoy a detour to the fine playground on a peninsula in the lake below. Otherwise, turn right and follow the road, which crosses a ravine and then turns south. Pass a road leading right to the group tent camping area; then make a right just after and follow a road past the large group picnic shelters. Go around a yellow gate to some soccer fields and follow the road along the south side of the fenced earthworks back to your starting point, 1.0 mile from the Yucaipa Regional Park Trailhead.

trip 7.15 Crafton Hills: Grape Avenue Trail

Distance	4.7 miles (loop)
Hiking Time	2 hours
Elevation Gain	1,000'
Difficulty	Moderate
Trail Use	Dogs allowed, suitable for mountain biking, suitable for equestrians
Best Times	October–April
Agency	Crafton Hills Open Space Conservancy
Optional Map	USGS *Yucaipa* 7.5'

DIRECTIONS From the 10 Freeway, take Exit 83 north/east for Yucaipa Boulevard. Proceed 2.9 miles, and then veer left onto Oak Glen Road. In 2.6 miles, turn left onto Bryant Street. In 1.1 miles, turn left onto Grape Avenue. In 0.5 mile, park on the residential street. The trailhead is marked with a small sign on the south side of the road, just before you reach a house at 34889 Grape Ave.

This hike explores the east end of the Crafton Hills, with good views into Oak Glen and San Gorgonio Wilderness. The first part of the trail leads behind a neighborhood to East Reservoir. The trail then climbs to the Crafton Hills backbone and loops around before returning. This area burned in the 2013 Mill Fire, so watch for the process of regeneration in the fire's aftermath.

From the trailhead, follow the narrow path southwest into the chaparral. Even though the trail backs up against a row of houses, the dense trees give you an immediate sense of entering the wilderness. In 0.3 mile, climb to a ridge marked by a metal tower. Stay right at a fork and descend behind a house 0.2 mile to an access road below a dam. Follow the trail 0.3 mile up to the right (east) end of the dam, where you meet the paved dam-access road. Follow the well-marked trail, which heads west overlooking East Reservoir for 0.1 mile to a signed junction with the 38 Special Trail on the right. This loop ascends the left trail and returns on the 38 Special on the right.

Follow the left trail 0.6 mile as it switchbacks up to a junction where it rejoins the 38 Special Trail. From here, you can continue west for a mile to Zanja Peak before you return; otherwise, head down the right fork on the north side of the hills. The first section has multiple paths, giving you the option of switchbacking or descending straight down the ridge.

In 0.2 mile, veer right at a fork and hike across the head of a canyon, then down another ridge overlooking Mill Creek; then switchback into a canyon and arrive at a paved road in 0.9 mile. Turn right and hike up the road 0.2 mile until you can pick up another trail on the right that follows an old road cut 0.4 mile back up to the junction above East Reservoir. Then return the way you started.

East Reservoir

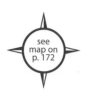

see
map on
p. 172

trip 7.16 Crafton Hills: Hilltop Trail

Distance	7 miles (out-and-back)
Hiking Time	3 hours
Elevation Gain	1,200'
Difficulty	Moderate
Trail Use	Dogs allowed, suitable for mountain biking, suitable for equestrians
Best Times	October–April
Agency	Crafton Hills Open Space Conservancy
Optional Map	USGS *Yucaipa* 7.5'

DIRECTIONS From the 10 Freeway, take Exit 83 north/east for Yucaipa Boulevard. Proceed 1.6 miles, and then turn left onto Sand Canyon Road. In 0.3 mile, turn right at Campus Drive into Crafton Hills College. In 0.4 mile, where the road bends left, look for free trailhead parking on the right.

This hike follows the crest of the Crafton Hills from their southwest terminus at Crafton Hills College to the high point at Zanja Peak (3,543'). You can follow the gently graded fire road, or choose to hike the steep strenuous trail that undulates along the very tops of the hills. This hike offers fine views and a good workout.

From the trailhead, a short spur on the right leads to the Three Hawks Trail. Turn left and follow it up to join the Fire Road Trail on the ridgeline. Turn right and follow the fire road northeast, soon passing the Thunderbird Trail. At various junctures, you have a choice of staying on the easy road or taking steeper but shorter trails directly along the ridgetop. In about 3 miles, the trail runs alongside the road just below Zanja Peak; there are fine views along the ridge. Follow the trail 0.2 mile northeast to the summit, where you can take in the 360-degree panorama.

Return the way you came or, with a car or bicycle shuttle, explore more of the trail network lacing the Crafton Hills.

VARIATION

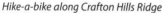

The Three Hawks and Thunderbird Trails can be combined to make a 2.3-mile loop with 600 feet of elevation gain.

Hike-a-bike along Crafton Hills Ridge

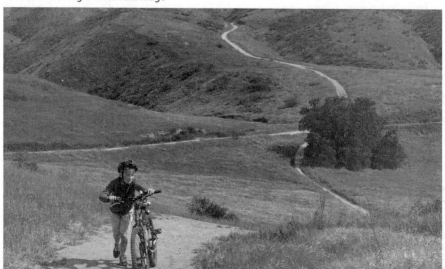

trip 7.17   El Dorado Ranch Park

Distance	3.5 miles (semiloop)
Hiking Time	2 hours
Elevation Gain	500'
Difficulty	Easy
Trail Use	Dogs allowed, good for kids, suitable for mountain biking, suitable for equestrians
Best Times	October–June
Agency	City of Yucaipa Parks and Recreation
Optional Map	USGS *Forest Falls* 7.5'

DIRECTIONS From the 10 Freeway, take Exit 85 for Oak Glen Road and follow it northeast 6.7 miles to El Dorado Ranch Park, on the left side of the road at 37216 Oak Glen Road.

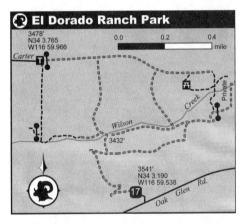

El Dorado Ranch Park is a 334-acre open-space preserve located along seasonal Wilson Creek, at the foot of Yucaipa Ridge. This area is especially appealing in the winter and spring, when you may find the creek running beside wildflowers or beneath snowcapped mountains. This trip describes a loop around the perimeter. A maze of trails crosses the center of the park, and you can visit several times to explore them all.

The Cahuilla and Serrano peoples once used this area and you might still recognize their trails and stone artifacts. Be sure not to disturb or remove artifacts. T. J. Wilson came to the area to establish a resort and developed the early water system in the 1860s. By the 1880s, the site was a ranch producing grain and honey. The Wildlands Conservancy and Yucaipa Valley Conservancy eventually acquired the land to protect the threatened alluvial sage scrub habitat, then donated it to the City of Yucaipa, which opened the park in 2014.

The trail, a broad dirt road, begins behind the picnic area and meanders down across a ravine, then down the steep lip into Wilson Creek. At the bottom of the grade, 0.6 mile from the start, turn right to make a counterclockwise loop. You'll encounter many road and trail junctions along the loop—stay right at each one to make the largest loop.

Hike east and then north; then stay right at a fork near Wilson Creek. Shortly beyond, come to ruins of an old water system near a gate where the dirt road exits the eastern end of the park into private lands. Turn left onto a trail that follows the fenceline and crosses riparian lands. Be alert for stinging nettles. On the far side of the creek, stay right at a T-junction of trails, and soon reach the east end of another dirt road that runs along the north edge of the property.

Follow this dirt road west, passing three roads on the left. The first leads to a picnic area

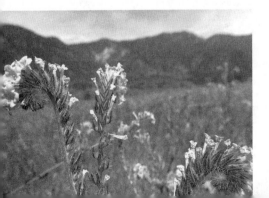

Phacelia blooms in March at El Dorado Ranch.

with hitching posts. Eventually, the road ends at a gate on the eastern end of Carter Street. This is an alternative trailhead for the park.

Turn left onto another narrow trail and follow it south along the western fenceline of the park. Just before Wilson Creek, pass a road on the left. Cross the creek and turn east near the foot of the bluffs. As you walk through the riparian zone, watch for both poison oak and *Rhus trilobata,* a three-leaved plant known as fake poison oak because it's easily confused with its hazardous cousin.

Soon rejoin the road. Turn right and then stay right at two more junctions to rejoin the path at the bottom of the grade where the loop began. Head back up the grade and to your vehicle.

trip 7.18 Bogart Park Loop

Distance	3.5 miles (loop)
Hiking Time	2 hours
Elevation Gain	600'
Difficulty	Easy
Trail Use	Dogs allowed, good for kids, suitable for equestrians
Best Times	September–May
Agency	Riverside County Regional Park and Open-Space District
Optional Map	USGS *Beaumont* 7.5'
Permit	$10 day-use fee required

DIRECTIONS From the 10 Freeway in Beaumont, take Exit 94 north for Beaumont Avenue. In 2.4 miles, turn right onto Brookside Avenue. In 0.8 mile, turn left onto Cherry Avenue. Proceed 1.5 miles to the park entrance, pay your day-use fee, and ask for the pamphlet describing the Nature Trail. The road's name changes to International Park Road. Continue 0.3 mile and park at the signed Oak Parking Area, on the left.

Bogart Park is a 414-acre parcel at the north end of Cherry Valley in the foothills of the San Bernardino Mountains managed by the Riverside County Regional Park and Open-Space District. The park offers hiking, picnicking, and camping along the oak-shaded banks of Noble Creek. It's beautiful in many seasons, especially in late March when the cherry trees blossom.

Bogart Park is a favorite destination among locals, but has faded into obscurity for most residents of Riverside County. Its origins lie in the Great Depression, when the community banded together to host a Japanese Cherry Blossom Festival. The first festival, held March 30, 1930, attracted 32,000 visitors to the tiny village of Beaumont. Dr. Guy Bogart, president of the Beaumont Rotary Club, went looking for a more suitable location for the next year's festival and identified the canyon that's now the site of the park. The government lacked the money to purchase the land, so 25 local businessmen joined together to buy the property for the county in time for the 1931 event. The land was named International Park, dedicated to international peace. Unfortunately, World War II and the Cold War soon ended the affection for Japan and hopes for world peace. In 1957, the county renamed the park in honor of Dr. Bogart.

The park, open 8 a.m.–sunset every day except Tuesday and Wednesday, features an elaborate system of poorly marked trails. This trip makes a counterclockwise loop around the park. Identifying all of the unmarked junctions is difficult, but as long as you stay on trails and don't veer far away from the paved road through the park, you'll eventually get where you want to go. Many long trails, popular among equestrians, veer off into the hills.

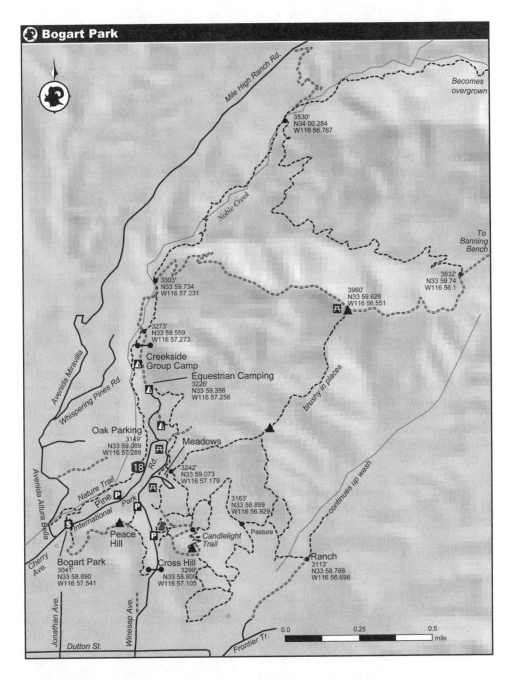

Turn back if you find yourself straying onto these trails, unless you're looking for a longer ramble. The trail map available at the entrance station is cute but has only the loosest relationship with the actual trails.

A sign at the southwest corner of the Oak Parking area indicates the start of the Nature Trail. Hike southwest on the trail past numbered signposts. The trail immediately splits, then soon rejoins to cross Noble Creek. It then splits again. The two branches run close by

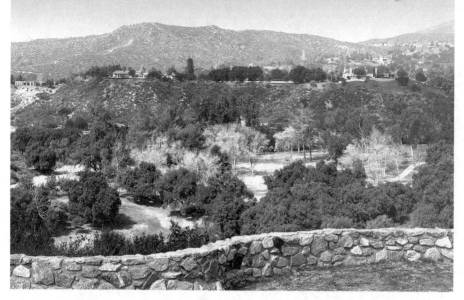

Views from Cross Hill

each other, so take either one. In 0.2 mile, the branches rejoin. You could follow the other branch back for a half-mile nature loop, but this trip continues straight. In 0.1 mile, turn left at a fork. Descend 0.1 mile to International Park Road by the entrance station. Cross the road and climb steeply up a trail on the south side 0.1 mile to reach a dirt road by a stable.

Turn left and follow the road 0.4 mile up to the top of David Starr Jordan Peace Hill, now marked with a green water tank. The hill was named for a former president of Stanford University, a peace activist and explorer of the wilderness. Join a trail that passes around the right side of the tank and descends to a paved park road just north of a gate in 0.3 mile.

Turn left and hike 0.1 mile up the road. Shortly before you reach the parking lot for a small lake, turn right onto a marked trail. The trail crosses the creek below a dam and then climbs steeply. Stay right at a fork; the left path descends to the lake. In 0.1 mile, reach a dirt road. Turn right and follow it 0.2 mile as it corkscrews up to the top of Cross Hill. A stone foundation marks the site where a large cross once stood. This hill offers the best views of the trip.

Descend the stone-lined Candlelight Trail that switchbacks down the north side of the hill to rejoin the road in 0.2 mile at a complicated five-way junction. A horse trail leads to the right (east). A dirt road makes a hairpin turn here, and both sides depart to the left (west). But this trip goes straight ahead on a trail to the north. In less than 0.1 mile, go left at a junction. In 0.2 mile, reach a four-way junction near the Meadows parking area. Families might enjoy turning left down to the Meadows, where a playground is located beside the field. This trip, however, goes straight to a T-junction near a paved road, then turns right.

Follow the trail north 0.7 mile, passing above a picnic area and campground, until you reach the equestrian campground. Turn right on a dirt road and hike through the Creekside Group Camp beneath the mature canyon oaks. Pass a gate indicating road closure; this

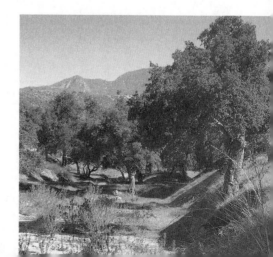

Oaks along Noble Creek

doesn't apply to foot traffic. In 0.3 mile, the road crosses Noble Creek. You could continue exploring farther upstream, but this trip makes a sharp left turn onto a trail that returns to the south on the west side of the creek. The trail forks, but both branches run parallel and rejoin near the south end of the campgrounds. In another 0.1 mile, arrive back at the Oak Parking where you began.

VARIATION

Those seeking a more strenuous (5.5-mile, 1,200' elevation gain) loop will enjoy starting at the equestrian campground and heading north up Noble Creek. In 1.4 miles, turn right at a T onto an abandoned roadbed and climb southeast to a saddle. Stay right again and follow a ridge west back down to Noble Creek.

---

trip 7.19   ## Simpson Park

Distance	3.6 miles (loop)
Hiking Time	2.5 hours
Elevation Gain	900'
Difficulty	Moderate
Trail Use	Dogs allowed, suitable for mountain biking, suitable for equestrians
Best Times	November–April
Agency	City of Hemet Parks Department
Optional Map	USGS *Hemet* 7.5'

DIRECTIONS From Highway 74 in Hemet, take Stanford Street south 0.8 mile. Turn right onto Crest Drive and then immediately left onto Vista Del Valle, which eventually becomes Rawlings Road. In 1.6 miles, bear right through the gate into Simpson Park. In 0.9 mile, park at a covered picnic area.

Simpson Park is a 483-acre wilderness park in the unincorporated Santa Rosa Hills south of Hemet. The hills—not to be confused with the nearby Santa Rosa Mountains or Santa Rosa Plateau—are dotted with interesting granite boulders and chaparral and

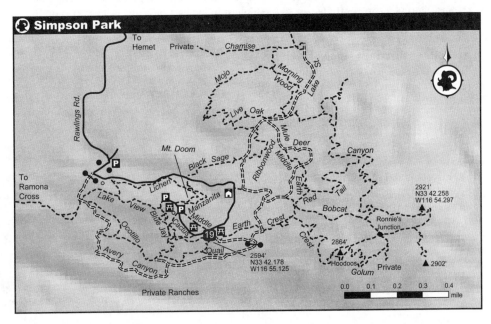

laced with an intricate web of trails that have become immensely popular with hikers and mountain bikers. Equestrians and jogging strollers use the dirt roads, and families enjoy scrambling on the rocks. This trip describes an outing to a high viewpoint, but a study of the map shows that many other loops between 1 and 15 miles are possible. Spring is an ideal time to visit as the park bursts into bloom. The park becomes dangerously hot in the summer. The park is open daily from 7 a.m. to 5 p.m. Beware that the automatic gates shut promptly at closing time and trap several visitors each week; park on Rawlings Road just outside the gate if you're unsure that you'll be out in time.

The hills are clad predominantly in chamise, mixed with buckwheat, thick-leaf yerba santa, brittlebush, and black sage. Trail signage is sporadic. To further complicate matters, a former city official randomly renamed the trails in 2007 after various plants, many of which are entirely inappropriate. Many trails extend onto public land beyond the park boundaries, but if you come to a NO TRESPASSING sign on a far-flung trail, you're encroaching on private land, so you should turn back. Studying the map will reveal countless enjoyable routes (avoid the steep and eroded Bobcat Trail); the description below highlights a fun loop through the eastern section.

From the east side of the picnic area, take the broad dirt road leading east. Immediately find a trail on the left, signed FOOT AND BICYCLE TRAFFIC ONLY. Both rejoin in 0.2 mile at the signed Crest Trail, locally known as the Slepski Trail in honor of Jeff Slepski, who has invested decades of volunteer labor to create and maintain the trail system.

Take the Crest/Slepski Trail east. Soon come to a fork; both paths soon rejoin but the left leg is shorter. Shortly after, pass the Red Tail Trail on the left and begin a set of switchbacks earnestly climbing the boulder-studded slopes. Enjoy magnificent views of four county high points: San Jacinto, San Gorgonio, San Antonio, and Santiago Peaks. In 0.9 mile from the picnic area, the trail tops out near Hoodoos (Peak 2,864'), a great place to rest and enjoy the view. Continue northeast 0.2 mile to a saddle known as Ronnie's Junction, commemorating a cyclist who loved these trails.

From here, the shortest option is to turn left (north) and follow the broad Upper Bobcat Trail 0.1 mile, then veer right at an unsigned fork onto the Canyon Trail. But a more interesting route is to continue east to the highest hill ahead, passing various trails on the right. A switchback brings you to a saddle just below the crest, from which you can take a climber's trail to the summit of Peak 2,921'. Take a rest and enjoy the stunning views of San Jacinto and San Gorgonio over the orchards of the valley. Then continue west to an unmarked junction with the aforementioned Canyon Trail, and turn right.

Descend the Canyon Trail, whose curves and obstacles are a mountain biker's delight. Various spurs fork off the main path, including the Red Tail Trail, which makes for an enjoyable alternate return. In 1.2 miles, the Canyon Trail ends at the broad dirt Lake Road. Turn left and follow it 0.4 mile up to the

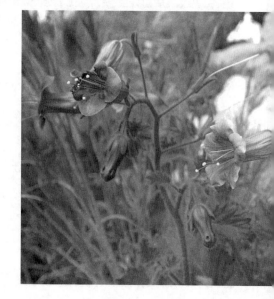

Canterbury bells (Phacelia minor)

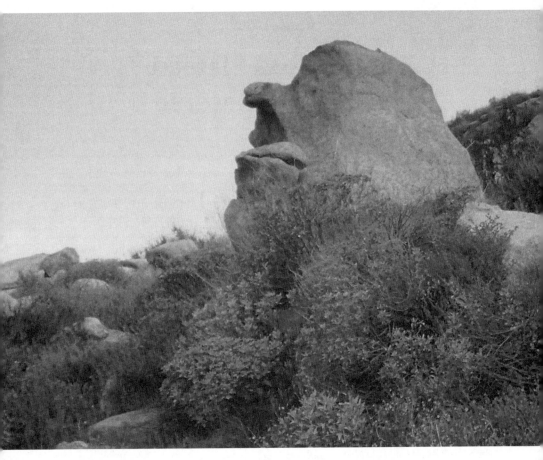

Gargoyle Rock

visitor center/park residence, and then stay left on paved Rawlings Road and continue 0.3 mile to the picnic area where you began.

VARIATION

For a 6-mile (1,000' elevation gain) grand tour visiting even more of the park's best features, start at the gate at the entrance to Simpson Park. Enter the park on the main road; then take the Lichen, Manzanita, Black Sage, Ribbonwood, Live Oak, Mojo, Morning Wood, Canyon, and Bobcat Trails to Ronnie's Junction; then turn hard right and take the Crest Trail to Hoodoos. Descend the Crest Trail; then turn left on the dirt road, pass through a gate, and follow the Avery Canyon Road, Quail, and Ocotillo Trails back to the entrance. Navigation is difficult on these often-unsigned trails, but everything eventually loops back so it's fine to stray from this suggested route.

chapter 8

Santa Rosa Plateau Ecological Reserve

If you've ever wondered what Southern California looked like before the arrival of European settlers, you can find out by visiting the Santa Rosa Plateau Ecological Reserve (not to be confused with the Santa Rosa Mountains covered in Chapter 12). The reserve is located at the southern end of the Santa Ana Mountains and is home to some of the finest remaining bunchgrass prairie in the state, along with endangered Engelmann oak woodlands, vernal pools, and chaparral. The best time to visit is in March or April after a wet winter, when the vegetation is lush, the pools and creeks are full, snowcapped mountains stand sentry above the horizon, and the wildflowers are in bloom. Birdsong carries playfully through the trees and on the breeze; you're likely to see raptors, coyotes, and smaller animals if you're quiet and watchful.

The 9,000-acre Santa Rosa Plateau Ecological Reserve is jointly managed by a public–private partnership involving The Nature Conservancy, the Riverside County Regional Park and Open-Space District, the California Department of Fish and Wildlife, the U.S. Fish and Wildlife Service, and the Metropolitan Water District of Southern California. The Nature Conservancy purchased half of the land in 1984 from a housing development company. The rest was intended for houses, shopping centers, and golf courses before it was purchased with government assistance in 1991–95. From vantage points where you can compare the

Aerial view of the Santa Rosa Plateau and Vernal Pool

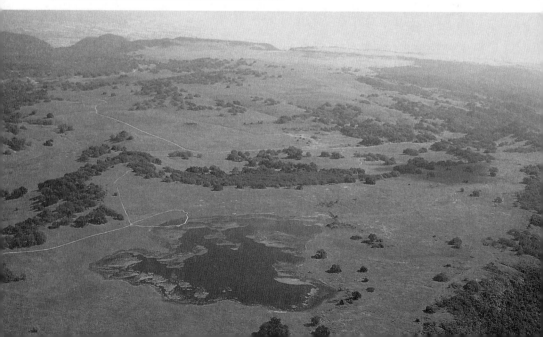

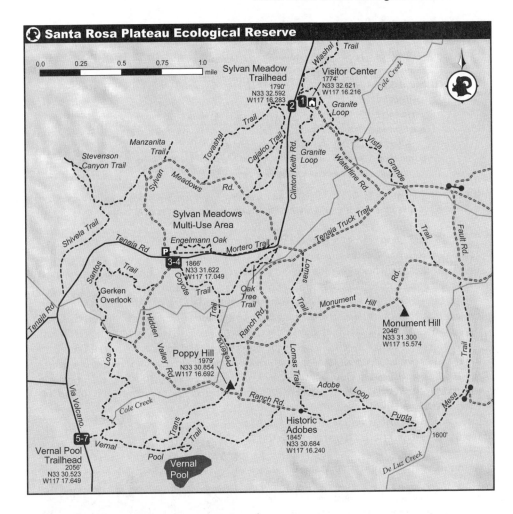

pristine reserve to the nearby hills scarred by ostentatious development, it's easy to appreciate some of the reasons why it was so important to set this land aside. Careful study of the lovely and endangered ecology reveals many more reasons to treasure the reserve.

The geology of the plateau contributes to its unique environment. Seven million years ago, this part of Southern California consisted of gently rolling hills. Volcanic eruptions filled the valleys with lava. You can see the eroded remnants of the lava flows in the mesas at the eastern edge of the park and in the basalt rocks around the vernal pools and tenajas (natural catch-basins). The pool floors are made of decomposed volcanic rock clay, which is nearly impermeable to water. Winter rains collect in the ponds and remain until they evaporate.

The reserve is open to the public daily from sunrise to sunset. The modest day-use fee ($4 adults, $3 kids ages 2–12) can be paid at the visitor center (open Tuesday–Sunday, 9 a.m.– 5 p.m.) or at the trailheads; park maps are also available at these locations. Do not disturb the plants, animals, and rocks within the reserve. Horseback and bicycle riding and dogs are allowed in the Sylvan Meadows multiuse area only. Trail runners enjoy all of the paths, which are relatively level and well marked. Visitors must remain on marked trails.

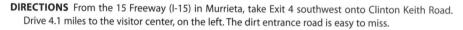

trip 8.1 Granite Loop

Distance	1.2–1.6 miles (loop)
Hiking Time	45 minutes
Elevation Gain	100'
Difficulty	Easy
Trail Use	Good for kids
Best Times	October–May
Agency	Santa Rosa Plateau Ecological Reserve
Optional Map	*Santa Rosa Plateau Ecological Reserve* or USGS *Wildomar* 7.5'
Permit	Day-use fee required (see page 183)

see
map on
p. 183

DIRECTIONS From the 15 Freeway (I-15) in Murrieta, take Exit 4 southwest onto Clinton Keith Road. Drive 4.1 miles to the visitor center, on the left. The dirt entrance road is easy to miss.

The Granite Loop is an easy introduction to the pleasures of the Santa Rosa Plateau Ecological Reserve. It tours three of the major ecosystems: oak woodlands, chaparral, and riparian zones. Benches along the way welcome you for a picnic, bird-watching, or quiet contemplation. This trip describes the loop in the clockwise direction.

The signed Granite Loop Trail begins at the north end of the parking area at the visitor center. It leads through chaparral 0.1 mile to an oak-shaded picnic area by the creek. If you have children along, be sure they stay in the clearing; the brush is infested with poison oak.

In another 0.2 mile, stay left at a signed junction; the unmarked path on the right cuts back to the visitor center. The trail leads through more chaparral encrusted in thick green lichen. In 0.2 mile, pass the Vista Grande Trail. Consider making a short detour to the left (east) on this trail to the Tenajas Overlook where, during wet years, you can admire a pool in Cole Creek. Watch for the Hammond two-striped garter snake, as well as Pacific tree frogs and southwestern pond turtles. Then return to the Granite Loop.

Immediately beyond the Vista Grande Trail, cross the dirt Waterline Road; then reach benches beneath a coast live oak patriarch. Beyond, pass piles of granite boulders and cross a branch of Cole Creek. Climb a small hill overlooking the visitor center, where you can see the contrast between the pristine reserve and the nearby hills scarred by development. Soon the loop ends at the south end of the visitor center parking lot.

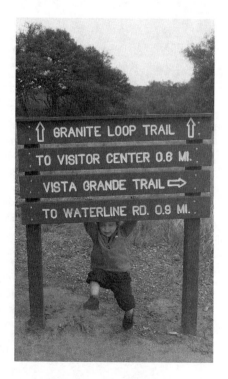

Signs are fun to play on.

trip 8.2   **Sylvan Meadows Loop**

see
map on
p. 183

Distance	4.5 miles (loop)
Hiking Time	2.5 hours
Elevation Gain	300'
Difficulty	Easy
Trail Use	Dogs allowed, suitable for mountain biking, suitable for equestrians
Best Times	October–May, especially March–April
Agency	Santa Rosa Plateau Ecological Reserve
Recommended Map	*Santa Rosa Plateau Ecological Reserve* or USGS *Wildomar* 7.5'
Permit	Day-use fee required (see page 183)

DIRECTIONS From the 15 Freeway in Murrieta, take Exit 4 southwest onto Clinton Keith Road. Drive 4.1 miles and park on the right (west) side of the road, opposite the visitor center entrance.

Sylvan Meadows is one of California's finest remaining native bunchgrass prairies. The meadow is dotted with magnificent oaks. The dirt Sylvan Meadows Road encircles the meadow. It's a designated multiuse trail, popular with equestrians and mountain bikers as well as hikers and joggers. The best time to visit is the spring, when the meadow is lush and the wildflowers are in bloom. This is also a good area for bird-watching. Ask at the visitor center for more information about birding.

From the trailhead parking, follow the Tovashal Trail west. In 0.2 mile, cross a bridge and come to a junction with the Cajalco Trail. Stay right on the Tovashal Trail. In 0.8 mile, reach a T-junction with Sylvan Meadows Road. Turn right and follow it around the meadow. In 0.3 mile, pass a signed turnoff for Manzanita Trail, which leads to the subdivision outside the reserve. Stay on the road and in another 0.2 mile, reach the Shivela Trail on the right.

VARIATION
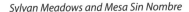
If you have time, a scenic detour into a lovely canyon is recommended here. Follow the Shivela Trail southwest 0.4 mile; then turn right onto a trail leading into the mouth of Stevenson Canyon. In 0.1 mile, the trail forks. Follow either side 0.3 mile up along a creek through the oak-shaded canyon where the forks rejoin; then return by the other fork, and retrace your steps to Sylvan Meadows Road. This variation adds 1.6 miles round-trip.

Sylvan Meadows and Mesa Sin Nombre

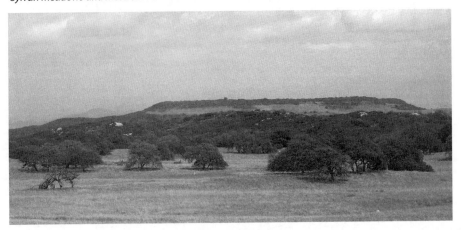

Continue along Sylvan Meadows Road past mistletoe-laden sycamores 0.5 mile to the Hidden Valley Trailhead. The Nighthawk and Mortero Trails lead east, parallel to Tenaja Road. Follow the Nighthawk Trail (which is set farther back from the road) 0.4 mile until it rejoins the Mortero; then continue another 0.4 mile east alongside the road to a junction.

Turn left onto Sylvan Meadows Road and go 0.5 mile to a junction with the Cajalco Trail. Turn right and follow it 0.8 mile back to the Tovashal Trail near the bridge. Then turn right again and return to the trailhead.

trip 8.3 Oak Tree Trail

see
map on
p. 183

Distance	2 miles (semiloop)
Hiking Time	1 hour
Elevation Gain	100'
Difficulty	Easy
Trail Use	Good for kids
Best Times	October–May, especially March–April
Agency	Santa Rosa Plateau Ecological Reserve
Recommended Map	*Santa Rosa Plateau Ecological Reserve* or USGS *Wildomar* 7.5'
Permit	Day-use fee required (see page 183)

DIRECTIONS From the 15 Freeway in Murrieta, take Exit 4 southwest onto Clinton Keith Road and drive 5.8 miles to the Hidden Valley Trailhead, on the left (south) side of the road. The trailhead is located shortly beyond where the road makes a sharp turn right (west) and becomes Tenaja Road.

The Santa Rosa Plateau is home to some of the last remaining Engelmann oaks. The majestic trees can live up to 300 years, and their many twisting limbs and gray-green leaves distinguish them from the more common coast live oaks. These spectacular oaks prefer to grow on mesas and foothills at least 20 miles inland from the ocean. Construction of subdivisions has led to the destruction of most of the native Engelmann oak woodlands, especially in the hills above Pasadena and Pomona. The Oak Tree Trail makes a short loop through a fine stand of Engelmann oaks along Cole Creek.

Look for two paths leading south from the Hidden Valley Trailhead. The Coyote Trail immediately branches left off Hidden Valley Road. Here, observant hikers may see coyotes and their prey intently engaged in the game of life.

Follow the Coyote Trail 0.5 mile through undulating grasslands to a junction. Turn left and follow the Trans-Preserve Trail 0.3 mile to the beginning of the Oak Tree Loop. You can then tour the 0.6-mile loop either clockwise or counterclockwise. When you're done, return the way you came.

trip 8.4 Los Santos Loop

see
map on
p. 183

Distance	5 miles (loop)
Hiking Time	2.5 hours
Elevation Gain	500'
Difficulty	Easy
Best Times	October–May, especially March–April
Agency	Santa Rosa Plateau Ecological Reserve
Recommended Map	*Santa Rosa Plateau Ecological Reserve* or USGS *Wildomar* 7.5'
Permit	Day-use fee required (see page 183)

Clouds over the Santa Rosa Plateau from the Los Santos Trail

DIRECTIONS From the 15 Freeway in Murrieta, take Exit 4 southwest onto Clinton Keith Road and drive 5.8 miles to the Hidden Valley Trailhead, on the left (south) side of the road. The trailhead is located shortly beyond where the road makes a sharp turn right (west) and becomes Tenaja Road.

The hills and meadows in the southwestern corner of the Santa Rosa Plateau are dotted with some of the stateliest Engelmann oaks in the reserve. This counterclockwise loop offers a scenic tour of the area along the Los Santos and Trans-Preserve Trails. Other highlights include the basalt Mesa de Colorado, Poppy Hill, and an optional short detour to the fascinating vernal pool. Quiet and observant hikers often see the coyotes and raptors that hunt in these hills.

Two paths lead south from the trailhead. Take the right fork, Hidden Valley Road. You'll return by the Coyote Trail later. The dirt road leads through a meadow. In 0.2 mile, turn right onto the narrow Los Santos Trail, which winds around and climbs a low ridge. In another 0.8 mile, reach a bench with terrific views at the Walter B. Gerken overlook, named for the former chairman of The Nature Conservancy. In 0.4 mile, the trail descends to another junction, where a connector path to the left leads back to Hidden Valley Road. Stay right and climb onto the Mesa de Colorado. As the soil becomes more volcanic in composition, the vegetation becomes noticeably different and varied. The prickly pear cacti produce spectacular flowers in late spring, but watch for poison oak if you stray from the trail.

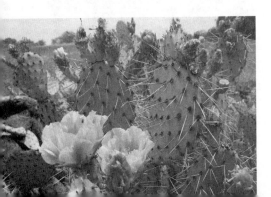

Cactus blooms along the Los Santos Trail.

In 1.1 miles, reach the Vernal Pool Trail, marking the halfway point of your hike. Turn left and go 0.3 mile to a junction with the Trans-Preserve Trail. In the spring, it's well worth taking a 0.2-mile detour onward to the big pool (see Trip 8.5) before you return via the Trans-Preserve Trail. In 0.8 mile, cross Hidden Valley Road and pass Poppy Hill, which ignites with California poppies in the spring. In another 0.8 mile, turn left onto the Coyote Trail and follow it the last half mile back to the Hidden Valley Trailhead.

trip 8.5   Vernal Pool

Distance	1.5 miles (out-and-back)
Hiking Time	45 minutes
Elevation Gain	100'
Difficulty	Moderate
Trail Use	Good for kids
Best Times	March–April
Agency	Santa Rosa Plateau Ecological Reserve
Optional Map	*Santa Rosa Plateau Ecological Reserve* or USGS *Wildomar* 7.5'
Permit	Day-use fee required (see page 183)

see map on p. 183

DIRECTIONS From the 15 Freeway in Murrieta, take Exit 4 southwest onto Clinton Keith Road and drive 6.9 miles; Clinton Keith becomes Tenaja Road along the way. At a stop sign, bear left onto Via Volcano. In another 0.8 mile, park along the left (east) side of the road at the Vernal Pool Trailhead.

In the southwest corner of the reserve is a shallow basalt basin that fills with water during the winter rains. Such vernal pools—so named because they usually hold an abundance of water in the spring—were once common in California, but more than 90% have been destroyed by development or agriculture. Vernal pools nourish a variety of endangered species. The Santa Rosa Plateau has some of the last remaining vernal pools. This one, the largest pool in the reserve, supports fairy shrimp, frogs, and waterbirds. One of the species of fairy shrimp is found nowhere else on Earth. Wildflowers encircle the pool and creep toward the center as the water evaporates in May. A short, well-marked trail leads to a boardwalk over the pool so that you can enjoy its wonders without trampling the fragile environment.

From the trailhead, hike east 0.1 mile to a junction. The Los Santos Trail forks off to the left (see Trip 8.4), but the Vernal Pool Trail continues straight. Hike through a meadow dotted with oaks; keep your eye out for the occasional small pool. In 0.3 mile, reach a second junction with the Trans-Preserve Trail, which also forks to the left. Continue straight 0.2 mile to the large vernal pool. Look for the boardwalk that leads over the pool. Interpretive signs explain some features of the site. Stay on the trail so that you don't disturb the sensitive wildlife.

Return the way you came. Or, for a longer walk, continue along the trail to the historic adobes (see Trip 8.6) or take a loop to the north toward Poppy Hill.

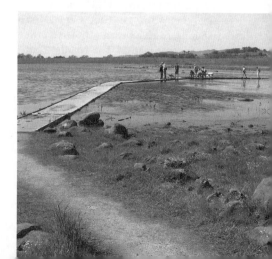

Vernal Pool boardwalk

trip 8.6   Historic Adobes

Distance	3.5 miles (out-and-back)
Hiking Time	2.5 hours
Elevation Gain	300'
Difficulty	Easy
Best Times	October–May, especially March–April
Agency	Santa Rosa Plateau Ecological Reserve
Recommended Map	*Santa Rosa Plateau Ecological Reserve* or USGS *Wildomar* 7.5'
Permit	Day-use fee required (see page 183)

see map on p. 183

DIRECTIONS From the 15 Freeway in Murrieta, take Exit 4 southwest onto Clinton Keith Road and drive 6.9 miles; Clinton Keith becomes Tenaja Road along the way. At a stop sign, bear left onto Via Volcano. In another 0.8 mile, park along the left (east) side of the road at the Vernal Pool Trailhead.

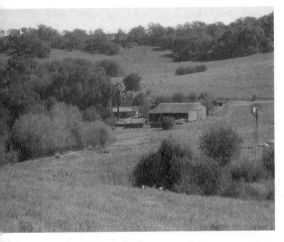

Santa Rosa Ranch

In 1846, Pio Pico, governor of California, granted the 48,000-acre Santa Rosa Rancho to Juan Moreno. Moreno built a ranch where he and his family grazed cattle. The small Moreno adobe is the oldest building in Riverside County, and the large Machado adobe, built later around 1855, is the second oldest. This hike visits the restored ranch, passing by way of the vernal pool and a shady creek. It's ideal in the spring, when the pool is full and the wildflowers are in bloom.

Follow the trail east 0.6 mile through meadows dotted with oaks to the large vernal pool (see Trip 8.5), staying right at junctions with the Los Santos and Trans-Preserve Trails along the way. This site is worth exploring, but stay on the marked trail and boardwalk to protect the endangered species living near the pool.

Continue along the trail 0.9 mile, dropping down through a band of chaparral to Ranch Road. Turn right and follow the road 0.1 mile to the historic ranch. Interpretive signs and a botanical garden walk explain the history and environment of the ranch.

VARIATION

For a scenic detour, continue east from the ranch toward the Punta Mesa Trail. In 0.5 mile, turn left at a sign for the Adobe Loop Trail. This trail leads back west along bubbling Adobe Creek beneath the oak canopy. Beware of the poison oak, which grows thick alongside the trail. Keep your eyes out for a tenaja, a pool formed by erosion along the stream. In another 0.5 mile, reach a T-junction with the Lomas Trail. Turn left and hike 0.1 mile back to the ranch.

Return the way you came, or explore an alternate route along the rich network of trails in this corner of the former Rancho.

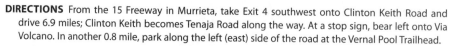

| trip 8.7 | **Santa Rosa Plateau Loop** |

Distance	11 miles (loop)
Hiking Time	6 hours
Elevation Gain	700'
Difficulty	Strenuous
Best Times	October–May, especially March–April
Agency	Santa Rosa Plateau Ecological Reserve
Recommended Map	*Santa Rosa Plateau Ecological Reserve* or USGS *Wildomar* 7.5'
Permit	Day-use fee required (see page 183)

see map on p. 183

DIRECTIONS From the 15 Freeway in Murrieta, take Exit 4 southwest onto Clinton Keith Road and drive 6.9 miles; Clinton Keith becomes Tenaja Road along the way. At a stop sign, bear left onto Via Volcano. In another 0.8 mile, park along the left (east) side of the road at the Vernal Pool Trailhead.

This trip offers a grand tour of the Santa Rosa Plateau including the vernal ponds, the historic adobes, and the volcanic mesas, culminating with a panoramic view from Monument Hill. If you have a full day to hike, this is a great way to see many of the diverse features in the reserve. The trail also features fine views of San Jacinto Peak, San Gorgonio Mountain, and Mount Baldy, the three tallest peaks ringing the Los Angeles Basin. Many variations let you shorten or lengthen the trip as you prefer. For example, you could start or end at the visitor center, and could extend the hike to include the Los Santos Loop (see Trip 8.4) and/or the Sylvan Meadows Loop (see Trip 8.2).

From the Vernal Pool Trailhead, hike 0.6 mile east through a meadow dotted with oaks, passing the Los Santos and Trans-Preserve Trails, to the big pool, which is full of water after winter's rains. After visiting the boardwalk along the pool, continue 0.9 mile to Ranch Road. Turn right (east) and hike 0.1 mile to the historic Santa Rosa Ranch, which is a good place to stop for a break.

Next, follow the Lomas Trail north along the west side of the ranch 0.1 mile to a gate marking the entrance to the Adobe Loop Trail. Turn right and follow the creek under the shady oaks 0.5 mile to a T-junction with the Punta Mesa Trail. Turn left (east) and follow the Punta Mesa Trail down through the chaparral to a small creek crossing; then continue up and north. Pass an intersection in 1.9 miles with Monument Hill Road and continue another 0.7 mile across a wide meadow to a junction with the Tenaja Truck Trail. The construction scars on the hills to the northwest show how fortunate it is that this pristine plateau was saved from development.

Turn left (west) and follow the dirt road 0.5 mile; then turn right and follow Waterline Road 0.7 mile toward the visitor center, passing oaks and granite boulders in the meadow. Shortly before you reach the visitor center, turn right on the Granite Loop Trail and go less than 0.1 mile; then turn right again on the Vista Grande Trail. The trail forks but both

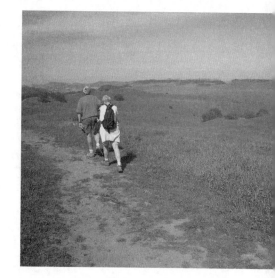

Hikers at Monument Hill

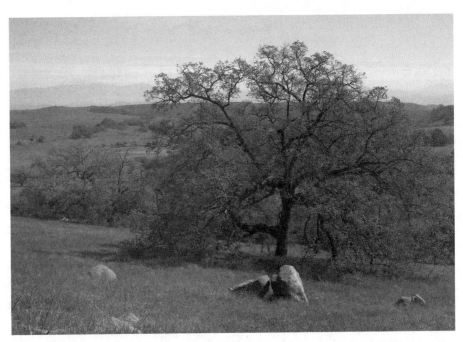

Oak grassland comprises much of the Santa Rosa Plateau.

branches rejoin shortly near a bridge over Cole Creek and a bench overlooking the tenajas. In 0.9 mile, cross the Tenaja Truck Trail again and continue 0.7 mile to a T-junction with Monument Hill Road. Turn right (west) and climb 0.4 mile to a spur trail that leads 0.1 mile to the summit of Monument Hill (2,046'), where you can take in views of the entire eastern half of the reserve that you've just explored.

Continue west along Monument Road, passing two junctions with the Lomas Trail, to reach Ranch Road in 1 mile. Turn left (south) and go 0.4 mile. At a junction near Poppy Hill, turn right (west) and hike 0.1 mile toward the hill; then turn left (southwest) on the Trans-Preserve Trail. Follow it 0.8 mile to a T-junction with the Vernal Pool Trail on Mesa de Colorado. Turn right (west) and retrace your steps 0.4 mile to where you began this big loop.

chapter 9

San Jacinto Mountains

The San Jacinto Mountains are the northernmost crest of the Peninsular Ranges, a spiny backbone that stretches roughly 900 miles from Southern California to the southern tip of the Baja California Peninsula. During the Cretaceous period, about 100 million years ago, magma welled up beneath the Earth's surface and slowly cooled, forming a vast expanse of granite called a batholith. The region was subsequently thrust upward by seismic activity along the San Andreas Fault. Millions of years of erosion have stripped off the overlaying rock, cutting deep canyons and revealing the spectacular granite of the San Jacintos.

Extending 30 miles from the 10 Freeway (I-10) to the Santa Rosa Mountains, the San Jacinto Mountains form the eastern wall of the greater Los Angeles Basin. Palm Springs nestles against the eastern side of the range; beyond lies the Coachella Valley and endless miles of the Colorado Desert. The mountain town of Idyllwild is perched on the western slope beneath Tahquitz Peak. San Gorgonio Pass, also known as Banning Pass, separates the range from the San Bernardino Mountains in the north. The range is also home to Southern California's second-tallest peak: San Jacinto's summit (10,834') towers nearly 2 vertical miles above Banning Pass.

The earliest known inhabitants of the San Jacinto Mountains and the surrounding deserts were the Cahuilla Indians. The Cahuilla routinely traveled into the mountains to hunt and to escape the summer heat. They first came in contact with the Spanish in 1774 when Juan Bautista de Anza was looking for an overland route between Monterey, California, and Sonora, Mexico. With the aid of Sebastián Tarabal, an Indian from the San Gabriel Mission who spoke Spanish and a number of native languages, Anza "discovered" the San Jacinto Valley, with the imposing snowcapped San Jacinto Mountains standing sentinel over the surrounding valleys and deserts. Under the aegis of the San Luis Rey Mission, cattle ranching was soon established in the San Jacinto Valley. Cattle ranching and sheep herding would come to dominate the San Jacinto landscape for the next 150 years.

Much like the Cahuilla before us, today's hikers escape the summer heat of the Coachella Valley by retreating to the mountains of San Jacinto. Where the Cahuilla had to negotiate the tricky granite mountainsides by foot to reach the cooler elevations, today's hikers only have to hop onto the Palm Springs Aerial Tramway, and in minutes they're whisked up among the cool breezes and whispering pines.

The tram offers a breathtaking ride in a rotating car up the rocky and steep Chino Canyon with awe-inspiring views of the Coachella Valley. The tram opened in 1963 after 17 years of bitter dispute between developers and conservationists. Even now, there are still serious concerns about the impact that hundreds of thousands of annual tram riders have on the wilderness; however, the tram station is undoubtedly the most popular trailhead for San Jacinto Peak.

The Palm Springs Aerial Tramway isn't the only attraction that lures people to the San Jacinto Mountains. Tahquitz Rock was the birthplace of technical rock climbing in Southern

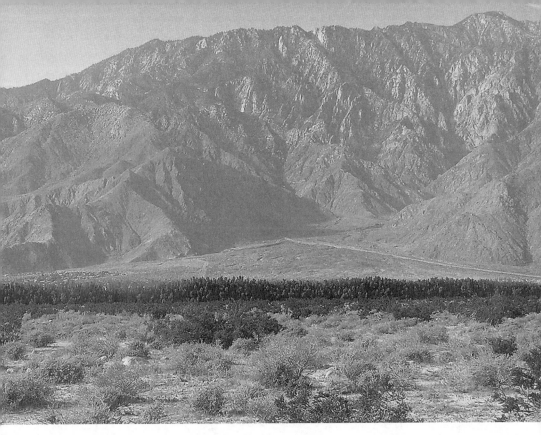

The San Jacinto Mountains from the Coachella Valley

California and remains a mecca for rock climbers. The modern system of rating climbs, now called the Yosemite Decimal System, was developed at Tahquitz.

The San Jacinto Mountains lie within Santa Rosa and San Jacinto Mountains National Monument, which includes both a state park and a federal wilderness area in its boundaries. Mount San Jacinto State Park and Wilderness encompasses the peak, the tram, and much of the high country. The San Jacinto Wilderness, administered by the U.S. Forest Service, extends north and south from the state park and includes Tahquitz and the Desert Divide as far south as Spitler Peak. The 280,000-acre monument was established by Congress in 2000 "in order to preserve the nationally significant biological, cultural, recreational, geological, educational, and scientific values found in the Santa Rosa and San Jacinto Mountains and to secure now and for future generations the opportunity to experience and enjoy the magnificent vistas, wildlife, land forms, and natural and cultural resources in these mountains and to recreate therein." Mary Bono Mack, who formerly represented the 45th Congressional District, spanning central and eastern Riverside County including the Coachella Valley, championed the bill designating the monument.

A wilderness permit is necessary for hiking anywhere within the state park or wilderness. The permit can be obtained from either the state park or Forest Service, depending on your entry location. At this writing, the quota for permits entering via the Devils Slide Trail from Idyllwild fills up in advance on summer weekends. Leashed dogs are allowed in the federal wilderness but not in the state park. Groups are limited to 12 in San Jacinto Wilderness and 15 in the state park.

Continued on page 196

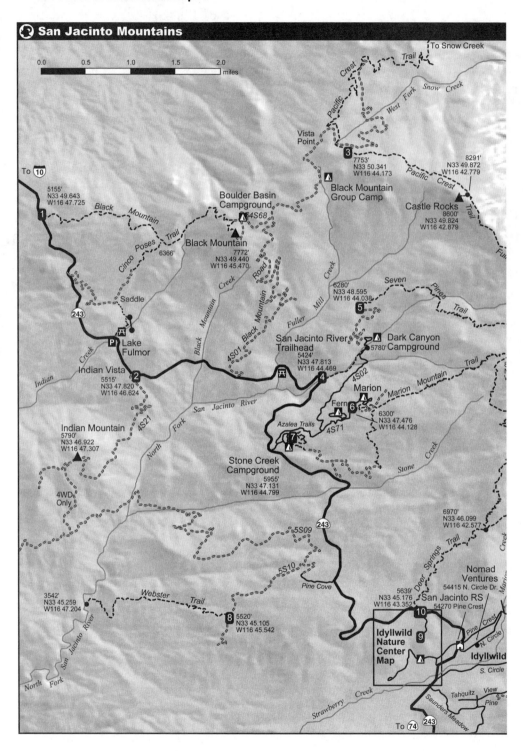

San Jacinto Mountains

0.0   0.5   1.0   1.5   2.0
miles

To Snow Creek

Trail

Pacific

Crest

West Fork

Snow Creek

Vista
Point

3 7753'
N33 50.341
W116 44.173

8291'
N33 49.872
W116 42.779

Pacific   Crest

To 10

5155'
N33 49.643
W116 47.725

Black   Mountain

1

Cinco Poses   Trail

6366'

Boulder Basin
Campground
4S68

Black Mountain

7772'
N33 49.440
W116 45.470

Black Mountain Road

Black   Mountain

Creek

Fuller

Mill

Creek

Black Mountain
Group Camp

Castle Rocks
8600'
N33 49.824
W116 42.879

Fu

Seven

6280'
N33 48.595
W116 44.038

5

Pines   Trail

Saddle

243

P Lake
Fulmor

Indian Vista

2

5515'
N33 47.820
W116 46.624

4S01

San Jacinto River
Trailhead

5424'
N33 47.813
W116 44.469

4

4S02

Dark Canyon
Campground
5780'

Marion

Marion   Mountain

Trail

Indian   Creek

Indian Mountain
5790'
N33 46.922
W116 47.307

San Jacinto River

North   Fork

4S21

Fern
6

Azalea Trails

7

4S71

Marion
6300'
N33 47.476
W116 44.128

Stone   Creek

4WD
Only

Stone Creek
Campground
5955'
N33 47.131
W116 44.799

243

6970'
N33 46.099
W116 42.577

5S09

5S10

Pine Cove

Deer   Springs   Trail

Creek

Nomad
Ventures
54415 N. Circle Dr.

3542'
N33 45.259
W116 47.204

Webster   Trail

8 5520'
N33 45.105
W116 45.542

5639'
N33 45.176
W116 43.352

San Jacinto RS
54270 Pine Crest

10

9

Pine Crest

N. Circle

North   Fork

San Jacinto River

Idyllwild
Nature
Center
Map

Idyllwild

S. Circle

Strawberry   Creek

Saunders   Meadow

Tahquitz   View

Pine

To 74   243

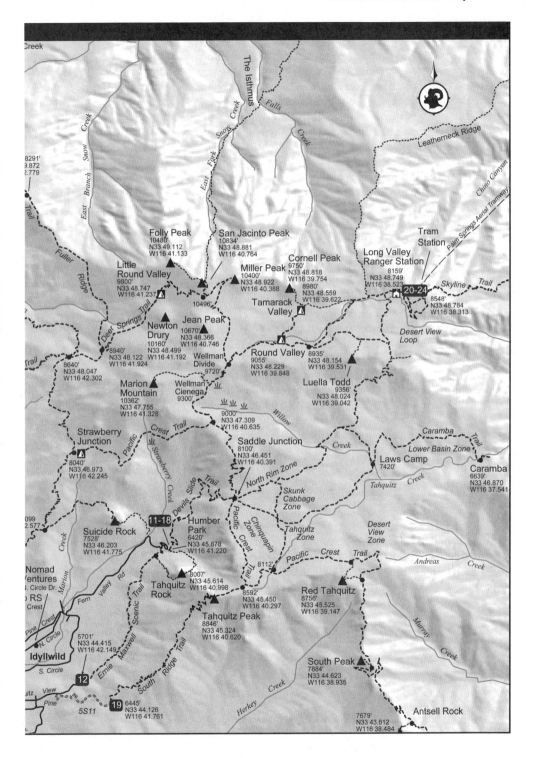

Leatherneck Ridge

Chino Canyon

The Isthmus

Falls

Snow Creek

East Fork

East Branch Snow Creek

Fuller Ridge

8291'
9.872
2.779

Trail

Palm Springs Aerial Tramway

Folly Peak
10480'
N33 49.112
W116 41.133

San Jacinto Peak
10834'
N33 48.881
W116 40.764

Tram
Station

Long Valley
Ranger Station
8159'
N33 48.749
W116 38.523

Little
Round Valley
9800'
N33 48.747
W116 41.237

Miller Peak
10400'
N33 48.922
W116 40.388

Cornell Peak
9750'
N33 48.818
W116 39.754

8980'
N33 48.559
W116 39.622

20-24

Skyline Trail

8548'
N33 48.784
W116 38.313

10496'

Tamarack
Valley

Deer Springs Trail

Newton
Drury
10160'
N33 48.499
W116 41.192

Jean Peak
10670'
N33 48.366
W116 40.746

Desert View
Loop

8940'
N33 48.122
W116 41.924

Wellman
Divide
9720'

Round Valley
9055'
N33 48.229
W116 39.848

8935'
N33 48.154
W116 39.531

8640'
N33 48.047
W116 42.302

Trail

Marion
Mountain
10362'
N33 47.755
W116 41.328

Wellman
Cienega
9300'

Luella Todd
9356'
N33 48.024
W116 39.042

9000'
N33 47.309
W116 40.635

Willow

Caramba
Trail

Strawberry
Junction
8040'
N33 46.973
W116 42.245

Crest Trail

Pacific

Strawberry Creek

Saddle Junction
8100'
N33 46.451
W116 40.391

Creek

Lower Basin Zone

Laws Camp
7420'

Tahquitz Creek

Caramba
6639'
N33 46.870
W116 37.541

North Rim Zone

099
2.577

Creek

Suicide Rock
7528'
N33 46.203
W116 41.775

11-18

Devils Slide Trail

Humber
Park
6420'
N33 45.878
W116 41.220

Pacific Crest Trail

Skunk
Cabbage
Zone

Chinquapin Zone

Tahquitz
Zone

Desert
View
Zone

Nomad
Ventures
l. Circle Dr.

o RS
Crest

Fern Valley Rd

Scenic Trail

Tahquitz
Rock

8007'
N33 45.614
W116 40.998

8112'

8592'
N33 45.450
W116 40.297

Pacific Crest Trail

Andreas Creek

Pine Crest
N. Circle

5701'
N33 44.415
W116 42.149

Maxwell Trail

Ernie Maxwell

Tahquitz Peak
8846'
N33 45.324
W116 40.620

Red Tahquitz
8756'
N33 45.525
W116 39.147

Murray Creek

Idyllwild

S. Circle

12

South Ridge Trail

Creek

South Peak
7884'
N33 44.623
W116 38.935

uitz View

Pine

5S11

19

6445'
N33 44.126
W116 41.761

Herkey Creek

7679'
N33 43.812
W116 38.484

Antsell Rock

Continued from page 193

A camping permit is required to stay overnight in either the state park or wilderness. The state park campgrounds are Round Valley, Tamarack Valley, Little Round Valley, and Strawberry Junction. The Forest Service has dispersed camping zones called Skunk Cabbage, Tahquitz, Chinquapin, North Rim, Lower Basin, and Desert View within the federal wilderness, labeled on this chapter's map; only Chinquapin, however, is currently open after the 2013 Mountain Fire left dangerous dead trees in the other zones. Dispersed camping is allowed in these zones at least 200 feet from trails, meadows, streams, and other campers. Larger groups will be assigned to established brown-post sites, and the Forest Service will give you a map. The camping permits must be obtained directly from the state park or the Forest Service, depending on where you plan to stay. A backpacking trip with nights in both zones requires separate camping permits. Many of these campgrounds and zones fill a month in advance during the summer, so plan ahead. Campfires are prohibited in all state and federal wilderness areas in the San Jacinto Mountains.

Water may be scarce in the summer and fall. On the west side, Bed Springs Crossing, 0.5 mile southwest of Little Round Valley, normally flows year-round even during drought. On the east side, Round Valley Camp has reliable water. Water might also be available at Wellman Cienega, Strawberry Cienega, and Tahquitz or Willow Creeks, but none are dependable year-round. Check with a ranger or haul your own water.

Camping permits for the state park can be obtained in person or by mail up to 56 days in advance from the Mount San Jacinto State Park Headquarters in Idyllwild, or in person from the Long Valley Ranger Station located west of the tram station. Hiking and camping permits for the federal wilderness can be obtained in person, by mail, or by fax from the San Jacinto Ranger Station in Idyllwild up to 90 days in advance. (See Appendix B.)

Nomad Ventures (951-659-4853), a well-equipped outfitter, is conveniently located at 54415 N. Circle Drive in Idyllwild, between the ranger station and Humber Park.

The elevation of San Jacinto Peak has been a subject of some discussion. The 1996 edition of the USGS *San Jacinto Peak* 7.5' topographic map erroneously lists the elevation at 10,804 feet. More recently, the elevation has been corrected to 10,834 feet. Some mountaineers argue that the survey benchmark sits 8 feet below the natural summit, so the true elevation of the peak should be 10,842 feet.

Note: The southern portion of the San Jacinto Wilderness burned in the July 2013 Mountain Fire. This 27,000-acre blaze was started by an electrical malfunction on private property in the Garner Valley and soon swept onto the Desert Divide. The federal government has sued the wealthy foreign landowner for $25 million to cover part of the cost of fighting the fire. At this writing, Tahquitz Valley and the Desert Divide north of the Spitler Peak Trail (see Chapter 10) are closed for recovery.

---

trip 9.1   ## Black Mountain

see map on p. 194

Distance	7 miles (out-and-back)
Hiking Time	4 hours
Elevation Gain	2,700'
Difficulty	Strenuous
Trail Use	Dogs allowed, suitable for backpacking
Best Times	May–October
Agency	San Bernardino National Forest (San Jacinto Ranger Station)
Recommended Map	Tom Harrison *San Jacinto Wilderness* or USGS *Lake Fulmor* 7.5'

DIRECTIONS From Banning, drive southeast on Highway 243 to the beginning of the Black Mountain Trail (2E35), at mile marker 243 RIV 16.75, 1 mile beyond Vista Grande Ranger Station. Turn left and drive 100 yards up a dirt road to the parking area.

Black Mountain (7,772') stands back from the bulk of San Jacinto on the northwest side. Not surprisingly, it offers fantastic views of the surrounding mountains and chaparral. The Forest Service takes advantage of these views with a fire lookout on the summit, staffed by volunteers. The lookout is open to visitors 9 a.m.–5 p.m. when the access road is open (typically Memorial Day–Labor Day). The volunteers are happy to share their mountain knowledge with hikers. The vigorous hike to the lookout makes for an enjoyable excursion through the forest and granite boulders typical in this mountain range. Backpackers must haul their own water; none is available at the Boulder Basin Campground.

Hike up the trail through bands of pine and oak forest and chaparral. Initially the climbing is steep, but it soon becomes more gradual on the boulder-strewn ridge. Cross a low divide into Hall Canyon; then contour across the head of the fern-filled canyon, where Indian Creek flows in the spring. Watch for a grove of sequoias that were planted here long ago. The nonnative but beautiful tree has some resemblance to incense cedar but is readily distinguished by its egg-shaped cones. Then climb steeply again to reach a spur of the Black Mountain lookout road just north of the summit.

Turn right and walk past a water tank; then follow a steep faint use trail up to the lookout tower on the top. If you lose your way, just choose your own route, avoiding the jumbo boulders along the way. Alternatively, descend the spur road east to the Boulder Basin Campground, turn right, and hike 0.5 mile up the gated dirt road to the lookout.

Return the way you came.

ALTERNATIVE FINISH

Another option is to make a one-way hike by arranging a car or bicycle shuttle at Boulder Basin Campground. To reach the campground from Highway 243, go 4.2 miles southeast from the Black Mountain Trailhead. Turn left (north) onto Black Mountain Road (4S01). Drive 4.8 miles up the good dirt road; then turn left onto 4S68 and proceed 0.4 mile to the campground.

VARIATIONS

The abandoned Cinco Poses Trail meets the Black Mountain Trail near the divide. Local users presently keep the chaparral cut back enough that the trail is passable and interesting for adventurous hikers. The distance and elevation are about the same as taking the main trail. One can park at the Lake Fulmor picnic area near mile marker 243 RIV 14.75; then follow the trail or dirt road along the north side of the lake 0.3 mile to a gate at the James Reserve, an ecological research station operated by the University of California. Turn left just before the fence and pick a steep cross-country path 0.4 mile up to a saddle, where you'll find an old logging road. Turn right and follow the road 0.5 mile to its end. Look closely for a faint trail headed up the slope,

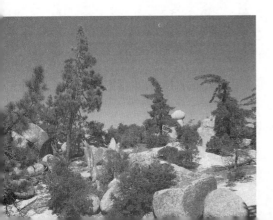

Boulders and pines from the Black Mountain Trail

which soon becomes a better path cut through the ceanothus, scrub oak, and manzanita. In 0.6 mile, reach the unsigned junction with the Black Mountain Trail.

Alternatively, one can walk or drive a high-clearance vehicle up the logging road 1.4 miles from its start near mile marker 243 RIV 16.00 to the aforementioned saddle.

---

trip 9.2   Indian Mountain

Distance	5.5 miles (out-and-back)
Hiking Time	3 hours
Elevation Gain	1,300'
Difficulty	Moderate
Trail Use	Dogs allowed
Best Times	October–June
Agency	San Bernardino National Forest (San Jacinto Ranger Station)
Recommended Map	Tom Harrison *San Jacinto Wilderness* or USGS *Lake Fulmor* 7.5'

DIRECTIONS From Banning, drive southeast on Highway 243 to the Indian Vista Overlook parking area, 0.6 mile past the Lake Fulmor picnic area and just past mile marker 243 RIV 14.00. The Indian Mountain Fire Road (4S21) begins just northwest of the overlook parking area.

Indian Mountain is perched amidst the chaparral on the western slopes of the San Jacinto Mountains. It's named for the nearby Indian Creek, which runs through the Soboba reservation. The approach along a fire road is unpleasantly hot in the summer, but on a crisp winter day, it offers a fine walk and an unforgettable view of snow-clad San Jacinto Peak towering above. Even if the fire road is blanketed by recent snowfall, the hike is straightforward as long as you have adequate footwear.

Follow the Indian Mountain Fire Road (4S21) down to a saddle and then up the east and south sides of Indian Mountain. When the road reaches its highest point immediately south of the summit, turn right and follow the partly overgrown trail to the summit boulders. Return the way you came.

Snowy San Jacinto from Indian Mountain

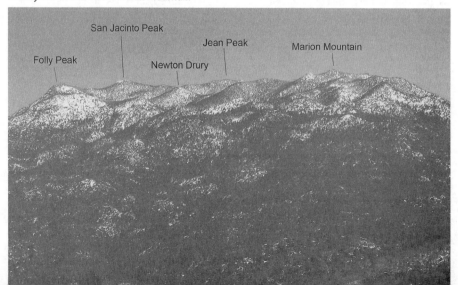

trip 9.3   San Jacinto Peak via Fuller Ridge

Distance	15 miles (out-and-back)
Hiking Time	8 hours
Elevation Gain	4,100'
Difficulty	Strenuous
Trail Use	Suitable for backpacking
Best Times	June–October
Agencies	San Bernardino National Forest (San Jacinto Ranger Station) and Mount San Jacinto State Park
Recommended Maps	Tom Harrison *San Jacinto Wilderness, Santa Rosa & San Jacinto Mountains National Monument,* or USGS *Lake Fulmor* and *San Jacinto Peak* 7.5'
Permit	San Jacinto Wilderness Permit required

see map on p. 194

DIRECTIONS From Highway 243, near mile marker 243 RIV 12.50, turn northeast up good dirt Black Mountain Road (4S01). After 4.8 miles, pass a side road on your left to Black Mountain Campground and fire lookout. Your road winds to the right through spectacular open forest dotted with giant granite boulders. It passes the entrance of the Black Mountain Group Campground after 1 mile, then a rocky outcropping on the left in another 0.8 mile featuring spectacular views of San Gorgonio Mountain and the pass below. Pass a junction with the Pacific Crest Trail, 0.7 mile beyond the outcrop; then turn right up a hill at a sign for the Fuller Ridge trailhead. Drive 0.2 mile and park in the clearing.

The Pacific Crest Trail (PCT) follows Fuller Ridge northwest from San Jacinto Peak. The long dirt road by which you arrived reaches the trail at 7,720 feet, the highest point to which you can drive on the mountain. This high trailhead might seem to offer an easy route to the summit, but the trail climbs up and down to bypass gendarmes on the rugged ridge, then makes a long detour south around Folly Peak to the Deer Springs area before climbing to the summit by way of Little Round Valley. On the way down, you make the same detour and the same downs and ups, resulting in a surprisingly demanding hike. Your hard work is rewarded with stunning views of Snow Creek carving the dramatic northwest face of San Jacinto. You're likely to enjoy solitude along this little-used section of the PCT.

Fuller Ridge from Black Mountain

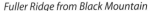

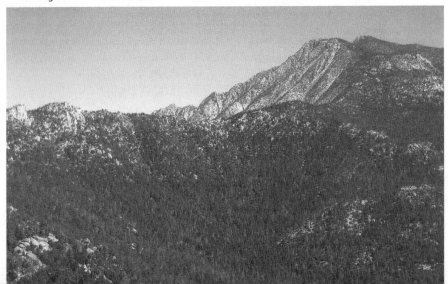

Backpackers with a camping permit from Mount San Jacinto State Park can stay at Little Round Valley Trail Camp; the quota often fills a month or more ahead of time on popular summer weekends. Water might be available at a stream in the meadow in Little Round Valley; it flows all year in wet years but can dry up in the summer during drought years. The most reliable creek in the area is Bed Springs Crossing, 0.5 mile southwest of Little Round Valley, but even this can dry up during severe drought. Ask the rangers about water before you go.

Hike on the PCT along the north side of Fuller Ridge through a rich forest of sugar pines and white firs. In 1 mile, pass a saddle on the right. A field of wild blue and red currants grows here, offering a tasty snack in late summer. Cross the state park boundary in 0.3 mile. In another 0.3 mile, the trail begins climbing steeply and then ascends a series of switchbacks.

VARIATION

Immediately before the first switchback, you may find a cairn on the right side marking a climber's trail up to the spires of Castle Rocks on the ridge. Despite the sheer cliffs atop much of Fuller Ridge, the highest point can be reached without any scrambling or bushwhacking if you care to make the optional detour. This excursion adds 300 feet of climbing in a steep 0.2 mile.

The trail reaches a saddle on the ridge. From here, there are terrific views of Snow Creek to the east and the forested slopes to the west. After passing the rocks, the trail contours south and crosses the headwaters of the San Jacinto River before reaching a junction with the Deer Springs Trail 5 miles from the start.

Turn left (northeast) and follow the Deer Springs Trail 1 mile to Little Round Valley Trail Camp, situated in a splendid bowl beside the creek. Then climb 1.3 miles to the saddle immediately south of San Jacinto Peak, turn left, and climb the last 0.3 mile to the summit.

Return the way you came, or make a longer loop on any of the other fine trails circling the mountain. Although a cross-country descent of upper Fuller Ridge by way of Folly Peak would appear to save substantial distance, the route involves unpleasant wading through a sea of manzanita and buckthorn.

trip 9.4 North Fork of the San Jacinto River

Distance	1.4 miles (out-and-back)
Hiking Time	1.5 hours
Elevation Gain	400'
Difficulty	Moderate
Best Times	March–November
Agency	San Bernardino National Forest (San Jacinto Ranger Station)
Recommended Map	Tom Harrison *San Jacinto Wilderness* or USGS *San Jacinto Peak* 7.5'

DIRECTIONS From Banning, drive southeast on Highway 243 to the signed North Fork of the San Jacinto River at mile marker 243 RIV 11.25, 0.7 mile past Fuller Mill Creek Picnic Area. The other end of the trail can also be reached from a bridge just south of the Dark Canyon Campground (see Trip 9.5), but parking is prohibited along this road.

The San Jacinto River is fed by small springs dotting the upper reaches of the mountain, which coalesce and flow down the west side. By the time it reaches Highway 243, it has grown into a modest but dependable stream tumbling down between boulders. In the springtime, the banks are lined with wildflowers. Water-loving trees hug the edge,

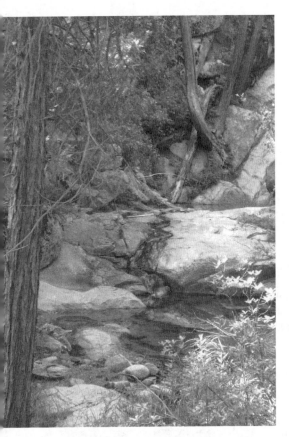

North Fork of the San Jacinto River

while oaks, incense cedars, and pines grow tall on the slopes above. This part of the river is a great place to take a saunter while visiting the Idyllwild area. Although this is a short hike, it becomes strenuous near the end because the trail can be steep and poorly defined. Wear boots with good traction.

The San Jacinto River is of special biological interest because it's one of the last populated habitats in the San Bernardino National Forest for the endangered mountain yellow-legged frog (*Rana muscosa*). Historically this was one of the most common frog species in Southern California and used to be found in virtually every year-round stream in the mountains, but it has been driven to near extinction in recent years. Because of the presence of this and other sensitive species, the Forest Service requires visitors to avoid water play, wading, rock-hopping, and fishing, and to stay 10 feet from the creek's edge. However, hiking the trail above the creek is still allowed. Watch for signs posted in the area with the latest information or check with the San Jacinto Ranger Station.

The unmarked trail begins on the south side of the highway bridge and leads east upstream. Frequent forks lead down to the water, but stay on the main trail. If it becomes indistinct, keep going and you'll soon find it again. Expect to encounter many downed trees. The shady canyon rings with birdsong. Wild thimbleberries and currants ripen along the trail in the summer, and moss beards the north-facing granite boulders.

Soon after passing an enormous old-growth ponderosa pine, the trail veers right to bypass some huge granite blocks, and it becomes steeper and harder to follow at times. At 0.7 mile, arrive at a bridge just south of the Dark Canyon Campground.

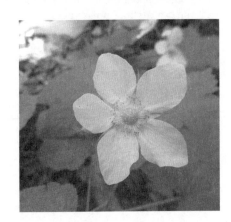

Thimbleberry flower

trip 9.5 Seven Pines Trail

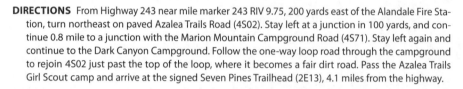

Distance	7 miles (out-and-back)
Hiking Time	4 hours
Elevation Gain	2,400'
Difficulty	Strenuous
Best Times	May–October
Agencies	San Bernardino National Forest (San Jacinto Ranger Station) and Mount San Jacinto State Park
Recommended Maps	Tom Harrison *San Jacinto Wilderness, Santa Rosa & San Jacinto Mountains National Monument,* or USGS *Lake Fulmor* and *San Jacinto Peak 7.5'*
Permit	San Jacinto Wilderness Permit required

see map on p. 194

DIRECTIONS From Highway 243 near mile marker 243 RIV 9.75, 200 yards east of the Alandale Fire Station, turn northeast on paved Azalea Trails Road (4S02). Stay left at a junction in 100 yards, and continue 0.8 mile to a junction with the Marion Mountain Campground Road (4S71). Stay left again and continue to the Dark Canyon Campground. Follow the one-way loop road through the campground to rejoin 4S02 just past the top of the loop, where it becomes a fair dirt road. Pass the Azalea Trails Girl Scout camp and arrive at the signed Seven Pines Trailhead (2E13), 4.1 miles from the highway.

The lightly traveled Seven Pines Trail climbs through the spectacular forests, creeks, and rock formations on the western slopes of San Jacinto. It's longer but less steep than the nearby Marion Mountain Trail (see Trip 9.6). This is a good place to escape when you'd like to contemplate the mountain in quiet and solitude.

From the trailhead, the Seven Pines Trail switchbacks up to the northeast, passing north of a small knob before turning south and descending to the San Jacinto River. This stretch of the river headwaters is home to the endangered mountain yellow-legged frog (*Rana muscosa*). To protect the frog and its habitat, the river and its banks are presently closed to all entry. However, crossing the river along the trail is still permitted. Beyond the river, the trail continues upward and twice crosses the intermittent creek flowing down from Deer Springs before arriving at the Pacific Crest Trail (PCT). Return the way you came.

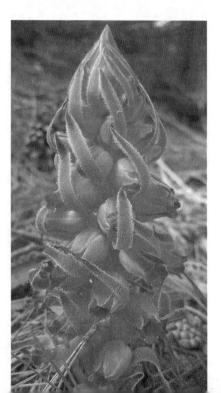

VARIATIONS————————————

Many other options are available for a longer trip. You can continue up to San Jacinto Peak. Or, with a 4-mile car or bicycle shuttle, you can descend the nearby Marion Mountain Trail. Note that the road between the two trails drops 600 feet to cross the San Jacinto River near Dark Canyon before climbing back up, so it's a vigorous bicycle ride in either direction.

Snow plant

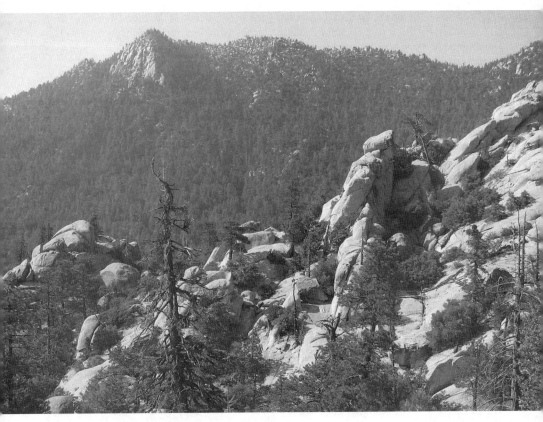

Western slopes of San Jacinto

trip 9.6   San Jacinto Peak via the Marion Mountain Trail

see map on p. 194

Distance	12 miles (out-and-back)
Hiking Time	7 hours
Elevation Gain	4,500'
Difficulty	Strenuous
Trail Use	Suitable for backpacking
Best Times	June–October
Agencies	San Bernardino National Forest (San Jacinto Ranger Station) and Mount San Jacinto State Park
Recommended Maps	Tom Harrison *San Jacinto Wilderness, Santa Rosa & San Jacinto Mountains National Monument*, or USGS *Lake Fulmor* and *San Jacinto Peak* 7.5'
Permit	San Jacinto Wilderness Permit required

DIRECTIONS From Highway 243 near mile marker 243 RIV 9.75, 200 yards east of the Alandale Fire Station, turn northeast on paved Azalea Trails Road (4S02). Stay left at a junction in 100 yards, and continue 0.8 mile to a junction with the Marion Mountain Campground Road (4S71). Turn right and follow this road 0.6 mile to the Marion Mountain Trailhead, located between Fern Basin and Marion Mountain Campgrounds.

The Marion Mountain Trail on the western flank of San Jacinto is the shortest route to the summit without taking the tram. This side of the mountain attracts relatively few hikers, so it's good for those seeking seclusion. Moreover, its short and direct route is ideal for springtime snow ascents of San Jacinto.

Backpackers with a camping permit from Mount San Jacinto State Park can stay at Little Round Valley Trail Camp; the quota often fills a month or more ahead of time on popular summer weekends. Water might be available at a stream in the meadow in Little Round Valley; it flows all year in wet years but can dry up in the summer during drought years. The most reliable creek in the area is Bed Springs Crossing, 0.5 mile southwest of Little Round Valley. Ask the rangers about water before you go.

The signed Marion Mountain Trail (2E14) starts across the road from the parking area and immediately begins switchbacking up the ridge through incense cedars, oaks, firs, pines, and manzanitas. In 0.4 mile, the trail crosses a dirt road leading left down to Marion Mountain Campground; it then passes an unmarked trail on the left down to the water tank by the campground. Just beyond a second road crossing, a signed trail on the right descends 2.8 miles to Stone Creek Campground.

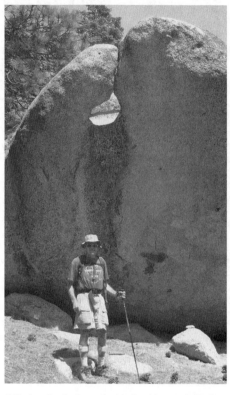

Window Rock along the Marion Mountain Trail

The Marion Mountain Trail continues up the north shoulder of the ridge, offering views into the headwaters of the San Jacinto River. At 1.25 miles, a rocky clearing 50 feet north of the trail offers unobstructed vistas. Shortly before you reach the Pacific Crest Trail (PCT), pass a peculiar gigantic boulder with a "window" near the top.

At 2.8 miles, reach the PCT and turn left. In 100 feet, pass a signed junction for the Seven Pines Trail that leads back down to Dark Canyon Campground (see Trip 9.5). Continue east and then north 0.5 mile, crossing the creek coming down from Deer Springs, to another junction where the Deer Springs Trail departs the PCT. Turn right and follow the Deer Springs Trail northeast to the pleasant camp at Little Round Valley (1 mile). This section involves difficult navigation when covered in snow because it can be difficult to pick out landmarks. Switchback another 1.3 miles up to the saddle between San Jacinto and Jean Peaks. Turn left and hike 0.3 mile up to the summit rocks of San Jacinto.

Return the way you came. Or, with a car or bike shuttle, explore any of the multitude of other fine trails girding the mountain.

trip 9.7   **Panorama Point**

see map on p. 194

Distance	0.8 mile (loop)
Hiking Time	20 minutes
Elevation Gain	100'
Difficulty	Easy
Trail Use	Dogs allowed, good for kids, wheelchair accessible
Best Times	May–October
Agency	Mount San Jacinto State Park
Optional Map	Tom Harrison *San Jacinto Wilderness* or USGS *San Jacinto Peak* 7.5'

DIRECTIONS From Highway 243 near mile marker 243 RIV 9.75, 200 yards east of the Alandale Fire Station, turn northeast on paved Azalea Trails Road. In 0.1 mile, veer right into Stone Creek Campground. Pay a use fee at the Iron Ranger; then drive to the top of the campground and park at the trailhead near site 16.

The San Jacinto area is peppered with delightful mountain campgrounds. Stone Creek Campground offers not only camping, but also a short nature trail to Panorama Point. The views from the point are now somewhat obscured by the fast-growing forest, but the trail is nevertheless pleasant and features excellent interpretive signs. Listen for the chickadees and keep an eye out for squirrels and lizards. The dirt path is wide and well graded, so sturdy wheelchairs can reach the vista. Call 800-444-7275 or see www.parks.ca.gov for campground reservations.

Walk north from the trailhead past the Panorama Point Trail sign. The trail is situated at nearly 6,000 feet, which is a transition zone in the forest. The manzanitas, oaks, ponderosa pines, and Coulter pines of the lower mountain begin giving way to sugar and Jeffrey pines. In 0.3 mile, reach an unmarked junction. Stay left and curve around 0.1 mile to Panorama Point. On a clear day, you can see all the way to the Pacific Ocean. Return to the junction and complete the loop back to the campground.

VARIATION

The 2.8-mile Stone Creek Trail climbs 800 feet from Stone Creek Campground up to Marion Mountain Campground. It passes the site of a historic sawmill en route. With a 1.5-mile car or bicycle shuttle, this trip can be done as a one-way excursion. Dogs and bicycles are prohibited on this trail.

The Stone Creek Trail crosses Mount San Jacinto State Park. Obtain a free day-use wilderness permit near the entrance of Stone Creek Campground. The trail starts at the southeast end of the campground near site 7. It leads east-southeast, following the path of a defunct nature trail. In 0.2 mile, reach a dirt logging road. Turn left and continue east 0.5 mile to a junction. Stay left again and climb 1.0 mile to a sign for the Stone Creek Trail. Turn left (north) onto the trail and reach Sawmill Flats in 0.1 mile. A disintegrating stone structure and heavy metal cables mark the site of the former mill. Continue north 1.0 mile to a junction with the Marion Mountain Trail and a dirt road (see Trip 9.6). Follow the dirt road down to the Marion Mountain Campground near site 11.

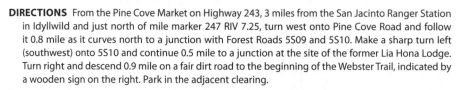

trip 9.8 **Webster Trail**

Distance	5 miles (out-and-back)
Hiking Time	3 hours
Elevation Gain	2,000'
Difficulty	Moderate
Trail Use	Dogs allowed
Best Times	October–June
Agency	San Bernardino National Forest (San Jacinto Ranger Station)
Recommended Maps	Tom Harrison *San Jacinto Wilderness* or USGS *Lake Fulmor* and *San Jacinto Peak* 7.5'

see map on p. 194

DIRECTIONS From the Pine Cove Market on Highway 243, 3 miles from the San Jacinto Ranger Station in Idyllwild and just north of mile marker 247 RIV 7.25, turn west onto Pine Cove Road and follow it 0.8 mile as it curves north to a junction with Forest Roads 5S09 and 5S10. Make a sharp turn left (southwest) onto 5S10 and continue 0.5 mile to a junction at the site of the former Lia Hona Lodge. Turn right and descend 0.9 mile on a fair dirt road to the beginning of the Webster Trail, indicated by a wooden sign on the right. Park in the adjacent clearing.

The Webster Trail plunges steeply down a ridge into the secluded canyon carved by the North Fork of the San Jacinto River. The river is a great place to take a dip on a moderately warm day and you'll likely have it to yourself. An ideal time to visit is shortly after a good rain in the spring, but don't underestimate the steep, shadeless climb on your return. Carry plenty of water and wear boots with good tread or use a hiking pole to help with the loose footing.

The Webster Trail is named for David G. Webster, who established an early ranch in the San Jacinto Valley and drove his cattle up to summer pastures along this trail in the 1870s and 1880s.

The trail descends westward along the ridge, briefly through a forest of Jeffrey pines and oaks, then down through chaparral. It makes a solitary switchback near the bottom to negotiate the final drop into the river canyon.

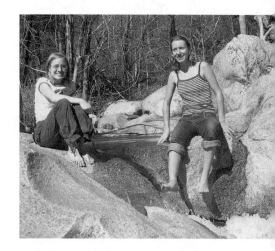

Hikers cool their feet at the North Fork of the San Jacinto River.

trip 9.9 **Idyllwild Nature Center Loop**

Distance	2.1 miles (loop)
Hiking Time	1.5 hours
Elevation Gain	600'
Difficulty	Moderate
Trail Use	Dogs allowed, good for kids
Best Times	All year
Agency	Riverside County Regional Park and Open-Space District

see maps on pgs. 194 & 208

Optional Maps Tom Harrison *San Jacinto Wilderness* or USGS *San Jacinto Peak* and
USGS *Idyllwild* 7.5'
Permit Day-use fee required ($4 adults, $3 kids ages 2–12)

DIRECTIONS From the San Jacinto Ranger Station, drive west 1 mile on High-way 243. Turn left (south) into the Idyllwild Nature Center. Pass through a gate and proceed 0.3 mile to the nature center parking at the end of the road.

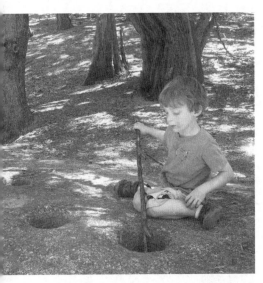

Grinding acorns in a metate near Lily Creek

The Idyllwild Nature Center is located on the west side of Idyllwild at the site of an ancient Cahuilla Indian village. It features nature programs, camping, picnicking, a short interpretive nature trail, and a longer loop trail. It's a good place to take a ramble, learn about mountain ecology, and enjoy fine views of Tahquitz Peak. The nature center is open Wednesday–Sunday, 9 a.m.–4 p.m., and sometimes Tuesdays. Begin your visit at the nature center to pay your day-use fee and pick up a map and trail guide. The exhibits at the nature center are unusually good and appeal to all ages. School and youth groups can arrange environmental education programs with advance notice.

Adjacent Idyllwild Park has a popular campground and picnic area; call 800-234-7275 for reservations. Although the park and nature center are both part of the Riverside County Parks system, they charge separate admission fees.

This loop begins behind the nature center. Follow a signed trail for the View Point and Campground southeast for 0.1 mile to the View Point atop a small hill, where you can enjoy a bench or admire the granite ramparts of Tahquitz Peak. The open forest is notable for gigantic treelike pink-bracted manzanitas (*Arctostaphylos pringlei* ssp. *drupacea*) as well as canyon live oaks and incense cedar, ponderosa pines, and Coulter pines. Continue 0.1 mile to a junction with a trail leading to the campground. Stay right and hike west 0.2 mile to an unmarked junction near a gigantic oak. The right fork leads back to the nature center, but take the left fork, cross Lily Creek, and reach a signed junction in 0.1 mile on the far side of the creek.

From here, make a loop. The easiest way to go is counterclockwise. Start up the right fork, variously labeled Summit Trail or Steep Trail. Follow the switchbacks 0.5 mile as they climb almost but not quite to the highest point of the hill at the edge of the park. The best views of the trip are found in this area. Follow marker posts down 0.5 mile to a four-way junction at the edge of the campground. Turn left and follow the Hillside Trail, which generally contours along the slope, passing some large granite blocks that are popular with boulderers. In 0.6 mile, arrive back at the junction beside Lily Creek.

Hike back across Lily Creek; then turn left to shortcut back. Go 100 yards to a T-junction; then turn right and go another 100 yards back to the nature center.

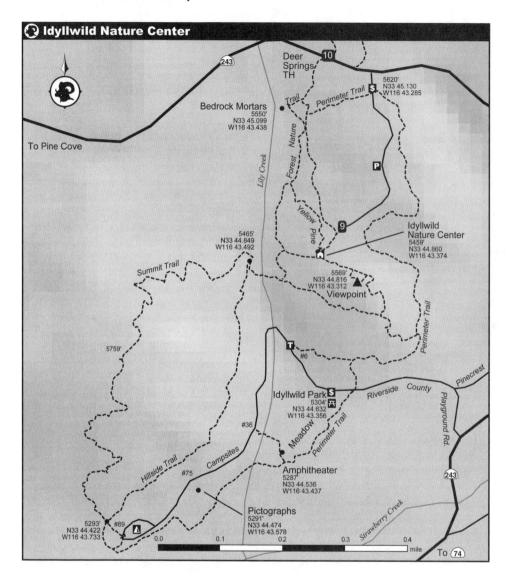

Idyllwild Nature Center

Deer Springs TH

10

243

5620'
N33 45.130
W116 43.285

S

Perimeter Trail

Trail

Bedrock Mortars
5550'
N33 45.099
W116 43.438

Nature

Forest

To Pine Cove

Lily Creek

P

Yellow

Pine

9

Idyllwild
Nature Center
5459'
N33 44.860
W116 43.374

5465'
N33 44.849
W116 43.492

Summit Trail

5569'
N33 44.816
W116 43.312
Viewpoint

Perimeter Trail

5759'

T
#6

Idyllwild Park
5304'
N33 44.632
W116 43.356

S

Riverside   County

Pinecrest

Playground Rd.

Meadow

Perimeter Trail

#36

243

Hillside Trail

Campsites

#75

Amphitheater
5287'
N33 44.536
W116 43.437

Strawberry Creek

5293'
N33 44.422
W116 43.733

#89

Pictographs
5291'
N33 44.474
W116 43.578

0.0   0.1   0.2   0.3   0.4

mile

To 74

VARIATIONS

The easy 0.7-mile Yellow Pine Forest Nature Trail starts at a sign in front of the nature center. Ten numbered posts are described in the trail guide, available at the nature center and the trailhead. One of the highlights of the trail is the bedrock mortars, called metates, where Cahuilla Indians ground acorns from black oaks.

The Perimeter Trail starts near the gate near Highway 243 at the north entrance to the Idyllwild Nature Center. Follow it east and then south 1 mile to the campground entrance road, just outside the fee station. Optionally, you can continue south past the amphitheater, negotiate a narrow section along a tributary creek, follow an easement outside the park fenceline to the southeast corner of the park, and then join the Hillside Trail and Nature Trail to make a return loop.

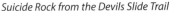

trip 9.10 **Suicide Rock**

Distance	7 miles (out-and-back)
Hiking Time	3.5 hours
Elevation Gain	1,900'
Difficulty	Moderate
Best Times	May–October
Agencies	San Bernardino National Forest (San Jacinto Ranger Station) and Mount San Jacinto State Park
Recommended Map	Tom Harrison *San Jacinto Wilderness, Santa Rosa & San Jacinto Mountains National Monument*, or USGS *San Jacinto Peak* 7.5'
Permit	San Jacinto Wilderness Permit required

see maps on pgs. 194 & 208

DIRECTIONS From the San Jacinto Ranger Station in Idyllwild, drive west 1 mile on Highway 243. Park on the right (north) side of the road, just west of the Idyllwild Nature Center entrance and just past a sign on your left pointing to DEER SPRINGS TRAILHEAD PARKING.

Suicide Rock sits atop the ridge overlooking Strawberry Valley, drawing rock climbers to test their mettle on its steep, clean, granite faces. According to legend, the rock gets its name from two young Native American lovers, who leapt from the top rather than obeying the chief's order to separate. The most straightforward route to the top of the rock is via the Deer Springs Trail from the western edge of Idyllwild.

The Deer Springs Trail itself (3E17) starts on the north side of the road 50 yards east of the parking area. Alternatively, walk up a steep unmarked path above the parking area 150 yards to a junction with the Deer Springs Trail near some power lines. Turn left and proceed uphill, joining the main trail.

The trail climbs north onto the ridge, through stands of huge treelike manzanita. As you gain altitude, the chaparral gives way to black oak and Jeffrey pine. In 2.3 miles, reach a signed junction and turn right onto the Suicide Rock Trail. The trail contours along the slope, then dips down to cross Marion Creek before climbing back up to Suicide Rock.

Suicide Rock from the Devils Slide Trail

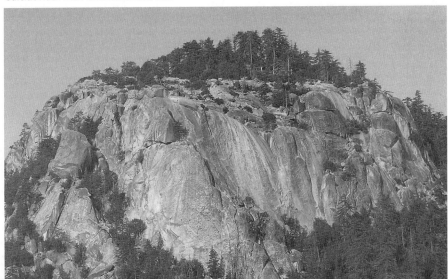

Enjoy the views, but take care that children don't stray too far from the trail. The cliffs roll off deceptively before dropping straight down. There is no safe way down to the east without a rope.

ALTERNATIVE FINISH

Return to the northwest end of Suicide Rock and find a climber's trail that descends the dirt slopes and drops down the steep hill to Fern Valley Road at the switchback below Humber Park. The trail can be difficult to follow in places, but with a car or bicycle shuttle, it makes for an interesting alternative route.

---

trip 9.11   Tahquitz Rock

see map on p. 195

Distance	2.2 miles (out-and-back)
Hiking Time	2 hours
Elevation Gain	1,600'
Difficulty	Moderate
Best Times	May–October
Agency	San Bernardino National Forest (San Jacinto Ranger Station)
Recommended Map	Tom Harrison *San Jacinto Wilderness, Santa Rosa & San Jacinto Mountains National Monument,* or USGS *San Jacinto Peak 7.5'*

DIRECTIONS From the San Jacinto Ranger Station on Highway 243, head northeast on Pine Crest Avenue. In 0.6 mile, veer right onto South Circle Drive. In 0.1 mile, turn left onto Fern Valley Road. After 1.7 miles, reach a small parking area for the Ernie Maxwell Scenic Trail. If you reach the large lot and restrooms at Humber Park, you've gone 0.1 mile too far.

Tahquitz Rock was the birthplace of technical rock climbing in the United States. In the 1930s, Robert Underhill brought modern rope techniques developed in the Alps back to Sierra Club members in California. The massive granite dome of Tahquitz Rock attracted immediate attention. In 1937, Dick Jones and Glen Dawson climbed the Mechanic's Route, which, with a rating of 5.8, was the most difficult route in America at the time. Since then, thousands of climbers have flocked to the rock's sheer walls to hone their skills. Fortunately for hikers, an easier route to the summit exists, involving some rock scrambling but no ropes.

Tahquitz Rock

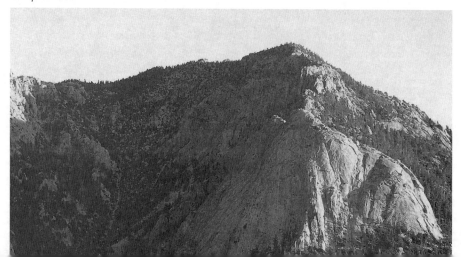

The United States Geographical Survey gave the formation the less imposing title Lily Rock in 1898, commemorating Lily Eastman, daughter of Dr. Sanford Eastman, one of the founding fathers of Riverside. However, the Tahquitz Rock name goes back far earlier to the Cahuilla people who occupied the region, and Tahquitz is the preferred name among rock climbers.

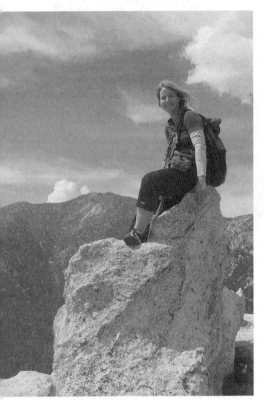

Hike south on the Ernie Maxwell Scenic Trail through a forest of oaks, white firs, incense cedars, and Jeffrey pines. Immediately descend to cross the east fork of Strawberry Creek; then round a bend and look for a signed steep climber's trail leading up the hill to your left, 0.2 mile. In 0.4 mile, reach a large boulder known to climbers as Lunch Rock. Pass around the right side to the base of Tahquitz Rock. Follow the climber's trail to the right around the south and east side of the rock; it can be difficult to follow in places but is worth finding because it avoids the worst of the bushes. When it tops out on a saddle directly east of the summit, climb third-class ramps and boulders to the summit of Tahquitz Rock, 0.5 mile. Descend exactly the way you went up, to avoid getting stuck on cliffs.

ALTERNATIVE FINISH

Once back to the saddle, you can also descend the north gully on another rough climber's trail and then follow a path along the East Fork of Strawberry Creek back to Humber Park.

Marion Mountain from Tahquitz Rock

trip 9.12 Ernie Maxwell Scenic Trail

Distance	5 miles (out-and-back)
Hiking Time	2.5 hours
Elevation Gain	700'
Difficulty	Easy
Trail Use	Dogs allowed
Best Times	May–October
Agency	San Bernardino National Forest (San Jacinto Ranger Station)
Recommended Map	Tom Harrison *San Jacinto Wilderness, Santa Rosa & San Jacinto Mountains National Monument,* or USGS *San Jacinto Peak* 7.5'

see map on p. 195

DIRECTIONS This trail can be accessed from either the south or north end. This description starts at the south end so that the hike is downhill on the way back. From Highway 243 near the south end of Idyllwild next to the Idyllwild School, turn east on Saunders Meadow Road. Note that Saunders Meadow forms a loop and intersects Highway 243 a second time farther south by the dump. Drive

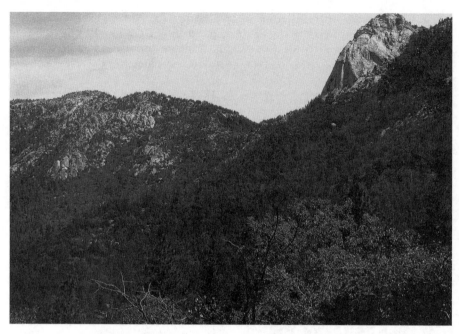

Tahquitz Rock and Strawberry Valley from the Ernie Maxwell Scenic Trail

0.8 mile, turn left (north) on Pine Avenue, go 0.2 mile, and turn right on Tahquitz View Drive. Proceed 0.5 mile, passing the South Ridge Road junction, to the signed Ernie Maxwell Scenic Trail. Parking is limited to a few wide spots along the road. The north end of the trail is just below Humber Park (see Trip 9.11).

The Ernie Maxwell Scenic Trail commemorates the founder of the *Idyllwild Town Crier* newspaper and longtime conservationist who greatly influenced the town of Idyllwild. This pleasant trail through the forest above town is a good place to take a stroll while visiting town.

Tahquitz Rock is prominently visible from the southern terminus of the trail. The path leads northeast through a forest of oaks, cedars, pines, and firs with occasional glimpses of Strawberry Valley and Suicide Rock through the woods. In the spring, you may see brilliant red snow plants poking up through the ground. In 2.5 miles, pass beneath Tahquitz Rock and reach the northern end at Humber Park. Return the way you came.

trip 9.13   Skunk Cabbage Meadow

Distance	6.5 miles (out-and-back)
Hiking Time	3 hours
Elevation Gain	1,700'
Difficulty	Moderate
Trail Use	Dogs allowed, suitable for backpacking
Best Times	May–October
Agency	San Bernardino National Forest (San Jacinto Ranger Station)

see map on p. 195

Recommended Map Tom Harrison *San Jacinto Wilderness, Santa Rosa & San Jacinto Mountains National Monument,* or USGS *San Jacinto Peak* 7.5'
Permit San Jacinto Wilderness Permit required

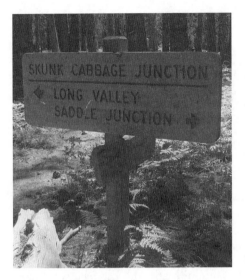

Skunk Cabbage Junction

DIRECTIONS From the San Jacinto Ranger Station on Highway 243, head northeast on Pine Crest Avenue. In 0.6 mile, veer right onto South Circle Drive. In 0.1 mile, turn left onto Fern Valley Road. Proceed 1.8 miles to the Humber Park Trailhead, at the road's end.

The Devils Slide Trail is the main trail out of Idyllwild. Cattle ranchers used to drive their herds up through the loose and dangerous slopes over thornbushes, boulders, and logs to summer pastures in Tahquitz Valley. The trail is now so well graded that some have rechristened it "Angel's Glide," but it nevertheless has a strenuous start if you're hiking with a heavy pack. On the far side of Saddle Junction is a fine conifer forest dotted with a few meadows. This trip leads to one of those meadows, with a pleasant camp centrally located for exploring the plethora of nearby trails. The Skunk Cabbage Meadow area is at the edge of the Mountain Fire burn zone.

The area beyond Saddle Junction is an appealing destination for an introductory backpacking trip. When you apply for your wilderness permit, you'll need to choose one of several camping zones in the area (Skunk Cabbage, Chinquapin, North Rim, or Tahquitz). The Forest Service will give you a map of campsites in your zone marked with brown posts; these tend to be excellent sites that can accommodate groups of up to 10. Tahquitz Creek may be dry in the summer; ask the ranger about water availability. Many brown-post sites are temporarily closed due to the 2013 Mountain Fire.

Take the Devils Slide Trail 2.5 miles to Saddle Junction. It climbs 1,700 feet from Humber Park to Saddle Junction. The ponderosa pines, incense cedar, and black oaks at Humber Park are soon replaced by canyon live oak and sugar pines as you climb. Jeffrey pines and white fir are also common, especially around Saddle Junction. As you pass the gullies with early-season creeks, watch for moisture-loving wildflowers, including columbine and scarlet monkeyflower. This is a good trail to observe four species of wild berries. From smallest to largest leaves, these include the Sierra gooseberry (with thorny stems and berries), the wax currant (with red berries), the Sierra currant (with blue berries), and the thimbleberry (with huge leaves and delicious red raspberry-like fruit).

Saddle Junction is a five-way junction. Take the signed fork leading northeast toward Skunk Cabbage Meadow and Willow Creek. Divinely perfumed azaleas grow by some of the springs adjacent to the trail. In 0.6 mile, turn right at another signed junction and hike 0.2 mile to the campsites near the meadow. Wilderness regulations require campsites to be at least 200 feet away from meadows. Water might be found between the junction and Willow Creek. Respect posted closure notices related to the Mountain Fire.

trip 9.14 Tahquitz Peak via Saddle Junction

Distance	8.5 miles (out-and-back)
Hiking Time	5 hours
Elevation Gain	2,400'
Difficulty	Strenuous
Trail Use	Dogs allowed, suitable for backpacking
Best Times	May–October
Agency	San Bernardino National Forest (San Jacinto Ranger Station)
Recommended Map	Tom Harrison *San Jacinto Wilderness, Santa Rosa & San Jacinto Mountains National Monument,* or USGS *San Jacinto Peak* 7.5'
Permit	San Jacinto Wilderness Permit required

see map on p. 195

DIRECTIONS From the San Jacinto Ranger Station on Highway 243, head northeast on Pine Crest Avenue. In 0.6 mile, veer right onto South Circle Drive. In 0.1 mile, turn left onto Fern Valley Road. Proceed 1.8 miles to the Humber Park Trailhead, at the road's end.

Tahquitz Peak (8,828') is the second major summit in the San Jacinto Mountains after San Jacinto itself. The summit overlooks Idyllwild and is guarded by dramatic granite buttresses, most notably Tahquitz Rock. Tahquitz Peak is named for a legendary evil Cahuilla shaman who eats the souls of the unwary. Hikers use several pronunciations, but the correct Cahuilla pronunciation is "**taw**-kwish."

The peak can be reached from either the north or south. This trip follows the more heavily traveled northern route, which starts from the popular Humber Park Trailhead. See Trip 9.19 for the route up the south ridge.

Backpackers with an overnight permit from the Forest Service can stay in the Chinquapin camping zone between Saddle Junction and Tahquitz Peak. Water may be unreliable in the summer and fall.

From Humber Park, hike 2.5 miles up the Devils Slide Trail to the five-way Saddle Junction, where you meet the Pacific Crest Trail (PCT). Take the rightmost fork and hike south on the PCT toward Tahquitz Peak, gradually climbing through the open forest. The trees become smaller and more weather-beaten as you climb. In 1.4 miles, reach the South Ridge Trail junction. Take it right (southwest) toward Tahquitz Peak 0.4 mile; then take a short spur up to the summit.

The Tahquitz Peak Fire Lookout is located on the summit, taking advantage of commanding views in all directions. The remote lookout is staffed during fire season by Southern California Mountains Foundation Fire Lookout Hosts who hike up to their airy post. The friendly and knowledgeable volunteers are happy to point out the sights and talk about the San Jacinto Mountains.

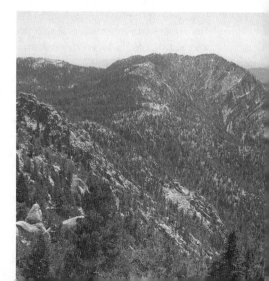

Tahquitz Peak from the north

trip 9.15 Caramba

Distance	14 miles (out-and-back)
Hiking Time	7 hours
Elevation Gain	3,300'
Difficulty	Strenuous
Trail Use	Dogs allowed, suitable for backpacking
Best Times	May–October
Agency	San Bernardino National Forest (San Jacinto Ranger Station)
Recommended Maps	Tom Harrison *San Jacinto Wilderness, Santa Rosa & San Jacinto Mountains National Monument,* or USGS *San Jacinto Peak* and *Palm Springs* 7.5'
Permit	San Jacinto Wilderness Permit required

see map on p. 195

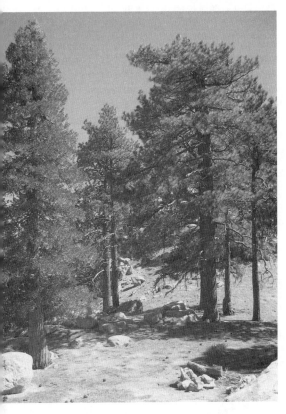

Caramba Camp

DIRECTIONS From the San Jacinto Ranger Station on Highway 243, head northeast on Pine Crest Avenue. In 0.6 mile, veer right onto South Circle Drive. In 0.1 mile, turn left onto Fern Valley Road. Proceed 1.8 miles to the Humber Park Trailhead, at the road's end.

Note: *This area burned in the 2013 Mountain Fire and remained closed at press time.*

Tahquitz Valley hangs on the southeastern slope of the San Jacinto Mountains, walled in by granite ridges. Tahquitz Creek flows down the gentle valley beneath the white firs and Jeffrey pines until it abruptly drops over a waterfall and plunges down Tahquitz Canyon to the desert near Palm Springs. Good campsites are found in the Lower Basin Zone, including one by the lip of the precipice. ¡Ay, caramba! is a Spanish expression of surprise, more recently popularized by Bart Simpson. Author John Robinson relates two stories of how the camp got its name. In one, cowboys camping on the rim were spooked by strange noises in the night. In another more prosaic story, the abrupt drop from Tahquitz Valley down to the desert shocked the travelers.

In 1916–17, Moses Gordon cut a remarkable trail from Palm Springs up Tahquitz Canyon to Caramba and on to Idyllwild to connect his winter home and summer cabin. He stayed at Caramba camp while building the trail. Unfortunately, the Gordon Trail has fallen into disrepair and now the upper reaches of Tahquitz Canyon are nearly impassable because of steep cliffs and heavy brush.

This trip offers a fine tour of Tahquitz Valley and impressive views down Tahquitz Canyon. It's a good backpacking trip, and you're likely to have camping to yourself even on a fine summer weekend where crowds flock to the less-remote camps on San Jacinto. Water sources are undependable in the summer, however, so check with the ranger before you go.

Grind your way 1,700 feet up the Devils Slide Trail 2.5 miles to the five-way Saddle Junction. Follow a signed trail southeast through the open forest toward Tahquitz Valley and Laws-Caramba. In 0.6 mile, pass a trail junction in Tahquitz Valley. Continue east another 1.6 miles to Laws Camp, where travel writer George Law built a stone summer cabin along Willow Creek in 1915. Beyond, the trail descends to another tributary creek, climbs, and then drops 2 miles to Caramba.

From the trail's end, you can wander a few yards downstream to the first Tahquitz Creek waterfall, which drops into Tahquitz Canyon. Better yet, scramble up the hillside east of camp for an unobstructed view down into the canyon. There is another beautiful campsite here, although you must haul water up from the creek.

VARIATION

South of Caramba are a pair of bumps on the ridge between Tahquitz and Andreas Canyons. The higher one (7,339') is unofficially known as Sam Fink Peak in honor of the Sierra Club leader who pioneered the trail along the Desert Divide; it's a fun excursion for campers with extra energy. Bring the USGS *Palm Springs* topo map for cross-country navigation.

Sam Fink Peak is reached from the ridge east of Caramba camp by taking a compass bearing on the saddle between the bumps and traveling half a mile cross-country to the saddle, then turning left (southeast) and hiking up to the summit for a spectacular view.

---

trip 9.16 Strawberry Valley Loop

Distance	10 miles (one-way or loop)
Hiking Time	5 hours
Elevation Gain	2,600'
Difficulty	Strenuous
Trail Use	Suitable for backpacking
Best Times	May–October
Agencies	San Bernardino National Forest (San Jacinto Ranger Station) and Mount San Jacinto State Park
Recommended Map	Tom Harrison *San Jacinto Wilderness, Santa Rosa & San Jacinto Mountains National Monument,* or USGS *San Jacinto Peak* 7.5'
Permit	San Jacinto Wilderness Permit required

see map on p. 195

Upper reaches of Strawberry Valley

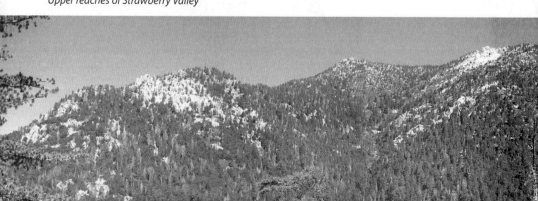

DIRECTIONS This loop hike near Idyllwild starts at Humber Park and ends at the Deer Springs Trailhead, requiring a 3.6-mile car shuttle. If you've brought just one vehicle, you can descend a climber's trail near Suicide Rock to return to Humber Park, but this demands some cross-country route-finding skill.

Leave a getaway vehicle at the Deer Springs Trailhead, 1 mile west of the San Jacinto Ranger Station in Idyllwild on Highway 243. The poorly marked trailhead is on the north side of the road, just west of the Idyllwild Nature Center entrance.

To reach Humber Park, go southeast down Highway 243 and turn left (northeast) onto Pine Crest Avenue, passing the San Jacinto Ranger Station in Idyllwild on your left. In 0.6 mile, veer right onto South Circle Drive. In 0.1 mile, turn left onto Fern Valley Road and proceed 1.8 miles to the Humber Park Trailhead, at the road's end.

Strawberry Creek carves a scenic valley out of the south slopes of Marion Mountain and the San Jacinto Ridge. The ridges are lushly forested and decorated with huge granite outcrops, including the famous Tahquitz and Suicide Rocks. This loop climbs the Devils Slide Trail to the east ridge, cuts across the north slopes of the valley, and descends the west ridge past Suicide Rock. Several fine campsites are located along the way.

The Devils Slide Trail (see Trip 9.13) climbs 1,700 feet from Humber Park over 2.5 miles to the five-way Saddle Junction, which delimits the west end of the splendid Tahquitz Valley. Creeks flow through the meadows and open forest, and there are good camping zones around Tahquitz Valley and Skunk Cabbage Meadow. If you have an extra day, consider spending the night in the valley and exploring the trails to Tahquitz Peak or the Caramba Overlook.

Turn left (north) at Saddle Junction and follow the Pacific Crest Trail (PCT) as it climbs the ridge. At a junction in 1.8 miles, turn left (west) and hike across the chaparral-clad slopes forming the north wall of Strawberry Valley. Enjoy magnificent views of Tahquitz and Suicide Rocks from this portion of the trail. Strawberry Creek flows down from its source high on Marion Mountain, and you may be able to refill water here, though the creek dries up in late summer. In 2.2 miles, come to the dry but spectacularly situated Strawberry Junction trail camp beneath the Jeffrey pines and to another trail junction just beyond. Camping permits for this site are issued by the Mount San Jacinto State Park rather than the Forest Service.

Turn left (south) and leave the PCT, joining the Deer Springs Trail instead. The pines and firs in this open forest are some of the most beautiful in Southern California. Follow the trail down the ridge 1.6 miles to the Suicide Rock turnoff. If a vehicle awaits at the Deer Springs Trailhead, continue straight down the ridge another 2.1 miles through a "forest" of giant manzanitas to the trailhead. The trail splits beneath some wires at the very end and the right path shortcuts down to the western trailhead parking.

ALTERNATIVE FINISH —————————————————————————————————

If you didn't arrange a shuttle, turn left at the Suicide Rock turnoff and hike 1.2 miles northeast up to the rock. This adds 600 feet of climbing to the trip. You may wish to continue all the way to the top to enjoy the view. However, the best descent begins back at the northwest end of the rock and skirts the cliffs. Take care not to head down Suicide Rock's sheer face, for obvious reasons. A climber's trail follows the base of the slabs to the east end of the rock, then drops down to Fern Valley Road. It can be difficult to follow at times and is quite steep in places. The route eventually meets Forest Haven Drive, then crosses Strawberry Creek and arrives at Fern Valley Road just below the water tanks, 1 mile down from the rock. Hike 0.3 mile up the road to the Humber Park lot.

see map on p. 195

trip 9.17 Idyllwild–Round Valley Loop

Distance	14 miles (loop)
Hiking Time	7 hours
Elevation Gain	3,600'
Difficulty	Strenuous
Trail Use	Suitable for backpacking
Best Times	May–October
Agencies	San Bernardino National Forest (San Jacinto Ranger Station) and Mount San Jacinto State Park
Recommended Map	Tom Harrison *San Jacinto Wilderness, Santa Rosa & San Jacinto Mountains National Monument,* or USGS *San Jacinto Peak 7.5'*
Permit	San Jacinto Wilderness Permit required

DIRECTIONS From the San Jacinto Ranger Station on Highway 243, head northeast on Pine Crest Avenue. In 0.6 mile, veer right onto South Circle Drive. In 0.1 mile, turn left onto Fern Valley Road. Proceed 1.8 miles to the Humber Park Trailhead, at the road's end.

John Robinson offers a marvelously poetic description of Round Valley in *San Bernardino Mountain Trails:*

> *Southeast from San Jacinto's lofty crown, nestled in high hanging valleys ringed by jagged spurs of white granite, is an enchanting wonderland of green. Here, suspended 8,000 feet above the desert, pines and firs grow tall and sturdy, lush meadows are waist-high with fern and azalea, lupines spot hillsides in their late-summer bloom of purple and pale mauve, and little singing streams flow clear and cold. In the heart of this high sylvan wilderness is Round Valley, an oval meadow of verdant grass, threaded by an icy-cold brook, surrounded by a dense forest of lodgepole pine. Here is the most popular trail camp in the San Jacinto high country, frequented by dozens of backpackers almost every summer and early fall weekend.*

This trip visits Round Valley the hard way, up the Devils Slide from Idyllwild and through Tahquitz Valley, offering a fine tour of the southeast side of San Jacinto.

Backpackers will need a camping permit from Mount San Jacinto State Park for Round Valley or from the Forest Service for the Chinquapin Zone. Water is fairly reliable at Round Valley and seasonal elsewhere along the route.

Follow the Devils Slide Trail 2.5 miles as it climbs 1,700 feet to the five-way Saddle Junction. Take the signed trail northeast toward Willow Creek and Long Valley. In 0.5 mile, pass a field of ferns and the signed turnoff for Skunk Cabbage Meadow. Continue east and drop down to cross Willow Creek; then climb to a trail junction on the north side of a rocky knob in another 1.5 miles. Take the north fork toward Long and Round Valleys. The trail climbs gradually before passing an intermittent creek on the way to a pleasant shady bench. Beyond, the trail switchbacks up toward the Hidden Divide. Watch for a rocky outcrop where you can scramble up for a fine view of Tahquitz Valley. Reach the saddle on Hidden Divide in 1.7 miles.

The main trail continues north and in 0.3 mile reaches another junction. If you like, you can take the right (north) fork, which leads to the Long Valley Ranger Station and tramway and curves back toward Round Valley, but it's shorter to head directly west 1 mile. Rejoin the trail from Long Valley continuing west and in 0.2 mile arrive at Round Valley, which is often filled with legions of happy campers who came the short way from the tram.

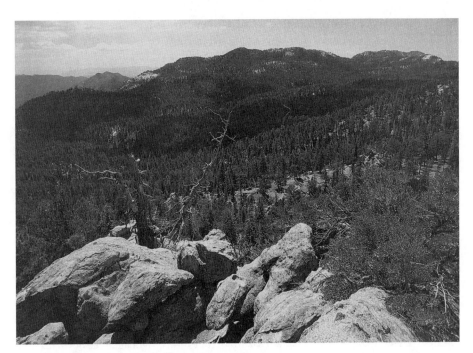

Tahquitz Valley from the south side of the Hidden Divide

Your route climbs steadily west 1 mile to the Wellman Divide, the highest point on the loop. Turn left and hike another mile past the seeping Wellman Cienega to reach a junction with the Pacific Crest Trail (PCT). Turn left again and hike 1.9 miles south down the ridge back to Saddle Junction; then follow Devils Slide Trail back to the trailhead.

trip 9.18 San Jacinto Peak from Humber Park

see map on p. 195

Distance	18 miles (loop)
Hiking Time	10 hours
Elevation Gain	4,500'
Difficulty	Strenuous
Trail Use	Suitable for backpacking
Best Times	June–October
Agencies	San Bernardino National Forest (San Jacinto Ranger Station) and Mount San Jacinto State Park
Recommended Map	Tom Harrison *San Jacinto Wilderness, Santa Rosa & San Jacinto Mountains National Monument,* or USGS *San Jacinto Peak* 7.5'
Permit	San Jacinto Wilderness Permit required

DIRECTIONS From the San Jacinto Ranger Station on Highway 243, head northeast on Pine Crest Avenue. In 0.6 mile, veer right onto South Circle Drive. In 0.1 mile, turn left onto Fern Valley Road. Proceed 1.8 miles to the Humber Park Trailhead, at the road's end.

This trip is my favorite tour of the San Jacinto Wilderness high country. This is a land of superlatives: the most dramatic granite faces, most beautiful conifer forests, and second-highest mountains in Southern California. Starting at Humber Park in Idyllwild, it makes a counterclockwise loop by way of Saddle Junction and over the Wellman Divide, then goes to the very pinnacle of San Jacinto Peak before descending through Little Round Valley and returning along the Pacific Crest Trail (PCT). It's a great way to get to know the San Jacinto Peak area. Beautifully situated camping zones along the route offer tempting backpacking options.

From Humber Park, take the strenuous Devils Slide Trail to Saddle Junction, climbing 1,700 feet in just over 2.5 miles. Along the way, enjoy spectacular views of Suicide and Tahquitz Rocks, which are swarming with bold climbers on pleasant days. Backpackers can find good camping zones south of Saddle Junction in the Chinquapin Zone, but our trip turns sharply left at Saddle Junction and joins the northbound PCT as it climbs the ridge overlooking Strawberry Valley.

In 1.9 miles, the trail reaches a junction. The PCT turns west toward Strawberry Junction (see Trip 9.16), but we continue north another mile past the swampy Wellman Cienega and up through chaparral and boulders to the Wellman Divide. Here another trail descends east to the campsites of Round Valley (dependable water) and down to the Palm Springs Aerial Tramway.

Continue north along the chaparral-clad east slope of Jean Peak. The prominent pyramid to the northeast is Cornell Peak (see Trip 9.22). After one big switchback, the trail reaches the saddle south of San Jacinto Peak in 2.4 miles. Turn right and hike north 0.3 mile to the granite summit boulders. Along the way, pass a stone hut, which offers emergency shelter (although it's not recommended in an electrical storm). The final yards to the summit involve hopping up the big talus.

After returning to the saddle, continue west and descend 1.3 miles to Little Round Valley, with splendid camping beneath the Jeffrey pines along a seasonal stream. This is about the halfway point of the trip, although all of the strenuous climbing is now behind you.

Descend the Deer Springs Trail southwest. In 0.5 mile, you'll cross a creek fed by Bed Springs, the most reliable water along this route, and in another half mile you rejoin the PCT. Follow it southwest 0.5 mile to junctions with the Seven Pines and Marion Mountain Trails, then south through a beautiful open forest of Jeffrey pines and white firs. In 2.3 miles, reach Strawberry Junction. A small dry trail camp with panoramic views is situated just east of the junction.

Here you have three return options: via the PCT, Suicide Rock, or Deer Springs. The 6.7-mile PCT option is the simplest choice, leading east across the head of Strawberry Valley, then turning south and retracing your earlier route to Saddle Junction and the Devils Slide Trail to Humber Park.

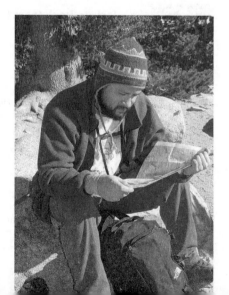

Consulting a map on the Wellman Divide

The 4.2-mile Suicide Rock option requires plenty of daylight and involves difficult cross-country travel that's recommended only for experienced hikers with light packs. Take the Deer Springs Trail south 1.8 miles; then turn left and follow the Suicide Rock Trail 1.0 mile to the 7,528-foot summit for an outstanding view. Retrace your steps to the northwest end of the rock, where you can find a climber's trail skirting the edge. Do not be tempted to descend the cliffs directly—there is no safe route without a rope. Follow the faint and often confusing climber's trail, which is occasionally marked with cairns. It passes along the base of the rock, then steeply descends a mile to Forest Haven Drive and back to Fern Valley Road. Hike uphill 0.4 mile back to Humber Park.

The Deer Springs option is the shortest but requires a car shuttle. Simply hike 4.1 miles down the ridge to the trailhead, located 1 mile west of the San Jacinto Ranger Station on Highway 243 in Idyllwild (see Trip 9.10).

---

trip 9.19   Tahquitz Peak via the South Ridge Trail

Distance	7 miles (out-and-back)
Hiking Time	4 hours
Elevation Gain	2,400'
Difficulty	Strenuous
Trail Use	Dogs allowed
Best Times	May–October
Agency	San Bernardino National Forest (San Jacinto Ranger Station)
Recommended Map	Tom Harrison *San Jacinto Wilderness, Santa Rosa & San Jacinto Mountains National Monument,* or USGS *San Jacinto Peak* 7.5'
Permit	San Jacinto Wilderness Permit required

see map on p. 195

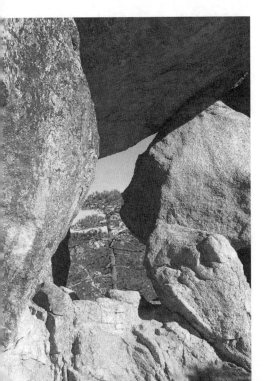

DIRECTIONS From Highway 243 on the south edge of Idyllwild next to Idyllwild School, drive up Saunders Meadow Road for 0.8 mile. Turn left on Pine Avenue, drive 0.2 mile, and then turn right on Tahquitz View Drive. After 0.3 mile, just before the road becomes dirt, turn right on South Ridge Road (5S11). Proceed 0.9 mile, passing several minor side roads, to the signed South Ridge Trail (3E08) parking area.

Tahquitz Peak (8,828') is the second major summit in the San Jacinto Mountains after San Jacinto itself. The summit overlooks Idyllwild and is guarded by dramatic granite buttresses, most notably Tahquitz Rock. The peak can be reached from either the north or south. This trip follows the shorter and more secluded route up the beautiful south ridge. See Trip 9.14 for the northern route.

Window on the South Ridge Trail

Follow the trail as it climbs to the crest of the ridge and then zigzags up the divide through rich forest. In 1.4 miles, pass a curious "window" in the rock framing a splendid view of the Desert Divide to the east. Continue through a field of massive boulders 0.3 mile to a flat clearing about halfway to your destination, a good rest stop. Beyond, you climb on the steep west face below the rocky ridge. Pass through chinquapin thickets, scattered lodgepole pines, and towering granite gendarmes. The views continue to open up, with Tahquitz Rock and the San Jacinto massif to the north; Suicide Rock and the San Gabriel Mountains to the northwest; Idyllwild and Santiago Peak to the west; and the Garner Valley, Desert Divide, and Toro Peak to the south. Just below the summit, reach a junction. Turn right and walk a short distance to the summit lookout, 3.6 miles from the start.

Tahquitz Peak Fire Lookout stands on the summit, taking advantage of the commanding views in all directions. The remote lookout is staffed during fire season by Southern California Mountains Foundation Fire Lookout Hosts who hike up to their airy post. The friendly and knowledgeable volunteers are happy to point out the sights and talk about the San Jacinto Mountains. Return the way you came.

ALTERNATIVE FINISH

For a terrific 11-mile loop, continue east to the Pacific Crest Trail (PCT), follow it north to Saddle Junction, descend the Devils Slide Trail, and hike back along the Ernie Maxwell Scenic Trail and South Ridge Road.

---

trip 9.20   Desert View Loop

Distance	1.6 miles (loop)
Hiking Time	1 hour
Elevation Gain	350'
Difficulty	Easy
Trail Use	Good for kids
Best Times	May–October
Agency	Mount San Jacinto State Park
Optional Map	Tom Harrison *San Jacinto Wilderness, Santa Rosa & San Jacinto Mountains National Monument*, or USGS *San Jacinto Peak 7.5'*

see map on p. 195

DIRECTIONS From Highway 111, 8.5 miles south of the 10 Freeway at the northern edge of Palm Springs, turn west up Tramway Road and drive 4 miles to Valley Station, the lower terminus of the Palm Springs Aerial Tramway. The tram operates daily, starting at 10 a.m. Monday–Thursday, and 8 a.m. Friday–Sunday and holidays. The last tram return is at 9:45 p.m. The tram closes for annual maintenance, typically in September. Check pstramway.com or call 888-515-TRAM for the most current information.

This family-friendly hike is an easy introduction to the pleasures of Mount San Jacinto State Park. It tours forest, meadow, and creek, as well as taking you to impressive vista points looking into the desert from the sheer east slopes of San Jacinto. There is a short Desert View Loop Trail and an even shorter

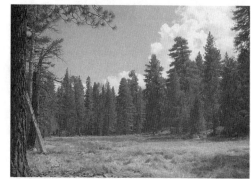

Desert View Nature Trail

Nature Loop Trail. Interpretive signs along the path explain some of the flora and fauna, while park volunteers periodically lead guided tours; ask at the Long Valley Ranger Station for more information. Kids may enjoy scrambling on the rocks and fallen logs; teach them not to trample the inviting but fragile meadow.

From Mountain Station, proceed 0.2 mile down the cement walkway to the Long Valley Picnic Area. Look for the sign marking the start of the Desert View Loop Trail to the left (south). If you reach the ranger station, you've gone 0.1 mile too far.

You can take the loop in either direction, but this description follows a counterclockwise direction. At a fork beyond the sign, veer right and cross a small bridge at the end of a meadow. Long Valley Creek runs through this area until August during a normal year, though it may dry up by July in a drought year. Look and listen for the many species of birds that inhabit the meadow and the adjoining forest of Jeffrey pines and white firs.

In 0.25 mile, the Nature Loop Trail veers left to loop back to the start, but the main Desert View Loop continues. In another 0.1 mile, come to a vista point above a granite dome. The loop curves around and climbs an open slope dotted with Jeffrey pines to a second vista point, where you can admire the Santa Rosa Mountains and Toro Peak on the skyline at the head of Palm Canyon. It then passes a third and fourth outlook with views into the desert. Occasionally the trail may become poorly defined, but choose the path that looks most heavily traveled. Pass a second junction with the Nature Loop Trail, and soon return to the start near the bridge.

trip 9.21 Round Valley

Distance	4.5 miles (out-and-back)
Hiking Time	2.5 hours
Elevation Gain	700'
Difficulty	Easy
Trail Use	Good for kids, suitable for backpacking
Best Times	May–October
Agency	Mount San Jacinto State Park
Recommended Map	Tom Harrison *San Jacinto Wilderness, Santa Rosa & San Jacinto Mountains National Monument,* or USGS *San Jacinto Peak* 7.5'
Permit	San Jacinto Wilderness Permit required

see map on p. 195

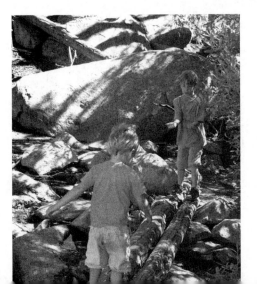

DIRECTIONS From Highway 111, 8.5 miles south of the 10 Freeway at the northern edge of Palm Springs, turn west up Tramway Road and drive 4 miles to Valley Station, the lower terminus of the Palm Springs Aerial Tramway. The tram operates daily, starting at 10 a.m. Monday–Thursday, and 8 a.m. Friday–Sunday and holidays. The last tram return is at 9:45 p.m. The tram closes for annual maintenance, typically in September. Check pstramway.com or call 888-515-TRAM for the most current information.

The Palm Springs Aerial Tramway provides rapid access to the high country in

Creek crossing on the trail to Round Valley

the Mount San Jacinto State Park Wilderness. From the tram station, it's an easy walk down to the Long Valley Ranger Station, then up along Long Valley Creek through the woods to the campground at Round Valley.

This is a popular destination in the summer for picnics, family campouts, and Boy Scout hikes. Winter brings easy access to snow, so this a great destination for cross-country skiers and snowshoers.

From the rear of the tram station, walk 0.3 mile west down to the Long Valley Ranger Station, passing the signed turnoff to the left for the Desert View Loop Trail. Get a wilderness permit at the ranger station and continue west. In 0.1 mile, arrive at another signed junction. The left trail leads to the Hidden Divide, but your trail continues straight ahead through the forest of pines and firs dotted with granite boulders. The Long Valley Creek nearby usually runs until August, though in a dry year it may stop in July. Look for a meadow with corn lilies before you reach another trail junction in 1.4 miles. A lateral trail turns hard left back toward the Hidden Divide, but the main trail again continues straight. Pass another meadow on the north side of the trail with good views of the pointy Cornell Peak beyond. In 0.4 mile more, arrive at the Round Valley Campground.

This is a good place to explore and have lunch. The spigot at the junction has reliable water but it should be treated. An outhouse is nearby. A trail leads north 0.5 mile to Tamarack Valley. Numerous fine campsites are scattered along side trails in Round and Tamarack Valleys. Return the way you came. Or, for a longer trip, continue up to San Jacinto Peak (see Trip 9.23) or Cornell Peak (Trip 9.22).

trip 9.22   Cornell Peak

Distance	6 miles (out-and-back)
Hiking Time	4 hours
Elevation Gain	1,400'
Difficulty	Moderate
Trail Use	Suitable for backpacking
Best Times	June–October
Agency	Mount San Jacinto State Park
Recommended Map	Tom Harrison *San Jacinto Wilderness, Santa Rosa & San Jacinto Mountains National Monument,* or USGS *San Jacinto Peak 7.5'*
Permit	San Jacinto Wilderness Permit required

see map on p. 195

DIRECTIONS From Highway 111, 8.5 miles south of the 10 Freeway at the northern edge of Palm Springs, turn west up Tramway Road and drive 4 miles to Valley Station, the lower terminus of the Palm Springs Aerial Tramway. The tram operates daily, starting at 10 a.m. Monday–Thursday, and 8 a.m. Friday–Sunday and holidays. The last tram return is at 9:45 p.m. The tram closes for annual maintenance, typically in September. Check pstramway.com or call 888-515-TRAM for the most current information.

Cornell Peak is an impressive pyramid-shaped peak with a rocky summit block overlooking Round Valley. This hike is relatively short but requires some cross-country navigation and some airy rock climbing at the very top. It is, by far, the most enjoyable summit in the San Jacinto area.

From the tramway station, descend to the Long Valley Ranger Station to get a wilderness permit; then hike west 2.2 miles to Round Valley (reliable water), and follow the side trail north 0.5 mile to the northernmost campsite in Tamarack Valley (see Trip 9.21). Along the way, keep an eye out for the distinctive peak and assess the best route to the top.

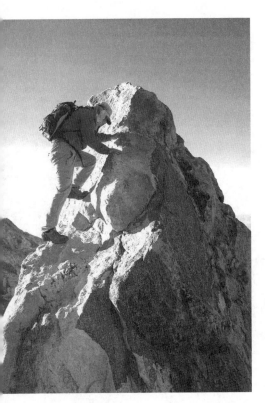

Cornell Peak's airy summit block

From Tamarack Valley, hike cross-country up steep slopes to the north, threading your way around bands of manzanita. You may find some use trails and animal paths, but it's hard to distinguish the best one from the others. Your goal is to reach the summit ridge between Cornell Peak and the rounded rock pile immediately to the east. Once on the ridge, turn west and follow it to the summit rocks.

The final 20 feet of climbing is tricky third class. Many hikers stop at the base rather than risk climbing the steep rock. The easiest ascent scales a wide crack with a chockstone, then shimmies along the summit block to the highest point. Getting down is harder than getting up.

VARIATIONS

If you wish to climb some more, there are two more small peaks nearby. The 9,520-plus-foot rock pile on the ridge just east of Cornell is locally known as Harvard Peak. The more interesting 9,360-plus-foot pinnacle southeast of Harvard Peak is called Yale Peak.

Descend the way you came, heading southeast until it's easy to walk down through the trees. Do not be tempted to head directly south or west from the summit—steep cliffs block all of these paths. Once off the summit, take a shortcut cross-country to the southeast to rejoin the main trail halfway back to Long Valley. The route follows a good use trail along the north bank of the north fork of Long Valley Creek. Rejoin the main trail in 0.6 mile at a switchback where the trail crosses the creek. Then follow the main trail 0.5 mile back to the Long Valley Ranger Station.

trip 9.23 San Jacinto Peak from the Palm Springs Aerial Tramway

Distance	10 miles (out-and-back)
Hiking Time	6 hours
Elevation Gain	2,600'
Difficulty	Strenuous
Trail Use	Suitable for backpacking
Best Times	June–October
Agency	Mount San Jacinto State Park
Recommended Map	Tom Harrison *San Jacinto Wilderness, Santa Rosa & San Jacinto Mountains National Monument*, or USGS *San Jacinto Peak* 7.5'
Permit	San Jacinto Wilderness Permit required

see map on p. 195

DIRECTIONS From Highway 111, 8.5 miles south of the 10 Freeway at the northern edge of Palm Springs, turn west up Tramway Road and drive 4 miles to Valley Station, the lower terminus of the Palm Springs

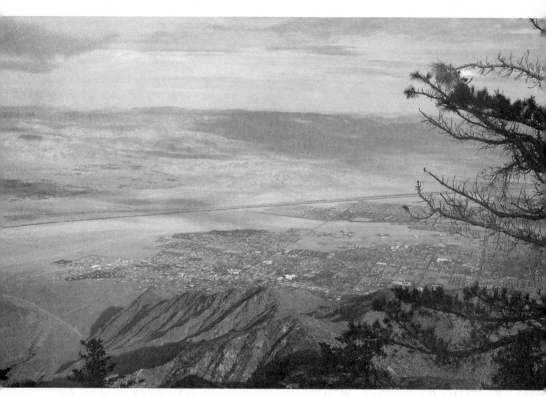

View of Palm Springs from the Aerial Tramway Observation Deck   Photo: Larry B. Van Dyke

Aerial Tramway. The tram operates daily, starting at 10 a.m. Monday–Thursday, and 8 a.m. Friday–Sunday and holidays. The last tram return is at 9:45 p.m. The tram closes for annual maintenance, typically in September. Check pstramway.com or call 888-515-TRAM for the most current information.

This is the easiest route to the summit of San Jacinto, but it's still a strenuous and rewarding hike.

From the tramway station, descend to the Long Valley Ranger Station to obtain a wilderness permit; then hike west 2.2 miles to Round Valley (see Trip 9.21). Continue 1 mile west to meet a trail junction on the Wellman Divide. Turn right (north) and gradually climb across the east face of Jean Peak through interminable fields of chinquapin; then switchback up to a saddle south of San Jacinto Peak in 1.7 miles. Turn right (north) and follow a trail 0.3 mile to the summit, passing an emergency shelter along the way. The cabin was constructed by the California Conservation Corps around 1933 and is cared for by volunteers; if you visit or must use it in a storm, leave it better than you found it. The final stretch involves scrambling up boulders to the summit rocks. For those who have hiked Half Dome in Yosemite National Park, this final stretch is reminiscent of the last part of the Half Dome Trail immediately below the cables.

Peer over the north edge of the summit to admire Snow Creek, which drops more than 8,000 feet to the desert below in scarcely 3 miles (see Trip 11.8). The precipice is especially impressive when covered with snow in the spring and early summer. Return the way you came.

trip 9.24 Seven Peaks of the San Jacinto Wilderness

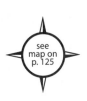

see map on p. 125

Distance	14 miles (loop)
Hiking Time	11 hours
Elevation Gain	5,400'
Difficulty	Very strenuous
Best Times	June–October
Agency	Mount San Jacinto State Park
Required Map	Tom Harrison *San Jacinto Wilderness, Santa Rosa & San Jacinto Mountains National Monument,* or USGS *San Jacinto Peak* 7.5'
Permit	San Jacinto Wilderness Permit required

DIRECTIONS From Highway 111, 8.5 miles south of the 10 Freeway at the northern edge of Palm Springs, turn west up Tramway Road and drive 4 miles to Valley Station, the lower terminus of the Palm Springs Aerial Tramway. The tram operates daily, starting at 10 a.m. Monday–Thursday, and 8 a.m. Friday–Sunday and holidays. The last tram return is at 9:45 p.m. The tram closes for annual maintenance, typically in September. Check pstramway.com or call 888-515-TRAM for the most current information.

This challenging trip explores all of the officially named summits of the San Jacinto high country; visiting the summits of Marion Mountain, Jean Peak, Newton Drury Peak, Folly Peak, San Jacinto, Miller Peak, and Cornell Peak. This excursion is primarily composed of cross-country hiking as opposed to traveling a well-used trail.

The high country here is as reminiscent of the Sierra Nevada as any location in Southern California. The Jeffrey pine and white fir forests give way to lodgepole and limber pines as you climb. San Jacinto's south-facing slopes are heavily overgrown with chinquapins, manzanitas, and buckthorns.

The central objective of this trip is to pick a path that minimizes the bushwhacking. Some of the summits involve stimulating third-class climbing on excellent granite. You should be intimately familiar with the area before you attempt this adventure. If you're doing it as a day hike, plan to take the 8 a.m. tram up. Bring a headlamp, and be sure to return before the tram closes at 9:45 p.m. Water sources along the route are unreliable, so carry at least 4 quarts.

From the tram station, hike down to the Long Valley Ranger Station and obtain a wilderness permit. Follow the trail to Round Valley and then up to Wellman Divide. The direct route from the divide to Marion Mountain is unbearably brushy. Instead, turn south and follow the trail 0.5 mile, descending several switchbacks to reach Wellman Cienega, in a huge field of ferns and corn lilies. Turn right (northwest) and pick a path up the unlikely-looking slope toward the saddle. This unfortunately involves tramping through the tall plants for a short distance; beware of rattlesnakes. Stay toward the right side of the corn lilies, and you'll

San Jacinto high country from Luella Todd Peak

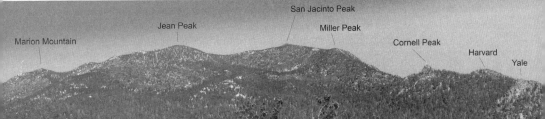

soon find a ducked climber's path where the chinquapin has been beaten down. This is crucial to the route; the alternatives are quite unpleasant. The route eventually shifts right onto a shallow ridge with Jeffrey and lodgepole pines mixed with chaparral, then bears left into a better-defined gully, and left again onto an open-forested slope that leads up to the saddle.

Marion Mountain is the westernmost high point along the ridge to your southwest. The top of the ridge is dotted with large boulders, so the best route is to contour west before you climb south. Again, you may find a ducked climber's trail. The summit boulders are immense; they can be climbed from the northeast by starting at a dead tree, scaling a short crack, jogging right, and then turning left again and ascending a third-class chimney. Marion has arguably the best view of any peak in the San Jacinto Mountains. The summit towers above the trees, offering a 360-degree panorama and a particularly good view of the next four peaks that you're about to climb. It's worth studying the map and planning your routes to Jean, Newton Drury, Folly, and San Jacinto.

The easiest path to Jean Peak is nearly a straight line, staying just west of Peak 10,388'. Navigation is tricky in the forest, but simply head for the high point after passing Peak 10,388'; there are no false summits near Jean. Although Jean is the second-highest peak in the area, views from it are obstructed by the forest.

Newton Drury Peak is the next destination. The peak was named for one of the most successful 20th-century American conservationists. He led the Save the Redwoods League of California, served for more than a decade as director of the National Park Service, and arranged the 1930 land swap with the Southern Pacific Railroad that created Mount San Jacinto State Park. The bump is puny for a man of such great stature, but it's covered in a beautiful limber pine forest and fine granite slabs. There is a shallow ridge connecting Drury to Jean. The south side of the ridge is brushy. The best route from Jean is to hike north toward a saddle before turning west toward Drury. Descend to another saddle immediately east of Drury; then scamper the short way up to the summit.

Folly Peak is another insignificant bump on the scenic and rocky Fuller Ridge, which drops northwest from San Jacinto. To reach Folly, return to the saddle east of Drury, and follow easy slopes northwest down to Little Round Valley Campground. You may find water here, though the source dries up early in the season in some years. Follow the San Jacinto Trail up seven switchbacks to the 10,000-foot contour, where you leave the trail and trudge north toward the ridge, weaving back and forth to avoid the worst of the chinquapin and boulders. Some bushwhacking is inevitable. There are several bumps on the ridge of nearly equal height to Folly Peak. Folly is the westernmost bump; below it, a boulder field drops down into the upper reaches of Snow Creek.

Follow the ridge from Folly up to San Jacinto. You may find a climber's trail in places just south of the ridgeline. The tectonic forces that thrust upward and shattered these massive granite blocks to build San Jacinto are nearly inconceivable. On a pleasant summer afternoon, you're very likely to surprise day hikers relaxing on the summit.

Follow the trail down from San Jacinto, past the emergency shelter, heading south to the saddle and then northeast to a major switchback. Miller Peak is scarcely a stone's throw away. Take an easy walk up and across a sandy clearing before you scramble up the dark summit boulders. The bump on the ridge is named for Frank A. Miller, the founder of Riverside's famous Mission Inn. He was a prominent advocate of Boy Scouting and world peace. The peak was dedicated in 1936 by 22 Scout troops that simultaneously ignited bonfires atop summits all over Southern California. A plaque on the summit commemorates Miller and the Scout Oath.

Follow the San Jacinto Trail south to Wellman Divide and back down to Round Valley. A historic trail once shortcut directly down to Tamarack Valley, but it was closed to protect a sensitive deer fawning area. If daylight permits, continue on to Cornell Peak. This dramatic granite pyramid is the lowest but most exhilarating of the seven summits. From Round Valley, follow the trail north to Tamarack Valley; then pick a path among the numerous use trails up to the top (see Trip 9.22). The summit register is located immediately below the summit rocks. Climbers will enjoy the third-class scramble up a crack and an airy shimmy to the highest block. Descend the way you came; staying too far east leads to some tricky climbing.

For your return, hike east cross-country from Tamarack Valley to shortcut back to the main trail. The route follows a good use trail along the north bank of the north fork of Long Valley Creek. It rejoins the main trail in 0.6 mile at a switchback where the trail crosses the creek. Then you follow the main trail 0.5 mile back to the Long Valley Ranger Station, and finally stumble up the paved walkway to the tram.

VARIATIONS

This loop obviously has many possible variations, and you may add or subtract peaks according to your tastes. Jean Peak can also be reached without too much bushwhacking by climbing its northeast slope from the San Jacinto Trail or by running the ridge from San Jacinto.

The west ridge of Folly Peak looks like a convenient shortcut down to the Pacific Crest Trail (PCT) on Fuller Ridge, but it's not recommended because of heavy brush.

The 9,520-plus-foot rock pile immediately east of Cornell is locally known as Harvard, and the more attractive 9,360-plus-foot summit southeast of that is called Yale.

Peak 9,356' on the Hidden Divide is sometimes called Luella Todd or Landells Peak, and features a grand view of San Jacinto's east side.

Taking a breather on San Jacinto Peak

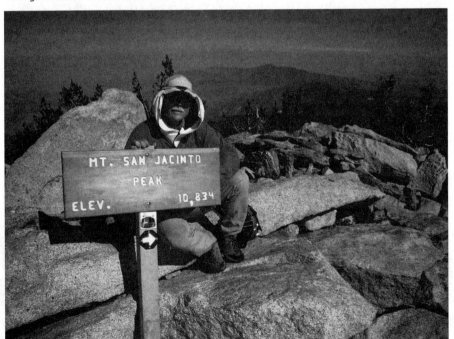

chapter 10

Desert Divide

The Desert Divide is a remote and lonely mountainous backbone running south from San Jacinto and Tahquitz Peak to Highway 74. It overlooks the tranquil Garner Valley to the west and the deep Palm Canyon to the east. The northern section is rugged, studded with massive granite outcrops, while the southern section is rounded and gentler.

Much of the divide is covered in dense chaparral. The legendary Sam Fink, a Santa Ana fire captain and Sierra Club leader, spent nearly a decade in the 1960s and 1970s chopping a route along the crest of the divide. The Pacific Crest Trail (PCT) now follows much of the Sam Fink Trail's original route. Constructing the PCT along the divide required three years of drilling, blasting, and cutting, making it the most difficult stretch to build in Southern California. The well-engineered trail now offers hospitable access to this formerly inaccessible country.

The Desert Divide is a great place to visit if you're seeking solitude. It can be suitable for hiking year-round, but tends to be hot in the summer, and sometimes the northern exposures are icy well into the spring. If you plan to visit the higher elevations before the middle of April, an ice ax and crampons may be necessary.

The entire Desert Divide is within the Santa Rosa and San Jacinto Mountains National Monument, which was established by Congress in 2000. The portions of the Desert Divide north of Fobes Saddle are in San Jacinto Wilderness. A wilderness permit is required to enter wilderness areas. The permits can be obtained in person or by mail, at no charge, from the San Jacinto Ranger Station in Idyllwild. At this writing, the Devils Slide Trail is the only trailhead with a quota.

On April 29, 2008, a thoughtless hiker discarded a lit cigarette on the trail. The resulting Apache Fire burned 784 acres on Apache Peak and the upper reaches of Murray and West Palm Canyons. More than 700 firefighters hiked in and chopped their way through dense chaparral to contain the blaze.

Then in July 2013, a spark from an electrical equipment failure ignited the Mountain Fire. The fire swept onto the Desert Divide and consumed more than 27,000 acres between Cedar Spring and Tahquitz Valley. The PCT took major damage along the rugged divide. At this writing, it remains closed between the Spitler Peak Trail and Tahquitz Peak.

Desert Divide from the east

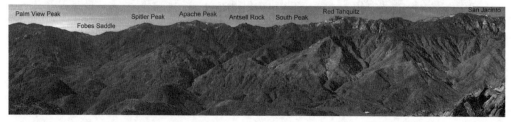

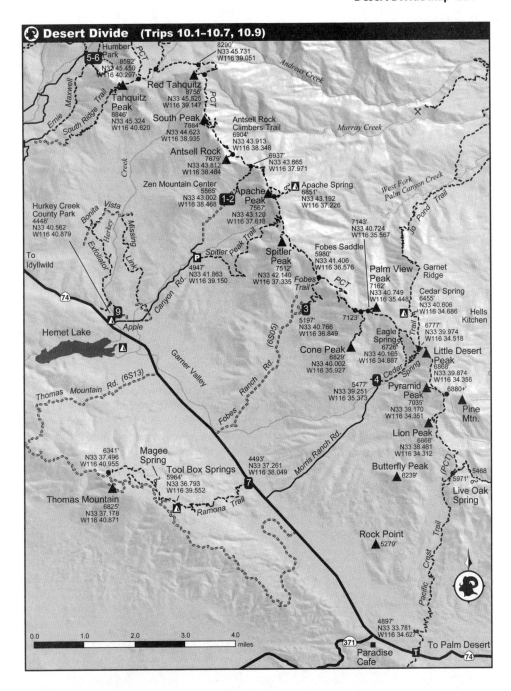

Desert Divide (Trips 10.1–10.7, 10.9)

Humber Park
5-6
8592'
N33 45.450
W116 40.297

PCT

8290'
N33 45.731
W116 39.051

Andreas Creek

Red Tahquitz
8756'
N33 45.525
W116 39.147

Tahquitz Peak
8846'
N33 45.324
W116 40.620

South Peak
7884'
N33 44.623
W116 38.935

PCT

Antsell Rock Climbers' Trail
6904'
N33 43.913
W116 38.348

Murray Creek

Ernie Maxwell

South Ridge Trail

Antsell Rock
7679'
N33 43.812
W116 38.484

6937'
N33 43.665
W116 37.971

Creek

Zen Mountain Center
5565'
N33 43.002
W116 38.468

Apache Peak
1-2
7567'
N33 43.120
W116 37.618

Apache Spring
6851'
N33 43.192
W116 37.226

West Fork
Palm Canyon Creek

Hurkey Creek County Park
4448'
N33 40.562
W116 40.879

Bonita Vista

Hurkey

Missing Link

Exfoliator

Spitler Peak Trail

P
4947'
N33 41.863
W116 39.150

Spitler Peak
7512'
N33 42.140
W116 37.335

Fobes Trail

Fobes Saddle
5980'
N33 41.406
W116 36.576

7143'
N33 40.724
W116 35.567

Pond Trail

Palm View Peak
7162'
N33 40.749
W116 35.448

Garnet Ridge

To Idyllwild

74

9

Apple

Canyon Rd.

(6S05)

3
5197'
N33 40.766
W116 36.849

7123'

PCT

Cedar Spring
6455'
N33 40.606
W116 34.686

Hells Kitchen

6777'
N33 39.974
W116 34.518

Hemet Lake

Garner Valley

Ranch Rd.

Cone Peak
6829'
N33 40.002
W116 35.927

Eagle Spring
6726'
N33 40.165
W116 34.887

Cedar Spring Trail

Little Desert Peak
6868'
N33 39.874
W116 34.356

Thomas Mountain Rd. (6S13)

Fobes

5477'
N33 39.251
W116 35.373

4
Pyramid Peak
7035'
N33 39.170
W116 34.351

6880'

Pine Mtn.

6341'
N33 37.496
W116 40.955

Magee Spring

Tool Box Springs
5964'
N33 36.793
W116 39.552

4493'
N33 37.261
W116 38.049

7

Morris Ranch Rd.

Lion Peak
6868'
N33 38.461
W116 34.312

Butterfly Peak
6239'

(PCT)

5468

5971'

Live Oak Spring

Thomas Mountain
6825'
N33 37.178
W116 40.871

Ramona Trail

Rock Point
5279'

Pacific Crest Trail

0.0   1.0   2.0   3.0   4.0
miles

371

4897'
N33 33.781
W116 34.627

Paradise Cafe

To Palm Desert

74

| trip 10.1 | **Antsell Rock** |

Distance	4 miles (out-and-back)
Hiking Time	4 hours
Elevation Gain	2,300'
Difficulty	Strenuous
Best Times	April–June, October–November
Agency	San Bernardino National Forest (San Jacinto Ranger Station)
Recommended Maps	Tom Harrison *San Jacinto Wilderness, Santa Rosa & San Jacinto Mountains National Monument,* or USGS *Idyllwild* and *Palm View Peak* 7.5'
Permit	San Jacinto Wilderness Permit required

see map on p. 231

DIRECTIONS From Highway 74, 3.4 miles southeast of Mountain Center and just before mile marker 074 RIV 62.75, turn left (east) onto Apple Canyon Road. Proceed 3.3 miles to the road's end at Pine Springs Ranch. Immediately before you enter the ranch, veer right onto a good private dirt road leading to the Zen Mountain Center. In 1.1 miles, park in a small dirt lot on the left just before you enter the Zen Center.

Note: *This area burned in the 2013 Mountain Fire and remained closed at press time.*

Antsell Rock is the jewel of the Desert Divide. Edmund Perkins, of the USGS, named it for an artist at the Keen Camp Resort who was painting the peak. Antsell Rock stands high above the divide, and its stony buttresses make an impressive sight from most directions. It's also one of the few mountaineers' peaks in Southern California requiring more than the usual plodding to reach the third-class summit. While this trip is short, it certainly isn't easy.

Access to the Desert Divide is plagued by private property inholdings within the San Bernardino National Forest. However, the Zen Mountain Center graciously allows hikers to cross its property and follow a spectacular trail that leads directly to the divide. Please help retain this privilege by being a courteous trail user. Avoid bringing large groups or large numbers of vehicles. Keep your voice down while crossing the center so as not to

Antsell Rock after the Mountain Fire

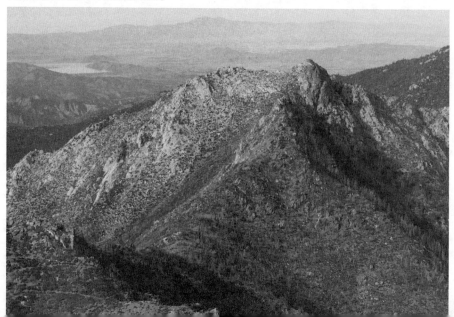

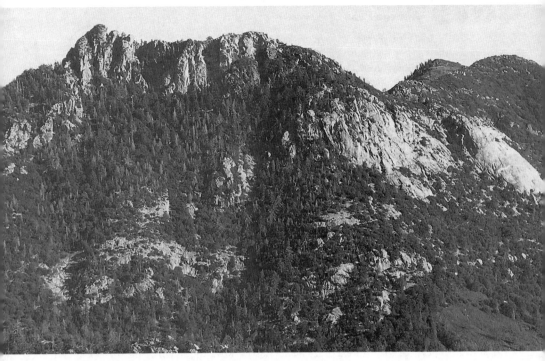

Antsell Rock from the south ridge of Tahquitz Peak

disturb meditation. Dogs are prohibited. This trail isn't shown on topographic maps and isn't regularly maintained.

From the parking area, continue up the dirt road through the gate. Stay left at a fork by the office, then left again at a fork near the cabins. Continue up the dirt road toward the low point on the Desert Divide. In 0.3 mile, pass two water tanks. The unsigned trail begins here where the road switchbacks. It follows the spectacular canyon along a seasonal creek beneath enchanting incense cedars and black oaks. In 0.1 mile, a spur on the right leads to the creek while the main trail begins climbing steeply to the left. Watch for Coulter pines with their enormous cones. The trail ascends the chaparral-clad slopes and reaches the crest in another 0.8 mile.

Turn left (west) and follow the Pacific Crest Trail (PCT) along the northeast side of Antsell Rock. In 0.5 mile, look for a gully marked with cairns in a grove of black oaks. A use trail up this gully leads to the summit of Antsell Rock. The jaunt is only 0.3 mile as the crow flies, but involves 800 feet of strenuous climbing. The steep and loose gully leads up to a prominent notch to the right of the rocky peak. The summit register can be found in this notch, so those uncomfortable with rock scrambling may stop here. For one of the more delightful mountaineering experiences in Southern California, continue up to the true summit. Scramble up a weakness in the rock above the notch, and then go left around the corner to another tree-filled gully leading to the rocky summit ridge. Some third-class climbing is required.

Return the way you came. Or, for a longer trip, continue southeast on the PCT to Apache Peak (see Trip 10.2).

trip 10.2   **Apache Peak**

see map on p. 231

Distance	6 miles (out-and-back), 8.5 miles (loop)
Hiking Time	5 hours
Elevation Gain	2,100'
Difficulty	Strenuous
Trail Use	Suitable for backpacking
Best Times	April–June, October–November
Agency	San Bernardino National Forest (San Jacinto Ranger Station)
Recommended Maps	Tom Harrison *San Jacinto Wilderness, Santa Rosa & San Jacinto Mountains National Monument,* or USGS *Idyllwild* and *Palm View Peak* 7.5'
Permit	San Jacinto Wilderness Permit required

DIRECTIONS From Highway 74, 3.4 miles southeast of Mountain Center and just before mile marker 074 RIV 62.75, turn left (east) onto Apple Canyon Road. In 2.6 miles, pass a turnout at the signed Spitler Peak Trailhead on the right. If you plan to make a loop trip, you may wish to leave a shuttle vehicle here. Continue 0.7 mile to the end of Apple Canyon Road at Pine Springs Ranch. Immediately before you enter the ranch, veer right onto a good private dirt road leading to the Zen Mountain Center. In 1.1 miles, park in a small dirt lot on the left just before you enter the Zen Center.

Note: *This area burned in the 2013 Mountain Fire and remained closed at press time.*

Apache Peak stands high on the Desert Divide, guarded on the north and west by sheer rock walls. Surprisingly, the summit itself is merely a rounded bump covered in chaparral. Whatever the peak may lack in rugged beauty, however, is compensated for by its 360-degree views of the entire Desert Divide, Santa Rosa Mountains, and Coachella and

Hikers on the PCT nearing Apache Peak

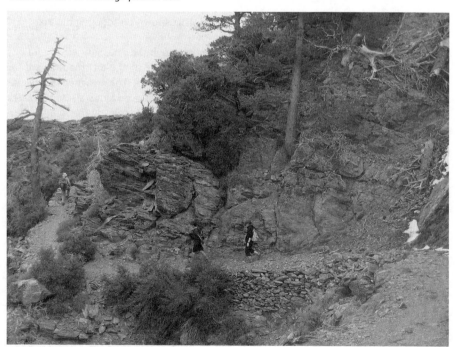

Garner Valleys. Backpackers will enjoy the nearby Apache Spring, with a reliable water source and good camping. The trip can be done as an out-and-back hike from the Zen Center or, with a short shuttle, as a loop down the scenic Spitler Peak Trail. Apache Peak is a seemingly strange name for the peak, which is located in the middle of Cahuilla Indian territory.

Access to the Desert Divide is plagued by private-property inholdings within San Bernardino National Forest. However, the Zen Mountain Center graciously allows hikers to cross its property and follow a spectacular trail that leads directly to the divide. Please help retain this privilege by being a courteous trail user. Avoid bringing large groups or large numbers of vehicles. Keep your voice down while crossing the center so as not to disturb meditation. Dogs are prohibited. This trail isn't shown on topographic maps.

From the parking area, continue up the dirt road through the gate. Stay left at a fork by the office, then left again at a fork near the cabins. Continue up the dirt road toward the low point on the Desert Divide. In 0.3 mile, pass two water tanks. The unsigned trail begins here where the road switchbacks. It follows the spectacular canyon along a seasonal creek beneath incense cedars and black oaks. In 0.1 mile, a spur on the right leads to the creek, while the main trail begins climbing steeply to the left. Watch for Coulter pines with their enormous cones. The trail ascends the chaparral-clad slopes and joins the PCT at the crest in another 0.8 mile.

Turn right (east) on the PCT and follow the trail as it climbs through the red cliffs. In 0.4 mile, round a corner at a rocky promontory to get your first views of Apache Peak. Follow a faint use trail onto the promontory for terrific views of the northern Desert Divide, San Jacinto massif, and the mountains and desert to the east.

Continue south 0.8 mile to reach the north slope of Apache Peak. The stately fir forest on this slope burned and now has been replaced by a buckthorn thicket. The trail loops around the east side of the peak. In 0.4 mile, where the trail reaches the summit plateau and abruptly turns left, look for a faint use trail leading through the chaparral toward the peak. Two hills are visible to the northwest; Apache Peak's highest point is the one on the left, 0.2 mile from the PCT. Enjoy the wide-ranging views from the top.

On the PCT, 100 yards south of the turnoff for the summit trail, is a sign marking a turnoff for Apache Spring. The year-round spring is located 0.5 mile northeast of the main trail and 500 feet down the slope. The Forest Service recommends boiling the water before drinking it. Several good camping sites sit on a knob just east of the spring, so this is a popular stop for PCT hikers. Return the way you came.

ALTERNATIVE FINISH

To make a worthwhile loop, continue 0.6 mile south from Apache Peak along the PCT to the saddle between Apache and Spitler Peaks. There are fine views to the east from the saddle into West Fork Canyon, over the Palisades on Garnet Ridge, and into the Santa Rosa Mountains. Follow the Spitler Peak Trail down as it makes gratuitously long and flat switchbacks through the oak and chaparral between the cliffs of the adjacent peaks. In 1 mile, reach a seasonal creek shaded by a diverse and gorgeous forest of incense cedars, Coulter pines, sugar pines, firs, and oaks. The trail then makes a long and gradual descent into the chaparral and crosses a splendid field of ribbonwood trees before reaching the paved road in another 3.7 miles. If you've left a car or bicycle here, your trip is complete. Alternatively, you can walk 1.8 miles up the road to the Zen Center Trailhead.

trip 10.3 Palm View Peak

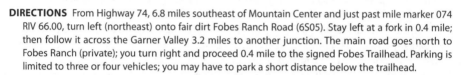

Distance	8 miles (out-and-back)
Hiking Time	5 hours
Elevation Gain	2,100'
Difficulty	Strenuous
Trail Use	Dogs allowed
Best Times	October–June
Agency	San Bernardino National Forest (San Jacinto Ranger Station)
Recommended Map	*Santa Rosa & San Jacinto Mountains National Monument* or USGS *Palm View Peak* 7.5'

see map on p. 231

DIRECTIONS From Highway 74, 6.8 miles southeast of Mountain Center and just past mile marker 074 RIV 66.00, turn left (northeast) onto fair dirt Fobes Ranch Road (6S05). Stay left at a fork in 0.4 mile; then follow it across the Garner Valley 3.2 miles to another junction. The main road goes north to Fobes Ranch (private); you turn right and proceed 0.4 mile to the signed Fobes Trailhead. Parking is limited to three or four vehicles; you may have to park a short distance below the trailhead.

The Fobes Saddle and Palm View Peak offer a gentler hike to sample the pleasures of the Desert Divide. This southern region is lower in elevation, and is a good place to visit in the winter when the high country is buried under snow. Enjoy this hike for the journey more than for the destination. Palm View Peak itself is the least attractive part of the entire hike; the summit is lost in dense woods and offers neither palms nor views. This hike was lightly affected by the 2013 Mountain Fire.

From the trailhead, follow the seemingly never-ending switchbacks through the chaparral toward Fobes Saddle. This section of the trail passes through large stands of aptly named ribbonwoods (the bark hangs in shreds), also called red shanks (*Adenostoma sparsifolium*). In 0.5 mile, the trail forks; take the right fork. In another mile, reach the Pacific Crest Trail (PCT) junction at the Fobes Saddle on the crest of the divide.

Turn right and follow the PCT southeast, first on the east side of the ridge, then on the west, and finally switchbacking up the crest. The trail levels out and passes a small outcrop, then enters a clearing 2.4 miles from the saddle. Turn left and leave the trail, making a short cross-country excursion through white firs and black oaks to the summit of Palm View Peak. The proper departure point from the PCT can be difficult to identify because the summit is heavily wooded. If the trail starts to go downhill, you've gone too far. A small pile of rocks and a summit register mark the high point. Unfortunately, the peak is hemmed in by trees, so there are no views. Return to the clearing because the other sides of the summit are blocked by dense brush.

After enjoying the summit, retrace your steps to the car. There are many other peaks and trailheads along the Desert Divide, so numerous variations are possible if you bring a shuttle.

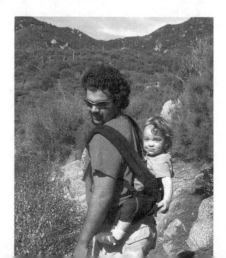

Happy hikers on Fobes Saddle Trail

trip 10.4   Cedar Spring

Distance	6.5 miles (out-and-back)
Hiking Time	3.5 hours
Elevation Gain	1,700'
Difficulty	Moderate
Trail Use	Dogs allowed, suitable for backpacking
Best Times	March–June, September–November
Agency	San Bernardino National Forest (San Jacinto Ranger Station)
Recommended Map	*Santa Rosa & San Jacinto Mountains National Monument* or USGS *Palm View Peak* 7.5'

see map on p. 231

DIRECTIONS From Highway 74, 8.6 miles south of Mountain Center in the Garner Valley and just beyond mile marker 074 RIV 67.75, turn left (northeast) onto paved Morris Ranch Road (6S53). Follow it up 3.7 miles, passing the Joe Sherman Girl Scout Camp, to the signed Cedar Spring Trailhead (4E17) on the right. The best parking is at a large lot on the east side of the road, 0.1 mile before you reach the trailhead.

Pacific Crest Trail (PCT) hikers on the lengthy Desert Divide depend on small springs as their only source of water. One of the most attractive of these is Cedar Spring, situated on the desert slopes east of the divide beneath a fine grove of incense cedars and black oaks. The best time to visit is in the spring, when the water is reliable, the temperatures are moderate, and the wildflowers are in bloom. This is a popular destination for Boy Scout troops.

Hike up the road from the parking area 0.1 mile to the signed Cedar Spring Trail (4E17) on your right. The first part of this trail follows a narrow fenced corridor through private prop-

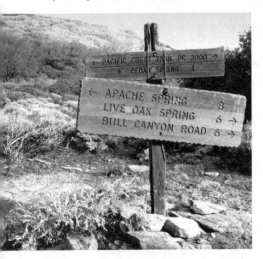

Saddle atop Cedar Spring Trail

erty; please respect the property owners by staying on the trail so that the path will remain open to hikers in the future. Pass through a gate at the start and close it behind you. The valley is filled with a diverse ribbonwood, manzanita, scrub oak, and yucca chaparral. Hike past a water tank and through a second gate in 0.4 mile, and then a third gate in another 0.4 mile. Just beyond, the trail turns left to join an old dirt road. In 0.2 mile, pass some picnic tables near the head of the valley as the road narrows back to a trail again. Here, the relentless switchbacks begin, climbing 1.3 miles to a saddle and four-way junction with the PCT.

The PCT crosses this saddle en route from Mexico to Canada, but our trail continues straight down the other side of the saddle through more chaparral. Parts of this area burned some time back, but the scrub oak is vigorously regenerating. Enjoy breathtaking views down into Palm Canyon and out over the Santa Rosa Mountains. In 0.9 mile, the trail abruptly rounds a bend and enters a shady grove where you can find Cedar Spring and plenty of fine campsites.

Return the way you came. There is 400 feet of climbing on the way back to the saddle.

VARIATION

Cedar Spring can also be reached from Palm Canyon by way of the arduous Jo Pond Trail (see Trip 11.15). The two trips can be combined into a lengthy one-way hike from the Garner Valley to Palm Canyon. Remember that the gate to Palm Canyon closes at 5 p.m.; plan to meet your getaway vehicle outside the gate unless you arrive before the gate closes.

---

trip 10.5   Northern Desert Divide

see map on p. 231

Distance	11 miles (one-way)
Hiking Time	6 hours
Elevation Gain	2,000' (without peaks)
Difficulty	Strenuous
Trail Use	Suitable for backpacking
Best Times	April–June, October–November
Agency	San Bernardino National Forest (San Jacinto Ranger Station)
Recommended Maps	Tom Harrison *San Jacinto Wilderness, Santa Rosa & San Jacinto Mountains National Monument* or USGS *San Jacinto Peak, Idyllwild,* and *Palm View Peak* 7.5'
Permit	San Jacinto Wilderness Permit required

DIRECTIONS Park a getaway vehicle at the Zen Mountain Center Trailhead; then drive a half hour back to the Devils Slide trailhead at Humber Park Trailhead. To reach the Zen Mountain Center Trailhead, take Highway 74 until you're 3.4 miles southeast of Mountain Center; then, just before mile marker 074 RIV 62.75; turn left (east) onto Apple Canyon Road. In 3.3 miles, reach the end of the paved road at Pine Springs Ranch. Immediately before you enter the ranch, veer right onto a good private dirt road leading to the Zen Mountain Center. In 1.1 miles, park in a small dirt lot on the left just be-fore you enter the Zen Center.

To reach Humber Park, drive back to Mountain Center and then north on Highway 243 to the San Jacinto Ranger Station (see the map on page 194). Turn right at the station onto Pine Crest Avenue. In 0.6 mile, veer right onto South Circle Drive. In 0.1 mile, turn left onto Fern Valley Road. Proceed 1.8 miles to the Humber Park Trailhead, at the road's end.

Note: *This area burned in the 2013 Mountain Fire and remained closed at press time.*

The northern stretch of the Desert Divide is one of the most rugged and spectacular ridges in Southern California. The well-built Pacific Crest Trail (PCT) runs along the divide,

Northern Desert Divide overlooking Garner Valley, with Antsell Rock on the right

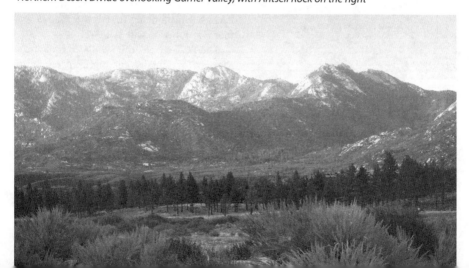

and offers fine hiking along this otherwise inaccessible terrain. This one-way trip starts in Idyllwild and ends in the scenic Garner Valley. Many variations are possible, including climbing some of the peaks along the way and extending the hike in either direction (see Trip 10.6).

Access to the Desert Divide is plagued by private property inholdings within the San Bernardino National Forest. However, the Zen Mountain Center graciously allows hikers to cross its property and follow a spectacular trail that leads directly to the divide. Please help retain this privilege by being a courteous trail user. Avoid bringing large groups or large numbers of vehicles. Keep your voice down while crossing the center so as not to disturb meditation. Dogs are prohibited. This trail isn't shown on topographic maps.

From Humber Park, hike 2.5 miles up the Devils Slide Trail to the five-way Saddle Junction, where you meet the PCT. Take the southeast fork 0.6 mile to Tahquitz Valley, where you can find the best camping available along this route. Turn south and hike 0.8 mile to meet the PCT in Little Tahquitz Valley.

Follow the PCT east along the forested north slope of Red Tahquitz Peak. In 1.4 miles, the trail rounds the east end of the mountain overlooking Andreas Canyon and turns south, marking the beginning of your adventures along the Desert Divide. Stands of Jeffrey pines, white firs, and incense cedars cling to the steep ridge. Hike south 1.8 miles across the head of Murray Canyon to South Peak. The trail skirts the peak on the east side, then switchbacks down the rocky slope and continues south toward the formidable obstacle of Antsell Rock. The PCT bypasses this difficult stretch on the northeast side by switchbacking down below the cliffs. In 2.1 miles, the trail enters a grove of black oaks at the base of a gully. Cairns mark a steep climber's trail up the gully to the summit (see Trip 10.1). But the PCT continues southeast another 0.5 mile to a saddle. The 2008 Apache Fire burned through the steep chaparral on the east side of the divide here.

From here, the easiest way off the divide is to descend the steep trail to the southwest, reaching the Zen Mountain Center in 1.2 miles.

ALTERNATIVE FINISH ——
Alternatively, continue along the PCT past Apache Peak, and follow the long but scenic Spitler Peak Trail down to Apple Canyon Road. See Trip 10.2 for directions to parking at the Spitler Peak Trailhead. This adds 5.7 miles to the trip.

——

trip 10.6   **Nine Peaks of the Desert Divide**

Distance	21 miles (without peaks), 27 miles (with nine peaks, one-way)
Hiking Time	11–15 hours
Elevation Gain	5,700' (without peaks), 9,000' (with nine peaks)
Difficulty	Very strenuous
Trail Use	Suitable for backpacking
Best Times	April–June, October–November
Agency	San Bernardino National Forest (San Jacinto Ranger Station)
Required Maps	Tom Harrison *San Jacinto Wilderness* (covers only northern part of route), *Santa Rosa & San Jacinto Mountains National Monument,* or USGS *San Jacinto Peak, Idyllwild,* and *Palm View Peak* 7.5'
Permit	San Jacinto Wilderness Permit required

see map on p. 231

DIRECTIONS Park a getaway vehicle at the Cedar Spring Trailhead; then drive a half hour back to the Devils Slide Trailhead at Humber Park. To reach the Cedar Spring Trailhead from Highway 74, 8.6 miles south of Mountain Center in the Garner Valley and just beyond mile marker 074 RIV 67.75, turn left (northeast) onto the paved Morris Ranch Road (6S53). Follow it up 3.7 miles, passing the

Joe Sherman Girl Scout Camp, to the signed Cedar Spring Trailhead (4E17) on the right. (If you reach Morris Ranch, you've driven 0.25 mile too far.) The best parking is at a large lot on the east side of the road, 0.1 mile before you reach the trailhead.

To reach Humber Park, drive back to Mountain Center and then north on Highway 243 to the San Jacinto Ranger Station (see the map on page 192). Turn right at the station onto Pine Crest Avenue. In 0.6 mile, veer right onto South Circle Drive. In 0.1 mile, turn left onto Fern Valley Road. Proceed 1.8 miles to the Humber Park Trailhead, at the road's end.

Note: *The Desert Divide burned in the 2013 Mountain Fire and remained closed from Tahquitz Valley to the Spitler Peak Trail at press time.*

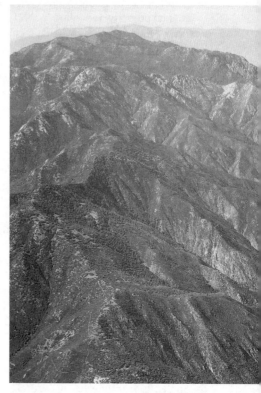

Aerial view of the Desert Divide from the south. Fobes Saddle is in the foreground, with San Jacinto at the far end and the tall ridge of San Gorgonio looming on the horizon.

This challenging hike is one of the most rewarding in Southern California, offering a grand tour of the rugged and unique Desert Divide. It follows the Pacific Crest Trail (PCT) along the crest from Tahquitz Peak south to Cedar Spring, with optional excursions to nine nearby summits along the way: Tahquitz, Red Tahquitz, South Peak, Antsell Rock, Apache Peak, Spitler Peak, Palm View Peak, Little Desert Peak, and Pyramid Peak. The northern stretch is extraordinarily rugged, while the southern part becomes more gentle and rolling. It's especially enjoyable in April, when flowers are in bloom and when you may meet a parade of PCT thru-hikers starting their long northbound journeys. By the end of this trip, you're guaranteed to be tired, hungry, and fully satisfied. Good route-finding skills are essential to locate the easiest ways to many of the summits. There is no convenient water along this route, so bring at least 4 quarts on a cool day and more if it will be warm. A headlamp and enough clothing to survive an unplanned night out are also strongly advisable. Those looking for a somewhat easier trip through the best part of the Desert Divide with *only* four or five peaks may plan to exit the Spitler Peak or Fobes Trail instead (see Trips 10.2 and 10.3).

From Humber Park, hike 2.5 miles up the Devils Slide Trail to the five-way Saddle Junction, where you meet the PCT. Take the rightmost fork and hike south toward Tahquitz Peak, gradually climbing through the open forest. The granite slopes of Red Tahquitz come into view and the trees become smaller and more weather-beaten as you climb. In 1.4 miles, reach a junction with the South Ridge Trail. Follow this right toward Tahquitz Peak 0.4 mile; then take a short spur to the summit. From the top, study the granite-toothed Desert Divide leading south and the summits of Toro and Rabbit Peaks beyond; then return to the PCT.

Hike back east along the South Ridge Trail, pass the junction of PCT that you came in on, continuing east and then north on the PCT, descending in 0.8 mile to another junction with a side trail leading north to Tahquitz Valley. Continue 0.8 mile on the PCT as it leads east beneath the white north walls of Red Tahquitz, and pass just below and south of a small rocky knob; then in 0.2 mile more, come to a draw. This is one of the weaknesses in Red Tahquitz's defenses and the shortest way to the summit. Turn south and hike 0.3 mile uphill through the forest until you reach the mountaintop. Red Tahquitz sits on the border between the high-quality white granite of the San Jacinto–Tahquitz region and the band of distinctive red granite farther south. Although you may be tempted to take a shortcut down to the east, you're better off returning the way you came because the brush and cliff bands make an eastern descent difficult.

Follow the PCT east around a knob overlooking Andreas Canyon, then south across the head of Murray Canyon. The Desert Divide takes on its most rugged and interesting character between here and Apache Peak. Along the high part of the divide, Jeffrey pines, white firs, and incense cedars are common, though some chaparral also clings to the parched cliffs. In 2.4 miles, from Red Tahquitz pass along the east side of South Peak. At the corner where the trail turns west across the south side of the peak, look for a use trail, sometimes marked with cairns, that leads 0.1 mile up to the nearby summit.

The PCT switchbacks down the ridge, and the dark imposing hulk of Antsell Rock looms large ahead. The PCT drops to cross the east face below the cliffs. In 2.1 miles, look for a gully marked with cairns in a grove of black oaks. In this gully is a use trail to the summit of Antsell Rock. It's just 0.3 mile as the crow flies, but involves 800 feet of strenuous climbing. The steep and loose gully leads up to a prominent notch to the right of the rocky peak. The summit register can be found in this notch, so those uncomfortable with rock scrambling may stop here. But for one of the most fun mountaineering experiences in Southern California, continue up to the true summit. Scramble up a weakness in the rock; then go around the corner to another tree-filled gully that leads to the rocky summit ridge. Some third-class climbing is required. Return the way you came.

From the PCT continuing southeast in 0.5 mile, reach a saddle on the Desert Divide. Here, an unmarked trail leads up from the Zen Mountain Center in Apple Canyon (see Trip 10.1). Continue south on the PCT beneath the red battlements on the north wall of Apache Peak. The 2008 Apache Fire burned the east side of the Desert Divide in this area. From the junction with the Zen Mountain Center trail in 0.4 mile, consider following a use trail to a vista point atop the wall just before the trail rounds a corner. In another 0.8 mile, cross a burn zone on the north slope of Apache Peak. If you like, you can take a shortcut to the summit of Apache by bushwhacking up a gully to the skyline, then turning right and walking a few yards to the summit. Otherwise, follow the PCT as it loops 0.4 mile around the east side to reach the summit plateau of Apache Peak, where a faint use trail branches off. Two hills are visible to the northwest from the junction; Apache Peak's highest point is the one on the left, 0.2 mile from the PCT. The unimposing summit has terrific views.

In less than 0.1 mile farther south on the PCT, come to a signed junction with a trail leading east 0.5 mile and 500 feet down to the reliable Apache Spring. The Forest Service recommends treating water from this spring. A few tent sites with excellent views are available here.

Continue south on the PCT 0.6 mile to a junction with the Spitler Peak Trail coming up from Apple Canyon; this is an escape route if you have a vehicle parked below. Otherwise, Spitler Peak is the next challenge on the divide. It has two use trails marked with cairns. One climbs the serpentine north ridge from a point just south of the Spitler Peak Trail–PCT junction; the other rises almost straight up from a point 0.5 mile farther along the PCT, almost due east of the summit. It would be appealing to ascend the north ridge and descend to the east, but the summit is choked with vegetation and finding the eastern route from above can be difficult.

Spitler Peak marks the end of the rocky section of the Desert Divide. Farther south, the ridges and peaks are lower and more rounded. Pines and firs give way to oaks, manzanitas, buckthorns, and the striking ribbonwood. In 1.5 miles, reach Fobes Saddle, where a trail comes up from Fobes Canyon (another escape route). The PCT makes a long switchback, crosses over to the west side of the divide, and climbs 2.3 tedious miles to a flattish area. Palm View Peak is 0.2 mile to the east, hidden in a dense grove of oaks and firs. The summit is difficult to find because it's rather flat and concealed in the vegetation. If you begin to descend on the PCT, you've gone too far and now have a thicket blocking your path to the peak. The name is misleading; there are views of nothing but the trees you've just thrashed through. This is decidedly the least enjoyable peak on your route.

Return to the PCT and continue 1.4 miles southeast over some rolling hills and along a boulevard cut through the manzanita to reach the Cedar Spring Trail junction. If daylight and energy remain, follow the PCT 0.2 mile farther over the top of the unimpressive Little Desert Peak and 1 mile beyond to Pyramid Peak to round out your nine summits for the day. There is a climber's path up to the summit of Pyramid from the saddle south of Pyramid Peak. Then return to the Cedar Spring junction. Switchback down the Cedar Spring Trail to the southwest; then pass through a gate and reach some picnic benches in 1.3 miles. The trail becomes a dirt road for a while, then veers off to the right again and passes through several gates in a corridor between fenced properties. After a seemingly unending mile, complete your adventure at the signed trailhead.

ALTERNATIVE FINISH

Truly ambitious peak baggers can finish out the Desert Divide by following the PCT south past Pine Mountain and Lion Peak all the way to where the trail crosses Highway 74 at a signed trailhead. This stretch is 10.5 miles from the Cedar Spring junction, so it increases the total trip to 32 miles and 11 peaks. Pine Mountain has a ducked trail from the PCT that starts 100 yards north of the saddle at the south end of Peak 6,880'+ and leads over the small peak, then east to the saddle and up the southwest slope of Pine Mountain. The path can be horribly overgrown with chaparral unless somebody has trimmed the path recently. Many hikers skip the summit monolith, which involves moderate fifth-class climbing and a rappel descent on a 50-meter rope. Lion Peak has a climber's trail starting from the PCT at the saddle on the northeast side of the peak.

---

trip 10.7　**Thomas Mountain**

see map on p. 231

Distance	12 miles (out-and-back)
Hiking Time	7 hours
Elevation Gain	2,400'
Difficulty	Strenuous
Trail Use	Dogs allowed, suitable for backpacking, suitable for mountain biking, suitable for equestrians
Best Times	April–June, October–November
Agency	San Bernardino National Forest (San Jacinto Ranger Station)
Recommended Map	USGS *Anza* 7.5' (roads and trails have changed somewhat since the 1996 printing)

DIRECTIONS From Highway 74 in Garner Valley, 8.1 miles south of Mountain Center and just south of mile marker 074 RIV 67.25, turn west into the Ramona Trail parking area.

Optionally, cut the trip in half by arranging to leave a shuttle vehicle at the top: From Highway 74 at mile marker 074 RIV 64.25, about 3 miles north of the Ramona Trailhead, turn west onto fair dirt Thomas Mountain Road (6S13). Drive 7.4 miles up to the junction with 6S13C near yellow-post campsite 6, just north of the summit. Park wherever you won't obstruct traffic.

Thomas Mountain's long ridge forms the western side of the beautiful Garner Valley. It's perfectly situated to offer fantastic views of the Desert Divide and San Jacinto Wilderness. The lower slopes are covered in delightful stands of ribbonwoods. On the top of the ridge, cool breezes blow through the rich forest of Jeffrey pines, white firs, and incense cedars. Wildflowers are abundant in the spring and early summer. The mountain is named for Charles Thomas, a pioneer who founded a ranch in the valley in 1861. The valley was also known as Thomas Valley until the ranch was sold to Robert Garner, who gave the valley its present name.

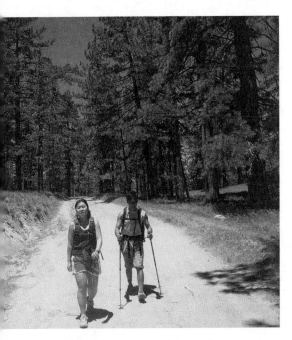

Hikers on Thomas Mountain Road

The Ramona Trail, named for the tragic heroine of Helen Hunt Jackson's novel, climbs to the ridge from Garner Valley. The dirt Thomas Mountain Road runs along the top of the ridge, providing access to numerous fine yellow-post camping spots and also offering an alternative descent if you choose to make a one-way hike.

The good trail (3E26) starts at the west end of the Ramona Trail parking area and switchbacks up the slope through stands of ribbonwoods, manzanitas, and mountain mahoganys. In 2.5 miles, the chaparral yields to forest on the upper flanks of the mountain. In another 1.0 mile, reach an unmarked fork. The main trail continues right, but a side trail leads left 100 yards up a draw to Tool Box Springs, shaded under the cedars and Jeffrey pines. The concrete trough here is suitable for watering stock, but is unappealing to hikers. Just above the spring is the quiet Tool Box Springs Campground located at the bottom end of a dirt road.

In 0.1 mile on the Ramona Trail, reach a second unmarked junction. Both trails lead to dirt roads and up to Thomas Mountain Road, but the right fork is the shorter way to go. In 0.2 mile, the right fork reaches a dirt road near yellow-post campsite 9. This trip follows the dirt road from here to the summit.

VARIATION

The trail crosses the dirt road at a trail marker by yellow-post site 9 and continues northwest. It can be hard to follow in places because it passes many unmarked cow paths. The first major cow path, 0.6 mile from the campsite, leads 0.1 mile down to Magee Spring, marked by a watering trough. The trail reaches Thomas Mountain Road in 2.1 miles at an unlabeled trail marker where the road makes a hairpin turn north of Thomas Mountain. Turn left and hike 0.2 mile back to 6S13C to rejoin the main route 0.4 mile below the summit.

Turn left up the road and follow it 0.3 mile to Thomas Mountain Road. Turn right and follow Thomas Mountain Road northwest along the ridge. Although hiking on a fire road might sound unappealing, the forest and wildflowers are delightful and the walking is pleasant. Pass yellow-post site 8, then a logging road on the left, and then yellow-post sites 7 and 6. In 1.8 miles, just beyond site 6, reach a road junction on the north side of Thomas

Mountain. Turn left and take the switchbacking road, 6S13C, 0.4 mile up to the summit of the mountain, where concrete foundations mark the site of the former fire lookout. From here, there are fabulous views south and west over Anza Valley and Cahuilla Mountain, and north to San Gorgonio, as well as the panoramas of the Desert Divide that you've enjoyed all along.

If you left a shuttle vehicle near the summit, your trip is done. Otherwise, return the way you came.

---

trip 10.8   ## Cahuilla Mountain

Distance	6 miles (out-and-back)
Hiking Time	3 hours
Elevation Gain	1,400'
Difficulty	Moderate
Trail Use	Dogs allowed, suitable for backpacking
Best Times	October–June
Agency	San Bernardino National Forest (San Jacinto Ranger Station)
Recommended Map	USGS *Cahuilla Mountain* 7.5'

DIRECTIONS From the 15 Freeway (I-15) in Temecula, take Exit 58 east onto Temecula Parkway (Highway 79) and, in 17 miles, turn left (north) onto Highway 371. In 11.25 miles, near mile marker 371 RIV 68.0 and a sign reading C A H U I L L A   M O U N T A I N   T R A I L 2E45, turn left (north) onto Cary Road, which in 1.8 miles curves left (west) and then right (north) and becomes Tripp Flats Road. At a signed junction in 1.8 miles, turn left onto good dirt Forest Road 6S22. Proceed 2.4 miles to the signed Cahuilla Mountain Trail (2E45), on your left, close to phone lines overhead. Park in the small clearing on your right.

Cahuilla (pronounced "ka-**wee**-ah") Mountain stands by itself, well to the west of the Desert Divide and Thomas Mountain, within the 5,575-acre Cahuilla Mountain Wilderness designated by Congress in 2009. It overlooks the Anza Valley and a Cahuilla tribal reservation. Although seldom visited today, it was the setting of Helen Hunt Jackson's famous 1884 novel, *Ramona,* about the injustices faced by Native Americans. At the height of the novel's popularity, tourists came by the wagonload to visit the scene and meet Ramona Lubo and visit the grave of her husband, Juan Diego. The novel is inspired by a true story. After a misunderstanding, a white man murdered Juan Diego, and a white judge acquitted the murderer. This is a good trip for those with a vivid imagination who can conjure up the events of the past and contemplate the current state of American justice. No wilderness permit is required, but groups are limited to 12 persons.

The well-built trail leads up the northeast side of the mountain through chamise chaparral. In 2.0 miles, it crosses to the west side and dips slightly, passing through a parklike forest of black oaks and Coulter pines. At 2.5 miles, pass a signed trail on the right leading 0.1 mile down a steep draw to a seasonal spring. The trail ends at the southeastern summit, which, at 5,635 feet, is the high point of the mountain.

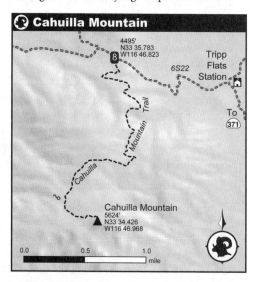

trip 10.9   Hurkey Creek

see map on p. 231

Distance	8 miles (loop)
Hiking Time	2.5 hours
Elevation Gain	900'
Difficulty	Moderate
Trail Use	Dogs allowed, suitable for mountain biking, suitable for equestrians
Best Times	March–June, September–November
Agency	Riverside County Regional Park and Open-Space District
Recommended Map	USGS *Idyllwild* 7.5'
Permit	Day-use fee required ($6 adults, $3 kids ages 2–12)

DIRECTIONS From Highway 74, 3.4 miles southeast of Mountain Center and just before mile marker 074 RIV 62.75, turn left (east) onto Apple Canyon Road. Then turn immediately left into Hurkey Creek Park. After paying a modest day-use fee and obtaining a park map, proceed 0.3 mile to the north end of the campground and park near the outhouse across from campsite 128.

Hurkey (sometimes spelled *Herkey*) Creek is a cool mountain stream flowing down from the granite ramparts of Tahquitz Peak. Riverside County has constructed a fine campground along the creek opposite Lake Hemet at the northern edge of the Garner Valley. A trail leads north from the campground, following the creek before connecting to a maze of other paths in the hills. This trip describes a loop that returns on another of the paths. The trip is a fine way to enjoy the splendor of the Desert Divide without enduring the steep climbs. It features a spectacular forest of ribbonwood and spring wildflowers. Some hikers will prefer making a shorter trip (up to 2 miles) out and back along the creek. Springtime is the ideal season to visit, when the creek is running and the days aren't yet too hot.

Campsites are available first-come, first-served or by reservation at 951-659-2050. Families with younger children will love the impressive park near the campground entrance. Showers are also available. Free camping can be found at a number of excellent yellow-post campsites just up Apple Canyon Road.

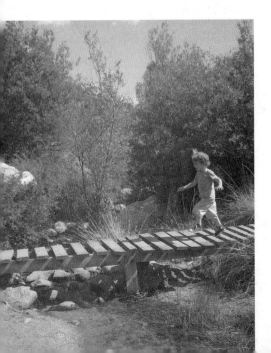

The trail, actually an old fire road, starts at an unmarked gate by site 130. It leads north along the west side of the creek past ribbonwood and Jeffrey pines. Numerous side paths bring you down to frolic by the water. A singletrack path soon crosses the trail. The left fork leads toward and parallels the highway. The right fork crosses the creek and loops around near the campground. This trip continues north on the main trail.

Continue to Bonita Vista fire road via a popular mountain bike route called Exfoliator. Turn right on Bonita Vista; then, shortly after you cross the main branch of Hurkey Creek, turn right on the Missing Link Trail and follow it back south. Hike through the lonely sagebrush country in an area known as

Hurkey Creek Trail

K Flat. From here, you can enjoy great views of the granite buttresses on Tahquitz Peak, Red Tahquitz, and the northern Desert Divide.

The trail passes beneath a canopy of giant ribbonwood plants; this section is known as the Tunnel of Love. When you reach a dirt road, turn left, then left again, and hike 0.4 mile to the paved Apple Canyon Road. This area is a tangle of dirt roads, but any road leading southeast will eventually get you to the pavement.

If you haven't prepositioned a bicycle or second vehicle, walk back to the trailhead. Turn left and follow Apple Canyon Road 1 mile back to Hurkey Creek Campground, passing the private Apple Canyon Center along the way. Then follow the campground road to your vehicle.

VARIATION

Hard-core mountain bikers will enjoy exploring the intricate network of fire roads and singletrack in the area. Riders flock to this area for the 24 Hours of Adrenaline and Idyllwild Spring Challenge races. A route map is available at mountainbikebill.com/images /trails/hurkeycreek/herkeycreekmap07.jpg.

trip 10.10 South Fork of the San Jacinto River

Distance	5 miles (out-and-back)
Hiking Time	2.5 hours
Elevation Gain	800'
Difficulty	Moderate
Trail Use	Dogs allowed, suitable for backpacking, suitable for equestrians
Best Times	October–May
Agency	San Bernardino National Forest (San Jacinto Ranger Station)
Recommended Maps	USGS *Blackburn Canyon* and *Idyllwild* 7.5'

DIRECTIONS On Highway 74 between Hemet and Mountain Center, park at the large Caltrans cinder bin lot at mile marker 074 RIV 56.60, on the south side of the road. The parking area is signed SOUTH FORK TRAIL 2E17.

Marion Mountain and Tahquitz Peak from the South Fork Trail

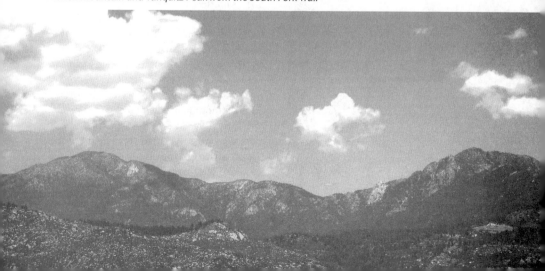

The South Fork of the San Jacinto River tumbles out of the Lake Hemet Reservoir and cuts a gorge down the west slopes of the San Jacinto Mountains south of Highway 74. The South Fork Trail (2E17) leads from the high-way over a low divide and down to the river. It's particularly attractive on a cool day in April or May when the chaparral and wildflowers are in bloom. The trail also draws fishermen to try their luck on this secluded portion of the river. Wildlife love the lushly vegetated banks, though the algae-filled pools aren't particu-larly appealing for water play. Congress passed the Omnibus Public Land Management Act of 2009, establishing the South Fork San Jacinto Wilderness to protect this land. No wilderness permit is presently required.

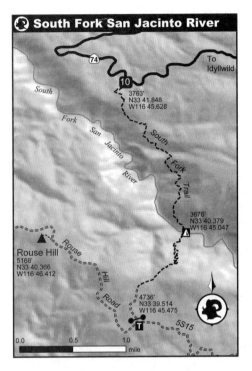

The trail starts at a post on the south side of the parking area. It then climbs 300 feet over 0.5 mile to reach the low ridge south of the highway. The slopes are covered in ribbonwood and other chaparral. Enjoy the views of Tahquitz Peak and Marion Moun-tain from the ridge.

The trail contours along the southwest-facing slopes for 1.6 miles, offering impres-sive views into the rugged canyon. Watch for quail along the trail and vultures circling overhead. This section would be oppressively hot in the summer. The rocky trail then abruptly drops the last 0.4 mile to the river. Stepping stones cross the river; they're usually straightforward, but they could be difficult during times of high flow. A few clearings that are large enough for tents can be found just up the hill on the far bank.

VARIATION

The South Fork Trail continues up to Rouse Ridge on the south side of the river. This is a "trail to nowhere," connecting only to a long, obscure, bumpy, and very scenic dirt road on the ridge. It may be attractive to those looking for a longer workout. Peak baggers also use the trail to access Rouse Hill, a fairly insignificant bump with fine views. Going all the way to Rouse Hill adds 6.6 miles round-trip with 1,800 feet of elevation gain.

The trail climbs steep switchbacks shaded under oaks and bigcone Douglas-fir. In 1.3 miles, it reaches an old jeep track on the ridge, now closed to motorized vehicles. Continue 0.4 mile to the junction with the Rouse Hill Road (5S15), which connects the Thomas Mountain Road to the Cranston Fire Station. If you wish to visit Rouse Hill, turn right and follow the road 1.6 miles to a turnout; then pick a path through the light brush for the last few hundred yards to the summit. Alternatively, you can shortcut part of the road by hiking over a hill to the west where the trail meets the jeep track.

chapter 11

Palm Springs and the Indian Canyons

Over time, the San Andreas Fault has thrust an enormous block of granite into the sky, forming the San Jacinto Mountains. Along the mountains' east and north faces, the elevation rises from below sea level in the Coachella Valley to 10,834 feet on San Jacinto Peak, forming the tallest vertical wall in the United States outside Death Valley. The Palm Canyon Fault, a spur of the San Andreas Fault system, slices a trench between the San Jacinto and Santa Rosa Mountains. The pulverized rock in the fault forms an impermeable layer. Desert streams that ordinarily run underground cannot penetrate this rock and are forced to the surface at a series of springs. Native California fan palm (*Washingtonia filifera*) oases are found here and in many of the nearby canyons.

Since ancient times, the Agua Caliente Band of Cahuilla ("ka-**wee**-ah") Indians has made its home in these canyons and in the nearby mountains, hunting and gathering the native animals and plants. Spanish missionaries brought farming, "civilization," and disease. A smallpox epidemic reduced the tribe to 70 individuals by the late 1800s.

In 1877, the Southern Pacific Railroad was completed, following a line near where the 10 Freeway presently runs. As an incentive for rail construction, the federal government

Palm Canyon and Murray Hill from the West Fork Trail

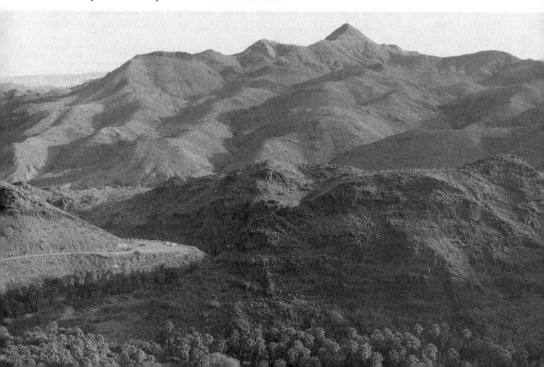

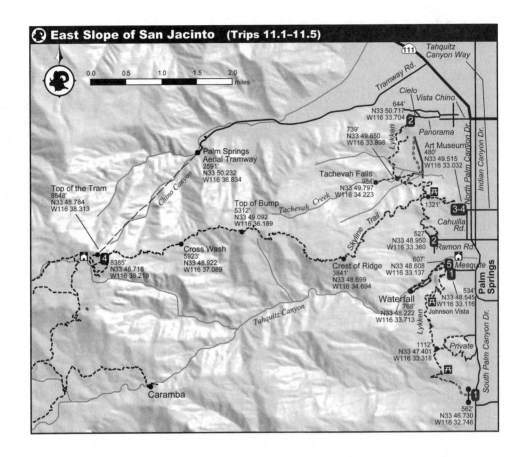

East Slope of San Jacinto (Trips 11.1–11.5)

granted Southern Pacific every other square mile section of land, forming a checkerboard extending 10 miles on either side of the tracks. Southern Pacific, in turn, began selling land to private owners.

In 1884, Judge John McCallum and his family became permanent settlers in the Palm Springs area. He built an irrigation canal from the Whitewater River to Palm Springs. Shortly after, hotels began to open, first catering to tuberculosis patients who sought the warm, dry weather and hot springs but soon drawing the rich and famous from all over the West. Golf courses and resorts followed.

By the 1980s, development reached a frenetic pace; the number of resorts and houses doubled in the decade and started to push into the pristine mountains. People became aware of the need to protect the wilderness for the enjoyment of future generations and for the survival of the desert bighorn sheep and other species. In 1990, portions of the area were designated as the Santa Rosa Mountains National Scenic Area under management of the Bureau of Land Management. In 2000, Congress established the Santa Rosa and San Jacinto Mountains National Monument, protecting 280,000 acres including most of the hills surrounding Palm Springs.

This chapter describes hikes around Palm Springs on the eastern desert flank of San Jacinto and in the Indian Canyons (see next page). Chapter 12 covers other hikes in the Santa Rosa Mountains, while Chapter 9 covers hikes near San Jacinto Peak, and Chapter 10 covers those along the Desert Divide overlooking Palm Canyon.

The Indian Canyons

The Agua Caliente Indian Reservation comprises lands both within and just outside of Palm Springs, as well as acreage within Santa Rosa and San Jacinto Mountains National Monument—more than 32,000 acres in all. Eight hikes in this chapter lie within the Indian Canyons, a part of the reservation that is open to the public for hiking. Four of these canyons—Andreas, Fern, Murray, and Palm—are clustered together just south of Palm Springs, while a fifth, Tahquitz, lies a few miles north, just off Palm Canyon Drive. Tahquitz Canyon has separate visitor facilities from the other four canyons, which are administered as one unit. ("Indian Canyons" is both the official name for the latter destination and the informal designation for all five canyons.)

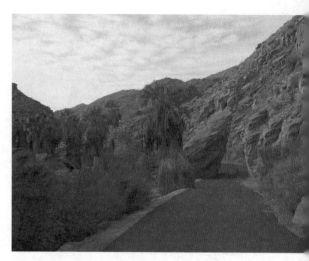

Entrance to Palm Canyon

At this writing, admission to Tahquitz Canyon (760-416-7044, tahquitzcanyon.com) costs $12.50 for adults and $6 for children ages 6–12; admission to the other four Indian Canyons (760-323-6018, indian-canyons.com) is $9 for adults, $7 for seniors and students, and $5 for kids ages 6–12. Admission fees support the maintenance of the excellent network of trails within the canyons.

You'll receive a trail map when you pay your admission at the Indian Canyons entrance station on South Palm Canyon Drive. Free digital maps in GIS and PDF formats, along with downloadable GPS tracks, are available at indian-canyons.com/trail_maps and tahquitz canyon.com/tahquitz_trail_maps.

At this writing, the Indian Canyons are open 8 a.m.–5 p.m. and Tahquitz Canyon 7:30 a.m.–5 p.m. Hours for both areas are daily October 1–July 4 and Friday–Sunday July 5–September 30. Note that during the heat of summer, only the shortest hikes are enjoyable. Mountain bikes are prohibited, partly due to the irresponsible behavior of a minority of riders in the past. Pets and rock climbing are also prohibited. The land is sacred to the tribe, so treat it as you would your own place of worship.

Tribal rangers lead short but informative hikes in Palm Canyon, Andreas Canyon, and Tahquitz Canyon; call for schedules. Wranglers from Smoke Tree Stables in Palm Springs also organize horseback excursions into Palm Canyon; for more information, call 760-327-1372 or visit smoketreeranch.com/smoketreestables.html.

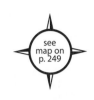

trip 11.1	**South Lykken Trail**

see
map on
p. 249

Distance	4.5 miles (one-way)
Hiking Time	2.5 hours
Elevation Gain	1,100'
Difficulty	Moderate
Best Times	October–April, day use only
Agency	Santa Rosa and San Jacinto Mountains National Monument
Optional Map	*Santa Rosa & San Jacinto Mountains National Monument* or USGS *Palm Springs* 7.5'

DIRECTIONS Leave a car or bicycle at the northern Mesquite Avenue Trailhead and then continue to the southern Palm Canyon Trailhead. To reach Mesquite Avenue from the 10 Freeway (I-10), take Highway 111 south into Palm Springs, where the road name changes to North Palm Canyon Drive. After about 12 miles, turn right onto Mesquite Avenue and go west 0.4 mile to the trailhead, where the road turns north toward the Tahquitz Canyon Visitor Center. The trailhead is at this corner, but the only parking is back down the hill along Mesquite Avenue just west of Palm Canyon Drive. Leave one vehicle here; then return to Palm Canyon Drive.

Turn right and continue south 0.5 mile. Most lanes turn left to become East Palm Canyon Drive, but stay right (straight) and continue on South Palm Canyon Drive 1.7 miles. Park at a turnout on the right (west) side of the road, 0.1 mile beyond Canyon Heights Drive.

The Lykken Trail is named in fitting tribute to Carl Lykken, a pioneering Palm Springs businessman and the city's first postmaster. The trail has two separate legs: South and North. Both start on the outskirts of Palm Springs, at city elevation. The trails ascend the slopes of the San Jacinto Mountains that border the city to the west, providing unparalleled views of Palm Springs and the Coachella Valley. From the ridges above the city, one can truly appreciate Palm Springs as a beautiful green oasis set against the forbidding Colorado Desert. Camping is prohibited along this trail.

The South Lykken Trail features a spectacular overlook from the curving lip of Tahquitz Canyon and also offers great views of the jets coming and going below you at Palm Springs International Airport. This trip can be done as a one-way hike. If you haven't arranged a car or bicycle shuttle, you can make a loop by taking a somewhat unpleasant 2.5-mile walk back on the shoulder of Palm Canyon Drive. For an out-and-back alternative, hike the first 3 miles to the dramatic Josie Johnson Vista; then retrace your steps.

VARIATION

For a longer one-way hike, join the North Lykken Trail (see Trip 11.2). The direct link between the two trails is conspicuously missing, but a brief detour on city streets will connect you to the other leg of the trail. Follow Mesquite Road east to Belardo Road; then go north to Ramon Road and back west.

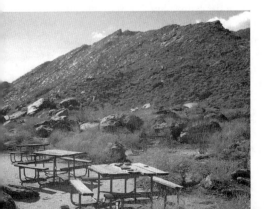

From the signed trailhead on the side of South Palm Canyon Drive, follow a closed gravel road east 0.4 mile along the north side of a wash to the signed start of the Lykken Trail. The footpath begins switchbacking

South Lykken Trail picnic tables

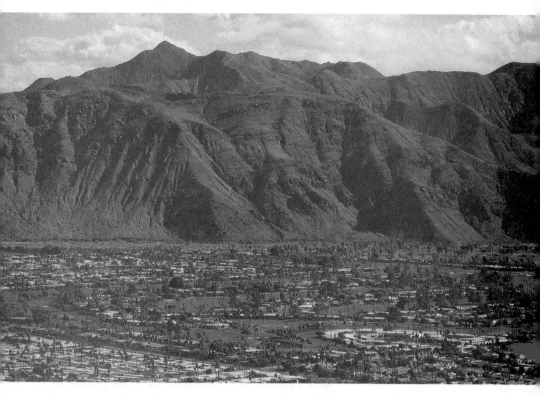

Murray Hill from South Lykken Trail

north up the toe of the mountain, reaching the Simone Kennett Vista Point in 0.7 mile. From here, there are memorable views of Palm Springs, Murray Hill, and the northern Santa Rosa Mountains, and Palm Canyon. The trail begins contouring north across the tilted slopes of San Jacinto. In 0.6 mile, it reaches a junction marked by a cairn, leading through private property to a residential neighborhood.

Continue north on the Lykken Trail from the junction another 1.4 miles past barrel and cholla cacti to picnic tables at the Josie Johnson Vista Park on the lip of Tahquitz Canyon. From here, there are impressive views down the steep walls of the canyon and out over the city. Aviation enthusiasts will also enjoy the steady stream of jets landing and departing from Palm Springs International Airport below.

The trail begins descending along the east rim of the canyon. In 0.1 mile, a spur trail leads left 100 yards to another impressive viewpoint on the canyon lip. This is a good place to admire Tahquitz Falls during the wetter months. The main trail switchbacks steeply down 1.3 miles farther to finish the south leg of the trail at Mesquite Avenue near the Tahquitz Canyon Visitor Center.

trip 11.2 North Lykken Trail

see map on p. 249

Distance	4 miles (one-way)
Hiking Time	2.5 hours
Elevation Gain	1,500'
Difficulty	Moderate
Best Times	October–April, day use only
Agency	Santa Rosa and San Jacinto Mountains National Monument
Recommended Map	*Santa Rosa & San Jacinto Mountains National Monument* or *Palm Springs* 7.5' (trail incompletely marked)

DIRECTIONS Leave a car or bicycle at the northern Cielo Drive Trailhead and then continue to the southern Ramon Road Trailhead. To reach Cielo Drive from the 10 Freeway, take Highway 111 south into Palm Springs, where the road name changes to North Palm Canyon Drive. After 9.7 miles, turn right (west) onto Vista Chino. In 0.2 mile, turn right onto Via Norte, proceed 0.1 mile, and turn left onto Chino Canyon Road. In 0.2 mile, turn left at a T and follow Panorama Road 0.3 mile; then stay left on Cielo Drive. In 0.1 mile, turn left on an unnamed spur to the trailhead parking between a tennis court and an impressive cactus garden.

To reach Ramon Road, return to Palm Canyon Drive and turn right. Continue south 2 miles, turn right (west) onto Ramon Road, and drive to the trailhead at the end.

The Lykken Trail is named in fitting tribute to Carl Lykken, a pioneering Palm Springs businessman and the city's first postmaster. The trail has two separate legs, designated South and North. Both start on the outskirts of Palm Springs, at city elevation. The trails ascend the slopes of the San Jacinto Mountains that border the city to the west, providing unparalleled views of Palm Springs and the Coachella Valley. From the ridges above the city one can truly appreciate Palm Springs as a beautiful green oasis set against the forbidding Colorado Desert. Camping is prohibited along this trail.

VARIATION

This trip can be done as a one-way hike with a car or bicycle shuttle. Alternatively, hike halfway, then descend the Museum Trail (see Trip 11.3) and follow Cahuilla Road 0.5 mile south back to Ramon Road.

Pick up the signed North Lykken Trail that soon begins climbing unrelentingly northwest. Barrel cacti cling tenaciously to the rocky soil. In 0.4 mile, reach a signed junction with another trail to the right that returns to the dirt road where you started. Stay left and continue up the Lykken Trail 0.9 mile to a second junction marked with a large cairn. The Museum Trail forks right and descends to the Palm Springs Art Museum (see Trip 11.3), but the Lykken Trail continues north.

In another 200 feet, at a sign painted on a boulder, the Skyline Trail forks to the left and climbs 8 arduous miles to Long Valley (see Trip 11.4), but the Lykken Trail again continues north, rounds the corner of the ridge, and

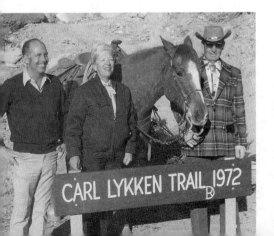

Dedication of the Lykken Trail, 1972: (left to right) then–Palm Springs Mayor Bill Foster, Jane Lykken Hoff (Carl Lykken's daughter), Scooter (Art Smith's horse), and Art Smith

Photo courtesy of Doug Evans, Desert Riders

switchbacks down to the valley floor in 1.1 miles. After completing the final switchbacks, look for an easy-to-miss trail junction. The right fork leads down to the spillway on a large levee and ends at a fence, but you stay on the left fork. In another 0.1 mile, reach a second junction near a huge boulder. Again, stay left rather than descending to the spillway.

VARIATION

In 100 yards, reach yet another unmarked junction. The left fork is a worthy side trip, although it's open for travel only from October to December to avoid disturbing bighorn sheep. It leads 0.4 mile up the narrow Tachevah Canyon to a spectacular slab topped by a lone palm tree. A thin waterfall trickles down the slab during the wet season. The rocky trail braids in and out of the wash and there are many ways to go. Beware of the long-thorned mesquite bushes near the end. Return to the junction after you've finished exploring.

The Lykken Trail continues north through the boulders at the wide mouth of the next canyon. It then climbs past creosote bushes and rounds a hill. Avoid the unmarked side trail on the right, which leads into private property belonging to the Riverside County Flood Control District. Instead, stay on the main trail, which once again climbs steeply up the next ridge to picnic tables at a flat area with fine vistas, then descends steeply to the north trailhead near Cielo Drive, 1.6 miles from Tachevah Canyon.

trip 11.3 Museum Trail

Distance	2 miles (out-and-back)
Hiking Time	1.5 hours
Elevation Gain	1,000'
Difficulty	Moderate
Best Times	October–April; by moonlight in the summer
Agency	Santa Rosa and San Jacinto Mountains National Monument
Optional Map	*Santa Rosa & San Jacinto Mountains National Monument* or USGS *Palm Springs* 7.5' (trail not marked)

see map on p. 249

DIRECTIONS From the 10 Freeway, take Highway 111 south into Palm Springs, where the road name changes to North Palm Canyon Drive. In 11.2 miles from the interstate, turn right (west) onto Tahquitz Canyon Way and go 0.2 mile; then turn right onto Museum Drive. There is no public parking at the Palm Springs Art Museum, but you may find limited parking on Museum Drive or in the public lot across from the museum.

Sunrise over the Santa Rosa Mountains and Palm Springs from the Museum Trail

The Museum Trail is a short but steep trail leading from the Palm Springs Art Museum up the western flank of San Jacinto. It offers great views of Palm Springs and is a popular exercise trail, either by itself or as a loop with the North Lykken Trail. Camping is prohibited along this trail.

The signed trailhead is in the northwest corner of the museum's northern parking lot. Immediately cross a private road. The trail switchbacks steeply up the hillside. Numerous unmarked shortcuts can be found along the way, but these paths increase erosion—try to stay on the most heavily used trail.

The trail climbs westward on the south side of the ridge 0.4 mile, then crosses over to the north side, descending 50 feet to bypass some rocks along the way. In another 0.4 mile, pass an outcrop and come to picnic tables near a four-way junction. Enjoy the magnificent views of saddle-backed Toro Peak at the head of Palm Canyon, the sheer sickle-shaped gorge of Tahquitz Canyon immediately south, the ridges and canyons of the Santa Rosa Mountains to the east, and the Little San Bernardino Mountains to the north, along with the city of Palm Springs immediately below.

ALTERNATIVE FINISH

Return the way you came. Or, if you prefer to make a loop with a more gradual descent, continue straight ahead 0.1 mile to a cairn marking the junction with the North Lykken Trail (see Trip 11.2). Turn left and descend the trail to Ramon Road; then follow Cahuilla Road north back to the Museum Trailhead. This option adds a mile of walking.

---

trip 11.4   ## Cactus-to-Clouds

Distance	10 miles (one-way)
Hiking Time	9 hours
Elevation Gain	8,000'
Difficulty	Very strenuous
Best Times	October–November
Agency	Santa Rosa and San Jacinto Mountains National Monument
Required Maps	Santa Rosa & San Jacinto Mountains National Monument or USGS Palm Springs and San Jacinto 7.5' (trail not marked)

see map on p. 249

DIRECTIONS If you plan to descend via the tram, you may wish to leave a vehicle at the Palm Springs Aerial Tramway station (or take a taxi/ride share back, though you may not have phone coverage here). From Highway 111, 8.5 miles south of the 10 Freeway at the northern edge of Palm Springs, turn west up Tramway Road and drive 4 miles to Valley Station, the lower terminus of the Palm Springs Aerial Tramway. The tram operates daily, starting at 10 a.m. Monday–Thursday and at 8 a.m. Friday–Sunday and holidays. The last tram returns at 9:45 p.m. The tram closes for annual maintenance, typically in September. Check pstramway.com or call 888-515-TRAM for the most current information.

To reach the trailhead, continue 3.2 miles south on Highway 111. The road name changes to North Palm Canyon Drive. Turn right (west) onto Tahquitz Canyon Way and go 0.2 mile; then turn right onto Museum Drive. There is no public parking at the Palm Springs Art Museum, but you may find limited parking on Museum Drive or in the public lot across from the museum.

Cactus-to-Clouds is a classic Southern California megahike. This trip describes the Skyline Trail portion, which has the greatest continuous elevation gain in the United States, climbing 8,000 feet up the sheer east ridge of San Jacinto from Palm Springs to the upper Aerial Tramway station. Most hikers stop at the station, but diehards continue on to bag the summit of San Jacinto. The Civilian Conservation Corps built the trail during the Great Depression. It had fallen into obscurity for decades, but is now heavily traveled.

The trail also features some of the most varied and interesting scenery and plant life found anywhere in Southern California. Camping is prohibited along this trail.

Some trail runners can make the enormous ascent in less than 5 hours, but a normal fit hiker should plan for double that. The trail is scorched by the sun at the bottom for most of the year and is covered in ice at the top after the first winter snows, so late fall is an ideal season for the climb. Several hikers have died on this route, and others have required rescue. Bring 4–6 quarts of water. After the first storm of the season, the upper part of the route is usually covered in snow and becomes unsuitable for hikers who don't already know the route and who lack ice ax, crampons, and adequate snow mountaineering experience.

The first mile of this hike climbs the Museum Trail (see Trip 11.3). The signed trailhead is in the northwest corner of the museum's northern parking lot. Immediately cross a private road. The trail switchbacks steeply up the hillside. Numerous unmarked shortcuts can be found along the way, but these paths increase erosion—stay on the most heavily used trail. The trail climbs westward on the south side of the ridge 0.4 mile, then crosses over to the north side, descending 50 feet to bypass some rocks along the way. In another 0.4 mile, pass a rock outcrop and come to picnic tables near a four-way junction with good views. Continue straight 0.1 mile to a cairn marking the junction with the North Lykken Trail (see Trip 11.2). Turn right and go 200 feet; then turn left where a sign painted on a rock indicates the trail to Long Valley. A sign near the start warns of the perils of the trail.

Follow the Skyline Trail 8.3 miles and another incredible 7,000 feet of elevation gain to reach Long Valley near the tram station. As you climb, observe how the vegetation transitions through many different zones. At the bottom, brittlebushes, creosote bushes, and barrel cacti are common. After climbing the ridge and east slopes, the trail momentarily levels out, then crosses to the right side of the ridge, offering great views into Tachevah Canyon to the north. The desert vegetation begins changing. Junipers, ribbonwoods, scrub oaks, valley cholla cacti, and Mojave yuccas start dotting the hillside. The trail briefly flattens again before gaining the crest of the ridge. After surmounting the next hill, the granite ramparts of the upper mountain come into view. You can pick out most of the route from here. Look for the prominent Coffman's Crag on the right side of the ridge; this is the largest monolithic rock on the east face. Eagle-eyed climbers may notice the Palm Springs Aerial Tramway passing immediately north of the crag. The trail follows the top of the narrowing ridge between Chino Canyon to the north and Tahquitz Canyon to the south, then switchbacks through the dense band of chaparral, then climbs into the forest and ascends the gully on the south side of Coffman's Crag.

The next stretch of desert vegetation is especially lush, with several species of yuccas dotting the landscape. Views of the dramatic upper ridge continue to improve. As the ridge narrows, you're briefly treated to breathtaking glimpses of the zebra-striped cliffs in Chino Canyon. At 6,000 feet, the trail crosses a dry wash above a small granite-slab waterfall. The vegetation abruptly changes to dense

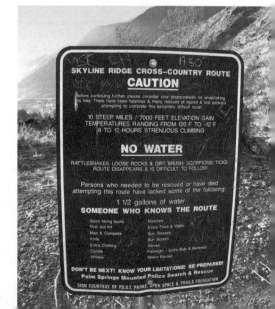

Dire warnings at the start of the Skyline Trail

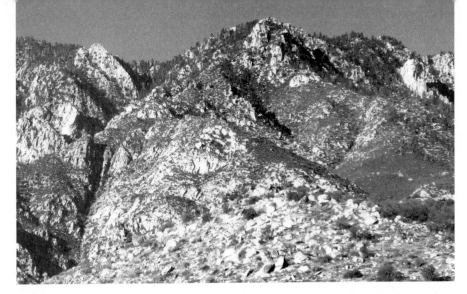

Upper Skyline Ridge

chaparral, including scrub oaks, manzanitas, and ribbonwoods. Travel would be horrendous were it not for the well-built trail snaking through the brush. In another 1,000 feet, Jeffrey pines begin to appear, followed by cedars and live oaks. Enjoy the impressive cliffs of Coffman's Crag as you pass directly alongside it; then suddenly pop over the lip of the ridge into the flat valley beyond.

You've now emerged onto the Desert View Loop Trail in Long Valley. From here, you have several options: you can return the way you came, take the tram down (a one-way ticket purchase is required), or get a wilderness permit and hike to the summit of San Jacinto. To reach the summit of San Jacinto, follow the directions in Trip 9.23. This adds 10 miles and 2,600 feet of elevation gain to your monumental adventure and typically demands a very early start. In 2005, *Backpacker* magazine cited this as one of the 10 most difficult day hikes in America. For the latter two options, follow the Desert View Loop Trail west and north to a signed junction with the paved trail coming down from the tramway. To reach the tram, turn right and hike up the switchbacks.

| **trip 11.5** | **Tahquitz Canyon** |

see map on p. 249

Distance	2 miles (loop)
Hiking Time	2.5 hours
Elevation Gain	350'
Difficulty	Easy
Best Times	September–May
Agency	Agua Caliente Band of Cahuilla Indians
Optional Map	*Tahquitz Canyon* map
Permit	Tahquitz Canyon admission fee required (see page 250)

DIRECTIONS From North Palm Canyon Drive 0.5 mile south of Ramon Road in Palm Springs (about 12 miles south of the 10 Freeway), turn west onto Mesquite Avenue. Follow Mesquite Avenue as it winds up to the Tahquitz Canyon Visitor Center at 500 W. Mesquite Ave.

Native peoples have inhabited Tahquitz Canyon for more than 3,000 years. According to Cahuilla Indian legend, Tahquitz was the tribe's first shaman. Tahquitz was powerful,

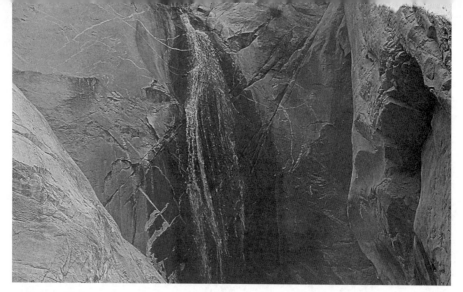

Tahquitz Falls

but he abused his might. Driven from the village by his people, he transformed himself into a green ball of fire and flew into the sky. Tahquitz then used his powers to harm others. Some members of the tribe still refuse to venture into Tahquitz Canyon alone. Hikers use several pronunciations, but the correct Cahuilla pronunciation is "**taw**-kwish."

The canyon was a countercultural haunt in the 1970s but has since been cleaned up and is now open to hikers 7:30 a.m.–5 p.m. Excellent 2.5-hour ranger-guided tours depart daily at 8 a.m., 10 a.m., noon, and 2 p.m. Schedules may change, so call 760-416-7044 or visit tahquitzcanyon.com for information and reservations. Admission to the Indian Canyons farther south may include a discount to Tahquitz Canyon, so if you'd like to explore both, consider visiting the Indian Canyons first.

The trail starts behind the Tahquitz Canyon Visitor Center and makes a figure-eight pattern up the canyon. On the guided hike rangers point out many native plants along the way that were used for food or medicine, including barrel and cholla cactus, creosote bush and brittlebush, mesquite, and cat's claw acacia. A stream flows most of the year in the upper portion of the canyon. The creek plunges over Tahquitz Falls at the top of the trail into a deep pool, 1 mile uphill from the visitor center. The Cahuilla people believe that this is a place of power that rejuvenates and energizes. After enjoying the waterfall, continue back along the loop trail.

trip 11.6 Desert Angel

Distance	1.6 miles (out-and-back)
Hiking Time	2.5 hours
Elevation Gain	1,200'
Difficulty	Moderate
Best Times	October–December (closed January–September)
Agency	Santa Rosa and San Jacinto Mountains National Monument
Required Maps	Tom Harrison *San Jacinto Wilderness, Santa Rosa & San Jacinto Mountains National Monument,* or USGS *Desert Hot Springs, Palm Springs,* and *San Jacinto 7.5'*

DIRECTIONS From the 10 Freeway, turn south on Highway 111 and proceed 5.5 miles, passing Windy Point and the mouth of Blaisdell Canyon. Park off the highway on your right, at the toe of the ridge.

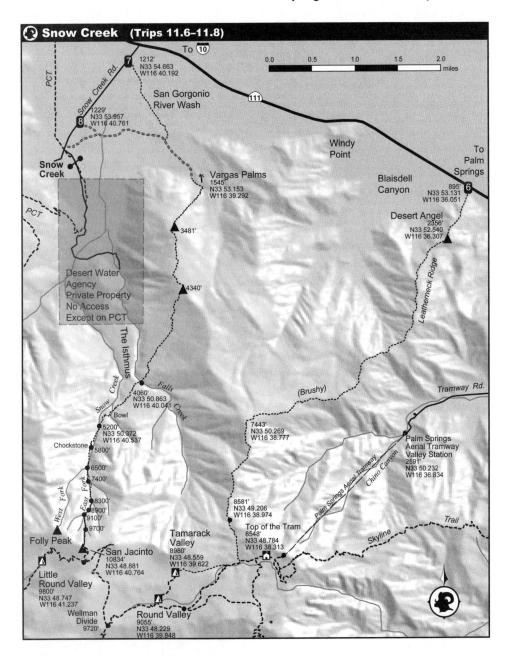

Snow Creek (Trips 11.6–11.8)

To (10)

7 1212'
N33 54.663
W116 40.192

San Gorgonio
River Wash

8 1229'
N33 53.957
W116 40.761

Snow Creek Rd.

PCT

Snow
Creek

Vargas Palms
1545'
N33 53.153
W116 39.292

Windy
Point

Blaisdell
Canyon

895' 6
N33 53.131
W116 36.051

To
Palm
Springs

Desert Angel
2356'
N33 52.540
W116 36.307

PCT

▲ 3481'

▲ 4340'

Desert Water
Agency
Private Property
No Access
Except on PCT

The Isthmus

Snow Creek

Falls Creek

4060'
N33 50.863
W116 40.041

Leatherneck Ridge

Bowl

(Brushy)

Tramway Rd.

5200'
N33 50.372
W116 40.537

Chockstone 5800'

7443'
N33 50.269
W116 38.777

Palm Springs
Aerial Tramway
Valley Station
2591'
N33 50.232
W116 36.834

6500'

7400'

West Fork

East Fork

8300'

8900'

9100'

9700'

Folly Peak ▲

8581'
N33 49.206
W116 38.974

Palm Springs Aerial Tramway

Chino Canyon

Tamarack
Valley
8980'
N33 48.559
W116 39.622

Top of the Tram
8548'
N33 48.784
W116 38.313

San Jacinto
10834'
N33 48.881
W116 40.764

Skyline

Trail

Little
Round Valley
9800'
N33 48.747
W116 41.237

Wellman
Divide
9720'

Round Valley
9055'
N33 48.229
W116 39.848

The long ridge off Highway 111 between Blaisdell and Chino Canyons is locally known as Leatherneck Ridge. The moderate cross-country scramble up the ridge to the first prominent hill, Desert Angel, is rewarded with fine views. Cross-country travel is legal only from October to December to protect the endangered Peninsular bighorn sheep.

From the toe of the ridge where you parked your car, climb onto the crest of the ridge and hike up the talus, slabs, and dirt to Desert Angel.

You could continue up Leatherneck Ridge all the way to the Palm Springs Aerial Tramway or San Jacinto. The hike to the tram is 8 miles with 9,000 feet of elevation gain. In August 2005, part of the ridge burned in a 5,000-acre brush fire started by careless campers in Blaisdell Canyon. The regrown chaparral makes part of the climb difficult and unpleasant.

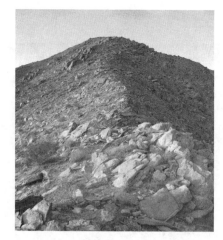

Desert Angel Ridge

trip 11.7　**Vargas Palms**

Distance	4.4 miles (out-and-back)
Hiking Time	2.5 hours
Elevation Gain	500'
Difficulty	Moderate
Trail Use	Dogs allowed
Best Times	October–April
Agency	BLM Palm Springs–South Coast Field Office
Optional Map	USGS *White Water* 7.5'

see map on previous page

DIRECTIONS From the 10 Freeway in San Gorgonio Pass, take Exit 111 south onto Highway 111. In 1.1 miles, turn right (southwest) onto Snow Creek Road. In 0.3 mile, park on the left (east) side of the road, near the mouth of a small wash.

As you drive along the 10 Freeway through San Gorgonio Pass, it's hard not to gawk at Snow Creek cutting a chasm down the dramatic north face of San Jacinto. But few travelers realize that several palm groves are also tucked away near the base of the mountain. This cross-country trip visits Vargas Palms, the largest of the oases. The route crosses an alluvial fan, dry washes, sand dunes, and boulder fields and is a great excuse to examine desert vegetation, especially during spring bloom.

Snow Creek is the dazzling granite-buttressed canyon to the south dropping 2 miles from the summit of San Jacinto to the desert floor. From the parking area, look southeast toward the first canyon left of Snow Creek. You'll see the Vargas Palms in a crease on the right edge of the canyon. It's critical to identify these and keep them in sight as you hike, because there is no trail. Pay attention to landmarks as you go so you'll be able to find your way back to your vehicle.

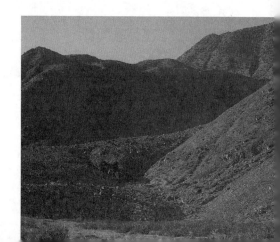

Vargas Palms Oasis, tucked in a crease below San Jacinto

A maze of washes and abandoned roads crisscrosses the desert, but it's too difficult to describe and follow a specific path to the palms. Instead, pick your own route toward the palms, weaving as necessary to avoid vegetation. You'll pass creosote, burrobrush, Mormon tea, cheesebush, and other desert scrub and grasses. In 0.8 mile, cross the broad wash of the San Gorgonio River and climb past indigo bushes onto a small sand dune. On the far side, you may find an old firebreak leading to an old road. Take this to its end at the base of a gully between the mountain and a hill covered with granite boulders and brittlebush.

Ascend the gully, hopping up the boulders as necessary. The odd red coloration on the rocks is fire retardant sprayed by aircraft fighting a wildfire. Your path soon ends at the Vargas Palms. In the wet season, you may find a small waterfall here.

Return the way you came. This can be difficult because of a lack of landmarks near the parking area. If you become disoriented, veer west until you reach Snow Creek Road; then follow it north back to the parking area.

trip 11.8	Snow Creek

see
map on
p. 259

Distance	12 miles (one-way)
Hiking Time	15+ hours
Elevation Gain	10,000'
Difficulty	Very strenuous, technical
Best Times	October, March–April
Agency	Mount San Jacinto State Park
Required Maps	USGS *White Water* and *San Jacinto Peak* 7.5'
Permit	San Jacinto Wilderness Permit required

DIRECTIONS This trip starts near the village of Snow Creek and ends at the Palm Springs Aerial Tramway Valley Station. You could leave a vehicle at the tram station, but you could also take a taxi or ride share 13 miles back to Snow Creek (though no cell signal may be available at the Valley Station).

To reach Snow Creek from the 10 Freeway near San Gorgonio Pass, take Exit 111 south onto Highway 111. In 1.1 miles, turn right onto Snow Creek Road. Proceed south 1.2 miles, and park by a pump station on the left. To get back to the trailhead from Valley Station, drive 4 miles down Tramway Road, turn left and take Highway 111 north 7.4 miles, and turn left onto Snow Creek Road.

Carved by the San Andreas Fault at San Gorgonio Pass, the north face of San Jacinto is the most impressive mountaineering site in the Inland Empire. Snow Creek cuts the face's rugged granite battlement, plunging 9,000 feet from the summit to the desert floor in only 3 horizontal miles. The climb up Snow Creek is a serious undertaking, suitable for experienced mountaineers accustomed to moving efficiently on difficult terrain. The ascent is most popular in the spring when the drainage is filled with well-consolidated snow, but may be dangerous if there are avalanche conditions or the snow is particularly icy. All avalanches on the north face of San Jacinto eventually pour down Snow Creek, producing a snow tongue that reaches 5,000–6,000 feet even in midspring. You may need to wait a week or longer after a snowstorm for the snow to consolidate. An ice ax and crampons are essential, and many parties bring a rope for a short rock pitch or to rescue companions who might fall through a snowbridge. The route can also be done in the fall, when it's a long scramble up talus and small waterfalls. Beware of rattlesnakes in the brush. Many rescues have occurred in this area. Navigation is challenging in any event, but substantially easier if you preload the track into your GPS. The tram closes at 9:45 p.m., so an early start and efficient movement are necessary. Most parties do the climb in a very long day with a predawn start because carrying overnight gear makes the trip even harder, but you can bivouac midway.

The Desert Water Agency (DWA) owns Section 33 of land at the mouth of Snow Creek and doesn't issue hiker permits. A security guard and dog enforce this restriction. This trip bypasses DWA land by way of the ridge above Vargas Palms, making an arduous climb even longer.

Your first goal is to reach the Vargas Palms oasis, 1.7 miles southeast of the pump station. A maze of abandoned roads, firebreaks, and washes starting on the north side of the pump station leads in this direction, and you might be able to follow it if you've loaded the track into your GPS; otherwise, expect some cross-country travel across the rough desert floor, fording Snow Creek along the way. This route to the oasis is more direct and easier in the dark but less scenic than the one in Trip 11.7. The roads end at a boulder-filled gully that you climb for 0.2 mile to the lowest palms in the oasis.

From Vargas Palms, turn right and climb the dirt ridge, which is steep but never difficult. The ridge is studded with granite boulders and graced with brittlebush, desert mallow, yerba santa, and spring wildflowers that gradually change as you ascend. Above Point 3,481', the angle decreases substantially. Continue to a saddle just beyond Point 4,340'.

The next challenge is a 1.4-mile traverse to Falls Creek. Descend slightly from the saddle. The best route, marked with occasional cairns, lies between the 4,000- and 4,200-foot contours, weaving to dodge the worst of the rock and brush obstacles. Reach a stand of ribbonwood shortly before the creek, climb briefly, and then drop down to cross the creek.

Travel becomes more difficult in the next segment as you cross above the "Isthmus" and ascend a bowl to enter Snow Creek above a pair of waterfalls. A surprisingly good climber's trail threads through the dense chaparral; the trail is occasionally hard to follow, but well worth the effort because the alternative is an awful bushwhack. Climb the slopes to join a tributary creek in the bowl; then follow it up until the tributary veers left at a cliff. The climber's trail resumes here, ascending steep slopes on the right under heavy tree cover.

Snow Creek Route

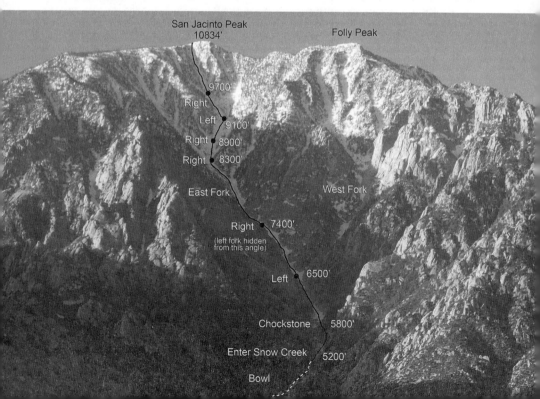

Follow the path up to the ridgeline and around boulders until you can easily descend into Snow Creek, where you'll find a small bivouac site at 5,200 feet.

The first and most significant obstacle in Snow Creek is a house-sized chockstone blocking the canyon at 5,800 feet. The chockstone is bypassed by climbing the wall to the right; the farther below the chockstone you start, the easier it is. Rock climbers will enjoy jamming an 80-foot 5.5 crack system, which starts 35 feet below the chockstone and ends at a prominent oak thicket. Otherwise, find a dirty third-class path at the lowest weakness on the right side of the canyon. If you take the latter route, you'll need to work your way up and left through a thicket of oaks until your path is blocked by a massive granite formation. Some route finding is required to discover a third-class path onto the rock from which you can traverse past the chockstone and follow a ramp back into the canyon.

In most years, continuous snow begins around here and you have an epic 5,000-foot snow climb ahead of you that concludes yards from the summit of San Jacinto. The angle is 25–35 degrees most of the way, steepening to about 40 degrees at the very top. It can be easy cramponing if conditions are ideal, or extremely dangerous if you face avalanche conditions, hard ice, thin snowbridges, or gale-strength winds; be prepared to evaluate conditions and turn around if necessary. Pay close attention to the many forks along the climb; the best route is frequently not obvious. At 6,500 feet, stay left in the West Fork of Snow Creek; the East Fork veers off to Folly Peak and requires difficult rock climbing in places. You may notice stunted limber pines growing in Snow Creek that can bend to endure the avalanches sweeping down the canyon. At forks at 7,400 feet, 8,300 feet, and 8,900 feet, stay right. At 9,100 feet, veer left; then, at 9,700 feet, stay right again in a couloir that tops out just left of the 10,834-foot summit. In the event of an emergency, you'll find a hut just below the peak.

A few hardy souls have skied or snowboarded back down Snow Creek, but most take the easy way out to the Palm Springs Aerial Tramway. In the fall, you can simply walk the 5-mile trail (see Trip 9.23), but in the spring it's easier to take a more direct 3-mile route east down the snow slopes, staying south of the rocky crest, passing Tamarack Valley, descending the North Fork of Long Valley Creek, and then reaching the ranger station and main trail up to the tram.

trip 11.9 Andreas Canyon

see map on next page

Distance	1 mile (loop)
Hiking Time	30–45 minutes
Elevation Gain	200'
Difficulty	Easy
Trail Use	Good for kids
Best Times	September–May
Agency	Agua Caliente Band of Cahuilla Indians
Optional Map	*Indian Canyons* map
Permit	Indian Canyons admission fee required (see page 250)

DIRECTIONS From the 10 Freeway, take Highway 111 south into Palm Springs, where the road name changes to North Palm Canyon Drive, then South Palm Canyon Drive. About 12.4 miles from the freeway, most lanes turn left to become East Palm Canyon Drive, but stay straight (south) to continue on South Palm Canyon Drive. Follow South Palm Canyon Drive 2.8 miles to the Indian Canyons tollgate. Beyond the gate, immediately turn right and follow Andreas Canyon Road 0.8 mile to its end at the Andreas Canyon parking area.

Andreas Canyon contains the world's second-largest California fan palm oasis and is the ancestral home of the Paniktum clan of the Agua Caliente Band of Cahuilla Indians.

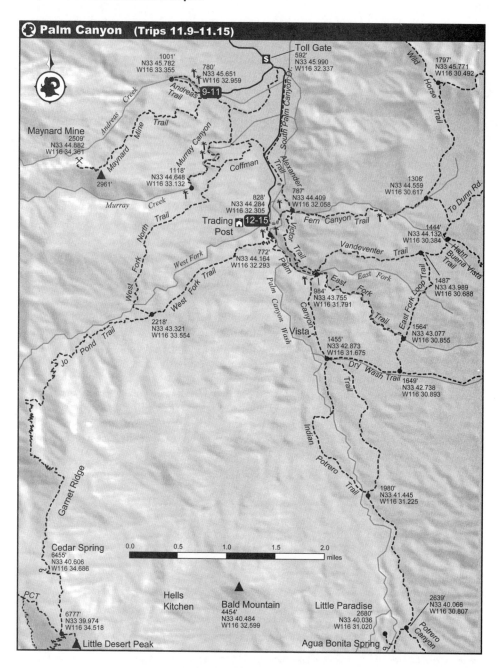

Palm Canyon (Trips 11.9–11.15)

Toll Gate
592'
N33 45.990
W116 32.337

1001'
N33 45.782
W116 33.355

780'
N33 45.651
W116 32.959

1797'
N33 45.771
W116 30.492

Andreas Trail

9-11

Wild Horse Trail

Andreas Creek

Maynard Mine
2509'
N33 44.882
W116 34.361

Maynard Mine Trail

Murray Canyon

Coffman

Alexander Trail

South Palm Canyon Dr.

1308'
N33 44.559
W116 30.617

To Dunn Rd.

2961'

1118'
N33 44.648
W116 33.132

787'
N33 44.409
W116 32.058

Fern Canyon Trail

1444'
N33 44.132
W116 30.384

Hahn Buena Vista Trail

Murray Creek

North Fork Trail

828'
N33 44.284
W116 32.305

Trading Post

12-15

Victor Trail

Vandeventer Trail

West Fork

772'
N33 44.164
W116 32.293

Palm Canyon

1487'
N33 43.989
W116 30.688

West Fork Trail

East Fork

East Fork

East Fork Loop Trail

West Fork Trail

984'
N33 43.755
W116 31.791

East Fork Trail

1564'
N33 43.077
W116 30.855

West Fork Trail

2218'
N33 43.321
W116 33.554

Palm Canyon Wash

Vista

1455'
N33 42.873
W116 31.675

Dry Wash Trail

1649'
N33 42.738
W116 30.893

Jo Pond Trail

Indian Potrero Trail

1980'
N33 41.445
W116 31.225

Garnet Ridge

0.0   0.5   1.0   1.5   2.0
miles

Cedar Spring
6455'
N33 40.606
W116 34.686

PCT

Hells Kitchen

Bald Mountain
4454'
N33 40.484
W116 32.599

Little Paradise
2680'
N33 40.036
W116 31.020

2639'
N33 40.066
W116 30.807

6777'
N33 39.974
W116 34.518

Little Desert Peak

Agua Bonita Spring

Potrero Canyon

This short trail follows Andreas Creek through the palm-filled canyon 0.5 mile, then returns along the south rim with views into the canyon. The Indian Canyons are open 8 a.m.–5 p.m. in season, and rangers lead interpretive hikes through the canyon Friday–Sunday at 1 p.m. Inquire at the entrance station for more information and to confirm times.

Before starting the hike, make sure to examine the rock mortars in which the Cahuilla Indians once ground their food; they're adjacent to the parking lot. The trail leads west from the parking lot along the creek beneath the dramatic metamorphic schist cliffs making up the north wall of the canyon. In 0.1 mile, steps lead down to the left to a seductively charming pool. Continue 0.4 mile to a fence marking the abrupt end of the trail. The trail then crosses the creek and climbs onto the south flank of the canyon where there are lovely views, and then returns to the parking area.

trip 11.10 Maynard Mine

Distance	5.5 miles (out-and-back)
Hiking Time	4 hours
Elevation Gain	2,400'
Difficulty	Strenuous
Best Times	October–April
Agency	Agua Caliente Band of Cahuilla Indians
Optional Map	*Indian Canyons* map
Permit	Indian Canyons admission fee required (see page 250)

DIRECTIONS From the 10 Freeway, take Highway 111 south into Palm Springs, where the road name changes to North Palm Canyon Drive, then South Palm Canyon Drive. About 12.4 miles from the freeway, most lanes turn left to become East Palm Canyon Drive, but stay straight (south) to continue on South Palm Canyon Drive. Follow South Palm Canyon Drive 2.8 miles to the Indian Canyons tollgate. Beyond the gate, immediately turn right and follow Andreas Canyon Road 0.8 mile to its end at the Andreas Canyon parking area.

Jim Maynard established a small tungsten mine on the narrow ridge between Andreas and Murray Canyons during World War II. This trip makes a steep climb to the mine site, offering a vigorous workout and sweeping views. Go on a cool day. The Indian Canyons are open 8 a.m.–5 p.m.

From the parking area, hike south across a bridge over Andreas Creek. Immediately beyond, the road turns left, but a sign marks the Maynard Mine Trail leading straight. The trail passes through a grove of honey mesquite and then switchbacks unrelentingly up the brittlebush-covered slopes. In 2.5 miles, it passes along the north side of Peak 2,961'. The trail then plunges almost 500 feet down the narrow ridge to the west to its signed terminus.

Maynard Mine

Turn right and walk about 100 feet down the north slope toward Andreas Canyon to the site of Maynard's excavation. You'll find the small adit in the hillside above a clearing. The gasoline engine nearby was brought to the site in pieces on muleback.

trip 11.11 Murray Canyon

Distance	4 miles (out-and-back)
Hiking Time	2 hours
Elevation Gain	500'
Difficulty	Moderate
Trail Use	Suitable for equestrians
Best Times	October–May
Agency	Agua Caliente Band of Cahuilla Indians
Optional Map	*Indian Canyons* map
Permit	Indian Canyons admission fee required (see page 250)

see map on p. 264

DIRECTIONS From the 10 Freeway, take Highway 111 south into Palm Springs, where the road name changes to North Palm Canyon Drive, then South Palm Canyon Drive. About 12.4 miles from the freeway, most lanes turn left to become East Palm Canyon Drive, but stay straight (south) to continue on South Palm Canyon Drive. Follow South Palm Canyon Drive 2.8 miles to the Indian Canyons tollgate. Beyond the gate, immediately turn right and follow Andreas Canyon Road 0.8 mile to the Andreas Canyon parking area. Turn left, cross a bridge, pass the Bent Palm Picnic Area, and park at the Murray Canyon Trailhead in 0.2 mile.

Murray Canyon is named for the Scottish rancher Welwood Murray, who founded the Palm Springs Hotel in 1887 and brought attention to the area as a spa and resort. The canyon cuts a groove down the rugged eastern slope of the Desert Divide. The trail ends at the Seven Sisters, a series of stone pools with a 12-foot waterfall. Murray Creek runs through the winter and spring. The trail crosses the creek a dozen times, and the rocks can be slippery so a trekking pole is helpful; this trip isn't recommended for those unsure of their balance. Murray Canyon is one of my favorite hikes of its length in the area. The falls are a great destination for a picnic, but don't expect to find solitude on this popular trail. The Indian Canyons are open 8 a.m.–5 p.m.

Follow the trail south across the desert at the base of a ridge past brittlebushes and creosote. In 0.2 mile, pass the Andreas Canyon South Trail on your left. In another 0.5 mile, make a switchback down to cross Murray Creek at a palm oasis. On the far side, pass another junction on the left with the West Fork North Trail. In 0.3 mile, reach the mouth of Murray Canyon.

The trail follows the winding canyon, repeatedly crossing the creek. The California fan palms and honey mesquite bushes growing along the creek were important sources of food for the Cahuilla Indians. You may see debris from a 2013 flood that swept down the canyon after the Mountain Fire. In 0.4 mile, reach a junction on the left with the Coffman Trail, which leads over the ridge out of the canyon. Just beyond, find a hitching line. Equestrians should leave their horses here because the last 0.5 mile of the canyon is unsuitable for riding. After negotiating some steep climbs and slick rocks, arrive at the waterfall at trail's end.

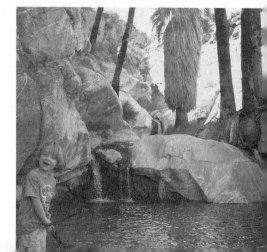

Waterfalls in Murray Canyon

see
map on
p. 264

trip 11.12 **Lower Palm Canyon**

Distance	2.6 miles (loop)
Hiking Time	1.5 hours
Elevation Gain	500'
Difficulty	Easy
Trail Use	Good for kids
Best Times	September–May
Agency	Agua Caliente Band of Cahuilla Indians
Recommended Map	*Indian Canyons* map or *Santa Rosa & San Jacinto Mountains National Monument*
Permit	Indian Canyons admission fee required (see page 250)

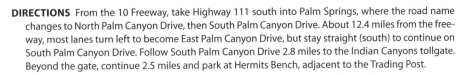

DIRECTIONS From the 10 Freeway, take Highway 111 south into Palm Springs, where the road name changes to North Palm Canyon Drive, then South Palm Canyon Drive. About 12.4 miles from the freeway, most lanes turn left to become East Palm Canyon Drive, but stay straight (south) to continue on South Palm Canyon Drive. Follow South Palm Canyon Drive 2.8 miles to the Indian Canyons tollgate. Beyond the gate, continue 2.5 miles and park at Hermits Bench, adjacent to the Trading Post.

Palm Canyon contains the world's largest California palm oasis and is the ancestral home of the Atcitcem Clan of the Agua Caliente Band of Cahuilla Indians, who have lived here for countless centuries. The oasis is one of the most spectacular sights in the Palm Springs vicinity. If you can see only one of the many oases described in this book, choose Palm Canyon. The tribe charges a modest admission fee, which supports rangers and trail maintenance. Palm Canyon extends 15 miles all the way up to Highway 74 high in the Santa Rosa Mountains, but the first mile has many of the best sights. This loop starts at the road's end, follows the floor of the canyon south 1 mile through the palms, and then returns via the Victor Trail along a ridge overlooking the canyon. The Indian Canyons are open 8 a.m.–5 p.m.

There is a fine view of Palm Canyon from the trailhead near the Trading Post. Follow the Palm Canyon Trail, which switchbacks down into the canyon to the south. You can enjoy a snack at the picnic tables beneath the magnificent trees. As you explore, keep an

Lower Palm Canyon

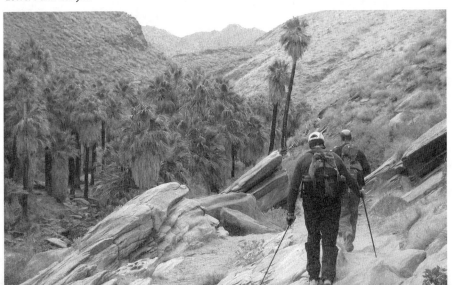

eye out for the stone mortars where Cahuilla women once ground their food near the stream's edge.

In 0.2 mile, reach a signed junction with the West Fork Trail at the south end of the main oasis. Continue south on the Palm Canyon Trail along the stream, passing a warm spring. At 1 mile, come to a second large oasis and a complex trail junction. Palm Canyon continues south. If you want a longer ramble, you can follow it as far as you choose before you return. But this loop turns hard left and joins the Victor Trail, which climbs onto the ridge immediately east of Palm Canyon. Watch for trail signs and take care not to mistakenly follow the Vandeventer or East Fork Trails instead. The stunning Victor Trail was dedicated in 1974 in memory of John Victor, father of the dedicated Desert Rider, Laine Victor.

The vegetation abruptly changes as you climb out of the canyon. Teddy bear cholla and barrel cacti are scattered among the creosote bushes and brittlebushes on the dry hillsides. The rocky trail leads north for a mile, overlooking Palm Canyon, then descends to another junction with the Fern Canyon and Alexander Trails. Turn left (west) and follow a trail across the creek. At the next junction with the Palm Canyon Trail, turn right and climb to the Trading Post parking area.

trip 11.13   Fern Canyon

see map on p. 264

Distance	6.5 miles (loop)
Hiking Time	3 hours
Elevation Gain	1,000'
Difficulty	Moderate
Trail Use	Suitable for equestrians
Best Times	October–May
Agency	Agua Caliente Band of Cahuilla Indians
Recommended Map	*Indian Canyons* map or *Santa Rosa & San Jacinto Mountains National Monument*
Permit	Indian Canyons admission fee required (see page 250)

DIRECTIONS From the 10 Freeway, take Highway 111 south into Palm Springs, where the road name changes to North Palm Canyon Drive, then South Palm Canyon Drive. About 12.4 miles from the freeway, most lanes turn left to become East Palm Canyon Drive, but stay straight (south) to continue on South Palm Canyon Drive. Follow South Palm Canyon Drive 2.8 miles to the Indian Canyons tollgate. Beyond the gate, continue 2.5 miles and park at the Trading Post.

Crossing Palm Canyon to reach the Fern Canyon Trail

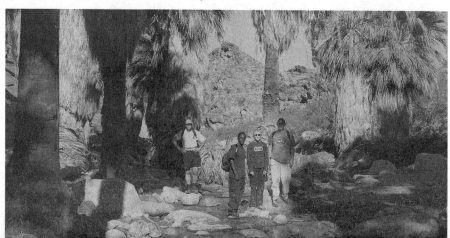

Fern Canyon is named for a wall where seeping water once supported a vertical garden of maidenhair ferns. In this drier time, there are fewer ferns, but the canyon is still home to a pleasant oasis. This loop hike is a good way to see many of Palm Canyon's most notable attractions with only a moderate amount of hiking. In addition to the sandy wash and oasis of Fern Canyon, this trip features views down into the huge Palm Canyon oasis and a ridge hike through fields of barrel and teddy bear cholla cacti. The Indian Canyons are open 8 a.m.–5 p.m.

From the parking area, walk east on a gated dirt road to a kiosk marking the start of the Fern Canyon, Victor, and Alexander Trails. Follow the trail north and east to a T-junction. The right fork leads to the main Palm Canyon oasis, but this trip turns left, crosses Palm Canyon, and climbs over a low ridge to a four-way junction at a bend in Wentworth Canyon, 0.4 mile from the parking area. The Victor Trail leads to the right. The Alexander Trail, used mostly by equestrians, leads left. But this trip goes straight ahead up Wentworth Canyon, which is now better known as Fern Canyon.

The Fern Canyon Trail follows the sandy wash east up the canyon. It then briefly leaves the wash and climbs steeply up a ridge before dropping down to the fern wall near another small oasis. The trail also affords good views of Murray Hill to the north.

Reach a series of signed junctions with connector trails. At each junction, stay right and wind around to the south, then west. Pass the Wild Horse Trail, Dunn Road Trail, Hahn Buena Vista Trail, and East Fork Loop Trail as you climb out of the wash and onto a broad ridge studded with spectacular cactus. Your trail changes its name to Vandeventer, and finally descends to a trail junction above a large palm oasis.

You can choose either of two paths back to the Trading Post. The 1-mile Palm Canyon Trail follows the canyon bottom through the enormous oasis, while the 1.6-mile Victor Trail follows the east rim of the canyon and offers sweeping vistas.

To take the Palm Canyon Trail (see Trip 11.12), turn left, walk 220 feet to a second junction; then turn right and descend Palm Canyon for a mile. At a picnic area in the main oasis, follow a path up the hill to the Trading Post.

To take the Victor Trail, turn right and follow the trail along the ridgeline 1.2 miles, then down into a dry wash where you reach a junction with the Fern Canyon and Alexander Trails where you started this trip. Turn left (west) and follow signs 0.4 mile back to the Trading Post.

trip 11.14   Pines-to-Palms

see map on p. 264

Distance	15 miles (one-way)
Hiking Time	7 hours
Elevation Loss	3,500'
Difficulty	Strenuous
Trail Use	Suitable for backpacking, suitable for equestrians
Best Times	October–March
Agency	Agua Caliente Band of Cahuilla Indians
Required Maps	Santa Rosa & San Jacinto Mountains National Monument or USGS Palm View Peak, Butterfly Peak, and Toro Peak 7.5'
Permit	Indian Canyons admission fee required (see page 250)

DIRECTIONS This trip requires a car shuttle between Pinyon Pines and the Trading Post. Unfortunately, the Indian Canyons are open only 8 a.m.–5 p.m., so unless you can arrange for somebody else to pick you up or you leave your car outside the tollgate, you must hike quickly.

Position one car where you'll emerge at the Trading Post. From the 10 Freeway, take Highway 111 south into Palm Springs, where the road name changes to North Palm Canyon Drive, then South Palm

Canyon Drive. About 12.4 miles from the freeway, most lanes turn left to become East Palm Canyon Drive, but stay straight (south) to continue on South Palm Canyon Drive. Follow South Palm Canyon Drive 2.8 miles to the tollgate at the entrance to the Indian Canyons. Notify the ranger at the gate if you expect that you might be out after 5 p.m. Beyond the gate, continue 2.5 miles to the Trading Post.

To reach the upper trailhead, return to the tollgate, backtrack north 2.8 miles on South Palm Canyon Drive, and turn right (east) onto East Palm Canyon Drive, which becomes Highway 111. Go east-southeast 11 miles to Highway 74; then turn right and follow Highway 74 south for 18 miles. Just past mile marker 074 RIV 77.85, turn right onto Pine View Drive and proceed 0.2 mile to the end of the paved road. This shuttle takes about 45 minutes.

Palm Canyon should be on the to-do list of every serious Southern California hiker. The canyon separates the San Jacinto Mountains and Desert Divide on the west from the Santa Rosa Mountains on the east and offers magnificent scenery in all directions. This trip follows the Palm Canyon Trail from the pinyon pines of the mountains down through the Seussian plant life of the Upper and Lower Sonoran Zones. The enormous palm oasis at the bottom of the trail is a fitting conclusion to the long but rewarding day. Some hikers prefer doing this trip in the uphill direction for more exercise. This can also be done as a backpacking trip, but camping isn't allowed in the northern half of the canyon, which lies within Agua Caliente Indian Reservation land. The boundary between National Forest and Agua Caliente land is about a mile north of Agua Bonita Spring.

Hells Kitchen from Middle Palm Canyon

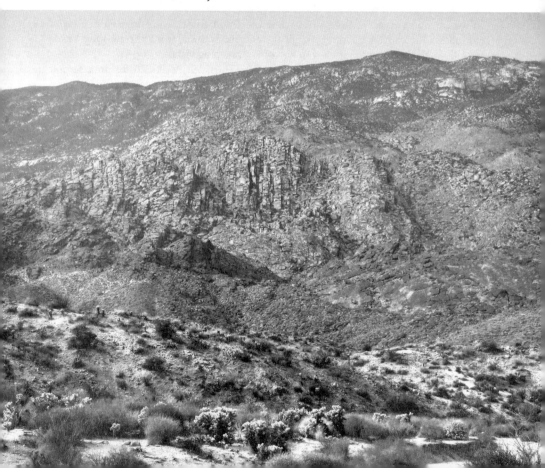

See the Toro Peak map on page 298 for details about the southern end of the trail. From the parking area on Pine View Drive, walk north up a dirt road. In 0.1 mile, veer right onto a trail that may be signed PINES TO PALMS. Hike north through ribbonwood chaparral, enjoying the sweeping views of the upper reaches of Palm Canyon. Watch for Mojave and whipple yucca and several species of prickly pear cactus. In 1.3 miles, reach a signed four-way junction. A dirt road leads right. A trail leads left down into the bottom of Palm Canyon, while jeep tracks lead straight north along the ridge past a marble mine. (This marble is readily recognized by its white color and sandpaper-like texture.) The ridge route north is faster and preferable because the canyon trail is overgrown and more difficult to follow.

The trail hugs the rolling ridgeline, then switchbacks northeast down into Omstott Canyon. Turn left and follow the trail down the canyon. (If you're doing this hike in the opposite direction, beware: this junction can be hard to spot. It's easy to miss the point where the trail leaves Omstott Canyon. If you find yourself wandering up the canyon bottom, you've missed the turnoff.) Go around a bend and rejoin the canyon bottom trail at a post on the floor of Palm Canyon, 2.5 miles from where the trails originally forked. Cat's claw acacia, desert willow, Gander's cholla, and hedgehog cactus are common in this area.

The next stretch of trail along Palm Canyon is narrow and faint in places. This land is used for cattle ranching and several gates control the cattle; close them behind you. The unmaintained Live Oak Canyon Trail once started up the first canyon to the northwest, but it burned and portions have completely vanished. The Dutch Charlie Trail then cuts east to Dunn Road, and soon after, the faint and unmaintained Oak Canyon Trail (4E03) veers off southwest through the mesquite, rounds a bend to Hidden Falls, and eventually joins the Live Oak Canyon Trail. However, this trip continues north on the main Palm Canyon Trail.

The next section of the trail is notable for the abundance of yuccas that grow here. In 2 miles, reach a signed junction. Agua Bonita Spring is on the canyon bottom below to the west. Water is available here much of the year. Look for bedrock mortars where the Cahuilla once ground their food.

VARIATION ───────────────────────────────

Adventurous hikers may scramble down to the creek at Agua Bonita and walk upstream for a few dozen paces until they're able to trudge up the west slope, then turn right and follow a rocky draw north to Little Paradise. Unfortunately, it would be better called Paradise Lost—all that remains after the 1980 Palm Canyon Fire are a dead palm tree and some prickly bushes.

A third of a mile past Agua Bonita Spring, the Potrero Canyon Trail veers off to the right. Stay in Palm Canyon as it becomes deeper and takes on a rugged appearance. The rocks on the west side have a scalelike look as if they once belonged to a gigantic stone reptile; this area is known as Hell's Kitchen. In another 2 miles, come to a junction with the Indian Potrero Trail. Both Indian Potrero and Palm Canyon Trails lead north, one on each side of Palm Canyon, and both are enjoyable. The Indian Potrero and Palm Canyon Trails rejoin in 2 miles at a junction with the aptly named Dry Wash Trail, which leads east; the Palm Canyon Trail continues north. By now, the lush vegetation of the upper canyon has given way to teddy bear cholla and brittlebush.

In 1.0 mile past the Dry Wash Trail, come to an enormous palm oasis at the junction with the Victor, Vandeventer, and East Fork Trails. Stay left on the Palm Canyon Trail for another mile, passing many more palms before you climb to the Trading Post.

see
maps on
pgs. 264
& 231

trip 11.15 Jo Pond Trail

Distance	16 miles (out-and-back), 11.5 miles (one-way to Cedar Spring Trailhead)
Hiking Time	9 hours (out-and-back)
Elevation Gain	6,200'
Difficulty	Strenuous
Trail Use	Suitable for backpacking, suitable for equestrians
Best Times	October–November, March–April
Agency	Agua Caliente Band of Cahuilla Indians
Recommended Map	*Santa Rosa & San Jacinto Mountains National Monument* or USGS *Palm View Peak 7.5'*
Permit	Indian Canyons admission fee required (see page 250)

DIRECTIONS From the 10 Freeway, take Highway 111 south into Palm Springs, where the road name changes to North Palm Canyon Drive, then South Palm Canyon Drive. About 12.4 miles from the freeway, most lanes turn left to become East Palm Canyon Drive, but stay straight (south) to continue on South Palm Canyon Drive. After paying your admission fee at the Indian Canyons tollgate, drive south 2.5 miles and park at the end of the road at the Trading Post.

If you're doing a one-way hike, start by arranging to leave a second vehicle at the Cedar Spring Trailhead. Return to the tollgate, backtrack north 2.8 miles on South Palm Canyon Drive, and turn right (east) onto East Palm Canyon Drive, which becomes Highway 111. Go east-southeast 11 miles to Highway 74; then turn right and follow Highway 74 south, west, and back north 28 miles to Garner Valley. Near mile marker 74 RIV 67.75 and immediately after Riverside County Fire Department Station 53, turn right (northeast) onto paved Morris Ranch Road (6S53) and follow it 3.7 miles, passing the Joe Sherman Girl Scout Camp, to the signed Cedar Spring Trailhead (4E17) on the right. (If you reach Morris Ranch, you've driven 0.25 mile too far.) The best parking is at a large lot on the east side of the road 0.1 mile before you reach the trailhead. The drive between the trailheads takes about 75 minutes. (See Trip 10.4 and the map on page 231.)

The Salton Sea and Santa Rosa Mountains from the Jo Pond Trail

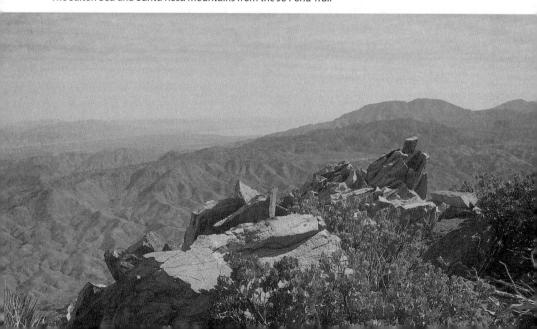

The Jo Pond Trail, completed in 1994, connects Palm Canyon to the Desert Divide, relentlessly climbing Garnet Ridge to Cedar Spring. Considered one of the most spectacular trails in the region, it's named not for a body of water but for Josephine Rose Pond, a Palm Springs socialite, philanthropist, and member of the Desert Riders, a longstanding equestrian club that built and helps maintain the present-day Indian Canyons trail network.

Beyond its length and steepness, the trail presents substantial logistical challenges. The tollgate at the Indian Canyons is open only 8 a.m.–5 p.m., so hiking up and back demands speed as well as stamina. By arranging a car shuttle from the Cedar Spring Trail, you can slightly shorten the trip and avoid the knee-pounding descent, but you must still leave time for the drive back to retrieve your vehicle before the gate is locked. Let a tribal ranger know about your plans, because a search is initiated if vehicles are still present when the gate closes. If you're unsure of your ability to get back in time, notify the tribal rangers before 5 p.m. at 760-323-6018. Also pay special attention to the weather conditions: while Palm Canyon is roasting under an unrelenting sun, the Desert Divide may be covered in snow and ice. The north-facing Garnet Ridge holds snow at surprisingly low altitudes after a winter storm. An ice ax and crampons may be necessary if the upper part of the trail is icy.

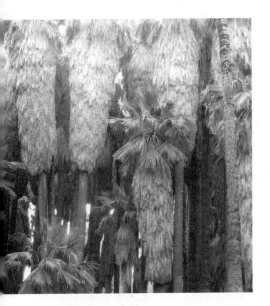

Palm Canyon Oasis

From the trailhead, look southwest and identify the massive Garnet Ridge extending toward you from the Desert Divide. The prominent cliffs on the ridge are called the Palisades. Hike south from behind the Trading Post on the Palm Canyon Trail, descending into the enormous palm oasis in Palm Canyon. In 0.2 mile, reach a signed junction at the south end of the oasis. Turn right and switchback up the West Fork Trail. Good views of Palm Canyon and of the pointy Murray Hill open up as you climb. The boulders prominently show desert varnish, a mixture of clay with iron and manganese oxide formed by chemical reactions on the surface of hot dry rocks. The hills are studded with barrel and cholla cacti. The trail climbs to the rim of the canyon and in 2 miles arrives at a signed junction.

Take the left fork, which is the start of the Jo Pond Trail. The trail is less used and takes more care to follow. It follows a creek for another mile before it gradually veers away from the canyon and onto the toe of Garnet Ridge. Watch how the vegetation zones change from cactus to chaparral as you switchback up the ridge. Eventually, the grade relents as you gain the upper portion of the ridge and you cross fields of red rocks amidst the manzanitas. The trail next enters an open forest of black oaks and white firs, then arrives at Cedar Spring. The spring usually has water in the wetter months, and there's room to camp beneath the shady trees. At this point, you've hiked 8.2 miles and gained 5,900 feet of elevation.

If you left your car at the Trading Post, retrace your steps. Alternatively, if you have a car shuttle, hike south another mile and 300 feet up to the crest of the Desert Divide, to a four-way junction. Take the Cedar Spring Trail (see Trip 10.4) straight ahead, going southwest 2.3 miles down to your vehicle.

chapter 12

Santa Rosa Mountains

The Santa Rosa Mountains tumble south and east from Palm Springs toward the Salton Sea. The deep Palm Canyon separates the Santa Rosas from the San Jacinto Mountains. Toro Peak (8,716') crowns the range and is clad in a white snowy mantle for most of the winter. At first glance, the range might appear hot, dry, and desolate, but closer inspection reveals the Santa Rosas to be undiscovered gems of Southern California: the mountainsides are dotted with marvelous cacti and are home to the endangered Peninsular bighorn sheep (*Ovis canadensis nelson*). Whether you have an hour at sunrise to jog the hills or a day in the fall or winter to trace ancient Indian footpaths across this remote wilderness, you'll come to love this range more with each visit.

Congress established the Santa Rosa and San Jacinto Mountains National Monument in 2000 to protect the outstanding natural and cultural resources of these mountains and to provide enduring opportunities for recreation. Spanning 280,000 acres, the land is administered by a wide variety of governmental agencies, the Agua Caliente Band of Cahuilla Indians, and private landowners. In general, the Forest Service is responsible for the higher mountains, the Bureau of Land Management is responsible for the desert regions, and the Agua Caliente Band is responsible for Palm Canyon. Major portions of the Santa Rosa and San Jacinto Mountains are designated wilderness areas.

This chapter focuses on hikes in the Santa Rosa Mountains. The range is split by Highway 74. North of the highway, an extensive trail network provides access from the Coachella Valley. The Desert Riders, an active equestrian organization, constructed many of the trails. Some trails trace the routes once followed by the Indians who crossed the mountains in search of food and commerce. The publication of the *Santa Rosa & San Jacinto Mountains National Monument* trail map in 2008 was a watershed event for hikers.

South of Highway 74 are the biggest peaks, notably Toro and Rabbit. The top of Toro Peak is on private tribal land and is closed to the public, but it's of little interest anyway because it has been bulldozed flat to mount a large antenna farm that's accessible by road. Rabbit Peak, on the other hand, is as wild and difficult as any peak in Southern California, and draws a steady flow of hardy hikers wishing to test their desert mettle. A few ancient Indian footpaths cross the wild country in the southern Santa Rosas and are described in this chapter.

The Santa Rosa Mountains are one of the remaining homes for the endangered Peninsular bighorn sheep. An estimated 900–1,000 of the majestic but shy animals roam the rocky

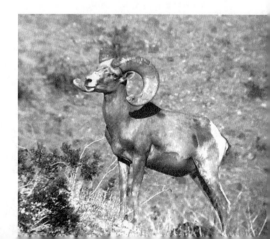

Peninsular bighorn sheep
Photo reprinted with permission of the Bighorn Institute

desert slopes. Count yourself fortunate if you catch a fleeting glimpse of one during a season of hiking in these mountains. Their numbers had been steadily declining as human development encroached on their habitat; sustained efforts in recent years are starting to reverse this decline. Government agencies, including the U.S. Fish and Wildlife Service, the Bureau of Land Management (BLM), and the California Department of Fish and Wildlife, are researching ways to better protect the sheep. For more information about the Peninsular bighorn sheep, visit bighorninstitute.org.

Most established trails are open year-round. A few trails that pass sensitive watering spots for bighorn sheep are closed during the hot season, June 1–September 30. In the lower elevations outside the national forest, cross-country travel and camping are allowed only October 1–December 31 to avoid disturbing sheep during lambing season and the hot months. Dogs are prohibited on most trails because the sheep fear them as predators. Motorized vehicles are prohibited in the wilderness areas and on Dunn Road. In general, hikers are encouraged to stay on established trails to minimize disturbing the desert and wildlife. You may notice damage done by hikers creating unauthorized social trails and by cutting switchbacks; please practice Leave No Trace ethics.

The Colorado Desert around the Coachella Valley is one of the hottest and driest zones in the United States. The Santa Rosa Mountains are similarly hot and dry; they're best visited from late fall through early spring. When much of the Inland Empire shivers under gloomy clouds or rain, the Santa Rosas are usually sunny and mild, perfect for hiking. Nevertheless, be ready for any weather. The desert is known for rapid changes of weather, and for rare but intense showers that will chill the unprepared and unleash flash floods down the narrow canyons. During hotter parts of the year, many of the shorter Santa Rosa hikes are still ideal at dawn, at sunset, and by full moon.

For more information, contact the Santa Rosa and San Jacinto Mountains National Monument Visitor Center. The visitor center also organizes hikes and wildflower walks; call for the current schedule of activities.

trip 12.1 Garstin Trail

Distance	2.5–3.6 miles (out-and-back or loop)
Hiking Time	2 hours
Elevation Gain	1,000'
Difficulty	Moderate
Trail Use	Suitable for equestrians
Best Times	October–April
Agency	Santa Rosa and San Jacinto Mountains National Monument
Optional Map	*Santa Rosa & San Jacinto Mountains National Monument* or *Palm Springs* 7.5' (trail not marked)

see map on p. 279

DIRECTIONS From the 10 Freeway (I-10), take Highway 111 south into Palm Springs, where the road name changes to North Palm Canyon Drive, then South Palm Canyon Drive. Most lanes turn left to become East Palm Canyon Drive, but stay straight (south) and continue on South Palm Canyon Drive 1.9 miles. Turn left onto East Bogert Trail and follow it 0.9 mile over the bridge across Palm Canyon Wash; then immediately turn left onto Barona Road and park at the end.

Continued on page 278

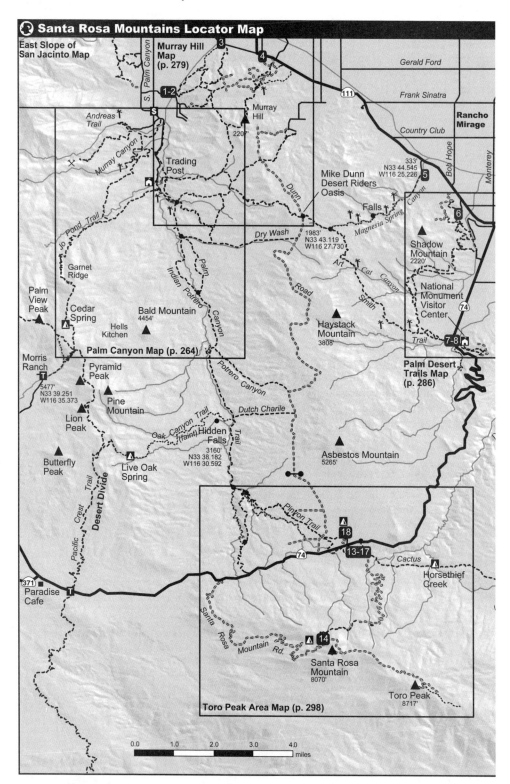

Santa Rosa Mountains Locator Map

East Slope of
San Jacinto Map

Murray Hill
Map
(p. 279)

3

4

111

Gerald Ford

Frank Sinatra

Rancho
Mirage

1-2

Andreas
Trail

S

Murray Canyon

S. Palm Canyon

Murray
Hill

2207'

Country Club

Bob Hope

Monterey

Trading
Post

Jo Pond Trail

Garnet
Ridge

Mike Dunn
Desert Riders
Oasis

333'
N33 44.545
W116 25.226

5

Falls

Dunn

Magnesia Spring

6

Canyon

Shadow
Mountain
2220'

Dry Wash

1983'
N33 43.119
W116 27.730

Art

Cat

Canyon

National
Monument
Visitor
Center

74

Palm
View
Peak

Cedar
Spring

Indian

Potrero

Palm

Bald Mountain
4454'

Hells
Kitchen

Canyon

Palm Canyon Map (p. 264)

Road

Smith

Haystack
Mountain
3808

Trail

7-8

Palm Desert
Trails Map
(p. 286)

Morris
Ranch

5477'
N33 39.251
W116 35.373

Pyramid
Peak

Pine
Mountain

Lion
Peak

Butterfly
Peak

Oak Canyon Trail
(faint)

Live Oak
Spring

Potrero Canyon

Dutch Charile

Hidden
Falls

3160'
N33 38.182
W116 30.592

Trail

Asbestos Mountain
5265'

Pacific

Crest

Trail

Desert Divide

Pinyon Trail

18

74

13-17

Cactus

Horsethief
Creek

371

Paradise
Cafe

Santa

Rosa

Mountain Rd.

14

Santa Rosa
Mountain
8070'

Toro Peak
8717'

Toro Peak Area Map (p. 298)

0.0   1.0   2.0   3.0   4.0
miles

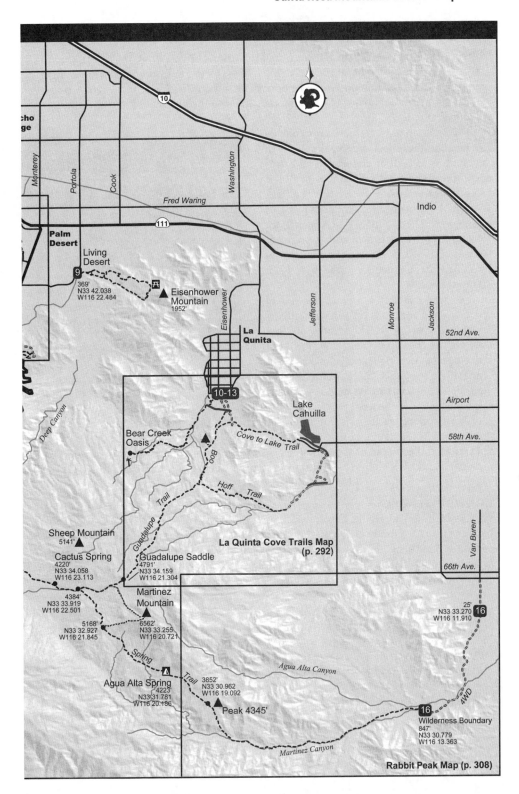

10

Monterey
Portola
Cook
Washington
Fred Waring
Indio

111

Palm Desert

Living Desert

9
369'
N33 42.038
W116 22.484

Eisenhower Mountain
1952'

Eisenhower

La Qunita

Jefferson
Monroe
Jackson
52nd Ave.

10-13

Lake Cahuilla

Airport

58th Ave.

Deep Canyon

Bear Creek Oasis

Cove to Lake Trail

Boo

Hoff   Trail

Guadalupe   Trail

Van Buren

Sheep Mountain
5141'

Cactus Spring
4220'
N33 34.058
W116 23.113

Guadalupe Saddle
4791'
N33 34.159
W116 21.304

La Quinta Cove Trails Map
(p. 292)

66th Ave.

4384'
N33 33.919
W116 22.501

Martinez Mountain

25'
N33 33.270
W116 11.910
16

5168'
N33 32.927
W116 21.845

6562'
N33 33.255
W116 20.721

Spring

Agua Alta Canyon

Trail
3852'
N33 30.962
W116 19.092

4WD

Agua Alta Spring
4223'
N33 31.781
W116 20.186

Peak 4345'

16
Wilderness Boundary
847'
N33 30.779
W116 13.363

Martinez Canyon

Rabbit Peak Map (p. 308)

Continued from page 275

The Garstin Trail is a short but steep trail that climbs from Palm Canyon Wash up to a stunning plateau beneath Murray Hill. It offers a vigorous workout and great views of the San Jacinto Mountains. It can be done as an out-and-back hike or a slightly longer loop. Or you can link to any of the numerous trails on the plateau for an endless variety of longer rambles.

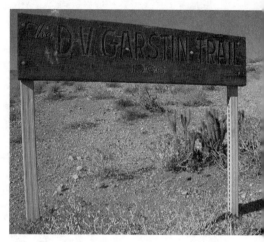

Top of the Garstin Trail

The trails in this area are conveniently located near the Smoke Tree Stables. Many of the trails were built by and named for members of the Desert Riders. The Garstin Trail is named for trail boss D. V. Garstin. The Henderson Trail is named for past president Earl Henderson. The Shannon Trail is named for Shannon Corliss, daughter of past president Ray Corliss. All of the trails are steep; beginning riders are better off staying in Palm Canyon Wash.

The trail starts at a post at the end of Barona Road and leads east. In 150 yards, it reaches a signed fork. The Henderson Trail veers left and heads northeast along the toe of the ridge, but turn right and follow the Garstin Trail up steep switchbacks hewn from the hillside. Your efforts are rewarded by steadily widening views to the west.

Shortly before reaching the top of the hill, the trail forks. Both paths run parallel and rejoin in 0.1 mile; the right fork follows the ridgeline and is recommended for its views. (This fork and merge aren't shown on the map; the two parallel paths run too close together to distinguish.) Soon after, 1.2 miles from the start, come to a major junction with the Berns Trail on top of the ridge. Many hikers turn around here.

ALTERNATIVE FINISHES

Hikers desiring a somewhat longer walk have two options:

For the first, continue straight 0.1 mile on the Berns Trail to another intersection with the Shannon Trail, then 0.1 mile farther to a high point on Smoke Tree Mountain that offers outstanding 360-degree views. From here, either return the way you came or descend the Shannon Trail (0.9 mile); then turn left and follow the Henderson Trail 1.0 mile back to the start.

For the second, turn right and follow the Garstin Trail 0.5 mile to its end, passing two unmarked connector trails to the left along the way. There is a large sign for the Garstin Trail at the four-way junction at the end. Turn right and follow the unmarked Thielman Trail 1.0 mile southwest down to a dirt road near two water tanks. Turn right on the road and continue 0.3 mile down to a gate at the end of the paved Ridgemore Drive in the posh Andreas Hills neighborhood. Follow this road down to its end; then make a right onto Andreas Hills and another right onto Bogert. Shortly before the bridge, turn right onto Barona Road to regain the trailhead. This variation involves 0.6 mile of walking through the neighborhood.

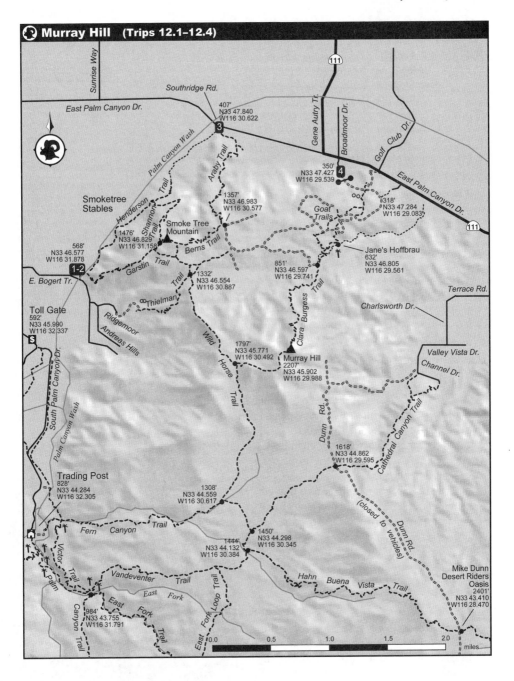

Murray Hill (Trips 12.1–12.4)

Sunrise Way

Southridge Rd.

East Palm Canyon Dr.

407'
N33 47.840
W116 30.622

3

Gene Autry Trl.

Broadmoor Dr.

Golf Club Dr.

East Palm Canyon Dr.

350'
N33 47.427
W116 29.539

4

111

Smoketree
Stables

Palm Canyon Wash

Araby Trail

Henderson Trail

Shannon Trail

1357'
N33 46.983
W116 30.577

Goat
Trails

318'
N33 47.284
W116 29.083

1476'
N33 46.829
W116 31.158

Smoke Tree
Mountain

Berns Trail

568'
N33 46.577
W116 31.878

1-2

E. Bogert Tr.

Garstin Trail

851'
N33 46.597
W116 29.741

Jane's Hoffbrau
632'
N33 46.805
W116 29.561

1332'
N33 46.554
W116 30.887

Clara Burgess Trail

Charlsworth Dr.

Terrace Rd.

Toll Gate
592'
N33 45.990
W116 32.337

S

Thielman

Ridgemoor

Andreas Hills

Wild Horse Trail

1797'
N33 45.771
W116 30.492

Murray Hill
2207'
N33 45.902
W116 29.988

Valley Vista Dr.

Channel Dr.

South Palm Canyon Dr.

Palm Canyon Wash

Dunn Rd.

Cathedral Canyon Trail

1618'
N33 44.862
W116 29.595

Trading Post
828'
N33 44.284
W116 32.305

1308'
N33 44.559
W116 30.617

(closed to vehicles)

Dunn Rd.

Fern Canyon Trail

1450'
N33 44.298
W116 30.345

1444'
N33 44.132
W116 30.384

Mike Dunn
Desert Riders
Oasis
2401'
N33 43.410
W116 28.470

Victor Trail

Vandeventer Trail

East Fork Loop Trail

East Fork

Hahn Buena Vista Trail

Palm Canyon Trail

984'
N33 43.755
W116 31.791

East Fork Trail

0.0   0.5   1.0   1.5   2.0

miles

trip 12.2　Murray Hill

Distance	7 miles (out-and-back)
Hiking Time	5 hours
Elevation Gain	1,700'
Difficulty	Strenuous
Trail Use	Suitable for equestrians
Best Times	October–March
Agency	Santa Rosa and San Jacinto Mountains National Monument
Recommended Maps	*Santa Rosa & San Jacinto Mountains National Monument* or USGS *Palm Springs and Cathedral City* 7.5' (trail not marked)

see map on previous page

DIRECTIONS From the 10 Freeway, take Highway 111 south into Palm Springs, where the road name changes to North Palm Canyon Drive, then South Palm Canyon Drive. Most lanes turn left to become East Palm Canyon Drive, but stay straight (south) and continue on South Palm Canyon Drive 1.9 miles. Turn left onto East Bogert Trail and follow it 0.9 mile over the bridge across Palm Canyon Wash; then immediately turn left onto Barona Road and park at the end.

Prominent from many directions, the pyramid-shaped Murray Hill offers panoramic views across the Santa Rosa Mountains. It's best climbed on a clear, cool day. Its rather diminutive name belies the fact that Murray Hill is a steep and strenuous peak that challenges and rewards the intrepid explorer. Murray Hill is named for the Scottish rancher Welwood Murray, who founded the Palm Springs Hotel in 1887 and drew attention to the area as a spa and resort. Murray Hill can be approached from the west, north, or south. This trip describes the western approach via the Garstin and Wild Horse Trails, but one can make an enjoyable longer loop or one-way trip in combination with the other routes.

The trail starts at a post at the end of Barona Road and leads east. In 150 yards, it reaches a signed fork. The Henderson Trail veers left and heads northeast along the toe of the ridge, but turn right and follow the Garstin Trail up steep switchbacks hewn from the hillside. Your efforts are rewarded by steadily widening views to the west.

Shortly before reaching the top of the hill, the trail forks. Both paths run parallel and rejoin in 0.1 mile; the right fork follows the ridgeline and is recommended for its views. Soon after, 1.2 miles from the start, come to a junction with the Berns Trail on top of the ridge.

From here, Murray Hill is clearly visible looming to the southeast. Your goal is to reach the Wild Horse Trail, which climbs the western ridge of the peak. Unfortunately, this area contains a maze of poorly marked trails. Turn right and head toward Murray Hill. In 0.3 mile, stay right at a fork. Just beyond, at a four-way junction with the Thielman Trail, go straight onto the Wild Horse Trail.

Follow the Wild Horse Trail 1.2 miles up the ridge to a junction. The right fork drops

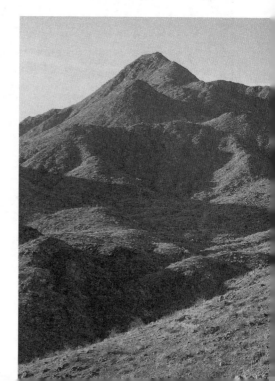

Murray Hill from the north

down to Fern Canyon, but this trip stays left onto the Clara Burgess Trail, which follows the spectacular ridgeline 0.8 mile to the summit of Murray Hill. Return the way you came.

ALTERNATIVE FINISHES

Alternatively, descend to the north or south. The Clara Burgess Trail leads 1.4 miles north to a large metal sign marking its start near a wash. From here, you can turn left and follow a system of dirt roads back to the Garstin Trail, or continue down the wash to Jane's Hoffbrau Oasis and the confusing network of Goat Trails (see Trip 12.4). If, instead, you return to the Wild Horse Trail (sometimes faint) and go south 1.6 miles, you can reach the Fern Canyon Trail (see Trip 11.13). The Fern Canyon Trail leads back to the Trading Post in Palm Canyon. If you don't have a ride waiting there, you can slog about 3 miles down the sandy Palm Canyon Wash back to the Garstin Trailhead.

---

trip 12.3   Araby Trail

Distance	3.2 miles (out-and-back), 4.6 miles (loop)	
Hiking Time	2–3 hours	
Elevation Gain	1,000'–1,400'	
Difficulty	Moderate	
Trail Use	Suitable for equestrians	
Best Times	October–April	
Agency	Santa Rosa and San Jacinto Mountains National Monument	
Optional Map	*Santa Rosa & San Jacinto Mountains National Monument* or USGS *Palm Springs* 7.5' (trail not marked)	

see map on p. 279

DIRECTIONS From the 10 Freeway, take Highway 111 south into Palm Springs, where the road name changes to North Palm Canyon Drive, then South Palm Canyon Drive. The road veers left and the name changes to East Palm Canyon Drive. Go 2.2 miles on East Palm Canyon Drive, cross a bridge over wide Palm Canyon Wash, and turn right at a sign labeled SOUTHRIDGE/RIMCREST. Make an immediate right and park in a dirt lot. **Note:** *Do not continue driving up the private road.*

The Araby Trail climbs the canyon overlooking the modernistic Bob Hope estate on the southern edge of Palm Springs and offers close-up views of the comedian's sprawling ridgetop compound. The Palm Springs International Airport is nearby, and you're likely to see the private jets of the rich and famous landing and departing as you hike. The hike also offers an accessible taste of the Santa Rosa Mountains with their rocky canyons, steep slopes, and fragile vegetation. The Araby Trail is a popular exercise hike for locals because it's short, steep, and close to town. The area is also a favorite of equestrians, especially the Desert Riders, who built many of the trails. The Santa Rosa Mountains are a bighorn sheep sanctuary, so dogs aren't allowed. The trail is closed from dusk to dawn.

From the car, walk 100 feet up the private road to the signed Araby Trail on the left. The first part of the trail leads above a trailer park and below a row of homes—please respect the owners and don't stray from the trail. After passing above a pool area in the trailer park, the trail forks. The left fork descends to the trailer park. Take the marked right fork, which switchbacks up. It passes near a bend in the private road; then, a faint trail leads left 150 feet to a small hill with great views over Palm Springs and up to the Bob Hope estate and the mountains above. The main trail continues up the west slope of the canyon toward the estate, then cuts across the floor of the canyon over to the east slope. It climbs steeply up to gain the ridge at the head of the canyon, where large signs mark the junction with the Berns Trail. Climb the small hills to your left or right for a grand view. The homes, trees,

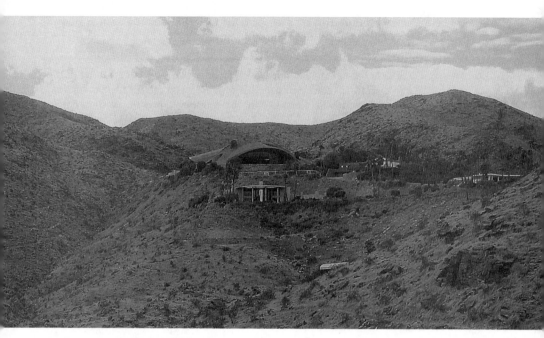

Bob Hope's estate from the Araby Trail

and golf courses of Palm Springs sprawl across the valley to the north. The steep slopes of San Jacinto tower into the sky to the west. And the pointy desert summit of Murray Hill draws your eye as you look southward into the Santa Rosa Mountains. At this point, you've hiked 1.6 miles and climbed 1,000 feet. Enjoy the scenery and retrace your steps to the car.

ALTERNATIVE FINISH

For a 1.5-mile longer loop, turn right and walk 100 feet to a large metal sign indicating the start of the Berns Trail. At the sign, a short trail to the right leads up a hill with a good view, but the main Berns Trail stays left, switchbacks westward down into a canyon, and then switchbacks up the hill on the other side. The trail continues westward atop a low ridge with views southwest into the Indian Canyons. Pass an unmarked junction leading south to the Wild Horse Trail and climb another small hill (Smoke Tree Mountain) marked with a huge cairn, 0.9 mile and 400 feet up from the end of the Araby Trail. This portion of the trail is notable for its assortment of barrel and cholla cacti. Beyond the hill is another signed junction. Turn right (north) onto the Shannon Trail; the Garstin Trail leads down to the southwest (see Trip 12.1).

The Shannon Trail descends northward along the ridge just west of the Bob Hope estate and provides more views of the elaborate compound. It then switchbacks down the west slope of the ridge to a junction with the Henderson Trail (1 mile). Turn right (northeast) again and follow the Henderson Trail 0.5 mile past a house down to the valley floor. Cross a paved road to reach the huge Palm Canyon Wash (dry most of the year). Turn right and walk 0.6 mile northeast along the sandy floor of the wash toward the bridge where East Palm Canyon Drive crosses the wash. Immediately before you reach the bridge, exit the right side of the wash and climb to your car.

trip 12.4 Jane's Hoffbrau Oasis

Distance	2 miles (out-and-back)
Hiking Time	1 hour
Elevation Gain	700'
Difficulty	Moderate
Trail Use	Suitable for mountain biking, suitable for equestrians
Best Times	October–March
Agency	Santa Rosa and San Jacinto Mountains National Monument
Optional Map	*Santa Rosa & San Jacinto Mountains National Monument* or USGS *Cathedral City* 7.5' (trail not marked)

see map on p. 279

DIRECTIONS From East Palm Canyon Drive (Highway 111) in Palm Springs, 0.2 mile east of Gene Autry Trail, turn south onto Broadmoor Drive. Park along the street or in the dirt at the south end, taking care not to block the gate.

Tucked away in the sheer-walled Eagle Canyon scarcely a stone's throw from Palm Springs, Jane's Hoffbrau Oasis is certain to surprise and delight. It's named for Jane Lykken Hoff, a former president of the Desert Riders equestrian group. The oasis is located near the unmarked tangle of roads and bike paths called the Goat Trails, so it requires some navigational skills to locate. This trip follows the dirt road for ease of navigation, but if you're a repeat visitor, the narrow trails are shorter, steeper, and fun to explore.

Hikers have access to the trail, so walk past the misleading NO TRESPASSING signs on the gate at the trailhead. Hike up the gated dirt road past spur roads and water tanks to a saddle with good views of San Jacinto, 0.5 mile from the start. The dirt road forks here and rejoins in 0.2 mile; the right branch has more views. Then curve around a hill to the south and take the first trail on the left that drops into Eagle Canyon.

Follow this trail 0.2 mile to a point immediately overlooking Jane's Hoffbrau Oasis. Turn left and switchback down to the oasis on the canyon floor. You can't order a pastrami sandwich here, but you can enjoy your own snacks beneath the palms or beside a dry waterfall. Return the way you came.

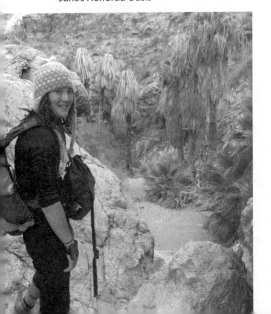

Jane's Hoffbrau Oasis

ALTERNATIVE FINISHES

Explore Eagle Canyon or some of the Goat Trails. Those desiring a longer hike can continue up Murray Hill (see Trip 12.2). The Clara Burgess Trail to Murray Hill starts farther up Eagle Canyon. You can return to the trail just above the oasis and follow it southwest. If you enjoy scrambling, you can head directly up the canyon floor. This involves third-class climbing up a dry waterfall above the oasis, followed by easier scrambling up short dry falls higher in the canyon.

see map on p. 276

trip 12.5   Magnesia Spring Falls

Distance	2.5–12 miles (out-and-back or one-way)
Hiking Time	1–6 hours
Elevation Gain	Variable
Difficulty	Easy–strenuous
Best Times	October–December
Agency	Santa Rosa and San Jacinto Mountains National Monument
Required Map	*Santa Rosa & San Jacinto Mountains National Monument* or USGS *Rancho Mirage 7.5'*

DIRECTIONS This trip starts at Mountain Park in Rancho Mirage. From Highway 111 between Country Club Drive and Bob Hope Drive, turn south onto Mirage Road. Follow it 0.4 mile until the road turns left; then make an immediate right into a signed parking area for Mountain Park next to Rancho Mirage Elementary School.

Magnesia Spring Canyon is one of the least known of the Santa Rosa Mountains' many gems. The gorgeous gorge is continually interesting, with a series of dry waterfalls and palm oases. Although there is no trail, the canyon has largely been scoured clean of tedious obstacles so walking is relatively easy. However, the canyon forks repeatedly, and hikers must pay close attention to stay on route; a GPS can be handy. This area is part of the Magnesia Spring Ecological Reserve and is closed January 1–September 30 to protect the bighorn sheep that frequent the area, so plan to visit during the three-month window when it's open. The canyon is subject to flash floods, so don't go when there's even the most remote chance of rain.

There are at least three interesting options that a hiker might choose. Families may wish to go to Lower Magnesia Falls for a 2.5-mile round-trip with 200 feet of elevation gain; this is

Lone palm at the mouth of Magnesia Spring Canyon

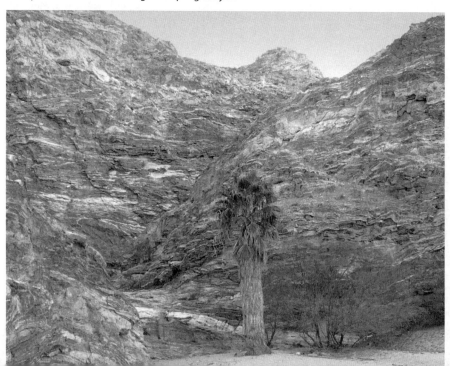

a fun destination for kids who like to scramble on rocks. Those wanting to see all the major features of the canyon can continue all the way to the base of Upper Magnesia Falls, then turn around, for a 6.5-mile round-trip with 1,100 feet of gain that will take about 5 hours. Well-conditioned hikers seeking an outstanding adventure can follow the canyon all the way to its junction with the Art Smith Trail (see Trip 12.7) and take this trail down to Highway 74, where you've arranged a 6-mile car or bicycle shuttle or ride share. This option is 12 miles with 3,000 feet of elevation gain and takes about 7 hours.

From the parking area, return to the corner of Mirage Road and follow a signed path along the flood-control channel 0.1 mile southwest. Cross a gated bridge on the right into Mountain Park and continue through the park. You'll encounter many poorly defined trails in the park, but take anything leading southwest up the canyon. In 0.8 mile, reach a fence just before a flood-control dam. An old sign for the Magnesia Spring Ecological Reserve warns NO TRESPASSING, but hikers without dogs nevertheless have permission to enter October–December. Climb over the flood-control dam, continue across the basin, and pass the left edge of a fenceline at the mouth of Magnesia Spring Canyon in 0.2 mile.

Walk to the lone palm tree where the canyon turns left and narrows. The high walls of Precambrian or Paleozoic metasedimentary rock date back to a long-lost shallow sea. You'll see a guzzler here, and plenty of scat from the bighorn sheep and other animals that come to drink. The canyon immediately welcomes you with a 12-foot dry waterfall that's easy to climb. Just around the corner is Lower Magnesia Falls, a 50-foot waterfall; it's not difficult to scale unless wet. Kids will enjoy testing their courage on the sloping slab, and this is a good turnaround point for a family hike.

Otherwise, continue up past several more dry falls to a grove of palms where the canyon widens. The action never stops as you climb yet more small falls and pass a second palm grove. Watch for a minor canyon on the left, but stay straight in the main canyon. In another 0.5 mile, reach a major split (**N33° 43.487' W116° 26.607'; 994'**). The right fork becomes choked with gneiss boulders, but this trip takes the left fork that ascends a 10-foot wall to another palm grove. (When in doubt on this trip, follow the fork with the palm trees!)

A hundred yards past the last palm and just before the canyon turns right, look for a cairn marking a use trail climbing the right wall of the canyon. Peer around the corner to view Middle Magnesia Falls, a huge dry waterfall with a hardy palm growing halfway up. This obstacle is passable only by serious rock climbers with proper gear, so hikers should return to the cairn and follow a steep use path 180 feet vertically to a ridge, from which you can drop back down into the canyon above the waterfall.

The section of canyon beyond hasn't been scoured as clean, and your progress is slowed as you have to work your way around boulders and brush. In 0.5 mile, the canyon is blocked yet again by the even larger and more vertical Upper Magnesia Falls (**N33° 43.301' W116° 26.948'; 1,385'**). This is a good turnaround point for an out-and-back trip because you've seen the highlights of the canyon.

To continue upcanyon, bypass the falls via a talus slope on the left side. After a 200-foot climb, make a level 0.1-mile traverse until you can reenter the canyon without losing elevation. Work your way around a mesquite patch to another split in the wash (**N33° 43.229' W116° 27.023'; 1,556'**). Stay right in the main fork, and walk through a palm grove and then a second grove that's the longest in the canyon. At a split in a sandy section of the wash (**N33° 43.192' W116° 27.440'; 1,814'**), stay right and continue toward yet more palms. Scramble up the last easy sloping slab waterfall. In 0.1 mile more, reach a sign where the Art Smith Trail enters the sandy upper section of Magnesia Spring Canyon. If you've left a getaway vehicle at the Art Smith Trailhead, you can turn left and follow the trail 6.8 miles out to complete a superb tour of the northern Santa Rosa Mountains.

trip 12.6   **Bump and Grind Trail**

Distance	4 miles (loop)
Hiking Time	2 hours
Elevation Gain	1,100'
Difficulty	Moderate
Trail Use	Suitable for mountain biking, suitable for equestrians
Best Times	All year, but hot in summer
Agency	Santa Rosa and San Jacinto Mountains National Monument
Optional Map	*Santa Rosa & San Jacinto Mountains National Monument* or USGS *Rancho Mirage* 7.5' (trail not marked)

DIRECTIONS From Highway 111 in Palm Desert between Bob Hope Drive and Fred Waring Drive, turn south onto Painters Path. Proceed 0.5 mile to the trailhead and park on the side of the road behind Desert Crossing Shopping Center, taking care to observe the parking restrictions.

The Bump and Grind Trail, also known as the Mirage Trail, is an extremely popular trail because it's so conveniently located in town and offers a vigorous workout over a short distance. On a pleasant weekend, you're likely to meet hundreds of hikers and joggers getting their exercise on the trail, which climbs the northern flank of Shadow Mountain. The upper portion crosses the Magnesia Spring Ecological Reserve, and dogs aren't allowed. Some portions of the trail are quite steep, so shoes with good tread are recommended. Many social trails have developed in this area; please minimize your impact by staying on the main trail (as best as you can recognize it).

The loop begins at the Mike Schuler Trailhead. To make a counterclockwise loop, take the right fork. Climbing beneath the impressive varnished granite outcrops, the trail travels up well-built switchbacks to a notch on a ridge. Creosote bushes and brittlebushes cling to the sunbaked and sparsely vegetated hills. Continue across the next canyon above a nursery to reach the next ridge, 0.9 mile from the start. Here, you meet a dirt road, whose cut forms a deep scar on the slope.

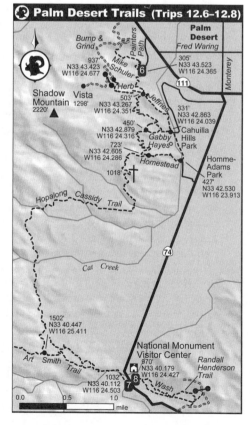

The road rises up from the former trailhead in Rancho Mirage. This portion was named Bump and Grind by the cyclists who toil up the hill. Several side trails shortcut bends in the road. On a clear day, you'll enjoy splendid views over the Coachella Valley. San Jacinto and San Gorgonio to the west are capped with snow in the winter and spring. The Little San Bernardino Mountains to the north form a wall on the edge of Joshua Tree National Park. Countless bright green golf courses dot the arid Palm Springs region. In another 0.9 mile, the road turns hard right and reaches a gate.

In 2011, the California Department of Fish and Game banned travel beyond this

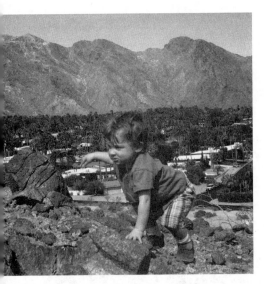

Rocks and palms from the Bump and Grind Trail above Rancho Mirage

gate to avoid disturbing the Peninsular bighorn sheep in the ecological reserve. The California State Assembly took the unusual step of overriding the Fish and Game Department in 2013, opening the trail May–January, while leaving it closed February–April during lambing season. If you're hiking during open season, you can continue up 0.5 mile to a vista point with outstanding views of the Coachella Valley and Shadow Mountain. Hiking beyond this vista point is prohibited year-round.

Return to the gate and turn onto the unlabeled Herb Jeffries Trail, named for the African American star of western films. The trail reaches a ridge, where you can admire the extensive network of trails covering the hills like a spider web. The rocky hills above the Art Smith Trail are clearly visible to the south, with Toro Peak and Martinez Mountain in the background. Traverse above a sheer face and switchback down the steep ridge. In 0.6 mile, reach a confusing four-way junction.

Take the leftmost branch, which is the bottom end of the Hopalong Cassidy Trail, named for one of America's best-known movie and television cowboy heroes. Cassidy and Jeffries were both once Palm Desert residents. The trail leads 0.6 mile back to the trailhead where you started.

VARIATIONS

The rightmost branch of the four-way junction is the Hopalong Cassidy Trail. It leads along the hillside 8 miles to join the Art Smith Trail (see Trip 12.7). Along the way, it passes the Gabby Hayes Trail, which leads down to Cahuilla Hills Park, and the Homestead Trail, which leads down to Homme-Adams Park. It then passes the Stone Eagle Golf Course and a large lighted cross before detouring around the Bighorn development. Some junctions are unsigned, and a variety of confusing social trails have developed. Navigating this area requires a map and a good sense of direction. The center branch is a continuation of the Herb Jeffries Trail, which leads 0.7 mile down to Cahuilla Hills Park.

---

trip 12.7	**Art Smith Trail**

see maps on pgs. 279 & 286

Distance	6–16 miles (out-and-back)
Hiking Time	3–8 hours
Elevation Gain	1,300'–3,300'
Difficulty	Moderate–strenuous
Trail Use	Suitable for mountain biking, suitable for equestrians
Best Times	October–March (closed June 15–September 30)
Agency	Santa Rosa and San Jacinto Mountains National Monument
Recommended Map	*Santa Rosa & San Jacinto Mountains National Monument* or USGS *Rancho Mirage* 7.5' (trail not marked)

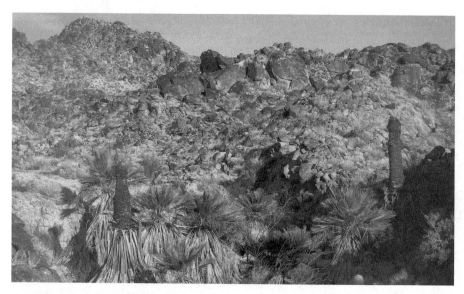

Oasis along the Art Smith Trail

DIRECTIONS The Art Smith Trailhead is on Highway 74, south of Palm Desert. It can be reached by exiting the 10 Freeway at Monterey (Exit 131) and driving south across Highway 111, where the road becomes Highway 74. It can also be reached directly from Highway 111 or by driving through the Garner Valley from Hemet. In any case, the trailhead is 4 miles south of Highway 111 on the west side of the road, directly across from the Santa Rosa and San Jacinto Mountains National Monument Visitor Center.

The Art Smith Trail, named in 1977 for the late longtime trail boss of the Desert Riders who was responsible for the development of numerous routes in these mountains, is the gem of the northern Santa Rosas, offering a grand tour through the heart of the wilderness. The trail features outrageous cacti, outlandish rock formations, several small palm oases, and a chance to commune with the desert. Despite its length and the rugged terrain, the trail gains less elevation than might be expected. Those looking for an action-packed jaunt along the most interesting segment of the trail can hike 3 miles out past palm oases to a vista point, then return. For a longer hike, go all 8 miles to the end at Dunn Road, then return. Or better yet, with a car shuttle, connect to the Hahn Buena Vista Trail and follow it down to Fern and Palm Canyons.

This area is frequented by the endangered Peninsular bighorn sheep. Dogs are prohibited at all times. The Art Smith Trail is closed from June 1 to September 30 west of its intersection with the Hopalong Cassidy Trail to protect bighorn sheep during the hot season. The trail once started up Dead Indian Canyon, but this area has been closed and the trail rerouted to protect a water source for the sheep.

The signed Art Smith Trail begins at the north end of the parking lot. Follow it north along the levee 0.2 mile to a fenceline. Turn left and walk another 0.2 mile until you reach the first of many Bureau of Land Management signposts marking the route. Switchback up the hill 0.2 mile to the top. In 0.7 mile, reach a signed junction where the Hopalong Cassidy Trail forks off north to Homme-Adams Park and the Art Smith Trail continues west.

Continue west up a hill through desert agaves and barrel cacti. The trail levels out amidst granite boulders varnished brown by centuries of exposure to the desert. In 0.6 mile, it reaches the first palm oasis. Watch for a granite boulder with a shallow metate on the north side of the trail beside a palm tree. In another 0.6 mile, it climbs to another oasis and con-tours northwest along the flank of flat-topped Haystack Mountain. Then, 0.4 mile beyond, it crests a small hill from which you can see the Salton Sea glittering beyond the ridge to the east. You've now traveled 3 miles; this is a good turnaround point if you're looking for a short jaunt through the most scenic sections of the trail.

Continue west on the Art Smith Trail, reaching more palms in the dry Cat Creek wash in about 2 miles. You're in the heart of the Santa Rosa Mountains, out of sight of civilization, of the teeming hordes, malls, golf courses, and galleries that sprawl across the Coachella Valley. In another 2 miles, enter a long sandy wash at the upper end of Magnesia Spring Canyon (see Trip 12.5). Continue through a narrow canyon; then exit the wash on the right. Follow the trail to the crest of a small ridge, where you're treated to panoramic views to the west. Look for Dunn Road, a wide swath cut across the mountain range from north to south. Descend 0.2 mile through vast fields of agaves to reach the Mike Dunn Desert Riders Oasis, a grandiose name for a motley collection of weathered picnic tables and a broken-down bulldozer. Dunn used the bulldozer in the 1960s and 1970s to tear this road through the Santa Rosa Mountains. This marks the end of the Art Smith Trail, 8.2 miles from the start. Return the way you came.

ALTERNATIVE FINISHES

With a car shuttle or ride share, you can link up with other trails for an outstanding one-way hike.

Proceed straight onto the scenic Hahn Buena Vista Trail and explore the magnificent network of trails near Palm Canyon (see Trip 11.13). Depending on your route, this involves at least 6 miles of hiking, mostly downhill. Be sure to reach the Trading Post before Palm Canyon closes at 5 p.m.

Another option is to turn right and follow Dunn Road and the Cathedral Canyon Trail down to Cathedral City (see the Murray Hill map on page 279). To reach this trailhead from Highway 111 in Cathedral City, turn south onto Cathedral Canyon Drive. At a T-junction in 0.5 mile, turn right onto Terrace Road. Then turn left onto Paradise Way in 0.5 mile, right onto Valley Vista Drive in another 0.5 mile, and left onto Channel Drive in 0.3 mile. Meet a vehicle at the end of Channel Drive.

---

trip 12.8 Randall Henderson Loop

see map on p. 286

Distance	1.2–2.2 miles (loop)
Hiking Time	1–1.5 hours
Elevation Gain	300'–450'
Difficulty	Easy
Trail Use	Good for kids
Best Times	All year, but hot in summer
Agency	Santa Rosa and San Jacinto Mountains National Monument
Recommended Map	*Santa Rosa & San Jacinto Mountains National Monument*

DIRECTIONS The Randall Henderson Loop starts at the Santa Rosa and San Jacinto Mountains National Monument Visitor Center on Highway 74 south of Palm Desert. The trailhead can be reached by exiting the 10 Freeway at Monterey (Exit 131) and driving south across Highway 111, where the road becomes Highway 74. It can also be reached directly from Highway 111, or by driving through the Garner Valley from Hemet. In any case, the visitor center is 4 miles south of Highway 111 on the east side of the road. Park in the first lot, closest to the trailhead. If the visitor center is closed, park across the highway at the Art Smith Trailhead.

The Randall Henderson Loop explores the valley above the Santa Rosa and San Jacinto Mountains National Monument Visitor Center. It's convenient for visitors looking for a short hike; it has fine views and a variety of interesting cacti. On a quiet day, you're likely to see rabbits, lizards, and other small desert animals. The visitor center periodically arranges naturalist-guided hikes in the cooler months; call ahead for a schedule. Ask for a free brochure describing interpretive points along the loop. The trail was named for a longtime Palm Desert resident who published *The Desert Mountain* from the 1930s through the 1960s. Henderson's exploration, journalism, and vision were instrumental to the development of Palm Desert.

Cutoff trails allow you to choose from among three possible loops: the 1.2-mile Wash Loop, the 1.7-mile Cholla Loop, or the 2.2-mile Canyon Loop. Either of the first two options are recommended; the last adds a less interesting segment on a dirt road.

Start at the signed Randall Henderson Trail. The trail splits in 150 yards. Take the left fork to begin the Wash Loop. This is a good area in which to enjoy the desert plants. Smoke trees grow in the washes and creosote bushes are common. Cat's claw acacia may catch up the

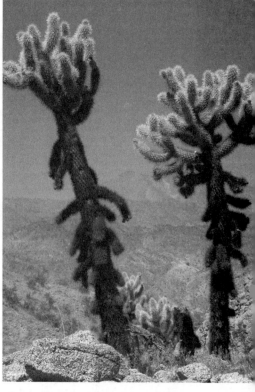

Haystack Mountain between two teddy bear chollas, from the Randall Henderson Trail

unwary hiker. Different species of cacti prefer different altitudes and soils. Watch for silver, pencil, Gander's, and teddy bear chollas in the lower elevations, and beavertail and barrel cacti higher up.

The trail leads up a wash, bypassing a small dry waterfall. In 0.6 mile, reach a cutoff on the right; take this if you want to do the shorter Wash Loop. Otherwise, continue another 0.4 mile to a second junction where you can return on the Cholla Loop. The 0.7-mile walk back includes a stretch on a ridge and through another wash. Watch for views across the highway to a palm oasis in Dead Indian Canyon and Haystack Mountain beyond.

trip 12.9   Living Desert Zoo and Gardens

Distance	5 miles (loop)
Hiking Time	2.5 hours
Elevation Gain	800'
Difficulty	Easy
Trail Use	Good for kids
Best Times	October–April
Information	Living Desert
Recommended Map	*Living Desert* (free at entrance)
Permit	Living Desert admission fee ($19.95 adults, $17.95 seniors age 62+, $9.95 kids ages 3–12)

see map on p. 277

DIRECTIONS From the 10 Freeway, take Exit 131 south on Monterey Avenue and go 6 miles to Highway 111 in Palm Desert. Turn left (east) and proceed 1 mile to Portola Drive. Turn right (south) and go 1.5 miles to the signed entrance of the Living Desert Zoo and Gardens.

The Living Desert is a combination zoo and botanical garden in Palm Desert. Besides the zoo and garden, hikers will enjoy the wilderness trail system that leads east from the Living Desert grounds up onto the flank of Eisenhower Mountain. This trip features good views of the Coachella Valley and surrounding mountains.

At this writing, the Living Desert is open daily October 1–May 31, 9 a.m.–5 p.m. Summer hours (when it's too hot for enjoyable hiking) are reduced to 8 a.m.–1:30 p.m. Ask for a brochure at the entrance showing the trails.

From the Living Desert entrance, walk east past the gift shop and model train display, then north past the bighorn sheep hill to the signed start of the wilderness trail system.

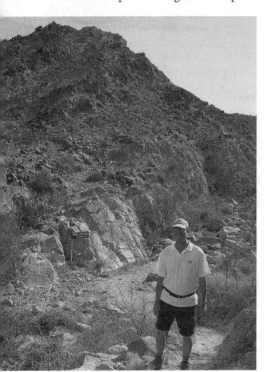

tem. The trail features numerous interpretive signs, including an exhibit marking the San Andreas Fault line. In 0.1 mile, pass the short Inner Loop Trail on the left that circles back to the start. In another 0.4 mile, pass the Middle Loop Trail on the left.

Soon after, the trail enters a rocky wash. In 0.8 mile, watch for a sign indicating where the trail exits the canyon bottom on the left.

Eventually, climb onto the side of Eisenhower Mountain, turn north, and reach a sheltered picnic ground at the halfway point. On a clear winter day, there are spectacular views of the snowcapped San Jacinto and San Gorgonio Mountains high above the golf courses and sprawling development in the Coachella Valley.

The trail turns west and descends back to the Living Desert grounds. Enjoy the botanical garden and other attractions of the Living Desert before you depart.

Hiker on the Living Desert Wilderness Trail

---

trip 12.10   **Bear Creek Oasis**

see map on next page

Distance	9 miles (out-and-back)
Hiking Time	5 hours
Elevation Gain	2,400'
Difficulty	Strenuous
Trail Use	Suitable for equestrians
Best Times	October–March
Agency	Santa Rosa and San Jacinto Mountains National Monument
Recommended Maps	*Santa Rosa & San Jacinto Mountains National Monument* or USGS *La Quinta* and *Martinez Mountain* 7.5' (trail not marked)

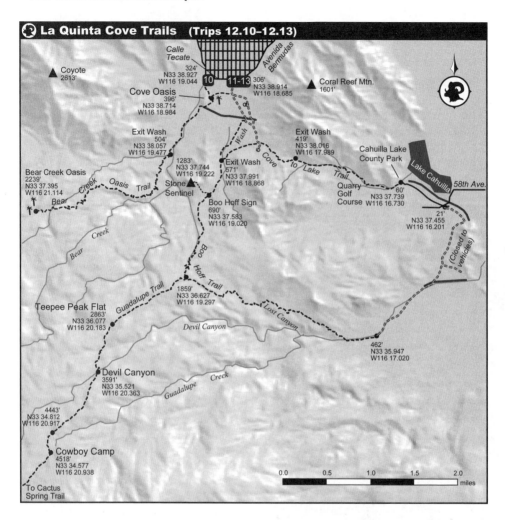

La Quinta Cove Trails (Trips 12.10–12.13)

Calle Tecate
324'
N33 38.927
W116 19.044

Avenida Bermudas

Coyote
2613'

10 **11-13** 306'
N33 38.914
W116 18.685

Coral Reef Mtn.
1601'

Cove Oasis
396'
N33 38.714
W116 18.984

Exit Wash
504'
N33 38.057
W116 19.477

Wash

Exit Wash
419'
N33 38.016
W116 17.989

Cove to Lake Trail

Cahuilla Lake
County Park

Lake Cahuilla

58th Ave.

1283'
N33 37.744
W116 19.222

Exit Wash
571'
N33 37.991
W116 18.868

Bear Creek Oasis
2239'
N33 37.395
W116 21.114

Bear Creek Oasis Trail

Stone Sentinel

Quarry
Golf
Course

60'
N33 37.739
W116 16.730

21'
N33 37.455
W116 16.201

Boo Hoff Sign
690'
N33 37.583
W116 19.020

Bear Creek

(Closed to vehicles)

Boo Hoff Trail

1859'
N33 36.627
W116 19.297

Guadalupe Trail

Teepee Peak Flat
2863'
N33 36.077
W116 20.183

Devil Canyon

Lost Canyon

462'
N33 35.947
W116 17.020

Devil Canyon
3591'
N33 35.521
W116 20.363

Guadalupe Creek

4443'
N33 34.812
W116 20.917

Cowboy Camp
4518'
N33 34.577
W116 20.938

To Cactus
Spring Trail

0.0   0.5   1.0   1.5   2.0
miles

DIRECTIONS From the 10 Freeway, take Exit 137 south onto Washington Street, proceed 1.3 miles, and then turn right onto Eisenhower Drive. Follow it as it curves to the left and eventually ends in 3.7 miles at Avenida Bermudas. Turn right; in 0.2 mile, Avenida Bermudas turns right again (west) and becomes Calle Tecate. Continue 0.5 mile to the end, where Calle Tecate meets Avenida Madero, and park on the street.

Nestled among the canyons of the parched Santa Rosa Mountains, lush oases form where underground water is forced to the surface. The Bear Creek Oasis is hidden high on the slopes above the La Quinta Cove. This

Stone Sentinel from Bear Creek Canyon Ridge (see Trip 12.12)

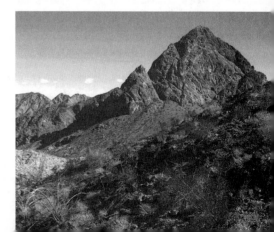

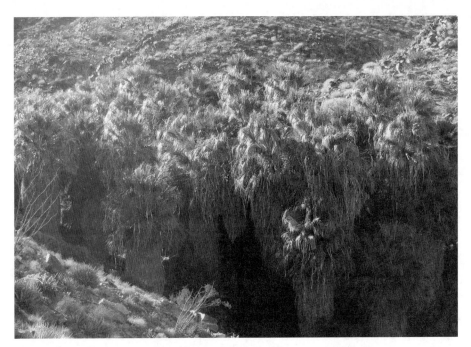

Bear Creek Oasis, hidden among cholla-covered hills

hike passes through a sandy wash and up the ridge along the dramatic Bear Creek Canyon through veritable gardens of cacti before abruptly rounding a corner and ending at the oasis. The upper portion of this route is closed from June 1 to September 30 to protect the bighorn sheep's access to water during the hot season.

A signed trailhead for Cove Oasis is located on the south side of the road. Hike south on the broad dirt path, reaching the Cove Oasis in 0.2 mile. The date palms at this park were a private gift to the city celebrating the Coachella Valley date industry; 90% of the US date supply comes from Coachella Valley.

Identify the prominent Stone Sentinel (Peak 1,283') directly south of Cove Oasis. Your first goal is to hike up the Bear Creek wash right (west) of this peak. Pass around the south side of a hill adjacent to the oasis and then around the west end of a levee to drop into Bear Creek. Follow the sandy dry wash south until you reach the Bear Creek Oasis Trail exiting on the west side and climbing onto Bear Creek Ridge. Several use paths veer off too soon—the correct trail is heavily used and departs the wash near the mouth of a major side canyon near trail signs. Hikers also enjoy continuing up the wash, so don't be distracted by the footprints and miss the turnoff. The Bear Creek Oasis Trail is closed beyond this point in the summer.

The trail parallels the wash and then crosses a minor canyon before gaining a ridge with dramatic views into Bear Creek Canyon. This region of the Santa Rosa Mountains supports diverse species of cacti, including pencil cholla, teddy bear cholla, barrel cactus, and beavertail cactus. As you ascend, the Salton Sea and Joshua Tree National Park come into view. Eventually, veer north away from Bear Creek Canyon and continue up the ridge to cross the upper reaches of a tributary creek. Soon after, arrive at the densely vegetated Bear Creek Oasis tucked away in a small canyon high on the mountainside, 4.5 miles from the start.

After exploring the area, return the way you came.

`trip 12.11` ## Boo Hoff Loop

Distance	12 miles (loop)
Hiking Time	8 hours
Elevation Gain	2,200'
Difficulty	Strenuous
Trail Use	Suitable for equestrians
Best Times	October–March
Agency	Santa Rosa and San Jacinto Mountains National Monument
Recommended Maps	*Santa Rosa & San Jacinto Mountains National Monument* or USGS *La Quinta* and *Martinez Mountain* 7.5' (trail not marked)

see map on p. 292

DIRECTIONS From the 10 Freeway, take Exit 137 south on Washington Street and drive south into La Quinta past Highway 111. Alternatively, from Highway 111, turn south onto Washington Street. Proceed 1.3 miles south of Highway 111; then turn right onto Eisenhower Drive. Eisenhower curves to the left and eventually ends in 3.7 miles at Avenida Bermudas. Turn right; in 0.2 mile, Avenida Bermudas turns right again (west) and becomes Calle Tecate. Park in the Top of Cove dirt lot near this corner.

The view south from the La Quinta Cove resembles an alien landscape. A maze of twisting canyons cuts through the serrated ridges. Ocotillos and cacti dot the hillsides. The Boo Hoff Trail, named in 1979 for a longtime member of the Desert Riders, follows a historic Indian footpath through this curious wilderness. This hike makes a remarkable loop: It starts in the La Quinta Cove, climbs onto the north slopes of towering Martinez Mountain, and then turns east and descends beside Devil Canyon. The path then leads to Lake Cahuilla before returning to the cove on the Morrow Trail.

Teddy bear cholla and the Salton Sea from the Boo Hoff Loop

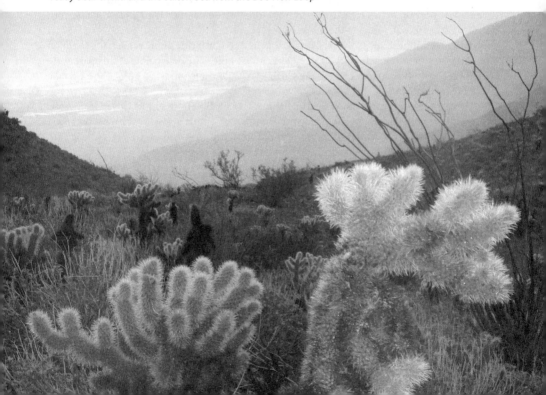

From the trailhead, look south and identify Stone Sentinel (Peak 1,283') standing alone 1.5 miles away. Your first goal is to pass left of this peak. There is a maze of trails and roads in the area, but unfortunately no direct trail leads to this point. Begin walking south from the parking area on a dirt road. In 0.2 mile, it forks in three directions. The trail to the right leads to Cove Oasis, but you choose the road in the middle, passing on the west (right) side of two water tanks. In another 0.4 mile, reach the top of a levee.

From the levee, descend through a gate on a right-veering service road, and then turn right at the base. In a few dozen yards, watch for a post indicating that the Boo Hoff Trail leaves the road and heads south directly up a wash. The next 0.4 mile in the broad wash is ill defined, but eventually the wash narrows as it approaches Stone Sentinel. Watch for another post directing you out of the wash and along the eastern base of Stone Sentinel. In 0.5 mile, drop back into the wash. Continue up it 0.3 mile, ignoring the use trails that might tempt you out, until you reach a large metal sign marking the Boo Hoff Trail.

The Boo Hoff Trail leaves the wash and abruptly begins climbing a shallow ridge overlooking the east fork of Bear Creek (usually dry). The slopes are dotted with ocotillos and chollas. Occasionally, you'll see traces of an old jeep road that once led up here, but stay on the established trail. As you gain elevation, the dominant cactus species visibly change. Pass the wilderness boundary in 1.5 miles. In another 0.1 mile, reach an unmarked trail junction that's critical but easy to miss. The right fork follows the Guadalupe Trail up into the remote wilds of the Santa Rosa Wilderness (see Trip 12.13), but this trip veers left and begins descending eastward.

Impressive views of the Salton Sea are framed by the mountains as you hike down the ridge. In 0.8 mile, the trail dips into a wash and then promptly climbs out the other side. Don't miss the exit, and continue down the wash. Soon you can look down into Lost Canyon on the right (south). Unnamed on the USGS *Martinez Mountain* 7.5' map, it's the northwestern tributary of Devil Canyon. In another 0.4 mile, the trail dips again into a small wash that feeds into Lost Canyon. Cross the wash and continue following the trail 1.6 miles down to the desert floor, where another large metal Boo Hoff sign marks the end of the trail.

Hike down the wide wash 0.3 mile to the wilderness boundary, marked with a sign and a former parking area. A jeep road leads northeast from here; it's open for horses and hikers. In 1.0 mile, stay left at a junction with a second jeep road. Just beyond, cross a levee. There is a maze of trails and old roads through the next part of the hike, but stay on the main dirt road, which is usually marked with trail signs. Your goal is to pass the dramatic hills ahead on their west side and then, at their north end, squeeze between a housing development and a levee until you reach a paved road at a Y-junction (1.2 miles). Then take Cahuilla Park Road 0.7 mile northwest to Lake Cahuilla Recreation Area.

The Cove to Lake Trail begins at the northwest corner of the park at the base of the mountains. Look for a sign reading DOGS PROHIBITED; cross the dike and hike west to another sign reading MORROW TRAIL. This trail leads west 1.6 miles, hugging the base of the hills north of The Quarry at La Quinta golf course. It sometimes stays in the wash and sometimes climbs the toe of the ridge; there are several ways to go, all of which rejoin. When possible, choose the trail on the ridge rather than in the wash. As the wash enters a narrow canyon, be alert for a cairn and trail leading out on the left (south) side. If you reach the dead end of the canyon in a steep bowl, you've gone 0.2 mile too far. The trail climbs out of the canyon and reaches an improbable saddle. Then it descends 0.3 mile to a dirt road below a water tank (where you may have started if you stayed on trail at the beginning of the hike). Turn right (north) and follow the road 1.0 mile back to the trailhead.

see
map on
p. 292

trip 12.12   **Stone Sentinel**

Distance	4.4 miles (out-and-back)
Hiking Time	3 hours
Elevation Gain	1,000'
Difficulty	Strenuous
Best Times	October–December
Agency	Santa Rosa and San Jacinto Mountains National Monument
Recommended Map	*Santa Rosa & San Jacinto Mountains National Monument* or USGS *La Quinta 7.5'*

DIRECTIONS From the 10 Freeway, take Exit 137 for Washington Street and drive south into La Quinta past Highway 111. Alternatively, from Highway 111, turn south onto Washington Street. Proceed 1.3 miles south of Highway 111; then turn right onto Eisenhower Drive. Eisenhower curves to the left and eventually ends in 3.7 miles at Avenida Bermudas. Turn right; in 0.2 mile, Avenida Bermudas turns right again (west) and becomes Calle Tecate. Park in the Top of Cove dirt lot near this corner.

Mountaineers exploring the La Quinta Cove can't help but admire a small but striking peak at the south end of the cove. Peak 1,283', locally known as Stone Sentinel, has only one moderate route to the summit, and even this route involves a pitch of stimulating third-class rock climbing on an exposed ridge. This route ascends a gully on the southeast side. Many would-be climbers have erred by starting up too soon and have found themselves separated from the high point by a sheer cliff. This route involves cross-country travel and hence is closed January–September to avoid disturbing bighorn sheep.

The best place to begin the cross-country ascent is from the large metal BOO HOFF TRAIL sign on the south side of the peak. To get there from the parking area, begin as with Trip 12.11: Walk south from the parking area on a dirt road. In 0.2 mile, take the middle fork. In another 0.4 mile, reach a levee, pass a gate, and follow a dirt road down and to the right. Immediately reach a Boo Hoff Trail marker post on the left pointing you up a wash. Follow the wash toward the peak 0.5 mile; then exit the wash on the right side where the trail resumes along the base of Stone Sentinel. In another 0.5 mile, the trail drops back into the wash. Continue 0.3 mile, passing misleading use trails emerging from the wash, until you reach the large metal BOO HOFF TRAIL sign on the right side of the wash.

Leave the Boo Hoff Trail at the sign, and pick a path to the notch. The peak on the left is the high point.

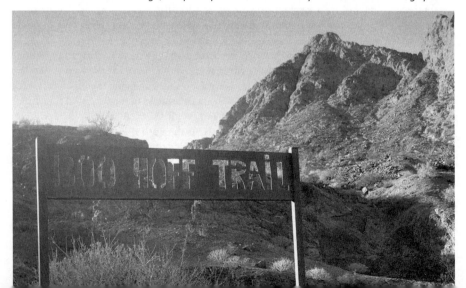

From the sign, identify the prominent notch on the skyline of Stone Sentinel. Leave the trail and pick a path past ocotillo and barrel cactus across the slopes and up a gully leading to the notch. Beware that the gully is full of loose rock. From the notch, turn left and ascend an exposed catwalk to the peak. The crux is a steep slab where some climbers may want a belay.

trip 12.13 Guadalupe Trail

see maps on pgs. 277, 292, & 298

Distance	14 miles (one-way)
Hiking Time	8 hours
Elevation Gain	5,100'
Difficulty	Strenuous
Trail Use	Suitable for backpacking
Best Times	October–December
Agency	Santa Rosa and San Jacinto Mountains National Monument
Required Maps	*Santa Rosa & San Jacinto Mountains National Monument* or USGS *La Quinta, Martinez Mountain* and *Toro Peak* 7.5' (trail not marked)

DIRECTIONS The Guadalupe Trail is a one-way hike from the La Quinta Cove to the Sawmill Trailhead in Pinyon Pines with a 40-minute car shuttle. Position a getaway vehicle at the Cactus Spring/Sawmill Trailhead. This is reached from Highway 74 by turning south at mile marker 74 RIV 80.50 onto Pinon Flats Transfer Station Road (7S09). Go 0.3 mile to the Sawmill Trail parking area, on the left.

To reach the starting point, backtrack north 15 miles on Highway 74; then turn right on Highway 111 in Palm Desert and drive 6 miles east. Turn right onto Washington Street and proceed 1.3 miles south; then turn right onto Eisenhower Drive. Eisenhower curves to the left and eventually ends in 3.7 miles at Avenida Bermudas. Turn right; in 0.2 mile, Avenida Bermudas turns right again (west) and becomes Calle Tecate. Park in the dirt Top of Cove dirt lot near this corner.

The Guadalupe "Trail" is a cross-country route following an old Indian path through the heart of the Santa Rosa Mountains from the desert to the pines. The first part follows the Boo Hoff Trail, but the middle travels up a faint Indian footpath past Devil Canyon and Guadalupe Creek before rejoining the Cactus Spring Trail on the west side of Martinez Mountain. The Guadalupe Trail is strenuous and demands advanced route-finding skills, but also offers tremendous rewards to experienced hikers who undertake its challenge.

Martinez Mountain and Teepee Peak from the Guadalupe Trail

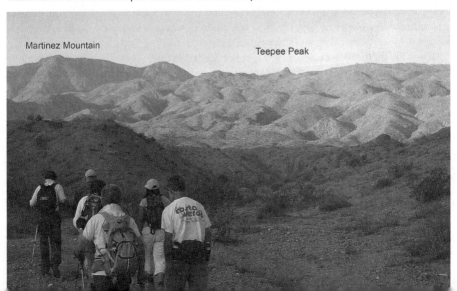

Martinez Mountain

Teepee Peak

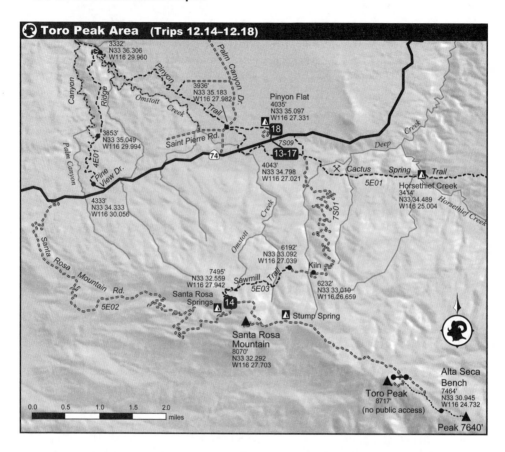

Many desert plant species, ranging from ocotillo and cactus, to agave and yucca, to pinyon pine, are represented. Each of these species favors a specific band of elevation. The route passes an old cowboy camp, and sharp-eyed hikers may note old Indian artifacts along the way. Please leave what you find for the enjoyment of future hikers. It's helpful to wear gaiters to protect yourself from occasional brush and to carry pliers in case of an unfortunate encounter with a cholla cactus. The best way to do this hike is with a friend or group who knows the way; failing that, a GPS or exceptional map reading skills are necessary.

From the trailhead, look south and identify Stone Sentinel (Peak 1,283') standing alone 1.5 miles ahead. Your first goal is to pass left of this peak. There is a maze of trails and roads in the area, but unfortunately no direct trail leads to this point. Begin walking south from the parking area on a dirt road. In 0.2 mile, it forks in three directions. The trail to the right leads to Cove Oasis, but you take the road in the middle, passing on the west (right) side of two water tanks. In another 0.4 mile, cross the top of a levee. Despite NO TRESPASSING signs to the contrary, hikers are allowed past the gate.

From the levee, descend through a gate on a right-veering service road, and then turn right at the base. In a few dozen yards, watch for a post indicating that the Boo Hoff Trail leaves the road and heads south directly up a wash. The next 0.4 mile in the broad wash is ill defined, but eventually the wash narrows as it approaches Stone Sentinel. Watch for another post directing you out of the wash and along the eastern base of Stone Sentinel. In 0.5 mile, drop back into the wash. Continue up it 0.3 mile, ignoring the use trails that might tempt you out, until you reach a large metal sign marking the Boo Hoff Trail.

Again, survey the territory in front of you. The biggest mountain ahead is Martinez Mountain, which is prominent from much of the eastern Santa Rosas. To the right is a spire on the skyline locally known as Teepee Peak. Your next goal is to follow the trail to the base of Teepee Peak.

The Boo Hoff Trail leaves the wash and abruptly begins climbing a shallow ridge overlooking the east fork of Bear Creek (usually dry). The slopes are dotted with ocotillos and chollas. Occasionally, you'll see traces of an old jeep road that once led up here, but stay on the established trail. As you gain elevation, the dominant cactus species visibly change. Pass the wilderness boundary in 1.5 miles. In another 0.1 mile, reach an unmarked trail junction that's critical but easy to miss. The left fork continues on the Boo Hoff Trail descending east toward the Salton Sea (see Trip 12.11), but this trip veers right on the Guadalupe Trail and continues climbing.

Teddy bear chollas soon become the dominant cactus. Soon after, hike through a canyon full of agaves and come to a flat site at the base of Teepee Peak, 1.2 miles from the junction. This site was once used by the Cahuilla Indians who lived in the area; it's a good place to take a break and explore.

In another 0.5 mile, reach a brush-choked canyon. Follow a faint path along the rocks on the right side until you can cross on a good trail and switchback up the far side. It's well worth your effort to find the trail. In 0.8 mile, reach a small plateau with a rocky point at the east end of the shelf. This was once another Indian camp. The trail becomes hard to follow here. Work your way south across the brushy bottom of Devil Canyon; then regain a faint ducked trail on the far side. Continue up a ridge, aiming for the saddle to the right of the pinyon-clad Martinez Mountain. Hike southwest up a shallow ridge on the right side of the Guadalupe Creek Canyon. Soon the trail becomes indistinct again; enter the Guadalupe Creek drainage and head for the saddle. Shortly below the saddle, arrive at Cowboy Camp, marked with a rusted cast-iron stove and assorted detritus. About 200 feet above the camp, you may sometimes be able to obtain murky water from a small spring. Continue 0.6 mile up the canyon and along a sandy wash to reach the saddle, 7.6 miles from the trailhead.

Look southwest and identify Toro Peak, the antenna-studded high point of the Santa Rosa Mountains. Hike toward Toro Peak until you enter a wash; follow the wash southwest and then west until you reach a wooden post marking the intersection with the Cactus Spring Trail in 1.3 miles. This intersection is easy to overlook, but very important.

Turn right and follow the Cactus Spring Trail west. Pass Cactus Spring (a grassy spot north of the trail where water rarely flows now) and, in 2.4 miles, reach the cottonwood-shaded camp at Horsethief Creek, the only reliable water source on the trip. Continue west past some historic mining operations and in another 2.2 miles reach a dirt road. Continue west 0.2 mile to the Sawmill Trailhead.

trip 12.14   Sawmill Trail

Distance	16 miles (out-and-back)
Hiking Time	8 hours
Elevation Gain	3,900'
Difficulty	Strenuous
Trail Use	Dogs allowed, suitable for backpacking
Best Times	October–November, March–April
Agency	Santa Rosa and San Jacinto Mountains National Monument
Recommended Map	*Santa Rosa & San Jacinto Mountains National Monument* or USGS *Toro Peak* 7.5'

DIRECTIONS From Highway 74 at mile marker 74 RIV 80.50, turn south onto Pinon Flats Transfer Station Road (7S09). Go 0.3 mile to the Sawmill Trail parking area, on the left.

Optionally, arrange a second vehicle or bicycle at the top of the trail to do a one-way hike (or do the hike downhill). To reach the top, continue 3.6 miles west on Highway 74 to the fair dirt Santa Rosa Truck Trail (7S02), near mile marker 74 RIV 77.00. Turn left (south) and follow the mountain road 8.7 miles to the signed start of Trail 5E03, near a bend and a side road. This is 0.5 mile above the turnoff for Santa Rosa Springs Campground.

From the Sawmill Trail parking area, walk east along a dirt road, staying right at an immediate fork. In 0.2 mile at a signed junction with the Cactus Spring Trail, stay right on Sawmill Road (7S01 to Sawmill Trail 5E03). Follow this road 5.4 miles as it switchbacks unforgivingly up a chaparral-covered ridge.

Ribbonwoods and cacti give way to manzanitas and scrub oaks as you ascend. Watch for Steller's jays, quail, and birds of prey along the way. Views of the Pinyon Pines community, Deep Creek's convoluted canyon, Sugarloaf and Asbestos Mountains, and the Desert Divide and San Jacinto become more expansive as you climb. The rough road is usually passable by 4WD vehicles if you'd prefer to drive this part and shorten the hike.

At the top of the Sawmill Road is an old charcoal kiln. Two faint roads continue. The left one reaches a reliable spring in 0.1 mile, but this trip follows the jeep tracks to the right that contour for another 0.4 mile. Where they peter out, look for a signed trail marker for Trail 5E03. This trail crosses the headwaters of Omstott Creek, which flows down the mountainside much of the year from the Stump Spring area. Vegetation becomes momentarily lush along the banks of the creek, then fades to chaparral again before entering a band of black oaks. Not far beyond, climb into the mature forest of Jeffrey pines, white firs, and incense cedars that crowns the upper reaches of the Santa Rosa Mountains. The trail makes final switchbacks before reaching Santa Rosa Truck Trail (7S02), 2.4 miles from the end of the jeep tracks.

From here, you can return the way you came. Alternatively, if a vehicle is parked at the top, your work is complete. The purist may choose to continue up to the summit of Santa Rosa Mountain. (8,070'). This adds 500 feet of elevation gain. Either follow the dirt road to the top, or pick a cross-country route directly up the steep forested ridge.

Charcoal kiln at top of Sawmill Road

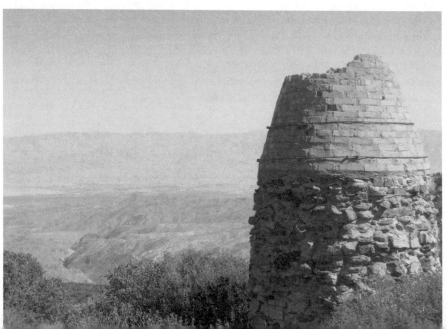

trip 12.15 Horsethief Creek

Distance	4.5 miles (out-and-back)
Hiking Time	2.5 hours
Elevation Gain	900'
Difficulty	Moderate
Trail Use	Dogs allowed, suitable for backpacking, suitable for equestrians
Best Times	October–March
Agency	Santa Rosa and San Jacinto Mountains National Monument
Recommended Map	*Santa Rosa & San Jacinto Mountains National Monument* or USGS *Toro Peak* 7.5'
Permit	Sign in at the wilderness box

see map on p. 298

DIRECTIONS From Highway 74 at mile marker 74 RIV 80.50, turn south onto Pinon Flats Transfer Station Road (7S09). Go 0.3 mile to the Sawmill Trail parking area, on the left.

Between Highway 74 and Toro Peak is a high bench covered in chaparral and sliced by rugged canyons. Horsethief Creek flows through one of these canyons throughout the wet season. Alongside the creek is a small campsite shaded by cottonwoods. The trip to the creek is one of the few moderate hikes in this remote region of the Santa Rosa Mountains. According to legend, rustlers made their hideout here in the 19th century as they preyed upon honest folk in San Diego and San Bernardino.

This trail is a botanist's delight, with more than 200 species. Hikers must beware of all things sharp and pointy. You'll observe four species of prickly pear cactus (Mojave, Vasey's, beavertail, and pancake), three species of cholla (Gander's, cane, and teddy bear), and Engelmann's hedgehog cactus. Nolina, Mojave yucca, and desert agave grow in plenty, and you'll occasionally have to dodge cat's claw acacia. The larger trees include ribbonwood, pinyon pine, and juniper; medium shrubs include sugarbush and scrub oak.

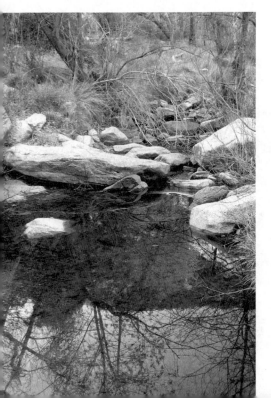

The signed Cactus Spring Trail (5E01) starts at the east end of the parking lot. Walk along the dirt road, staying right at an immediate fork. In 0.2 mile, turn right and then immediately left onto the signed Cactus Spring Trail. Sign in at the wilderness box. Hike through fields of prickly pear cactus, agave, manzanita, and ribbonwood, and pass some old dolomite mining structures. An ominous sign warns you to BE PREPARED FOR HAZARDOUS CONDITIONS BEYOND THIS POINT. In 0.9 mile, you'll reach the wilderness boundary. The trail descends through colorful hills and canyons. In another 1.2 miles, the trail drops down into the canyon of Horsethief Creek.

You can enjoy a picnic or spend the night here. Explore up or down the rough canyon alongside Horsethief Creek. Then return the way you came.

Horsethief Creek

trip 12.16   Cactus Spring Trail

see maps on pgs. 277 & 298

Distance	21 miles (one-way)
Hiking Time	11 hours
Elevation Gain/Loss	3,000'/7,000'
Difficulty	Very strenuous
Trail Use	Suitable for backpacking
Best Times	October–March
Agency	Santa Rosa and San Jacinto Mountains National Monument
Required Maps	*Santa Rosa & San Jacinto Mountains National Monument* or USGS *Toro Peak, Martinez Mountain, Clark Lake NE,* and *Valerie* 7.5'
Permit	Sign in at the wilderness box

DIRECTIONS This is a long one-way hike requiring a 1-hour car shuttle. Position one vehicle at the south end of Van Buren Street amid the farms northwest of the Salton Sea. This trailhead can be reached from Highway 111 in Indio by driving 10 miles south on Jackson Street, then 1 mile east on 66th Avenue. Turn right onto good dirt Van Buren Street and thread your way past fields for 1.0 mile to its end at a Bureau of Land Management marker. If you have a high-clearance vehicle, you can continue 4.0 miles on a sandy and sometimes confusing road/wash to the wilderness boundary.

Drive the second vehicle back to Highway 111; then head 10.5 miles west to Highway 74, then 15 miles south to mile marker 74 RIV 80.50. Opposite the Pinyon Flats Campground road, turn left (south) onto Pinon Flats Trans Station Road (7S09). Go 0.3 mile to the Sawmill Trail parking area, on the left.

The Cactus Spring "Trail" is one of the wildest routes in the Santa Rosa Mountains, following an old Indian path from the forested heights around Martinez Mountain down rugged Martinez Canyon to the date palm groves near the Salton Sea. The first half follows an established but sometimes faint trail; the second requires cross-country navigation skills. Long pants and gaiters are recommended because of the brush in Martinez Canyon and the perpetual cactus hazards.

Cactus Spring Trail

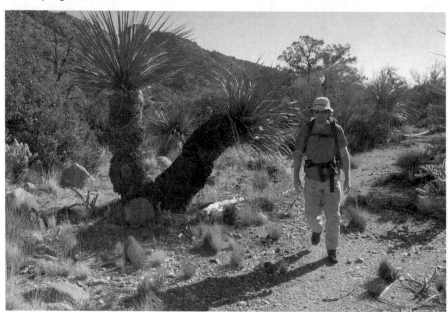

The signed Cactus Spring Trail (5E01) starts at the east end of the Sawmill Trail parking lot. Walk along the dirt road, staying right at an immediate fork. In 0.2 mile, turn right and then immediately left onto the signed Cactus Spring Trail. Sign in at the wilderness box. Hike through fields of prickly pear cacti, agaves, manzanitas, and ribbonwoods, and pass some mining structures. In 0.9 mile, reach the wilderness boundary. The trail descends through colorful hills and canyons. In another 1.2 miles, reach Horsethief Creek, where a campsite is shaded with cottonwoods. Beyond this point, the trail is less used and sometimes requires attention to follow. Climb out of the canyon and in 0.6 mile enter a sandy wash. Watch for posts marking the entrance and exit of washes. In another 1.9 miles, look for Cactus Spring on the left (north) side of the trail. The spring is easy to miss; it's now just a grassy area that occasionally offers a trickle of water. This is one of the most sacred areas for the Cahuilla Indians who live in this area. Observant explorers may find bedrock mortars for grinding food, smooth rock dance floors, and pictographs and petroglyphs.

The trail continues southeast toward the looming Martinez Mountain. In 0.7 mile, pass a post where the Guadalupe Trail veers off to the left side of Martinez Mountain (see Trip 12.13). The Guadalupe Trail is a cross-country route, and you're likely to miss it unless you're familiar with the area. The Cactus Spring Trail curves around the right side of Martinez Mountain through a pinyon pine forest, passing over a 5,168-foot saddle that marks the high point of the route, 6.9 miles from the start.

Beyond this point, the trail becomes even less distinct, but it's marked with cairns and is worth your while to find. Be especially alert when crossing washes in order to locate the trail on the far side. In 2.5 miles, the trail reaches the signed Agua Alta Spring campsite on the south side of Martinez Mountain. The campsite, complete with hitching post, is a few hundred feet up the canyon north of the trail. The spring, in the dense grass above the campsite, is undependable.

VARIATION

From Agua Alta Spring, some hikers prefer to descend Agua Alta Canyon to rejoin Martinez Canyon near the bottom. This is also a very difficult journey.

Beyond the spring, the path traverses southeast across Pinyon Alta Flat and drops into Martinez Canyon. It's marked with the occasional cairn but is so seldom used that few traces remain. The best way to navigate is to look for the prominent rocky Peak 4,345' to the southeast. The trail passes just right of the peak before following a steep ridge that drops down to the junction of Martinez and Tahquitz Canyons, 2.8 miles from Agua Alta Spring.

VARIATION

Intrepid explorers can walk up Martinez Canyon 1.2 miles to the two-room Jack Miller Cabin, built of stone in the 1930s. The miner's cabin, also called the Martinez Canyon Rockhouse, was placed on the National Register of Historic Places in 1999.

Your navigation problems are over, but the hiking is no easier. The Martinez Canyon Trail once descended Martinez Canyon, but it's no longer maintained and few traces are left. Boulder-hop eastward 5 miles. Where springs flow, the narrow canyon is choked with reeds that are difficult to push through. Eventually, the canyon widens and Agua Alta Canyon joins in from the northeast. Finally, reach the wilderness boundary, where jeep tracks lead 4 miles out of the canyon and north past fields to Van Buren Street.

trip 12.17 Martinez Mountain

see maps on pgs. 277 & 298

Distance	17 miles (out-and-back)
Hiking Time	10 hours
Elevation Gain	4,300'
Difficulty	Strenuous
Trail Use	Suitable for backpacking
Best Times	October–April
Agency	Santa Rosa and San Jacinto Mountains National Monument
Recommended Maps	*Santa Rosa & San Jacinto Mountains National Monument* or USGS *Toro Peak* and *Martinez Mountain 7.5'*
Permit	Sign in at the wilderness box

DIRECTIONS From Highway 74 at mile marker 74 RIV 80.50, turn south onto Pinon Flats Trans Station Road (7S09). Go 0.3 mile to the Sawmill Trail parking area, on the left.

Imposing from the north but less dramatic from the west, Martinez Mountain (6,560+') is the fourth-highest point in the Santa Rosa Mountains after Toro, Santa Rosa, and Rabbit. The mountain was named for a Cahuilla village in the vicinity. The lightly visited summit requires a long and strenuous cross-country approach through the spectacular desert gardens of the Santa Rosa Wilderness. Martinez Mountain is a worthy undertaking for hikers with the experience, conditioning, and outlook to enjoy such desert peaks. Undeveloped camping opportunities can be found along much of the route, including by the wash at the base of the mountain and on sandy clearings on the summit plateaus beneath the shelter of pinyon pines and granite boulders. The trip requires excellent navigational skills, and a GPS can be helpful. Long pants, gaiters, and trekking poles are all recommended.

The signed Cactus Spring Trail (5E01) starts at the east end of the parking lot. Walk along the dirt road, staying right at an immediate fork. In 0.2 mile, turn right and then immediately left onto the signed Cactus Spring Trail. Sign in at the wilderness box.

The trail leads southeast, past the ruins of the historic Dolomite Mine, down into the cottonwood-shaded Horsethief Creek, and then up out of the canyon and along dry washes. Watch for a zone of rough white marble in the wash before you climb over a low

Martinez Mountain summit route: ascend the gully to the rightmost saddle.

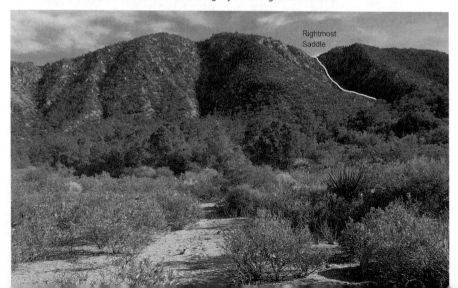

Rightmost Saddle

saddle. In another 0.6 mile, watch for a wooden post marking the trail where it crosses a wash. Cactus Spring is the sometimes-damp spot 40 yards up the wash.

In another 0.7 mile, the trail meets another wash coming from a low area to the east between Martinez and Sheep Mountains, due north of Point 4,996'. This unmarked and easy-to-miss spot is the head of the Guadalupe Trail and the recommended departure point for Martinez Mountain. Use your topo map or GPS waypoint to identify this spot. Walk up the wash. In 0.9 mile, after passing a spur ridge, it will turn right and veer south toward Martinez Mountain.

This is a good place to size up your route ahead. Martinez Mountain is the high point to the southeast with three prominent saddles. The wash you're following will take you to the rightmost saddle. Initially wide and sandy, it soon becomes a narrow and rocky gully, marked with an astonishing and unnecessary number of cairns. After a strenuous ascent, emerge from the gully and look for cairns leading up and left onto the summit ridge. The high point is a tall granite rock pile 0.2 mile east of the top of the wash. It's most easily climbed by looping around the left side of the formation to a third-class weakness on the rear. You may find the summit register in a crevice at the base of the weakness. If you're using a GPS, beware that Garmin's database incorrectly indicates the summit 0.2 mile farther north near the 6,562 label on the topographic map.

If you prefer not retracing your steps, you can descend the west ridge of the peak to rejoin the very faint Cactus Spring Trail at a saddle. Pick a path through the boulders and pines along the summit plateau to the top of the west ridge. You'll likely find occasional ducks along the ridge, and with care, you can avoid bushwhacking and rock scrambling. In 1 mile, rejoin the trail and follow it north 1.4 miles to the wash where you originally left the trail.

VARIATION

Sheep Mountain is another named high point in the Santa Rosa Mountains, 1.4 miles north-northeast of Cactus Spring but not hidden behind lower hills. Dedicated peak baggers can reach it by departing at Cactus Spring and hiking over Peak 4,678' and Peak 5,067'. The summit sees about a dozen parties a year. Then return to near Peak 5,067' and follow a maze of ridges and washes southeast to rejoin the route up Martinez Mountain. This detour adds about two hours of strenuous cross-country travel to the trip.

---

trip 12.18   **Pinyon Trail**

see map on p. 298

Distance	8.5 miles (out-and-back, or a cross-country loop)
Hiking Time	5 hours
Elevation Gain	1,400'
Difficulty	Moderate
Trail Use	Dogs allowed, suitable for mountain biking, suitable for equestrians
Best Times	October–April
Information	Santa Rosa and San Jacinto Mountains National Monument
Required Map	*Santa Rosa & San Jacinto Mountains National Monument* or USGS *Toro Peak 7.5'*

DIRECTIONS From Highway 74 at mile marker 74 RIV 80.50, turn north onto Pinyon Drive. In 0.1 mile, reach the entrance to Pinyon Flats Campground. Unless you're staying at the campground, park on the shoulder of Pinyon Drive.

The Pinyon Trail (5E02) is an alternative route into Palm Canyon originating from Highway 74. It was constructed by the Coachella Valley Trails Council in the 1990s. Starting at the Pinyon Flats Campground, it leads across a magnificent plateau covered with ribbonwoods, cacti, yuccas, and, of course, pinyon pines. It features great views of Santa Rosa Mountain and the southern Desert Divide. It's easy to get lost in this part of the desert, so this trip isn't recommended for beginning navigators. Adventurous hikers can make a loop, returning by the Palm Canyon Trail or Omstott Creek. For those wanting a truly wild backpacking trip from the Salton Sea to Palm Springs, the Pinyon Trail makes the critical link between the Cactus Spring Trail and Palm Canyon.

The trail starts next to the PINYON FLATS CAMPGROUND sign and leads north along the west side of Pinon Road 0.1 mile, then turns left and heads west. It generally follows the fence line marking the boundary between U.S. Forest Service and private land and, in another 0.6 mile, reaches a pair of trail markers where the trail crosses the dirt Palm Canyon Drive (private). This is a critical junction; be sure to depart this junction to the northwest on a signed trail rather than accidentally taking one of the power-line roads or other dirt roads.

ALTERNATIVE START

An alternative start for this trip begins at the Sawmill Trailhead (see Trip 12.14), but it's difficult to follow. Hike west from the Sawmill Trail parking area across the road to the signed Ribbonwood Equestrian Campground Road. In 0.1 mile, where the campground road veers left, continue straight onto a trail at an unlabeled trail post. The equestrian trail braids repeatedly. In 1.0 mile, reach an equestrian tunnel passing beneath Highway 74. On the far side, the trail again braids countless times. If all goes well, you'll arrive in 0.6 mile at a trail marker where the Pinyon Trail crosses good dirt Palm Canyon Drive. Neither path is named at this intersection. If all doesn't go well, you'll nevertheless eventually intersect Palm Canyon Drive by hiking northwest.

The Pinyon Trail leads into the badlands of the Santa Rosa Mountains. Erosion has gouged the plateau with gullies that progressively deepen to canyons as you head north. The unusual ribbonwood trees are the dominant vegetation, but a wealth of sharp and pointy desert flora are sprinkled amidst the ribbonwoods.

In 1.1 miles, reach a cairn where an unmarked footpath comes in from the right, but stay straight on the main trail. (This footpath, handy for locals, leads north 0.3 mile to the west

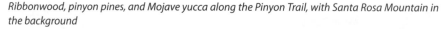

Ribbonwood, pinyon pines, and Mojave yucca along the Pinyon Trail, with Santa Rosa Mountain in the background

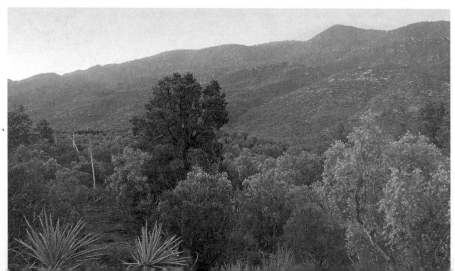

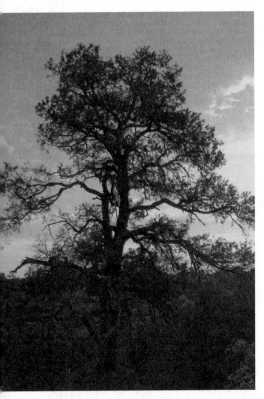

Pinyon pine at dawn on the Pinyon Trail

end of Pinesmoke Road) The trail begins to wind in and out of minor canyons, and then makes a steep series of switchbacks to drop into Omstott Creek. It climbs back up onto the hill beyond, then drops back into Omstott Creek at an unmarked junction with the Palm Canyon Trail. The junction is on the bottom of the canyon directly opposite the point where the Palm Canyon Trail begins switchbacking out of the canyon. This point is 3.6 miles from Palm Canyon Drive. The junction is hidden by bushes, so locating the Pinyon Trail from below would be difficult unless you know to look for it where the Palm Canyon Trail leaves the canyon floor. Return the way you came.

ALTERNATIVE FINISH ——————————

You can make a loop returning up the Palm Canyon Trail or Omstott Creek.

The Palm Canyon Trail switchbacks up onto a ridge and, in 3.5 miles, reaches Pine View Drive by Highway 74, 2.7 miles west of Pinon Road (see Trip 11.14). This is an enjoyable hike, especially if you've arranged a vehicle at Pine View Drive so that you don't have to trudge back along the highway.

The Omstott Creek route is shown on the National Monument map but is only for hardy cross-country travelers. It follows the canyon floor, roughly parallel to the Pinyon Trail. While most of the hike is on an easy sandy creekbed, some sections are seriously overgrown and require pushing through dense brush. Watch out for rattlesnakes and for bees that are drawn to the damp creekbed. The lower part of the canyon features some magnificent pancake prickly pear cacti tenaciously rooted in the rock walls. In 3.3 miles, exit the canyon where it splits in two directions, and becomes hopelessly choked with brush. Walk south across the desert to reach the dirt Saint Pierre Road near some houses. Turn left (east) and follow the road 0.4 mile to Palm Canyon Drive. Turn left (northeast) and continue 0.1 mile to the signed junction where the Pinyon Trail crosses the road. Turn right onto the Pinyon Trail and return to Pinyon Flats Campground.

---

trip 12.19   **Rabbit Peak from the Salton Sea**

see map on next page

Distance	16 miles (out-and-back)
Hiking Time	12–14 hours
Elevation Gain	6,800'
Difficulty	Very strenuous
Trail Use	Suitable for backpacking
Best Times	October–December (closed during the rest of the year)
Agency	Santa Rosa and San Jacinto Mountains National Monument
Required Map	USGS *Rabbit Peak* 7.5'

DIRECTIONS From the eastbound 10 Freeway in Indio, take Exit 145 south onto the 86S Expressway. Drive south 12 miles; then turn right (west) onto 66th Avenue. In 1.1 miles, turn left onto Pierce Street, which ends at Harrison Street in 5.3 miles. Turn left onto Harrison Street, then right onto 78th Avenue in 0.6 mile, and then left onto Fillmore Street in another 1.0 mile. Follow Fillmore Street 0.5 mile to its end near some citrus groves.

Rabbit Peak (6,640+') is the toughest mountain in Southern California to climb, even when you ascend by the easiest route. Anchoring the south end of the Santa Rosa Mountain crest, it requires climbing more than 6,000 feet of rugged trailless terrain from

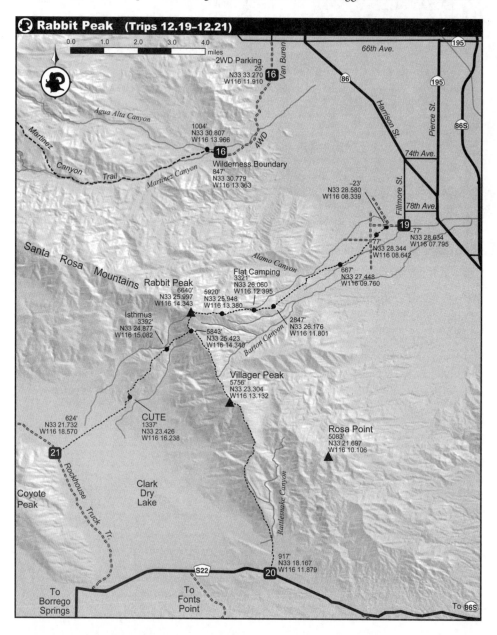

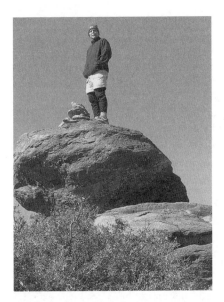

Rabbit Peak summit rocks

any direction. The rewards include fine views of the Salton Sea and Santa Rosa Mountains, close interaction with the full gamut of desert vegetation, and a great physical workout. The three most common routes on the mountain are this one from near the Salton Sea, an ascent of similar difficulty from Clark Lake to the west (see Trip 12.21), and a tremendously long climb up the south ridge over Villager Peak (see Trip 12.20). These routes can be done as two-day backpacking trips, but the trade-off is that you must haul all your water. A few hardy souls have traversed the entire spine of the Santa Rosa Mountains from Toro Peak to Rabbit and on down over Villager Peak; this route is reportedly 24 arduous cross-country miles with patches of awful bushwhacking and involves 11,000 feet of elevation gain despite running the ridge in the net downhill direction.

The system of roads, levees, and ranches around the start of this trailhead has changed since the USGS map was printed, and the navigation across the desert floor in the dark can be the crux of the route-finding challenge. Indeed, this area is developing rapidly and the network of roads may change again by the time you read this. Access from this side involves cross-country travel through bighorn habitat in the National Monument, which is permitted only October 1–December 31. Your first goal is to identify the long ridge between Alamo and Barton Canyons leading up Rabbit Peak. This is easiest to do in the daylight. The ridge is at a bearing of 230 degrees from the trailhead. A GPS receiver and extra batteries are helpful to record the route in the event that you retrace it after dark. Headlamps are indispensable for any route on Rabbit Peak.

From your vehicle, respecting the NO TRESPASSING signs on the citrus groves, walk south past a gate at the end of Fillmore Street; then immediately turn right (west) and follow a road on a levee between two citrus groves. In 0.4 mile, the levee veers right where two washes converge. Follow the left wash as it continues west. In 0.1 mile, turn left (south) at the west end

Rabbit Peak between Alamo and Barton Canyons. Note the lower approach ridge pointing down toward the trailhead.

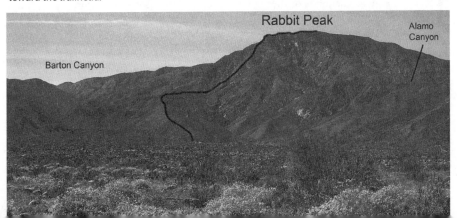

of a grove. Follow the wash a few yards; then scramble up the west side into the desert, where you'll find faint traces of an old dirt road leading toward Rabbit Peak. Follow it southwest.

Soon you'll begin seeing white cairns along the path. (The white rocks show up well by headlamp on a nighttime descent, but this section is nevertheless challenging and tedious to follow in the dark.) In 0.4 mile, cross a wash and arrive at a metal post. The road ends here, but the trail continues, marked by more cairns. In another 2.8 miles, the trail switchbacks and climbs onto the south side of the base of the ridge. It gradually climbs along the side of the ridge to the ocotillo-studded crest. From here on, cairns are found sporadically but are difficult to consistently follow. Your goal is simply to go up along the path of least resistance. Pay attention to the route so you can locate the correct ridges on the descent.

The ridge climbs to a small saddle at 2,500 feet, ascends steeply, and then levels out into a jumbled field of boulders and agaves. Just west of Point 3,235' lie several clearings; these mark the halfway point and offer fine but exposed dry camping for those backpacking the mountain.

Farther west, cross a narrow isthmus between two canyons and begin climbing in earnest, gaining 2,600 feet in the next 1.1 miles. Pick your way around the innumerable cacti and agaves. Just before you reach the top, climb some Class 2 slabs and traverse an easy knife-edge rock ridge to reach the long hogsback of Rabbit Peak. Continue another 1.1 miles west through juniper and scrub oak country to the summit boulders at the extreme west end of the ridge.

Return the way you came or, with a car shuttle, descend to Clark Lake (see Trip 12.21).

---

trip 12.20   ### Rabbit and Villager Peaks

Distance	21 miles (out-and-back)
Hiking Time	14 hours
Elevation Gain	7,900'
Difficulty	Very strenuous
Trail Use	Suitable for backpacking
Best Times	October–March
Agency	Santa Rosa and San Jacinto Mountains National Monument
Required Maps	USGS *Fonts Point* and *Rabbit Peak* 7.5'

see map on p. 308

DIRECTIONS From the eastbound 10 Freeway in Indio, take Exit 145 south onto the 86S Expressway. Drive 35 miles, and turn right (west) onto the Borrego Salton Seaway (S22). Proceed 14 miles; then park in a turnout on the north side of the road adjacent to call box S22-319; this point is 0.1 mile west of mile marker 32 and directly opposite the Thimble jeep trail.

This is the most strenuous of the routes on Rabbit Peak described in this book, but it also involves the simplest route finding in the dark. It leads up the long crest of the Santa Rosa Mountains from the southern toe near the Borrego Salton Seaway, passing over Villager Peak en route to Rabbit. Bring headlamps and plenty of water; 6 quarts are merited on a cool day, more on a warm one.

From the parking area, identify the ridge to the north on the left (west) side of Rattlesnake Canyon. The Clark Fault has raised the interesting Lute scarp between the parking and the ridge. The scarp climbs gradually from the south but drops off precipitously on the north side. Hike across the desert toward the ridge, veering slightly right to remain east of the scarp. You may find ducks marking a path.

In 1.2 miles, gain the toe of the ridge. Look for switchbacks and a good use trail climbing unrelentingly. Watch for a spectacular display of cacti, ocotillos, and agaves. The rock

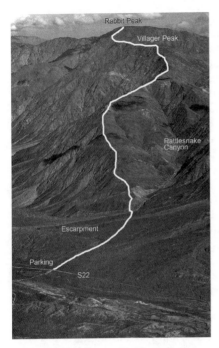

Aerial view of Rabbit and Villager Peaks from the south

sleeping circles were used by the Cahuilla people. Pass above a sheer face banded with white marble. After 5.8 miles of ridge walking, the use trail reaches the summit of Villager Peak (5,756').

If you have time and energy remaining, continue north 3.6 miles to Rabbit Peak. The undulating ridge involves 2,000 feet of ascent and 1,100 feet of descent that must be regained on the return. The use trail can generally be followed through the pinyon pines and scrub oaks to the summit of Rabbit, but if you lose the trail, simply pick the path of least resistance along the ridge.

Return the way you came. The ridge forks 1.8 miles south of Villager Peak, at an elevation of 4,400 feet. Be sure to stay right; the tempting left ridge lures hikers into the steep upper reaches of Rattlesnake Canyon. Once you reach the desert, finding your way back through the washes and boulders can be somewhat tricky at night. If you don't have a GPS, head south. The lights of passing vehicles show where the road lies, and the trailhead is near the closest point on the road.

SIDE TRIP

If you have extra time before or after the trip, consider taking a drive to Fonts Point for a fantastic view over the colorful Borrego Badlands. The Fonts Point Road begins 2.4 miles west of the Villager Peak Trailhead (0.5 mile west of mile marker 30) on S22. It follows a sandy wash and a 4WD vehicle is helpful, but ordinary passenger cars can usually navigate the wash with careful driving. Follow the wash 4 miles to the overlook.

---

trip 12.21   Rabbit Peak from Clark Lake

Distance	15 miles (out-and-back)
Hiking Time	12–14 hours
Elevation Gain	6,100'
Difficulty	Very strenuous
Best Times	October–March
Agency	Santa Rosa and San Jacinto Mountains National Monument
Required Maps	USGS *Clark Lake, Clark Lake NE*, and *Rabbit Peak* 7.5'

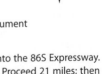

see map on p. 308

DIRECTIONS From the eastbound 10 Freeway in Indio, take Exit 145 south onto the 86S Expressway. Drive 35 miles, and turn right (west) onto the Borrego Salton Seaway (S22). Proceed 21 miles; then turn right (north) at the signed junction onto the Rockhouse Truck Trail; this point is 0.7 mile west of mile marker 27. This road becomes good dirt in 0.3 mile. In 1.2 miles, stay left at a fork. In 3.9 miles, park at a large turnout on the west side of the road just southeast of the Noll benchmark.

The western approach to Rabbit Peak from a point just north of Clark Lake is shorter but even steeper than the others. It crosses the Anza-Borrego Desert, which is justly famous for its remarkable cacti. Of all the trips in this book, this one offers the greatest opportunity to see all things sharp and pointy. Each plant occupies a distinctive habitat, and it's fascinating to watch the flora change as you climb. Clark Lake is named for Fred and Frank Clark, brothers who dug a well and established a cattle ranch at the playa here in 1891.

This trip is entirely cross-country, and not even cairns mark the trail. Carefully study your maps. Note the landmarks where you started near Coyote Mountain to assist your return, especially if the sun has gone down. A headlamp, GPS receiver, and spare batteries are helpful to find your way back to your vehicle at night.

From the parking area, look northeast and identify the major landmarks. Rabbit Peak is the highest point on the horizon. The long backbone of the Santa Rosa Mountains leads up from the south. The southernmost distinct high point is Villager Peak. Take a compass bearing of 50 degrees and identify a high point immediately north of Villager Peak. Walking on this bearing takes you to the south side of a ridge extending into the Clark Valley.

Follow the 50-degree bearing across the sandy desert floor past creosote bushes and pencil chollas. In 2.2 miles, reach the edge of the bajada, where walking becomes steeper and more difficult because of boulders and washes. Ocotillos, barrel cacti, and brittlebushes become common. Gain the toe of the ridge and pass the CUTE benchmark (1,337') in another 0.8 mile. Follow this poorly defined ridge up to Point 2719'. As you climb, look for teddy bear and valley chollas, beavertail cacti, small fishhook cacti, dense stands of desert agaves, and eventually junipers.

Continue northeastward up the ridge, which eventually narrows as it passes between two deep canyons. On this narrow isthmus are two small bivouac clearings with spectacular views. At this point, you've covered most of the distance but only half of the elevation gain. Follow the ridge northeastward toward the crest, gaining 2,300 feet in the next 0.8 mile. There is one short band of rock to negotiate, but most of the climbing is simply walking up steep dirt and easy talus. As you climb, reach zones of prickly pear cacti, Mojave yuccas, and nolinas.

Upon reaching the crest of the Santa Rosa Mountains at 5,800 feet, turn left (north). You may find a use trail, occasionally marked with cairns, on the east side of the crest. Pass over a small saddle; then make the final 800-foot ascent up slopes covered with pinyon pines and scrub oaks. Level out abruptly just south of the summit boulders.

Return the way you came or, with a car shuttle, take one of the other routes down (see Trips 12.19–20.) There are several clearings where people have camped on the hogsback east of the summit.

Clark Valley

Photo: Tony Condon

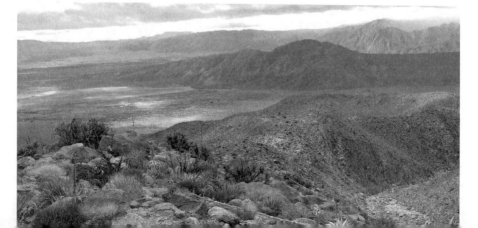

chapter 13

Colorado Desert

The Colorado Desert is a 7-million-acre portion of the Sonoran (Low) Desert encompassing most of southeastern California. The desert is bounded by the Peninsular Ranges on the west, the Gulf of Mexico on the south, the Colorado River to the east, and the Mojave Desert in Joshua Tree National Park and Mojave Trails National Monument to the north. This desert is lower and hotter than the Mojave, but benefits from the summer monsoon as well as winter rains, resulting in a unique biological community with many species found nowhere else.

This chapter covers a variety of areas in the Colorado Desert. The Mecca Hills Wilderness, on the northeast shore of the Salton Sea, has become extremely popular for its slot canyons and is covered in more depth below. Farther east along the 10 Freeway, the Orocopia, Chuckwalla, and Little Chuckwalla Mountains Wilderness areas see far fewer visitors but are worth a visit for their incredible desert vegetation and the historic Bradshaw Trail. The unique Stepladder and Mopah Mountains are even more remote but are well worth the effort to visit; they stand at the edge of the Mojave and Colorado Deserts but are covered in this chapter for simplicity.

Travelers with a 4WD vehicle will enjoy exploring the 65-mile Bradshaw Trail, which runs between the Salton Sea and Blythe past the Chuckwalla Mountains. This mostly graded dirt road was used during the gold rush from 1862 to 1877. Some notable sights include the dramatic Red Canyon Road, the Munz's cholla (California's largest cholla cactus, growing taller than a person and found only in this area), and the Hauser Geode Beds. Many gorgeous primitive camping options are available. Don't stray south of the road into the Chocolate Mountain Aerial Gunnery Range, where live bombing takes place.

Mecca Hills Wilderness

Fifteen miles southeast of Indio, near the north shore of the Salton Sea, the dusty town of Mecca sits amid lush fields of carrots, peppers, and artichokes; thick groves of oranges, pecans, and date palms; and row upon row of rich grape vines. The earliest people to inhabit Mecca were the Cahuilla Indians. Because they lived so far inland, these Desert Cahuilla had little contact with the colonizing Spanish who established missions in San Gabriel and San Diego.

Although the Desert Cahuilla had dug an extensive network of wells to support agriculture in the Coachella Valley, it wasn't until the late 19th century that Anglo-Americans considered developing the area for agriculture. In Mecca Hills' arid climate, it was the presence of water that led to the development of a railroad stop named Walters along the Yuma–Los Angeles rail line. Mecca's founder, R. Holtby Meyers, at the urging of his wife changed the town's name from Walters to Mecca because the desert climate and burgeoning date palm industry so closely resembled the famed holy city. Developers capitalized upon this connection and used the exotic images of Arabian oases to draw people to Mecca. It

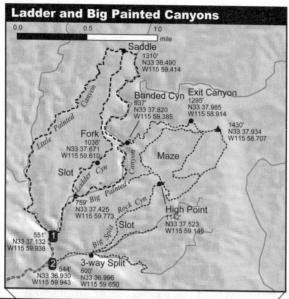

Ladder and Big Painted Canyons

0.0   0.5   1.0
mile

Saddle
1310'
N33 38.490
W115 59.414

Banded Cyn
937'
N33 37.820
W115 59.385

Exit Canyon
1295'
N33 37.985
W115 58.914

1430'
N33 37.934
W115 58.707

Fork
1036'
N33 37.671
W115 59.610

Little Painted Canyon

Slot

Ladder Cyn

Big Painted Canyon

Maze

759'
N33 37.425
W115 59.773

Rock Cyn

Slot

High Point
1142'
N33 37.523
W115 59.146

Big Split

1
551'
N33 37.132
W115 59.938

2
544'
N33 36.930
W115 59.943

3-way Split
600'
N33 36.996
W115 59.650

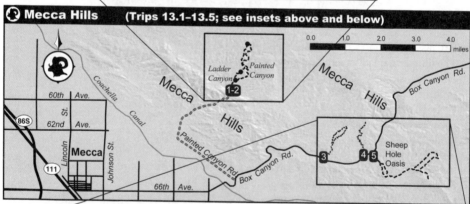

🧭 Mecca Hills   (Trips 13.1–13.5; see insets above and below)

0.0   1.0   2.0   3.0   4.0
miles

Mecca   Hills

Ladder Canyon   Painted Canyon

1-2

Mecca   Hills

Box Canyon Rd.

Coachella Canal

60th   Ave.

62nd   Ave.

86S

Lincoln St.

St.

Mecca

111

Johnson St.

66th   Ave.

Painted Canyon Rd.

Box Canyon Rd.

3

4 **5**

Sheep Hole Oasis

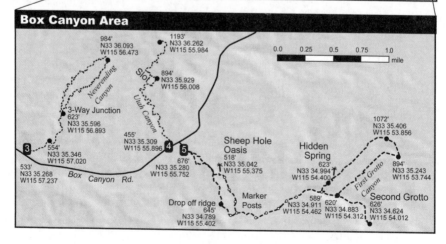

Box Canyon Area

984'
N33 36.093
W115 56.473

1193'
N33 36.262
W115 55.984

Slot

894'
N33 35.929
W115 56.008

Neverending Canyon

Utah Canyon

0.0   0.25   0.5   0.75   1.0
mile

3-Way Junction
623'
N33 35.596
W115 56.893

455'
N33 35.309
W115 55.896

4

5
676'
N33 35.280
W115 55.752

Sheep Hole Oasis
518'
N33 35.042
W115 55.375

Hidden Spring
623'
N33 34.994
W115 54.400

1072'
N33 35.406
W115 53.856

894'
N33 35.243
W115 53.744

First Grotto Canyon

Second Grotto
626'
N33 34.624
W115 54.012

3
554'
N33 35.346
W115 57.020

533'
N33 35.268
W115 57.237

Box Canyon Rd.

Drop off ridge
645'
N33 34.789
W115 55.402

Marker Posts

589'
N33 34.911
W115 54.462

620'
N33 34.883
W115 54.312

clearly worked; the area began to attract numerous family farmers. The completion of the Coachella branch of the All-American Canal in 1948 transformed small family farms into sprawling commercial fields.

Agriculture isn't the only lure in Mecca; the town lies beside a section of the San Andreas Fault zone that draws both professional and amateur seismologists. The seismic activity of the fault has thrust up a range of hills cut by a labyrinth of winding, narrow canyons, sandy washes, and caves, known locally as grottos. The violent upheavals that create the beautifully colored canyons of Mecca Hills Wilderness are the result of friction between the North American and Pacific plates along a spur of the San Andreas Fault. Much of the rock, which has been upturned and exposed by centuries of earthquakes, is more than 600 million years old. These rocks provide geologists and seismologists with valuable clues about the effects of temblors on the Earth's crust. Because of its unique geological formations, the United States Congress designated the Mecca Hills as a federally protected wilderness area in 1994.

Mecca Hills Wilderness is replete with flora and fauna that have adapted to the hostile desert environment. Yellow-bloomed palo verde trees densely populate the deep washes in the area. The Mecca aster, a violet-tinted flower resembling a daisy, grows only in this area and in Baja Mexico. Majestic ocotillos stand sentry on the tops of mesas and on the gentler slopes. Their branches typically burst forth in a flurry of vermilion blooms in late spring, adding yet another layer of rich color to the painted canyons in the area. The rare spotted bat, famous for having the largest ears of any North American bat, lives in Mecca Hills Wilderness. Desert tortoises and prairie falcons also call the area home. Bighorn sheep cross into Mecca Hills from the Orocopia Mountains looking for reliable sources of water at Sheep Hole Oasis and Hidden Spring Canyon.

Hikers in Ladder Canyon

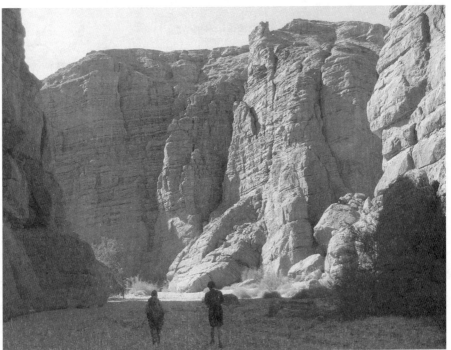

There are only a handful of established trails in Mecca Hills. This chapter describes the two most popular, Ladder Canyon and the Grottos, along with two cross-country routes exploring other spectacular canyons. However, inquisitive canyoneers will enjoy exploring the mazelike washes snaking through the colorful hills. Philip Ferranti's book *140 Great Hikes In and Near Palm Springs* is a handy reference for more canyon adventures in Mecca Hills.

The 1994 California Desert Protection Act designated much of the Mecca Hills as wilderness. No wilderness permit is required, but bicycles and motorized equipment are prohibited. Camping is allowed, with a maximum 14-day stay.

The pleasures of hiking in Mecca Hills include beautiful views of the Salton Sea. The Salton Sea lies in a basin more than 200 feet below sea level that was once connected to the Gulf of California until accumulated silt from the Colorado River cut the basin off and allowed the water to evaporate. The basin has refilled with water on many occasions. In the year 700, the Colorado River turned north and formed Lake Cahuilla, which lasted a thousand years, until the Colorado River changed direction once again, leaving the lake to evaporate over time. Subsequent outpourings of the river have occasionally created small salt lakes. In 1901, the California Development Company built a system of irrigation canals to divert the Colorado River to farm the Imperial Valley. A flood breached the canals, sending the river pouring into the basin for a year and a half. By the time the canals were repaired, the present Salton Sea had formed. It now covers 376 square miles and is the largest lake in California. The water evaporates rapidly but is replenished by agricultural runoff. This causes the salinity to steadily increase, imperiling the fish that live in the lake and the migrating birds that depend on the fish. On the other hand, if the lake were to completely dry up, it would leave a basin full of carcinogenic dust that would be whipped about the Coachella Valley by the strong desert winds. The Salton Sea clearly presents substantial environmental and economic challenges, but it's also a source of fascination and wonder. Consider detouring to visit it if you have extra time on a Mecca Hills trip.

trip 13.1 Ladder and Big Painted Canyons

see map on p. 314

Distance	4 miles (loop)
Hiking Time	3 hours
Elevation Gain	750'
Difficulty	Moderate
Trail Use	Good for kids
Best Times	October–April
Agency	BLM Palm Springs–South Coast Field Office
Recommended Maps	USGS *Mortmar* and *Cottonwood Basin* 7.5'

DIRECTIONS From the eastbound 10 Freeway (I-10) in Indio, take Exit 145 south onto the 86S Expressway and drive 10 miles to 62nd Avenue near the town of Mecca. Turn left on 62nd and drive east 2.2 miles to its end at Johnson Street; then turn right, proceed another 2 miles, and turn left onto 66th Avenue. The road name changes to Box Canyon Road and passes a signed turnoff for Painted Canyon Road. Turn left onto Painted Canyon Road. A sign indicates 4WD VEHICLES ONLY, but unless there have been heavy rains, the road is usually easily passable by low-clearance cars. Proceed 4.7 miles to the parking area in Painted Canyon. This parking area has seen a rash of vandalism, so be especially cautious not to leave valuables in your vehicle.

Ladder Canyon and Big Painted Canyon are highlights of the Mecca Hills and have become extremely popular. The path snakes through a steep-walled canyon, up several ladders, and through a narrow slot canyon. The ladders are usually maintained by volunteers, but assess the conditions for yourself before trusting your footing. Once you leave Ladder Canyon, you'll hike along the ridge, and find yourself surrounded by great views of Mecca Hills and

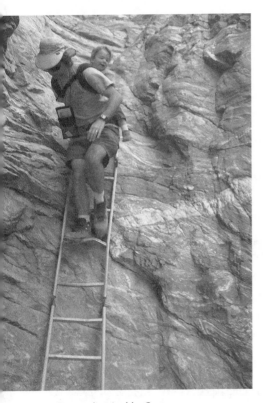

Descending Ladder Canyon
Photo: Cidney Scanlon

the Salton Sea. After the ridge, you'll descend into the aptly named Big Painted Canyon for your hike back.

From the parking area, begin hiking northeast up the wide canyon. Look for healthy palo verde trees, smoke trees, and ironwood growing in the bottom of the wash. In 0.5 mile, you'll come to a trail marker that points left toward the yawning boulder-strewn mouth of Ladder Canyon. Scramble into the side canyon and climb the ladders; then continue through the long narrow slot. After the canyon begins to open, stay right at a fork, 0.9 mile from the start. (Staying left here will also eventually get you to the ridge after a longer trek in the canyon.) In less than 0.1 mile, look for the first easy way to walk up the right slope of the canyon. Follow a use trail up the wall of the canyon; you'll need to negotiate a short but steep dirt wall partway up before you reach the ridge crest, 1 mile from the start.

Turn left at the top of the ridge and hike north. Enjoy the views into the canyons on both sides, but don't get too close to the edge because the sandy slopes drop off abruptly over tall cliffs. Soon you'll be able to see radio towers in the distance; follow the ridge toward these towers. In 1.1 miles, reach a saddle at the north end of the trail. To the left, you can see a dry waterfall near the head of Little Painted Canyon. The main trail turns right and drops into Big Painted Canyon.

Big Painted Canyon is a geologist's delight. Head down the canyon, staying right (downhill) at a junction. In 1.3 miles, watch for a ladder ascending the only notable tributary canyon on the left. The mouth of the canyon is brightly decorated with banded white, black, red, purple, and green rock. If you have time, this is a short and fun side trip with three more ladders to explore.

In another 0.3 mile, climb down another pair of ladders where the canyon narrows and drops. Reach the trail junction 0.5 mile farther, where you originally entered Ladder Canyon.

VARIATIONS

From the saddle at the north end of the ridge, you can also turn left and descend Little Painted Canyon. Though not as dramatic as Big Painted Canyon, it's a good option if you want to escape the crowds.

The white-and-black-banded tributary from Big Painted Canyon is also interesting to explore. After the three ladders, you can follow the sandy canyon floor for a mile, staying in the main canyon at all junctions. Eventually you can easily exit to the right near the head of the canyon and find cairns on a ridge. From the ridge, you can pick out an intricate and impossible-to-describe path over to Big Split Rock Canyon (Trip 13.2). Those exploring this route need a good sense of direction and a full day to explore. You stand a real chance of getting seriously lost—a GPS with a high-quality base map is very helpful, but it won't show all of the obstacles.

trip 13.2 Big Split Rock Canyon

Distance	2 miles (out-and-back)
Hiking Time	1.5 hours
Elevation Gain	400'
Difficulty	Moderate
Trail Use	Good for kids
Best Times	October–April
Agency	BLM Palm Springs–South Coast Field Office
Optional Map	USGS *Mortmar* 7.5'

see map on p. 314

DIRECTIONS From the eastbound 10 Freeway in Indio, take Exit 145 south onto the 86S Expressway and drive 10 miles to 62nd Avenue near the town of Mecca. Turn left on 62nd and drive east 2.2 miles to its end at Johnson Street; then turn right, proceed another 2 miles, and turn left onto 66th Avenue. The road name changes to Box Canyon Road and passes a signed turnoff for Painted Canyon Road. Turn left onto Painted Canyon Road. A sign indicates 4WD VEHICLES ONLY, but unless there have been heavy rains, the road is usually easily passable by low-clearance cars. Proceed 4.5 miles to the unmarked mouth of Big Split Rock Canyon on the right. If you reach the Ladder Canyon parking area at the end of the road, you've gone 0.2 mile too far.

Big Split Rock Canyon may well be the most fun slot canyon hike in California. Although shorter and less varied than the Ladder and Big Painted Canyons loop, it offers nonstop action in a very tight slot. This is a great hike for kids, but those who are broad shouldered may find it difficult, and claustrophobic hikers will not enjoy the trip. You'll likely be turning sideways in the squeeze section, so a small and light pack is preferable.

The sandy canyon is at first wide enough to support some vegetation, including smoke trees, cat's claw, creosote, and cheesebush. Watch for fascinating tapestries of dried mud on the walls. The canyon soon narrows and you hike up between the soaring walls. In 0.4 mile, come to a three-way split. The center canyon has a slot and the right canyon with the towering face leads to many branches, all of which are interesting to explore. But this trip takes the left canyon, the most action-packed of them all.

After passing a small slot canyon on the left, our canyon itself becomes a slot and passes under two sets of huge chockstones. In 0.3 mile, the tightest narrows begin. Squeeze through and find your way around various obstacles, including some chockstones that you must either climb over or crawl under.

A 10-foot dry waterfall marks a good turnaround point for those who don't like scrambling. However, you can continue into the upper canyon by stemming or chimneying up the short third-class pitch (possibly aided by a fixed rope). Various obstacles keep the hike interesting, and four ladders surmount more drop-offs. After the last and tallest ladder, the canyon widens again. You're now 1 mile into the canyon—a good turnaround point.

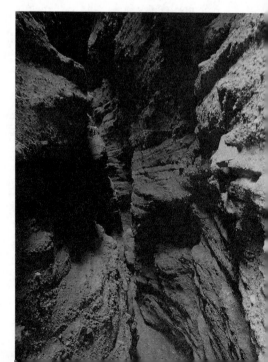

Narrows in Big Split Rock Canyon

VARIATION

Soon after the canyon widens, look for an arrow and/or cairn marking an exit from the canyon on the right. You can scramble up this gully and soon gain a ridge, following cairns 0.4 mile up to a local high point with views over the Mecca Hills. You could explore farther, but the terrain is very complicated, with sheer drops into impassable canyons, and it's easy to get disoriented up here.

trip 13.3   Never Ending Canyon

Distance	3.5 miles (loop)
Hiking Time	2 hours
Elevation Gain	500'
Difficulty	Easy
Trail Use	Dogs allowed
Best Times	October–April
Agency	BLM Palm Springs–South Coast Field Office
Recommended Map	USGS *Mortmar* 7.5'

see map on p. 314

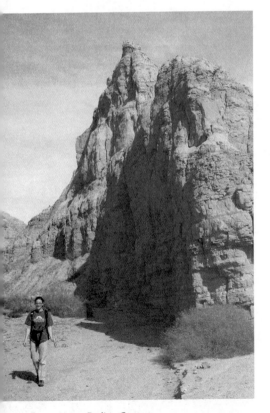

Never Ending Canyon

DIRECTIONS From the eastbound 10 Freeway in Indio, take Exit 145 south onto the 86S Expressway and drive 10 miles to 62nd Avenue near the town of Mecca. Turn left on 62nd and drive east 2.2 miles to its end at Johnson Street; then turn right, proceed another 2 miles, and turn left onto 66th Avenue. The road name changes to Box Canyon Road and passes a signed turnoff for Painted Canyon Road. Reset your odometer here. Drive on Box Canyon Road 3.4 miles past the Painted Canyon sign, and pull off onto a dirt road on the left. The beginning of the trail is marked by a line of large rocks blocking the dirt road.

Never Ending Canyon is a gorgeous hike between the colorful walls of the Mecca Hills. The hike leads you through two separate canyons, the second of which rejoins the first, leading you back to your car. You're rewarded by a breathtaking view when you reach the crest at the head of the canyons. Most of the hike follows trailless washes so cross-country navigation skills are necessary. Do not attempt this hike when rain threatens because the slot canyons are at risk of flash floods.

From your car, dirt roads lead east and north. Walk east down the larger road, passing the line of boulders. Follow the wash as it bends to the left near a damaged signpost, and enter the first canyon. Stay in the main wash when you encounter small side canyons. The trail will soon fork into two distinct trails on either side of a large formation near a rusty old icebox; continue into the left canyon. Follow this canyon and admire its unique sand and mud walls imprinted with fascinating water patterns. Soon you'll see an old, rusted car wreck. Avoid the smaller trail on the left, staying in the main canyon, and soon come to a three-way junction. Do not take the first smaller canyon on the far right. Instead continue your path in the middle canyon, winding around the right side of a prominent round-topped formation with interesting strata. (You'll return via the far left canyon.)

Stay in the larger canyon, avoiding smaller trails that branch off. Soon the canyon will narrow. Some fallen rocks and landslides may block your meandering path, but they're fun and easy to negotiate. Eventually the canyon opens up. At the head of the canyon ascend the rock field to the crest, and follow a path on the ridge crest outlined by rocks. The path leads to the left for a short distance to a cairn marking the high point. Take in the amazing view in all directions from the ridge.

Once you're finished enjoying the view, descend via the steep trail on the northwestern slope into the second canyon. The slope is easy enough to handle and free from imminent dangers, but it consists of loose dirt so take care not to slip. Follow the main wash downhill for the rest of your journey, taking time to admire the amazing walls that make Mecca Hills such a beautiful place to hike. You'll rejoin your previous trail at the three-way junction. From there retrace your steps back to your car.

---

trip 13.4 Utah Canyon

see map on p. 314

Distance	4 miles (out-and-back)
Hiking Time	2 hours
Elevation Gain	500'
Difficulty	Easy
Trail Use	Dogs allowed
Best Times	October–April
Agency	BLM Palm Springs–South Coast Field Office
Recommended Map	USGS *Mortmar* 7.5'

DIRECTIONS From the eastbound 10 Freeway in Indio, take Exit 145 south onto the 86S Expressway and drive 10 miles to 62nd Avenue near the town of Mecca. Turn left on 62nd and drive east 2.2 miles to its end at Johnson Street; then turn right, proceed another 2 miles, and turn left onto 66th Avenue. The road name changes to Box Canyon Road and passes a signed turnoff for Painted Canyon Road. Reset your odometer here. Drive on Box Canyon Road 4.9 miles past the Painted Canyon sign to the easy-to-overlook mouth of a canyon on the north, and park on the shoulder of the road. If you reach the Sheep Hole Oasis Trailhead marker on the south, you've gone 0.1 mile too far.

U tah Canyon, named for its resemblance to the colorful canyons of southern Utah, features brilliant rocks and narrow, winding passages. This hike is best done in the early morning or late afternoon when the sun highlights the intense reds, pinks, oranges, and mauves of the canyon walls.

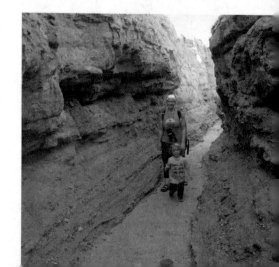

The Narrows in Utah Canyon

Hike north up a wide, sandy wash lined with sprawling mesquite and palo verde trees. The wash promptly branches; stay to the left. As you hike up the wash, the canyon narrows considerably. Creosote bushes spread their lanky branches lazily through the wash, often blocking the trail. Negotiate around them as you journey up the canyon, enjoying the twists and turns of the trail.

In 0.5 mile, the trail curves around an impressive mudfall (like rockfall, but made of dried mud). In another 0.7 mile, the canyon forks again. Bear left into a canyon that soon becomes a slot just wide enough for two to walk abreast. Beyond the narrows, the canyon reopens. Spindly stands of ocotillo grace the rocky slopes. Stay in the main wash as you pass several side canyons. In 0.4 mile, veer left at a major fork. The canyon soon ends in a small valley. Follow the slopes up to the ridge for a bird's-eye view of the multihued canyon systems winding down to the Salton Sea.

Return the way you came.

trip 13.5   The Grottos

Distance	7 miles (semiloop)
Hiking Time	5 hours
Elevation Gain	1,500'
Difficulty	Moderate
Trail Use	Dogs allowed
Best Times	October–April
Agency	BLM Palm Springs–South Coast Field Office
Recommended Map	USGS *Mortmar* 7.5'

see map on p. 314

DIRECTIONS From the eastbound 10 Freeway in Indio, take Exit 145 south onto the 86S Expressway and drive 10 miles to 62nd Avenue near the town of Mecca. Turn left on 62nd and drive east 2.2 miles to its end at Johnson Street; then turn right, proceed another 2 miles, and turn left onto 66th Avenue. The road name changes to Box Canyon Road and passes a signed turnoff for Painted Canyon Road. Reset your odometer here. Continue 5 miles to the signed Sheep Hole Oasis Trailhead, on the right.

The Grottos are two slot canyons nestled in the outlandishly colorful Mecca Hills. They've filled with giant boulders to form remarkable cave systems. Two palm oases bring further wonder to this unusual trip. If your time is limited, you can shorten the trip by visiting only one of the Grottos. Be sure to bring a flashlight; a helmet is also helpful. The terrain is complicated and is crisscrossed with a warren of trails, so a map and good navigational skills are essential. The main trail is almost always well used, so if the path becomes faint, you're probably on the wrong trail.

From the parking area, the Hidden Spring Trail leads into the canyon. You'll soon reach a fork; stay left, and follow the trail straight up the ridge to reach a hilltop with panoramic views of the Mecca Hills, the Salton Sea, and the Santa Rosa Mountains, 0.25 mile

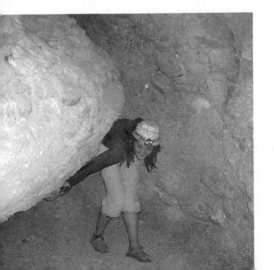

Second Grotto: not for the claustrophobic

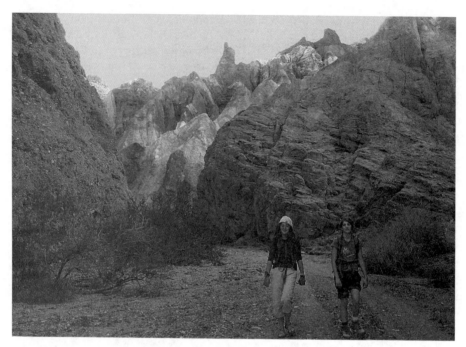

Hidden Spring Canyon below Second Grotto

from the start. Turn left and follow the crest of the ridge. You'll see the Sheep Hole Oasis below on your left, but pass the side trail leading down and continue south along the ridge until the main trail drops eastward into the canyon, 0.8 mile from the start. Cross the wash to a post; then continue east up a small side canyon to the top of a rise with another trail junction. Descend east into the large Hidden Spring Canyon. A series of posts marks the route northeastward up the sandy canyon floor. The canyon narrows and the walls become vertical; then they change into exotic purple, brown, and tan colors. The first canyon on your left after entering the narrows is home to Hidden Spring and is marked with a post. You'll later come down the canyon leading from Hidden Spring and return to this spot. The second canyon on the left is the entrance to the First Grotto, marked by a 6-foot-tall tree stump. You'll also return to this spot, so be sure that you can recognize it.

Continue east and then south up the main canyon to the very end, passing spires and battlements of green, pink, purple, red, and yellow sedimentary rock. Then turn left and enter a narrow slot canyon that's home to the Second Grotto. Explore the cave system until it ends at a 15-foot wall. Climbers will enjoy scrambling up the fourth-class conglomerate rock to the top, but our hike returns the way you came. Retrace your steps to the First Grotto Canyon.

Ascend First Grotto Canyon 0.4 mile until it becomes choked with boulders. Climb into their maw and pick your way through the cave system. Cross over to the left side of the canyon, walk a wooden plank, and descend into the tunnel. If the scrambling becomes difficult, you've gone off-route. After navigating through three stretches of caves, reach the upper portion of the canyon. Look for a steep jeep road cut through the canyon wall on the left. Ascend on the road until it levels out at a four-way junction; then turn left and follow the jeep trail as it crosses a wash and climbs another very steep hill. Beyond the hill, leave the jeep road at a faint trail leading left at a cairn. The trail heads west, then traverses a ridge southwest until the Hidden Spring Oasis comes into view on the left. As the ridge narrows to a knife-edge, follow a steep trail down to the oasis. After enjoying the palms, work your way down the narrow canyon back to the main Hidden Spring Canyon Trail at the post you passed earlier.

Turn right and retrace your steps out of the canyon, down the wide wash, and over the small rise. You may continue back up the ridge the way you came, or you may follow posts to Sheep Hole Oasis. At the oasis, beyond the topmost palm, a steep path climbs the left wall of the canyon to the ridgetop and rejoins the main trail.

trip 13.6   Black Butte

Distance	3 miles (out-and-back)
Hiking Time	2.5 hours
Elevation Gain	1,600'
Difficulty	Moderate
Best Times	October–April
Agency	BLM Palm Springs–South Coast Field Office
Required Map	USGS *Pilot Mountain* 7.5'

DIRECTIONS A 4WD vehicle is strongly recommended for this trip because of sand, steep berms, and occasional obstacles on the long dirt roads. From the 10 Freeway, take Exit 182 southeast onto fair dirt Red Cloud Mine Road. In 2 miles, come to a T-junction with Summit Road by train tracks. Turn left and, in 0.1 mile, stay left again to follow the power lines where Red Cloud Mine Road forks off Summit Road. In 1.8 miles, turn right onto the signed Gas Line Road, and continue following the power lines 7.8 miles. Turn left onto the Bradshaw Trail. Go 6.9 miles; then turn left onto a lightly used old mining road signed CM480. (This track is 0.4 mile east of an old structure along the south side of the Bradshaw Trail.) In 2.5 miles, reach a junction, where light-duty vehicles should park. Sturdy 4WD vehicles willing to risk scratched paint can turn right, cross a wash, and continue 1.0 mile to a signed junction with faint Road 481. Go straight and, in 0.3 mile, stay right at a fork; in another 0.3 mile, park at a wide spot before you enter a wash.

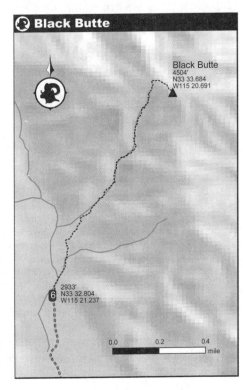

Black Butte

Black Butte
4504'
N33 33.684
W115 20.691

6 2933'
N33 32.804
W115 21.237

0.0   0.2   0.4
mile

Black Butte (4,504') is the high point of the Chuckwalla Mountains. The climb itself is short and not especially noteworthy save for the summit views, but this part of the Colorado Desert is remarkable and well worth the long drive. The drive passes through splendid fields of teddy bear cholla, barrel cactus, ocotillo, and Mojave yucca. Desert tortoise and bighorn sheep roam the wilderness. Some of the metamorphic rocks date back to Precambrian times. The peak is often done in combination with Chuckwalla Mountain (see Trip 13.7), making for a satisfying day. Only about a half-dozen parties sign the summit registers of these lonely peaks each year.

From the parking area, the peak is clearly visible on a bearing of 30 degrees, and a prominent gully leads up the mountain.

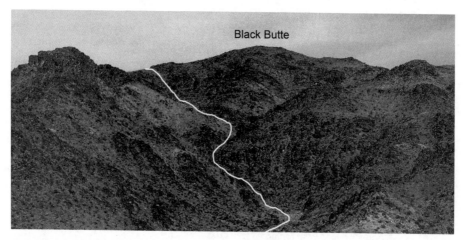

Black Butte

Black Butte summit route

Hike north into the gully and follow it up. In 0.7 mile, the gully narrows. Pick your way past nolinas and cactus up the banded metamorphic rock laced with feldspar crystals, ascending an easy dry waterfall. When the gully widens again and forks, the easiest route is up the leftmost fork to the ridgeline, where you can turn right and walk the last brief stretch to the summit.

Black Butte's summit offers outstanding views over the rugged Chuckwalla Mountains Wilderness to the Little San Bernardino Mountains, San Gorgonio, San Jacinto, the Orocopia Mountains Wilderness, the Santa Rosa Mountains, and the Salton Sea beyond the Chocolate Mountain bombing range.

trip 13.7   Chuckwalla Mountain

Distance	2.8 miles (out-and-back)
Hiking Time	2.5 hours
Elevation Gain	1,600'
Difficulty	Moderate
Best Times	October–April
Agency	BLM Palm Springs–South Coast Field Office
Required Map	USGS *Chuckwalla Spring* 7.5'

DIRECTIONS A high-clearance vehicle is required, and 2WD vehicles should be especially cautious of numerous sandy stretches. If you're visiting this peak by itself, the easiest access is from the 10 Freeway, 9.3 miles east of Desert Center. Take Exit 201 for Corn Springs Road and follow paved Chuckwalla Valley Road south-southeast 13 miles. Turn right (south) on good but sandy dirt Graham Pass Road, and drive 15.4 miles to a signed junction with a lightly used mining road signed 588. Take this road west 1.4 miles to a turnout just before the road veers left and descends into a wash. Park here.

If you're doing this hike in combination with Black Butte (see previous hike), take the road from Black Butte back to the Bradshaw Trail; then drive east on the Bradshaw Trail 14.7 miles to signed Graham Pass Road. Go north 0.3 mile and turn left onto a lightly used mining road signed 588, where you join the aforementioned directions.

Chuckwalla Mountain (3,446'), oddly enough, is the high point of the Little Chuckwalla Mountains, not of the nearby Chuckwalla Mountains. The peak looks rugged, but the climb is straightforward, with simple talus-hopping and the usual dodging of desert vegetation. It's especially recommended in combination with Black Butte (see Trip 13.6).

A highlight of the drive between the two hikes is the Munz's cholla cactus, a striking treelike species found on the Chuckwalla Bench and nowhere else. It has the smallest range of any cholla species in California. Some botanists believe the Munz's cholla is a hybrid resulting from a cross between teddy bear and silver cholla, both of which grow in the area, but it's easily recognized because it often grows to 6 feet in height, and around Chuckwalla Well much taller specimens are found. The cholla is named for Philip Munz, California's leading 20th-century desert botanist, who was

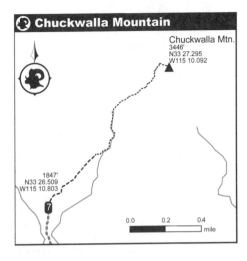

also the founding director of the Rancho Santa Ana Botanic Garden in Claremont.

The peak is named for chuckwalla lizards, a wide-bodied lizard that grows to more than a foot in length. When threatened, chuckwallas wedge themselves deep in rock crevices and inflate their lungs to avoid removal. Native Americans used a pointed stick to pop the lizard and collect it for food.

From the parking area, two abandoned mining roads lead northeast toward the peak. Take the left of the two and follow it up the alluvial fan. When the road peters out in 0.4 mile near the base of the mountain, walk a few paces right to enter the prominent wash that cuts the southwest face of the peak. Hike up the wash. Notice how the granite rocks on the slopes above are covered in thick red desert varnish, while the rocks in the wash have been weathered bare. In the late winter and spring, the desert lavender and brittlebush bloom. When the wash divides near a cluster of nolina, stay left. As you approach the summit ridge, the wash becomes ill-defined; pick your favorite way up to the ridge, and turn right and finish the short walk to the summit.

Chuckwalla Mountain summit route

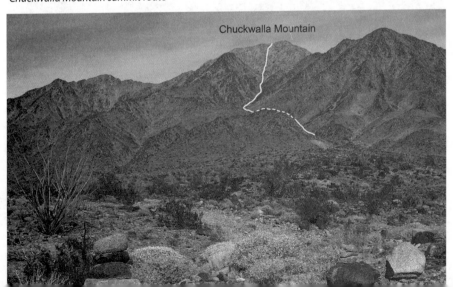

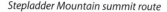

trip 13.8 Stepladder Mountain

Distance	10 miles (out-and-back)
Hiking Time	6 hours
Elevation Gain	1,300'
Difficulty	Strenuous
Best Times	October–April
Agency	BLM Needles Field Office
Required Map	USGS *Stepladder Mountains* 7.5'

DIRECTIONS This drive requires a 4WD vehicle, and you can expect scratches on your paint. From Vidal Junction, turn north onto US 95. Drive 36 miles to a point 0.7 mile north of mile marker 095 SBD 45, and turn left onto the NS202 gas pipeline road. The first part of this road has deep sand, but the rest is graded dirt. In 8.8 miles, pass high-voltage transmission lines and the NS056 Hightower service road. In another 0.5 mile, a post on the left marks the very faint BLM Road 254. Make a hard left and briefly follow the track down a wash before it veers right (south) into the desert. Take this poor, slow road 5.6 miles to the Stepladder Mountains Wilderness boundary, expecting possible vehicle scratches from close-growing vegetation. The Bureau of Land Management has moved this boundary marker in the past and might move it again. The drive from the highway will take about 1.5 hours.

If you're seeking a truly remote desert peak in the Inland Empire, you'll be hard-pressed to find a more interesting one than Stepladder Mountain (2,927'). The Stepladder Mountains are a low but rugged range whose highest peaks are composed of volcanic breccia. This trip climbs the high point, near the north end of the range. From a distance, the summit looks as if it might require technical climbing, but a handy system of ledges neatly zigzags up so that you scarcely need to remove your hands from your pockets.

One of the challenges of this trip may be finding your way back to your vehicle, which is hard to see from a distance in this featureless desert. A GPS is convenient, but if you prefer map and compass, record bearings to at least two prominent landmarks before you depart so that you can triangulate your return.

Stepladder Mountain summit route

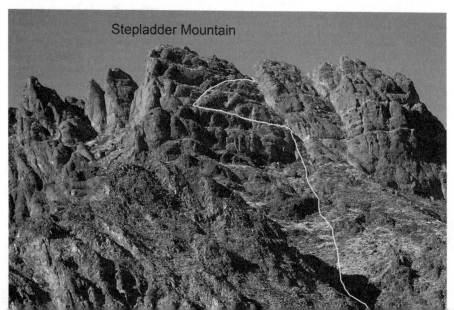

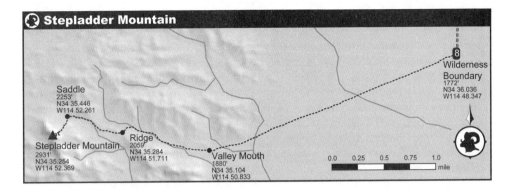

Stepladder Mountain

Saddle
2253'
N34 35.446
W114 52.261

Wilderness
Boundary
1772'
N34 36.036
W114 48.347

Stepladder Mountain
2931'
N34 35.254
W114 52.369

Ridge
2059'
N34 35.284
W114 51.711

Valley Mouth
1880'
N34 35.104
W114 50.833

0.0   0.25   0.5   0.75   1.0
mile

Look west and identify Stepladder Mountain on the skyline. The peak has two summits separated by a notch, and this trip climbs the left (southern) one, which is the highest. A row of volcanic hills stands between you and the mountain. Pick out the opening of a valley at the left end, by which you'll be able to work your way behind the hills and approach Stepladder. Hike toward the mouth of this valley on a bearing of 240 degrees, walking across flat bajada covered with creosote bushes, impressive buckhorn cholla cactus, and Mojave yucca. In places, you'll encounter ocotillo and beavertail, and barrel, and pencil cholla cactus.

In 2.8 miles, reach the mouth of the valley near a low hill labeled Point 595. After crossing lesser washes, find your way into the main wash heading west-northwest up the broad valley. The vegetation in the wash changes to brittlebush, cat's claw, desert lavender, and cheesebush, but the walking remains easy. The elusive desert tortoise inhabits this wilderness. In 1.0 mile, reach the first place where you could easily climb out of the left side of the valley. This spot is just before two small volcanic knobs. Climb over the low ridge and get a good look at your route ahead. The peak is directly to the west, and has two major clefts in the face. The left one leads to a notch between the north and south peaks. Your goal is to reach this notch; it's much easier than it looks. Once you've studied the peak, drop into the next valley to the west, which is situated at the foot of Stepladder.

Stepladder Mountain—note the approach valley to the left.

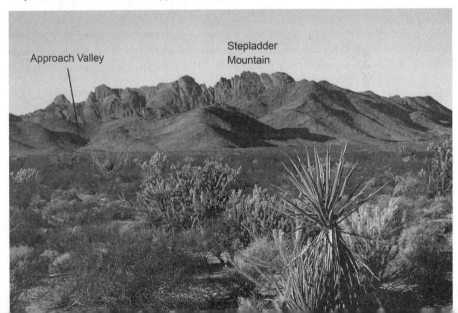

Approach Valley

Stepladder Mountain

The easiest way onto the mountain is to follow the wash up this second valley 0.7 mile to the saddle at its head, a quarter mile northeast of Stepladder Mountains. From here, turn left and pick your way up and to the left to get through a low row of cliffs; then continue up loose slopes to the cleft (**N34° 35.295' W114° 52.345'; 2,689'**). Watch for translucent white chalcedony rose crystals as you go (see Trip 13.9). The rock on the upper mountain is volcanic breccia, a type of conglomerate formed when volcanic rock fragments are cemented together with volcanic ash. The fragments range in size from limes to watermelons. Watch your holds because the ash matrix can be unstable. This portion of the mountain is reminiscent of the Crestone Range in Colorado.

The first 50 feet of the climb is easy, but as soon as it starts to look difficult, you'll see a broad ledge on the face to the left (**N34° 35.287' W114° 52.364'; 2,775'**). Walk south on this ledge almost to the south end of the face; then switchback and work your way back to the right on a higher ledge that brings you directly to the notch between the peaks (**N34° 35.281' 114° 52.378'; 2,888'**). Follow the easy ridge south to the summit. The views south over the serrated Stepladder Mountains to the Mopah Peaks is especially impressive.

trip 13.9 Mopah Point

Distance	8 miles (out-and-back)
Hiking Time	6 hours
Elevation Gain	2,000'
Difficulty	Strenuous
Best Times	October–April
Agency	BLM Needles Field Office
Required Maps	USGS *Mopah Peaks* and *Savahia Peak SW* 7.5'

DIRECTIONS From Vidal Junction, go north 12.3 miles on US 95 to a point 0.9 mile north of mile marker 095 SBD 21. Turn left onto BLM Road NS634. The road is normally passable by 2WD vehicles for the first 4.0 miles. 2WD vehicles should park at a large clearing with good camping options. High-clearance 4WD vehicles may continue across a sandy and rocky wash to another parking area at the well-marked wilderness boundary in 0.4 mile.

Mopah Point (3,530') is one of the most interesting summits in the Mojave Desert. Formed of weather-resistant rhyodacite, the peak and its neighbor Umpah are remnant plugs of Miocene-era volcanoes. Mopah has but one weakness in its 800-foot sheer cliffs, and this trip threads a path up this weakness. The route has some airy third class where many climbers will desire a rope. Highly prized by desert mountaineers, the peak nevertheless sees only about six groups a year signing the summit register. The peak is not labeled on the topographic map but is marked 1,076 (elevation in meters). It has two summits; this trip leads to the northern summit, which is slightly higher. The Mopah Peaks are a subrange of the Turtle Mountains and are part of the Turtle Mountains Wilderness.

The upper part of Mopah Point is visible from the trailhead, rising out of the desert like a clenched fist. From the wilderness boundary, walk west along a closed dirt road. The desolate desert offers little but creosote

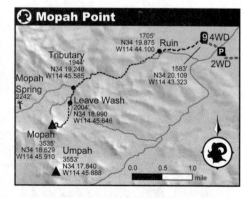

bushes and volcanic shrapnel. If you step off the road, you're likely to discover white translucent rocks with a ropey texture. These chalcedony roses are quartz crystals formed by volcanic processes, and the Mopah Range is one of the best places in the world to see them. Keen-eyed explorers may also discover jasper and agates. Remember that you're in a wilderness area; take only pictures, and leave the rocks for future explorers to enjoy.

In 0.9 mile, the road ends at a two-walled ruin at the mouth of a canyon. Continue southwest into the canyon, at first on the north edge, and soon in the broad sandy wash. Walking is easy as you pass typical desert vegetation including palo verde, cat's claw acacia, brittlebush, desert lavender, and cheesebush. Inspect the eroded walls to see the process of conglomerate rock formation in progress. Some holes in the conglomerate are homes to pack rats. Desert tortoises, bighorn sheep, mountain lions, and tarantulas are some of the other charismatic critters that a lucky hiker might observe here. Pass between recent basalt flows and then around the nose of a volcanic ridge that obscures the view of Mopah. Shortly beyond, at a spot 2.0 miles from the road end and just northwest of Hill 660+ m, watch for the first tributary wash on the south, concealed behind a grove of palo verde trees.

Take this tributary southwest about 0.3 mile; then climb out on the west side and survey the path ahead. The only weakness in Mopah's sheer walls is near the left skyline. Pick a path south-southwest toward this weakness, climbing steeply near the end. You might find ducks marking a route close to the base of the cliffs, but a lower route offers easier footing and less cat's claw. In 1.1 miles, pass through a notch at the weak area (**N34° 18.594' W114° 45.785';**

The forbidding face of Mopah Point

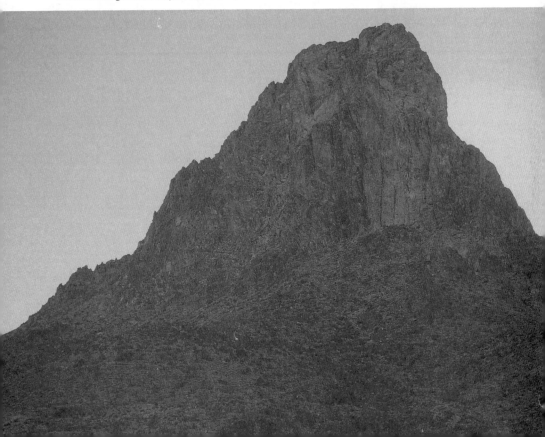

2,618'). From here up, watch for occasional ducks marking the climber's route, which takes the only easy path up the mountain.

Ahead, the slope opens into a broad chute. Work your way up and left to a second weakness by which you can surmount the lower cliff band (**N34° 18.589' W114° 45.872'; 3,090'**). Then follow a wide nolina-dotted shelf up and to the right until it ends beneath a roof (**N34° 18.615' W114° 45.861'; 3,192'**). Bypass the roof on the right via a 12-foot pitch of easy third-class climbing; then scramble up easier slopes. Just above an inconveniently situated cat's claw bush, take the left-most chute heading toward the skyline. Two more nolinas grow in the lower part of the chute. It's possible to climb the chute 50 feet to the skyline notch, but the upper third is rotten third-class rock, so you're better off taking the obvious exit halfway up on the right and winding your way around to meet the chute route on the back side of the ridge.

The next portion is the crux of the route. From a small platform (**N34° 18.645' W114° 45.869'; 3,371'**), climb a steep and exposed 8-foot wall. Rated class three, it's still sufficiently tricky and exposed that many climbers will want a rope, especially on the descent. With the difficulties now behind you, follow an easy ledge to the right, then up and left to the summit. Memorize the landmarks as you go, because it can be hard to find the right way back down.

Looking northwest from the summit, you'll see Mopah Spring near the head of the main canyon that you ascended. The oasis at this spring hosts the northernmost grove of California fan palms, and is an important watering hole for the flock of bighorn sheep that roam the Turtle Mountains Wilderness.

VARIATION

Umpah Point (3,553'/1,083 m), just to the south, is the true high point of the Mopah Range. This impressive pyramid would be a popular destination were it not for the even more remarkable Mopah. Some vigorous parties climb both in one day via a third-class route on the north face.

chapter 14

Desert Preserves

In recent years, the population explosion in Southern California has led to tremendous development in once-quiet communities near Banning Pass. Development has threatened to partition the desert and mountains into "islands" that disrupt traditional patterns of wildlife movement. The natural windblown movement of sand has also been disturbed by construction and off-road vehicles, threatening the fragile sand dune habitats. In response to these problems, a number of homegrown and national conservation groups have teamed with government agencies to purchase and preserve critical habitat. The groups have built fine trail systems so that hikers can enjoy these special places. This chapter describes trips in several of these preserves.

Big Morongo Canyon Preserve

Big Morongo Canyon, surrounded by cactus-studded desert, is the unlikely site of a lush wetland. Snowmelt from the San Bernardino Mountains flows underground through sandy soils until it encounters an earthquake fault in Big Morongo Canyon. The impermeable rock in the fault directs the water to the surface, creating an array of springs that support a marsh and grove of cottonwoods. Bighorn sheep and many other animals are drawn to the area for water and food, especially in the dry season. Birders from around the world flock to the preserve seeking rare species, especially during spring and fall migration. There are regularly scheduled bird walks; check bigmorongo.org for a calendar of events. The land around the preserve was seized from the Morongo band of the Serrano Indians in 1846, and was used for ranching until 1968, when 80 acres were acquired by The Nature Conservancy. Now it encompasses 31,000 acres and is administered by the Bureau of Land Management as an Area of Critical Environmental Concern and as part of Sand to Snow National Monument.

Coachella Valley Preserve

The 17,000-acre Coachella Valley Preserve, located northeast of Palm Springs and south of Joshua Tree, was established in 1986 to protect the sand dune habitat of the endangered Coachella Valley fringe-toed lizard. The preserve is managed by the non-profit Center for Natural Lands Management in partnership with the public agencies that own land on the preserve. The Coachella Valley Preserve's Visitors' Center is located on the San Andreas Fault. The crushed rock and clay in the fault are nearly impermeable to groundwater, directing the water to the surface and resulting in a series of springs that support spectacular palm oases in the midst of the parched desert. Unlike some other local palm oases that are fed by creeks, the numerous oases on the Coachella Valley Preserve are fed only from these earthquake seeps.

Before pioneers arrived in the Palm Springs area, the Coachella Valley was covered with nearly 100 square miles of sand dunes. The Coachella Valley fringe-toed lizard is specially adapted to sand dune habitat, with snowshoelike hind toes that give traction in the shifting sand. The lizard uses its shovel-like snout to burrow into the sand to avoid the extreme summer heat and to elude predators. In fact, the lizard has more adaptations than any other known species for survival in this extreme environment, where surface temperatures can reach 120°–140°F in the heat of the summer. Development projects and off-road vehicles have wiped out 95% of the lizard's dune habitat. The Coachella Valley Preserve system contains the Thousand Palms Oasis Preserve, along with two smaller satellite preserves, Whitewater and Edom Hill/Willow Hole. The preserve system protects some of the remaining dunes as well as the precious "sand source" areas of the hills that replenish the sand in the dune systems.

The Coachella Valley Preserve Visitors' Center is located in the Palm House in the second-largest grove of palms in the valley, known as the Thousand Palms Grove. For many years, the writer and naturalist Paul Wilhelm lived at this oasis. At the center, you can pick up a free brochure with map of the area, and can get hiking advice from the volunteer staff. More than 28 miles of hiking trails radiate through the desert to the other palm oases.

The preserve hours vary seasonally and the visitor center is closed in the summer. Docents offer guided hikes October–March. To protect the habitat, pets, camping, and smoking are prohibited. Stay on marked trails, and please don't stray into sensitive sand dunes or wetlands.

The Wildlands Conservancy

The Wildlands Conservancy, founded in 1995, has developed a grand vision of conservation and has been remarkably effective at carrying it out. By strategically purchasing private inholdings and other blocks at the edge of public lands, the conservancy has created an undeveloped corridor from San Gorgonio Mountain to Joshua Tree National Park. Some of its most notable properties include the 37,000-acre system of the Pioneertown Mountains Preserve, the Oak Glen Preserve, the Mission Creek Preserve, and the Whitewater Preserve.

A culmination of this effort was President Obama's designation of Sand to Snow National Monument in 2016, which links the San Gorgonio Wilderness and southeastern

Whitewater Canyon Ranger Station   Photo: Wildlands Conservancy staff

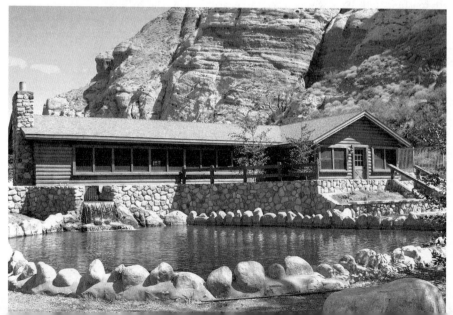

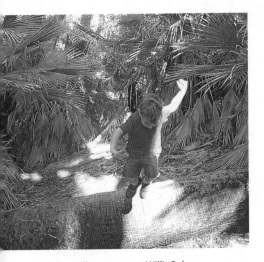

San Bernardino Mountains to the western edge of Joshua Tree National Park. The Conservancy contributed 60,000 acres to the new monument.

In 2001, the Conservancy also funded protection of 560,000 acres of desert farther east that are now part of Mojave National Preserve, Joshua Tree National Park, Mojave Trails National Monument, and various wilderness areas; many hikes in these areas are described in later chapters.

*Boundless energy at Willis Palms
(see Trip 14.3)*

trip 14.1   McCallum Nature Trail

Distance	2 miles (out-and-back)
Hiking Time	1 hour
Elevation Gain	100'
Difficulty	Easy
Trail Use	Good for kids
Best Times	October–March
Agency	Coachella Valley Preserve
Recommended Map	*Coachella Valley Preserve* map

see map on next page

DIRECTIONS From the 10 Freeway (I-10), take Exit 131 for Ramon Road and drive east (on the north side of the freeway) 4.5 miles. Turn left onto Thousand Palms Canyon Road and proceed 2.1 miles to the Coachella Valley Preserve visitor-center parking area, on the left.

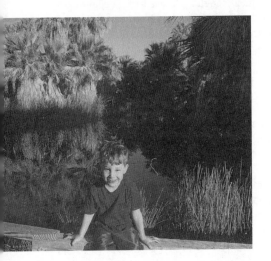

This self-guided nature walk brings you through the Thousand Palms Oasis Preserve, across the San Andreas Fault, and reaches the McCallum Grove of palms, where there is a pond and large sand dune. The trail departs from the Palm House Visitor Center in the midst of the Thousand Palms Oasis Preserve. This oasis has one of the world's largest groves of California fan palms (*Washingtonia filifera*), the only palm native to California. The palms grow to 60 feet and

Pond at McCallum Grove

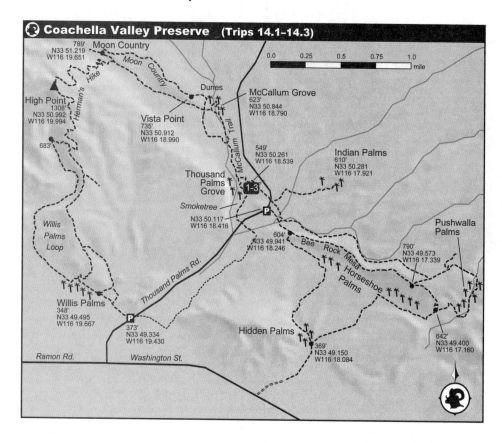

Coachella Valley Preserve (Trips 14.1–14.3)

live for about 250 years. Their fruit, produced in the spring, is important to birds and other animals in the oasis.

The brochure at the visitor center includes a map and guide to the sights along the way.

From the parking area, walk into the oasis and stop at the Palm House to pick up a map and check out the information on display. Continue through the grove to the beginning of the McCallum Trail, which crosses some wetlands on a boardwalk.

The trail then departs the north side of the grove and follows the edge of the wetlands through the desert. The Coachella Valley is shielded from moist air by the San Bernardino and San Jacinto Mountains, so it normally receives only 4–5 inches of rain per year. However, the rainfall is irregular; some years have virtually none, while others have brief but intense rains that cause flash flooding. You'll cross the San Andreas Fault, California's infamous earthquake fault. The fault is responsible for pushing up many of the bluffs and hills in this area. The unique geology of the fault zone keeps the water close to the surface, supporting numerous palm oases in the preserve.

In 0.2 mile from the start, a signed trail forks off to the right, leading directly back to the parking area. In another 0.3 mile, pass some private ranch houses. Stay on the trail, taking care not to disturb the residents. In another 0.3 mile, reach the south end of the McCallum Grove. The trail forks here and makes a loop. Take the right fork directly into the grove. Explore the palms, the pond, and the nearby sand dunes.

The oasis and pond are nourished by a spring. The pond is home to the desert pupfish, an endangered minnow-like fish adapted to shallow, salty desert pools. The pupfish burrows into the bottom of the pool and lies dormant during the cold winter; it becomes active in the spring and mates in the summer. The pupfish's habitat has been nearly eliminated through development, pollution, and the introduction of exotic species. Keep an eye out for the fish in the spring, but don't feed or disturb it. The sand dunes north of the oasis are built by strong winds that carry grains of sand for long distances. As the wind patterns shift and subside, the grains are deposited to form large piles. This preserve has been established to protect the dunes and fringe-toed lizard, so walking on the dunes is prohibited.

At the far end of the McCallum Grove, the trail loops around to return along the west edge of the grove. In 0.1 mile, pass a signed turnoff for Moon Country and the Vista Point (see Trip 14.3). This optional loop along a desolate ridge and back through a wash adds 2 miles to the hike and is recommended only on a cool day.

When you've finished exploring, return to the Thousand Palms Oasis Preserve. You can take a shortcut back to the parking area at the marked trail near interpretive post 5 shortly before you reach the oasis.

trip 14.2 Pushwalla, Horseshoe, and Hidden Palms Loop

Distance	6 miles (loop)
Hiking Time	4 hours
Elevation Gain	1,000'
Difficulty	Moderate
Best Times	October–March
Agency	Coachella Valley Preserve
Recommended Map	*Coachella Valley Preserve* map

DIRECTIONS From the 10 Freeway, take Exit 131 for Ramon Road and drive east (on the north side of the freeway) 4.5 miles. Turn left onto Thousand Palms Canyon Road and proceed 2.1 miles to the visitor-center parking area, on the left. If you don't plan to stop at the visitor center for a map, you can save a little walking by parking 0.3 mile back down Thousand Palms Canyon Road at a turnout on the east side.

Hikers on the ridge above Horseshoe Palms Grove

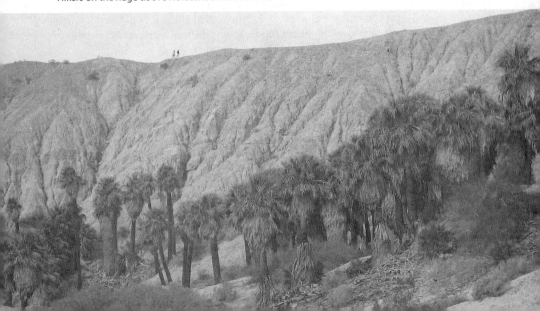

This loop hike offers a tour of the southeastern part of the Coachella Valley Preserve featuring three separate palm groves and expansive views from a narrow ridge. The diversity of scenery makes this my favorite moderate hike in the preserve. The Pushwalla Oasis is in a narrow canyon, so avoid this trip on rare rainy days when flash flooding is a hazard.

If you haven't already been to Coachella Valley Preserve, stop by the Palm House in the oasis next to the parking area and pick up a pamphlet with a map. Docents at the Palm House can tell you about current conditions and wildlife.

A sign on the south side of the visitor center parking lot indicates the start of the trail to the Pushwalla, Horseshoe, and Hidden Palms Oases. The trail leads through the desert and crosses Thousand Palms Canyon Road, then immediately reaches a signed junction. The left fork leads 0.5 mile to the Indian Palms Grove, but this trip takes the right fork, following frequent signposts. Keep your eyes open for steps cut up a steep hill onto Bee Rock Mesa. When you reach a large wash, turn right, hike a short distance along the wash, and exit the other side where the trail leads up the steps to the mesa. A sign at the top of the hill points left along the top of the ridge to Pushwalla Palms and right to Hidden Palms. This hike leads to Pushwalla, then returns via Hidden Palms to form a loop.

The trail follows the narrow and exposed crest of the ridge eastward for a mile. Here you'll find panoramic views of the desert, the mountains ringing the Coachella Valley, and the Horseshoe Palms to the south. At a signed trail junction at the end of the ridge, stay right and follow the trail down off the ridge to another junction. Stay left for Pushwalla Palms; you'll return to this junction later to take the other fork going to Horseshoe and Hidden Palms. Descend a narrow gully and arrive at the oasis in Pushwalla Canyon. In the wet months, a trickle of water is often found in the canyon bottom, though it's not suitable for drinking. Turn left and explore up the canyon to find the two main palm groves, 2.7 miles from the trailhead.

VARIATIONS

From here, you have several options. You may return the way you came. You may continue up the canyon 0.2 mile to reach a trail exiting the canyon to the left at the end of the oasis, near an old car wreck. This trail loops back to the junction on the end of the long ridge that you followed; it also offers the opportunity to walk back along the wash to the north of the ridge.

But if time permits, make a loop to visit the Horseshoe and Hidden Palms. Retrace your steps through the Pushwalla Oasis and up the narrow gully to the signed junction that you passed earlier. Go west toward the Horseshoe Palms, nestled at the foot of the ridge. The maze of trails through the valley can be confusing; follow the trail markers that eventually lead you onto an old jeep track down the middle of the valley.

After passing the Horseshoe Palms, come to a fork in the road at a hitching post. Take the right fork into the Hidden Palms Oasis. The road ends at a turnabout at the north end of the oasis and continues north as a trail before it eventually rejoins jeep tracks. (The network of trails through the desert can be confusing here; a map and navigation skills are important.)

At another fork beneath the power lines near the toe of the main ridge, take the right fork and return to the signed junction on Bee Rock Mesa. Descend the stairs and retrace your steps to the trailhead.

trip 14.3 Moon Country–Willis Palms Loop

Distance	8 miles (loop)
Hiking Time	4 hours
Elevation Gain	1,100'
Difficulty	Moderate
Best Times	October–March
Agency	Coachella Valley Preserve
Recommended Map	*Coachella Valley Preserve* map

see map on p. 334

DIRECTIONS From the 10 Freeway, take Exit 131 for Ramon Road and drive east (on the north side of the freeway) 4.5 miles. Turn left onto Thousand Palms Canyon Road, and proceed 2.1 miles to the visitor-center parking area, on the left.

Highly recommended for a second visit to Coachella Valley Preserve, this loop isn't as continuously remarkable as the Pushwalla Palms hike but it still has many intriguing points of interest, including the McCallum and Willis Groves, Moon Country, and impressive summit views.

From the parking area, stop by the Palm House in the Thousand Palms Oasis Preserve; then pick up the trail leading north to the McCallum Grove. In 0.2 mile, pass a spur on the right leading back to the parking area. Near some private residences in another 0.3 mile, pass a trail on the left shortcutting to Moon Country. It's well worth the minor extra effort to continue straight 0.3 mile to a Y-junction at the McCallum Grove oasis. The fork on the right leads on to the oasis; then you can return to the Y and take the left fork toward Moon Country.

In a minute, you'll see a spur on the right leading back to the oasis; then in 0.1 mile, come to a four-way junction atop a sandy rise. The path on the left is the shortcut mentioned earlier. The paths straight and to the right form the Moon Country Loop. This trip suggests the straight path along a wash because it's slightly shorter.

Follow the right side of the wash, which is occasionally marked with posts. Creosote, indigo, burrobrush, and cheesebush grow along the wash. In 0.9 mile, watch for a post on the left where the Herman's Hike trail begins switchbacking up the hill to the southwest.

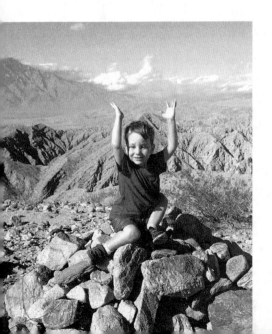

Pencil cholla joins creosote on the sparsely vegetated alluvial soil as views open up to San Gorgonio, San Jacinto, the Little San Bernardino Mountains, and contorted badlands immediately to the west. In 1.0 mile, reach a cairn marking the high point in the preserve.

Follow a desolate but scenic ridge south 0.9 mile to a minor saddle where you meet an abandoned roadbed. The Willis Loop veers right and drops into a canyon, but this trip takes the old road cut on the left that stays on the ridge. In 0.2 mile, pass an unsigned spur on the left where an abandoned road drops into a wash. In another 0.7 mile, come to a signed junction near the south end of the ridge. The road to the left is slightly shorter, but the far

High point on Herman's Hike

more scenic option is to pick up the trail on the right that descends 0.5 mile into the Willis Palms Oasis. After exploring the oasis, come to a signed junction with the Willis Loop. Head southeast 0.5 mile to reach the Willis Palms Trailhead on Thousand Palms Canyon Road.

Although you could walk back to the start on the shoulder of the road, that's neither scenic nor particularly safe. A more interesting but rather vaguely defined option is to continue southeast following occasional posts for Hidden Palms. Aim for a point just right of the south end of a prominent mesa. In 0.3 mile, reach a line of smoke trees in a wash near the base of the mesa. Turn northeast and follow the wash or base of the mesa 1 mile. Coachella Valley Preserve labels this as the Hidden Palms Loop Trail, but you'll find scant evidence of regular use. Near the north end of the mesa, watch for a post marking an abandoned road cut leading onto the mesa. Just north of here, a well-defined trail on the left leads 0.1 mile northwest to Thousand Palms Canyon Road. Cross the road and pick up the northbound Smoketree Ranch Trail, faint at first and better defined as you go, which stays east of the wash and returns you to Palm House in 0.3 mile.

---

trip 14.4   **Big Morongo Canyon Preserve**

Distance	0.6–10.0+ miles, depending on the route
Hiking Time	30 minutes–5 hours
Elevation Gain	Negligible
Difficulty	Easy–moderate
Trail Use	Good for kids, some wheelchair access
Best Times	October–May
Agency	Big Morongo Canyon Preserve
Recommended Map	*Big Morongo Canyon Preserve* map

DIRECTIONS From Highway 62 in Morongo Valley, 0.8 mile north of mile marker 062 SBD 1.00, turn east onto East Drive at a sign for Big Morongo Canyon Preserve. In 0.2 mile, turn left into the park entrance (11055 East Drive).

Marsh Trail boardwalk at Big Morongo

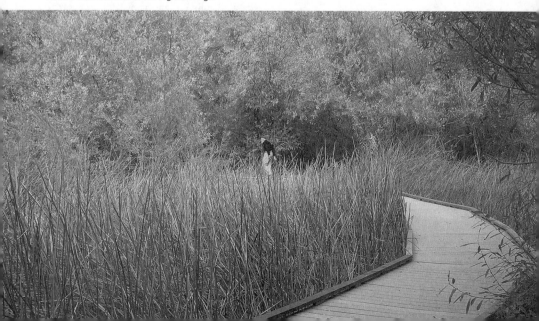

Big Morongo Canyon Preserve

Morongo
Valley
62

East Dr.

Desert
Willow
Trail

Trail

Mojave Dr.

2520'
N34 03.037
W116 34.234

4

Covington
Park

Yucca Ridge

Marsh
Trail

Overlook

Mesquite Trail

West Canyon Trail

Big Morongo Creek

Canyon Trail
(4 miles to
dead end)

0.0   0.1   0.2   0.3   0.4
mile

Numerous trails lace this preserve, and it's easy to choose as short or long a hike as you wish. There are benches and observation platforms along the way. All hikes start at the kiosk adjacent to the parking lot. Excellent maps are available here; take one and plan your excursion. The preserve is open 7:30 a.m.–sunset. Big Morongo is now part of the Sand to Snow National Monument.

The 0.6-mile Marsh Trail is not to be missed. Pick up a brochure at the kiosk describing 28 signed attractions along the wheelchair-accessible boardwalk. Hike the loop counterclockwise to follow the markers in order. Remarkably, this area burned in 1992, but large, fast-growing cottonwoods have already reached maturity and there are few signs of the destruction.

For a 1.7-mile hike offering views of more of the preserve, hike the north half of the Marsh Trail; then turn left onto the Desert Willow Trail. This trail zigzags along a path cut through the enormous honey mesquite trees. The protein-rich bean pods once formed an important part of the diet of many Indian bands. Beware of the long thorns! In 0.3 mile, turn right onto the Yucca Ridge Trail and climb up to the ridge. Unfortunately, this area was devastated in a June 2005 fire (started in a nearby private residence) that burned the splendid Mojave yuccas and cholla cacti that once dotted the hills. Recovery will not be nearly as fast as in the wet-lands below. Enjoy the views of the preserve, along with more distant views to San Gorgonio and San Jacinto, covered in snow through the winter and spring. At the end of the ridge, turn right onto the Mesquite Trail and follow it back down to the Marsh Trail.

VARIATION

For a longer workout, follow the Mesquite and West Canyon Trails to the Canyon Trail. The Canyon Trail leads south 4 miles, often following the remains of an old jeep route. The trail ends near the mouth of the canyon overlooking the Coachella Valley at a private land boundary. Retrace your steps the way you came. Including the walk to the start of the can-yon makes for an out-and-back hike of about 10 miles, or even more if you make a figure eight along some of the other trails.

---

trip 14.5 Pioneertown Mountains Preserve: Pipes Canyon Loop

Distance	6 miles (loop)
Hiking Time	3.5 hours
Elevation Gain	1,100'
Difficulty	Moderate
Trail Use	Dogs allowed
Best Times	October–May, day use only
Agency	The Wildlands Conservancy, Pioneertown Mountains Preserve
Recommended Map	USGS *Rimrock* 7.5'

DIRECTIONS From eastbound Highway 62 in Yucca Valley, 0.5 mile east of mile marker 062 SBD 10.00, turn left (north) onto Pioneertown Road. Drive through Pioneertown, which was built in 1946 as a set for western movies and now operates as a tourist attraction. In 7.6 miles, turn left onto good dirt Pipes Canyon Road. In 0.7 mile, stay right at a fork and continue 0.2 mile to the parking area.

Pipes Canyon is located west of Yucca Valley in the transition zone between the Mojave Desert and the San Bernardino Mountains. Pipes Creek is one of the few dependable streams in the area, and its lush riparian habitat is a critical resource for desert wildlife. Some say the canyon was named after an attempt by an early rancher to pipe water from the stream; another theory holds that the wind whistles musically through the rocks. South of the canyon are weird and wonderful geological features, including basalt hills and the aptly named Sawtooth Mountains. The land has been purchased by The Wildlands Conservancy to protect a corridor for wildlife to travel between the mountains, large conservation areas, and Joshua Tree National Park. The area is now part of the Conservancy's 20,000-acre Pipes Canyon Wilderness within the Pioneertown Mountains Preserve. This trip makes a scenic loop through the preserve, with an optional visit to Chaparrosa Peak.

This area was devastated by the lightning-triggered Sawtooth Fire in July 2006, which also burned portions of Pioneertown. It's now a good place to watch the process of regeneration. Unfortunately, most of the pinyon pines and majestic Joshua trees were burned beyond recov-ery, but many hardy nolinas have recovered and the scrub oak regrows rapidly.

From the ranger station near the parking area, hike west past a gate up a dirt road. In 0.2 mile, pass a second gate where the road narrows to a trail. The trail up Pipes Canyon

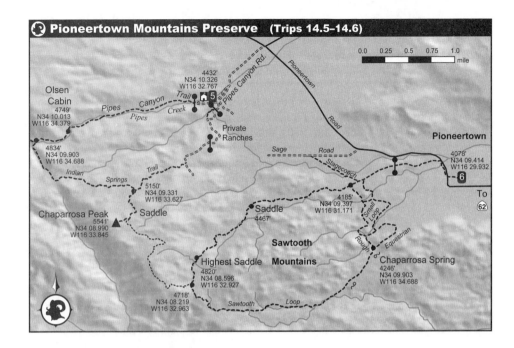

Pioneertown Mountains Preserve (Trips 14.5–14.6)

Olsen Cabin 4749' N34 10.013 W116 34.379

Pipes Canyon Creek

Pipes

4432' N34 10.326 W116 32.767

Trail

Pipes Canyon Rd.

Pioneertown Road

Private Ranches

Sage Road

Stagecoach

Pioneertown 4078' N34 09.414 W116 29.932

6

To 62

4834' N34 09.903 W116 34.688

Indian

Trail

Springs

5150' N34 09.331 W116 33.627

Chaparrosa Peak 5541' N34 08.990 W116 33.845

Saddle

Saddle 4467'

4185' N34 09.397 W116 31.171

Small Loop

Rough 6

Equestrian

Sawtooth Mountains

Highest Saddle 4820' N34 08.596 W116 32.927

Chaparrosa Spring 4246' N34 09.903 W116 34.688

4718' N34 08.219 W116 32.963

Sawtooth

Loop

leads along a section of year-round wetlands, where cottonwoods and desert willows fill the streambed and animals come for food and water. In another 1.6 miles, look for the ruins of the stone Olsen cabin on the northwest side of the creek. Swedish prospectors working the Onyx Mine during the Great Depression built this winter cabin.

Beyond the Olsen cabin, reach a signed turn in 0.4 mile at the first tributary canyon on the left (south). Be certain to take this route, called the Indian Springs Trail, rather than continuing up Pipes Canyon along traces of an old roadbed. On the Indian Springs Trail hike up the steep draw through ghostly stands of juniper and scrub to a saddle in 0.7 mile. Turn left (east) to begin a long, gradual descent. In 0.7 mile, a signpost marks the turnoff for Chaparrosa Peak on the right.

VARIATION

If you have the time and energy, this 1.4-mile round-trip to Chaparrosa Peak is well worth making and adds 500 feet of climbing. The trail leads south, curling around a volcanic hill to a

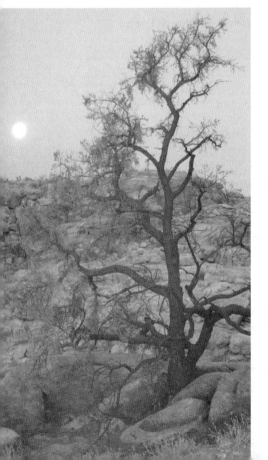

Burnt pinyon pine above Pipes Canyon

saddle on the ridge. It then veers right (southwest) along the ridge to the 5,541-foot summit. The peak's name contains the Spanish root *chaparro*, or scrub oak, which is a common species on these hills and is also the root of the English word "chaparral." From the summit, there are impressive views of the boulder-filled canyon to the south, San Jacinto, and the desert.

The main trail continues east from the Chaparrosa turnoff. There are excellent views along this stretch, including the volcanic mesas north of Pioneertown and the jagged Sawtooth Mountains to the south. In 0.8 mile, the trail ends at an old roadbed. Turn left and follow the roadbed down the ridge, passing around the right side of a locked gate. In another 0.8 mile, the roadbed turns right and leads toward private ranches, but you can follow a trail that leads 0.2 mile across a dry wash to rejoin another old roadbed near a gate beyond the ranches. Continue north another 0.2 mile near a former roadbed and gates to return to the trailhead parking.

SIDE TRIP

If time remains after your hike, movie buffs should consider stopping in Pioneertown. The town was built by the Hollywood movie industry after World War II as a set for westerns starring the likes of Gene Autry and Roy Rogers. Actors lived in the houses and ate at the saloons. Although it's used less frequently now for film, Pioneertown was saved from demolition and is now a living community, with a motel, restaurants, and theaters. You might catch a shootout on Mane Street each Saturday and Sunday at 2:30 p.m.

trip 14.6 Pioneertown Mountains Preserve: Sawtooth Loop

Distance	5–10 miles (semiloop)
Hiking Time	2.5–5 hours
Elevation Gain	500'/1,200'
Difficulty	Moderate–strenuous
Trail Use	Dogs allowed, suitable for equestrians
Best Times	October–April
Agency	The Wildlands Conservancy, Pioneertown Mountains Preserve
Optional Map	USGS *Rimrock* 7.5'

see map on previous page

DIRECTIONS From eastbound Highway 62 in Yucca Valley, 0.5 mile east of mile marker 062 SBD 10.00, turn left onto Pioneertown Road. Drive through Pioneertown, which was built in 1946 as a set for western movies and now operates as a tourist attraction. In 7.6 miles, turn left onto good dirt Pipes Canyon Road. In 0.7 mile, stay right at a fork and continue 0.2 mile to the parking area. Sign in at the ranger station; then return to Pioneertown. When Pioneertown Road abruptly turns left in the middle of town, make your first left onto good dirt Tom Mix Road. In 0.1 mile, park at the Post Office/Old Sheriff's Office.

The Sawtooth Mountains are a small but striking desert range between the San Bernardino Mountains and Joshua Tree National Park. A remarkable trail circles through the weird and wonderful rock formations. Visitors can choose between the 5-mile Small Loop and the full 10-mile Sawtooth Loop. Formerly known by equestrians as the Rim of the World Trail, this trail has been reworked and improved by The Wildlands Conservancy and AmeriCorps. Much of the area burned in the 2006 Sawtooth Fire and is in the process of regeneration. March and April are a particularly good time to enjoy the wildflowers and blooming cacti and nolina. Sharp-eyed visitors are likely to observe many reptiles on the rocks and fallen Joshua trees; watch for collared and horned lizards as well as the more common fence and side-blotched lizards.

Leave your vehicle in the middle of Pioneertown. Look for the OK Corral immediately to the west, and take a dirt road to the right of the corral that soon meets Pioneertown Road. Cross the road and find an unsigned trail on the far side that veers right and crosses a wash, then climbs onto a low ridge on the far side. Here you can watch the fire ecology in action. The wildflowers and scrub oaks benefit from the fire, but the burned yuccas are recovering very slowly. Follow the trail up this ridge to reach a gate beside a Wildlands Conservancy kiosk, 0.9 mile from the start. Continue west, passing an unsigned equestrian shortcut on the left and abandoned Stagecoach Road on the right, before you reach a signed junction in 0.5 mile where the Sawtooth Loop begins.

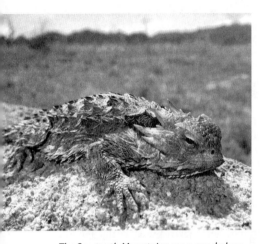

The Sawtooth Mountains are a good place to observe horned lizards.

For either the Small Loop or the full Sawtooth Loop, turn left and head south, crossing the wash again in 0.3 mile. On the far side, watch for marker posts where the Small Loop splits. The right branch is most interesting, wandering through the granite inselbergs of the Sawtooth Mountains. In 0.8 mile, come to another junction where a ROUGH TRAIL: HIKERS ONLY sign cautions equestrians to avoid the right fork.

If you're hiking the Small Loop, this is the point to circle back. Turn left and head northeast 0.1 mile to an easy-to-miss junction where the Small Loop departs the equestrian Sawtooth Loop. Then turn left again and follow the trail that parallels Chaparrosa Wash for a time, then turns left and drops back down to the northern Small Loop junction in 0.7 mile. Turn right here and retrace your steps to your vehicle.

If you're hiking the full Sawtooth Loop, you can take either the "rough" hiker trail or the longer equestrian trail. The boulders on the 0.2-mile rough trail won't bother most hikers, but equestrians must take the circuitous and less-scenic alternative, which rejoins in 0.8 mile near seasonal Chaparrosa Spring.

The trail now leads into the remote heart of the Sawtooth Mountains. Follow the canyon 1.5 miles south and west. When the trail starts to climb out of the canyon, look on the bottom of the wash for some huge unweathered light-gray boulders that tumbled down from the peak during the magnitude-7.3 Landers earthquake of 1992. As you climb, look back for more unweathered shattered granite on the slope.

Climb past a valley lush with nolina. In 1.2 miles, reach the tip of a major ridge. Peak baggers could depart here and follow the ridge cross-country up to Chaparrosa Peak (see Trip 14.5). This excursion is 1.7 miles each way with 800 feet of climbing. The Wildlands Conservancy may establish a trail here in the future.

In another 0.5 mile, the trail reaches a saddle marking the highest point along the Sawtooth Loop. It plunges into the next valley and crosses the wash, then climbs to a smaller saddle in another 1.0 mile. Here, turn east and, in 1.2 miles, reach the junction where the loop began.

trip 14.7 **Oak Glen Preserve**

Distance	1.8 miles (loop)
Hiking Time	1 hour
Elevation Gain	300'
Difficulty	Easy
Trail Use	Dogs allowed, good for kids
Best Times	All year
Agency	The Wildlands Conservancy, Oak Glen Preserve
Optional Map	USGS *Forest Falls* 7.5' (trail not shown)

DIRECTIONS The preserve can be reached from the west or from the south, or the two driving routes can be combined for a scenic tour through the foothills.

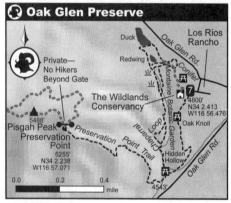

Coming from the west on the 10 Freeway in Yucaipa, take Exit 85 for Oak Glen Road and follow it northeast 10 miles into Oak Glen. Pass Oak Tree Village (with pony rides, animals, and other family attractions) and continue 1.1 miles to Los Rios Rancho at 39611 Oak Glen Road. Turn right and then right again into the parking area, across a bridge from the restaurant.

Alternatively, from the 10 Freeway in Beaumont to the south, take Exit 94 north onto Beaumont Avenue, which later becomes Oak Glen Road, and drive 9.2 miles to Los Rios Rancho at 39611 Oak Glen Road. Turn left and then right into the parking area.

Oak Glen, tucked away in the foothills below Yucaipa Ridge, is famous for its apple orchards and New England scenery. The Wildlands Conservancy has established its headquarters at Los Rios Rancho. Here you'll find the Southern California Montane Botanic Garden Trail, which leads through a historic orchard and evergreen forest to a pond and then along a creek. This family-friendly trail has special merits in the fall during apple-picking season, in the winter when the Yucaipa Ridge is blanketed in snow, and in the spring when the sweet scent of blooms draws butterflies to the orchards. Bring a picnic or purchase lunch and a locally baked apple pie at the adjacent restaurant. The first part of the trail to the pond is easily passable with a large-wheeled stroller.

The signed Montane Botanic Garden Trail starts at the northwest end of the parking lot. Follow a dirt road past the apple orchard and restrooms to the shady Cloud's Rest picnic area. Just beyond, a sign on the right indicates the California Conifers Trail, which parallels the dirt road and leads through a grove of giant redwoods and sequoias and native conifers. When the Conifers Trail rejoins the road, stay right and pass the Redwing Pond; then loop back between Duck and Redwing Ponds.

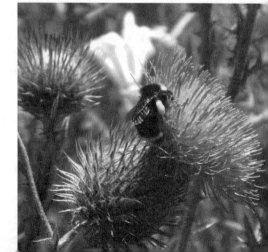

Wildflowers along the boardwalk attract bees and butterflies.

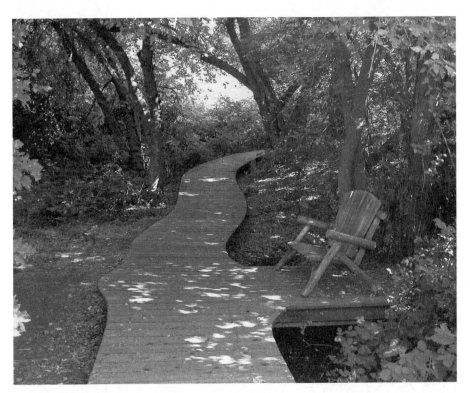

Oak Glen boardwalk   Photo: Wildlands Conservancy staff

Look for the floating dock in the Redwing Pond, where you can get close-up views of the waterfowl and fish.

From a junction below Redwing Pond, stay right and hike down through a forest of black oaks, and along a creek overgrown with thickets of invasive but delicious Himalayan blackberries. Pass a boardwalk on the left leading through the wetlands; families can loop back on the boardwalk for a pleasant and flat 1-mile hike. Signs identify the trees and bushes along the trail. Soon, reach a fork; the Stream Trail leads left, while the Chaparral Loop Trail leads right. Take either one; they soon rejoin. Then ford the creek at Reflection Pond and come to the Hidden Hollow picnic area at the south end of the preserve.

VARIATION

The signed Preservation Point trail departs from here and climbs onto the shoulder of Pisgah Peak. Hikers looking for a good workout may add this steep out-and-back trip, which climbs 800 feet over 0.8 mile. The manzanita and ceanothus burned in the 2009 Oak Glen III Fire and are presently recovering. The trail offers terrific views of Oak Glen and Yucaipa Ridge. The trail abruptly ends at a gate just below Pisgah Peak. Resist the temptation to trespass onto private land by the peak; thoughtless hikers have been creating tension between the landowners and Oak Glen Preserve.

Continue along the trail from Hidden Hollow as it climbs log steps out of the creek and back to Oak Knoll Park. Walk through the park and then continue through parking areas to the trailhead where you began.

trip 14.8   Whitewater Preserve to Mission Creek Preserve

Distance	7 miles (one-way)
Hiking Time	4.5 hours
Elevation Gain	900'
Difficulty	Moderate
Trail Use	Dogs allowed; suitable for equestrians (enter via Mission Creek)
Best Times	October–April
Agency	The Wildlands Conservancy, Whitewater Preserve
Recommended Maps	USGS *Whitewater, Catclaw Flat,* and *Morongo Valley* 7.5'

DIRECTIONS If you plan to make a one-way trip, you'll need to arrange a 15-mile car shuttle between Mission Creek Preserve and Whitewater Preserve. First, position one vehicle at the Mission Creek Preserve Trailhead. From the 10 Freeway, take Exit 117 north onto Highway 62 and drive 5 miles to mile marker 062 RIV 05.00; then turn left onto Mission Creek Road. The sign is easy to miss. Follow the good dirt road 2.3 miles, staying left at a junction, to its end at a gate.

To reach Whitewater Preserve, backtrack to the 10 Freeway and drive one exit (114) west to Whitewater Canyon Road. Exit north onto a frontage road that veers east; then immediately turn left (north) onto Whitewater Canyon Road and proceed 4.9 miles to the end of the road and the parking area for Whitewater Preserve.

This trip follows the Pacific Crest Trail (PCT) along two of the major waterways rushing down the southeast flank of San Gorgonio Wilderness. It offers outstanding mountain, river, and desert scenery. The best time to visit is in the spring after good rains when the wildflowers are in bloom. Animals large and small visit the canyons for the reliable water; this is a great place to watch for prints and scat. Consider bringing a pair of sandals for the river crossings because your feet are likely to get wet.

Whitewater Preserve and Mission Creek Preserve are both operated by The Wildlands Conservancy as part of the Sand to Snow National Monument. They border a portion of the San Gorgonio Wilderness and form the last link in a critical wildlife corridor stretching from the San Gabriel Mountains to the Nevada border. Former Secretary of the Interior Sally Jewell hiked this trail in May 2016 to celebrate the new monument.

The biggest river between the Mojave and the Colorado, the Whitewater pours out of the San Bernardino Mountains and flows through Palm Springs before emptying into the Salton Sea. The Whitewater Trout Farm, which operated for 65 years in Whitewater Canyon, was once a popular fishing destination but forbade hikers to cross its land and access the canyon upstream. When the trout farm closed, the land was slated for housing development.

The Wildlands Conservancy obtained the land in 2006 through a partnership with the Friends of the Desert Mountains and the Coachella Valley Mountains Conservancy. The Whitewater Preserve opened to the public in April 2008. The gate to the parking area is open daily, 8 a.m.–5 p.m. If you expect to exit later, ask at the ranger station for a combination to open the gate. There is a picnic area and a free campground (call for a reservation). Gas stoves are permitted, but wood fires are not. The trout

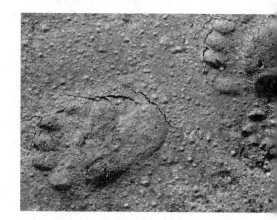

Bear tracks along the Whitewater River

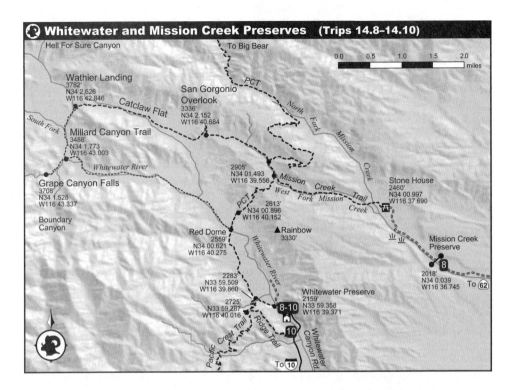

Whitewater and Mission Creek Preserves (Trips 14.8–14.10)

Hell For Sure Canyon

To Big Bear

0.0   0.5   1.0   1.5   2.0
miles

Wathier Landing
3782'
N34 2.626
W116 42.846

Catclaw Flat

San Gorgonio
Overlook
3336'
N34 2.152
W116 40.684

PCT

North Fork

Mission Creek

South Fork

Millard Canyon Trail
3488'
N34 1.773
W116 43.003

Whitewater River

2905'
N34 01.493
W116 39.556

Mission Creek

West Fork Mission Trail

Stone House
2460'
N34 00.997
W116 37.690

Grape Canyon Falls
3708'
N34 1.528
W116 43.337

2613'
N34 00.896
W116 40.152

Creek

Boundary
Canyon

Red Dome
2559'
N34 00.621
W116 40.275

▲ Rainbow
3330'

Whitewater River

Mission Creek
Preserve

8

2283'
N33 59.509
W116 39.860

2018'
N34 0.039
W116 36.745   To 62

2725'
N33 59.287
W116 40.016

Pacific Crest Trail

Ridge Trail

8-10

Whitewater Preserve
2159'
N33 59.358
W116 39.371

10

Whitewater Canyon Rd.

To 10

ponds are now closed to the public and are used for catch-and-release fishing programs for youths. The cliffs above the ranger station are made of fanglomerate, cemented remains of an old alluvial fan carried down from San Gorgonio. Raptors roost on these cliffs and bighorn sheep can be seen roaming the ledges.

Mission Creek is named for the Serrano band of Mission Indians who once roamed the San Bernardino Mountains. Many of the Serrano were forcibly relocated to Mission San Gabriel in 1834 by the Spanish missionaries. The American government again relocated the Serrano to a system of reservations in 1875, including one on Mission Creek. The land later passed into private hands before it was purchased by The Nature Conservancy; it was later turned over to The Wildlands Conservancy for management.

The preserve includes a group camping area at the Stone House. With a week's advance notice, visitors can get a permit and gate code to drive up to the Stone House, shaving 1.6 miles off the end of this hike. Call The Wildlands Conservancy for more information (see Appendix B, page 463).

This trip is worth the trouble of arranging a shuttle for a one-way hike, though you could also hike halfway or all the way and then return on foot. This trip follows part of the PCT, which continues all the way up to Big Bear Lake and beyond. The Whitewater River is a popular destination for families, who explore the first mile of the trail and play in the water (not recommended during times of peak runoff). The Whitewater Preserve lacks horse facilities and the trail crosses some sensitive wetlands, so equestrians are asked to access the area from the Mission Creek Preserve.

Before beginning this hike, inquire at the Whitewater Preserve Ranger Station about current trail conditions. The Whitewater River follows a broad wash and shifts its course after each major flood. Portions of the trail wash out from time to time. Crossing the river can be dangerous during times of peak runoff or during intense summer thunderstorms.

The trail starts on the north side of the parking area near a billboard with a map. The trail follows a rock-lined path between two palm trees. It then leads west, reaching the Whitewater wash in 0.2 mile. Along the way, it crosses an old jeep road leading north on the east side of the wash; don't be lured up this road. If the river hasn't flooded recently, you may find a marked trail across the wash. Reach a well-defined trail on the other side in 0.3 mile and follow it through a grove of desert willows 0.1 mile to a junction with the PCT at the mouth of a tributary canyon.

Turn right and follow the PCT upstream (north). In 1.4 miles, reach a corner where the Whitewater River begins to turn left. On the right side of the trail is a small volcanic lump called Red Dome. The PCT crosses the wash here. It can be difficult to follow, but you can pick it up again at a post in 0.4 mile at the mouth of a broad side-canyon on the far side. The trail then climbs northeast, passing brittlebushes, cat's claw acacias, and Mojave yuccas, and makes a few switchbacks to reach a saddle at the head of the canyon in 0.7 mile. A fence across the ridgeline delimits the boundary of the historic Whitewater Cattle Allotment.

The PCT then descends 0.6 mile into the West Fork of Mission Creek. Turn right onto a signed trail toward the Mission Creek Stone House. This trail has been rebuilt after the 2006 Sawtooth Fire. Watch for the beautiful green, purple, brown, and white formations in the sedimentary rocks overlooking the canyon. You may see coveys of quail running through the bushes.

In 1.9 miles, reach the junction with another canyon coming in from the left. A sign here indicates PCT 1.9 MILES. Hike east across the North Fork of Mission Creek. The trail may become indistinct in the wide wash but resumes in 0.2 mile at another trail marker. Beyond, 0.2 mile, reach the Stone House in Mission Creek Preserve. The building, picnic ground, and campground are open to the public and have information about the preserve and The Wildlands Conservancy.

After refreshing yourself, follow the good dirt road down the canyon. Pass the Painted Hills Wetlands where wild grape vines fill the creek beneath a magnificent cottonwood tree. In 1.6 miles, pass the ruins of the T Cross K Ranch, once a working ranch, which also hosted Hollywood stars looking for a desert retreat. Just beyond the ruins, reach the gate and parking area where you may have pre-positioned another vehicle.

trip 14.9 Whitewater Preserve: Canyon View Loop

Distance	3.7 miles (loop)
Hiking Time	2 hours
Elevation Gain	600'
Difficulty	Easy
Trail Use	Dogs allowed
Best Times	October–April
Agency	The Wildlands Conservancy, Whitewater Preserve
Optional Maps	USGS *White Water, Catclaw Flat,* and *Morongo Valley* 7.5'

see map on previous page

DIRECTIONS From the 10 Freeway between Highway 111 and Highway 62, take Exit 114 north for Whitewater Canyon Road. Follow a frontage road that veers east; then immediately turn left onto Whitewater Canyon Road and proceed 4.9 miles to the end of the road at the parking area for Whitewater Preserve.

The Whitewater River is the biggest river between the Mojave and the Colorado, pouring out of the San Bernardino Mountains and flows through Palm Springs before emptying into the Salton Sea. The river cuts a spectacular canyon down the southeast side of San Gorgonio.

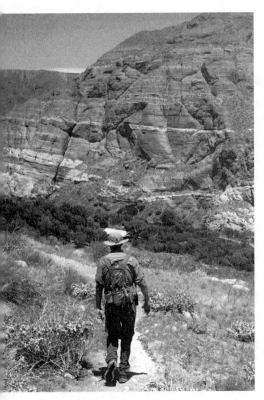

Descending the Ridge Trail into Whitewater Canyon

This hike starts at The Wildlands Conservancy's Whitewater Preserve and follows the Pacific Crest Trail (PCT) up to a ridge where there are great views of the canyon. It then descends the ridge and returns along the river's wide wash.

The Whitewater Trout Farm, which operated for 65 years in Whitewater Canyon, was once a popular fishing destination but forbade hikers to cross its land and access the canyon upstream. When the trout farm closed, the land was slated for housing development. The Wildlands Conservancy obtained the land in 2006 through a partnership with the Friends of the Desert Mountains and the Coachella Valley Mountains Conservancy. The Whitewater Preserve opened to the public in April of 2008.

The gate to the parking area is open daily, 8 a.m.–5 p.m. If you expect to exit later, ask at the ranger station for a combination to the gate. There is a picnic area and a free campground (call for reservations). Gas stoves are permitted, but wood fires are not. The trout ponds are now closed to the public, and are used for catch-and-release fishing programs for youths. The cliffs above the ranger station are made of fanglomerate, cemented remains of an old alluvial fan carried down from San Gorgonio. Raptors roost on these cliffs and bighorn sheep can be seen roaming the ledges.

This area was once home to an incredible assortment of spectacular cactus, especially in the nearby Devil's Garden. By the 1920s, it became fashionable to collect cactus to decorate private gardens in Southern California. Poachers soon stole most of the cactus from this area; you'll have to roam far from the beaten path to find the remaining stands. The problem was so severe that Minerva Hoyt of Pasadena organized a campaign that established Joshua Tree National Monument to protect a broad swath of desert vegetation. Collecting cactus from the wild is now illegal, but there is again a growing problem with "rustlers" stealing cactus to sell on the black market.

The trail starts on the north side of the parking area near a kiosk with a map. The trail follows a rock-lined path between two palm trees. It then leads west, briefly turns right along an old jeep road, and then turns left at a signed junction, reaching the Whitewater wash in 0.2 mile. If the river hasn't flooded recently, you may find a marked trail across the wash. Mulefat and desert willow are plentiful in the wash. Come to a well-defined trail on the other side leading to a junction with the PCT at the mouth of a tributary canyon.

Turn left (south) and follow the PCT as it switchbacks up the south wall of the canyon. The spring wildflowers can be quite diverse and impressive. In 0.7 mile, reach the top of the ridge where views open up to the south. The PCT continues south, but this trip goes to the left on the Canyon View Loop through a field of chamise. In 0.7 mile at the end of the ridge, the trail switchbacks down south-facing slopes covered in brittlebush.

The trail ends at Whitewater Canyon Road. Turn left and follow the road across the river; then watch for a signed trail on the left leading the final 0.4 mile back to the ranger station.

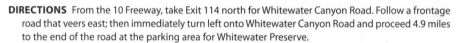

trip 14.10 **Whitewater Preserve: San Gorgonio Overlook**

Distance	11 miles (out-and-back), 14 miles (loop)
Hiking Time	5–8 hours
Elevation Gain	1,500'/2,000'
Difficulty	Moderate–strenuous
Trail Use	Dogs allowed (on leash)
Best Times	October–May
Agency	The Wildlands Conservancy, Whitewater Preserve
Recommended Maps	USGS *White Water* and *Catclaw Flat* 7.5'

see map on p. 347

DIRECTIONS From the 10 Freeway, take Exit 114 north for Whitewater Canyon Road. Follow a frontage road that veers east; then immediately turn left onto Whitewater Canyon Road and proceed 4.9 miles to the end of the road at the parking area for Whitewater Preserve.

This trip explores the remote country above Whitewater Preserve. Hikers have two options. The more moderate choice is to make an out-and-back trip on good trails to San Gorgonio Overlook, a bluff offering excellent views of the mountain's enormous east face. Adventurous souls looking for a strenuous hike will enjoy continuing along a partially overgrown jeep track all the way to the forks of the Whitewater River, then returning through the rocky wash. The latter option offers a short detour to frolic in Grape Canyon Falls. In the spring, the river runs strong and the desert is in blossom. Bring gaiters to keep the foxtail barley out of your socks.

Before leaving, sign at the Whitewater Preserve Ranger Station. Check with rangers about current conditions and the difficulty of river crossings. The loop is long and can be time consuming, so it's worth notifying the ranger that you might return late. The gate to

Enjoying a hard-earned watermelon at the Whitewater River

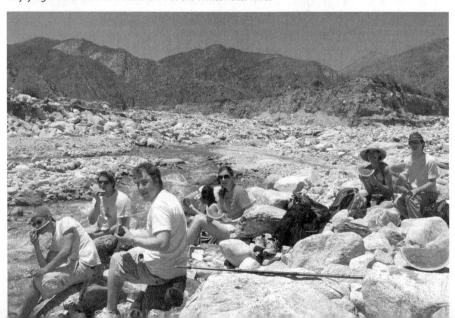

the parking area is open daily, 8 a.m.–5 p.m.; ask for the gate combination to exit in case you're late getting back. The loop involves some brush and lots of walking along unstable ankle-twisting boulders in the wash; bring gaiters and boots with ankle support, and don't do this one alone. Sandals are convenient if you'd like to cool off in the river.

From the signed trailhead, hike north between a pair of palm trees. Follow the rock-lined trail as it briefly merges with a dirt road before turning west and crossing the wash. Regular flooding makes it difficult to define a trail through the wash, but posts will help you navigate. Join the Pacific Crest Trail (PCT) at a signed junction near the west wall of the canyon, 0.6 mile from the trailhead. Follow the PCT north 1.4 miles past desert willows and brittle-bushes to a small volcanic knob called Red Dome.

The PCT crosses the Whitewater River wash here. Look north-northeast to pick out the closest canyon. Occasional posts and PCT trail markers may help you find your route, and logs or rocks may help you cross. The PCT resumes at the very left edge of the canyon in 0.4 mile. It passes desert vegetation including cactus, mesquite, and Mojave yucca, then switchbacks to reach an abrupt saddle at the head of the canyon in 0.7 mile. This portion of the trip offers great views of San Jacinto, whose north face is cut by the dramatic Snow Creek. Descend 0.6 mile to the floor of Mission Creek's West Fork, where you'll find a signed trail on the right leading to Mission Creek (see Trip 14.8).

This trip continues 0.4 mile north to a trail junction on the left. Here you leave the PCT. Hike west up a valley full of cat's claw acacias for 1.2 miles. San Gorgonio Overlook is atop a cliff at the head of the valley. This viewpoint offers a stunning look at the humongous mountain ahead.

If you're doing an out-and-back trip, this is your turnaround point. If you have time and energy to spare, continue along the old overgrown jeep track that makes a long switchback down into the next valley. This area burned in the 2006 Sawtooth Fire. A brushy road/trail continues west across Catclaw Flat. After crossing a dry creekbed, it steepens and reaches another saddle in 2.4 miles. From this saddle, you may see heavily overgrown traces of old jeep roads leading north and south. But our trail descends westward 0.3 mile to reach the Whitewater River canyon.

Wathier Landing is located in a grove of desert willows a few hundred yards north of the trail's end. All that remains are some old cinder blocks and junk from a hunters' camp. Inquisitive hikers with plenty of time may wish to detour north into the mouth of Hell For Sure Canyon, where an impressive waterfall can be found about 20 minutes up the canyon. But this trip turns south and follows the Whitewater River 0.5 mile to its confluence with the South Fork. Where possible, cross over to the southwest side of the river; then continue south 0.6 mile to the mouth of Boundary Canyon, which defines the eastern boundary of the San Gorgonio Wilderness.

The old Millard Canyon Trail once led into Boundary Canyon. It was almost wiped out in the Sawtooth Fire, but keen hikers may still see traces of it. Another beautiful waterfall is found at the mouth of Grape Canyon. To reach it, follow the faint Millard Canyon Trail southwest 0.5 mile to where the trail makes an abrupt switchback and climbs steeply north-west up the wall of Boundary Canyon. Grape Canyon Falls is located immediately south of this switchback. The trail used to continue to Kitching Peak, but is now heavily overgrown and not recommended.

Stills Landing was once located at the north end of Point 3,805' east of the mouth of Boundary Canyon. The area is now choked with trees and the site is difficult to find. It consists of a concrete slab and some vine-covered stones.

Continue east on the south side of the Whitewater River. This is a long and slow hike across the loose boulders filling the wash, but the scenery and river make it more enjoyable.

When your path becomes blocked by the mountainside, cross over to the north side, and then eventually return to the south side as the canyon bends to the right. Eventually, reach the PCT at Red Dome, 3.4 miles from the mouth of Boundary Canyon. Turn right and enjoy the stroll back to the trailhead.

trip 14.11   Dos Palmas Preserve

Distance	1 mile (loop)
Hiking Time	30 minutes
Elevation Gain	Flat
Difficulty	Easy
Trail Use	Dogs allowed, good for kids
Best Times	October–April
Agency	BLM Palm Springs–South Coast Field Office jointly with the Center for Natural Lands Management
Optional Map	USGS *Orocopia Canyon* 7.5'

DIRECTIONS From Highway 111 on the northeast side of the Salton Sea, directly opposite the Salton Sea State Recreation Area Visitor Center, turn east onto Parkside Drive. Go 1.8 miles to a T-junction; then turn right (south) onto Desert Aire Drive. In 0.4 mile, veer left onto good dirt Powerline Road. In 0.6 mile, turn left again onto Sea Breeze Drive. Proceed 1.7 miles to the trailhead parking, on the right side of the road immediately before a gate.

In 1862, William Bradshaw built the first "road" across the desolate deserts of Riverside County to the Colorado River, establishing a stage route from San Bernardino to the gold mines of La Paz, Arizona. His route followed a series of springs that friendly Native Americans had shown him. The best of these springs, a sparkling blue pool framed by twin palm trees, took the name Dos Palmas. The unlikely oasis in the midst of the alkali desert is nourished by water forced to the surface along the fractures of the San Andreas Fault. The twin trees have multiplied to hundreds, in three distinct groves. The oasis is now part

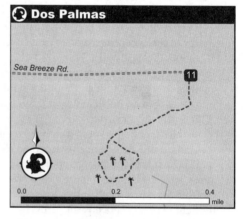

of the Bureau of Land Management's 20,000-acre Salt Creek Area of Critical Environmental Concern. The endangered desert pupfish can be found in pools within the preserve, and other threatened and endangered birds and lizards use the area. This trip makes an easy but scenic loop through the San Andreas grove of palms.

Consider a visit to the Salton Sea across Highway 111 or a drive along the Bradshaw Trail to round out your trip to this remote and fascinating corner of the desert. *Backcountry Adventures: Southern California,* by Massey and Wilson, is highly recommended for those considering the Bradshaw Trail or other 4WD excursions in the Inland Empire.

Hike along the signed San Andreas Trail, which is lined with rocks and timbers. In 0.3 mile, cross an old dirt road and enter the oasis. The trail loops through junglelike grove, crosses a bridge over a creek, and emerges at the dirt road. Turn left and walk 0.1 mile northwest along the road until you reach the San Andreas Trail. Turn right and return to the trailhead.

For a longer visit, you can also walk east past the gate and up the roads to Dos Palmas. The rancho is now closed, but the oasis is open to visitors on foot.

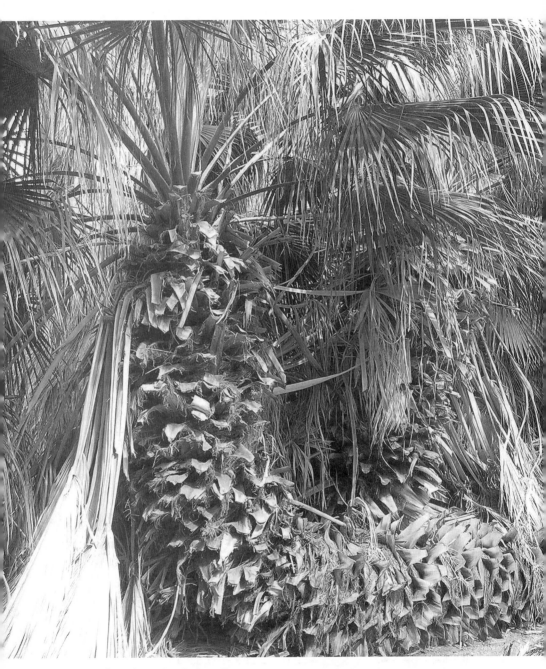

California fan palms at San Andreas Grove

chapter 15

Joshua Tree National Park: Park Boulevard

Joshua Tree National Park draws visitors from around the world to see its famous yuccas and outlandish geology. It's an international rock-climbing mecca where the author spent years dashing from climb to climb before noticing the fantastic hiking possibilities. The park is full of trails leading up mountains, to old mines, and through mazelike canyons, and it features many of the most interesting family-friendly hikes in the Inland Empire.

The Joshua Tree region is primarily composed of ancient Pinto gneiss (pronounced "nice") formed 1.6 billion years ago. More than 100 million years ago, molten rock forced its way upward and then slowly cooled to form large blobs of monzogranite about 15 miles underground. Earthquakes and stress from cooling caused the granite to crack, forming systems of horizontal and vertical joints. In wetter times, groundwater flowed through these cracks, eroding the sharp-cornered blocks into rounded boulders. Mountain-building action has lifted the rock and removed the upper layers, exposing the granite boulders. The boulders often form giant piles called inselbergs. On many hikes, you can see the contrast of the white monzogranite against the brown gneiss. The monzogranite is most striking in the Wonderland of Rocks, where the boulders form a formidable barrier to passage. The Geology Tour Road is another good place to explore these features. Trent and Hazlett's award-winning book *Joshua Tree National Park Geology* is a friendly introduction to the park's geological wonders.

The signature plant in the park is, of course, the Joshua tree. This many-armed yucca stands as tall as a house. The tree purportedly received its name from Mormon settlers who imagined the upstretched arms of Joshua leading the faithful to the Promised Land. John Frémont, the famous explorer and California's first senator, dubbed the Joshua tree "the most repulsive tree in the vegetable Kingdom." Millions of visitors to the park would likely quarrel with his ungenerous assessment. In more recent times, the curious tree has inspired

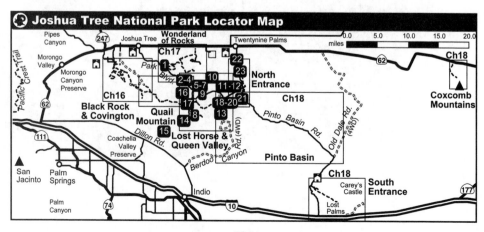

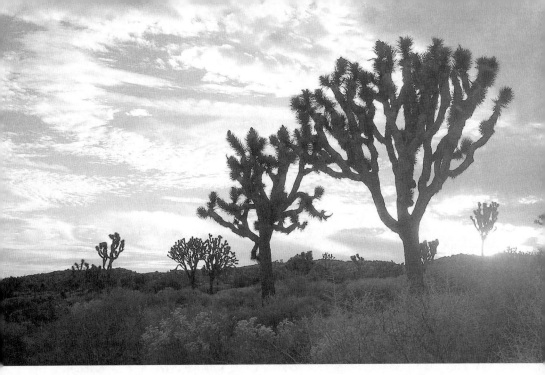

Joshua trees at sunset

the music of U2 and the art of Dr. Seuss. Joshua Tree is also an excellent place to find other spiky desert residents, especially the Mojave yucca and several species of cacti. In the spring of a good rain year, the whole desert bursts into glorious bloom.

Joshua Tree National Park lies at the border of two major ecosystems. The higher western end is part of the Mojave Desert, and tends to be slightly cooler and moister. The eastern end is part of the Colorado Desert, characterized by creosote bushes. Five "official" palm oases and a few smaller ones are scattered about canyons where water comes to the surface. Both deserts are full of spectacular cacti that pose a barbed threat to the unwary hiker.

Centuries ago, the land received more rainfall and Native Americans lived and hunted in the region. Even in the late 1800s, cattle ranchers were lured by reliable water. Soon, drought drove the ranchers away, and gold lust brought a flood of miners in their stead. Tourists were attracted to the exotic scenery, but also to poach the cacti, and to ignite the Joshua trees as giant torches. The park owes its formation largely to the efforts of Minerva Hoyt, who founded the International Deserts Conservation League and lobbied Franklin Roosevelt. In 1936, Roosevelt set aside 825,000 acres for Joshua Tree National Monument. Less than two decades later, mining interests chopped more than a quarter of the area out of the monument, but in 1994, Congress passed the Desert Protection Act that increased the area to 794,000 acres and changed Joshua Tree from a Monument to a National Park.

Joshua Tree offers all the services you'd expect in a National Park. Visitor centers, staffed by knowledgeable rangers, are located near the park entrances. The entrance fee at this writing is $25 per vehicle and $12 for cyclists and walk-ins. Numerous campgrounds can be found across the park; most are located near fascinating rock formations. Note that only Black Rock and Cottonwood Campgrounds have water, so plan to bring your own if going elsewhere.

See nps.gov/jotr for information and recreation.gov for campground reservations. Securing a campsite during the peak October–November and March–April seasons can be difficult. The Indian Cove and Black Rock Campgrounds accept reservations six months in advance, but the other campgrounds are first come, first served, and showing up late on Friday evening may not be sufficient to find a site for the weekend. The park has a dozen self-guided nature walks; these are good ways to learn about the unique environment here. Dogs and bicycles are prohibited on trails in the park but are permitted on the scenic backcountry roads.

Many hikers discover that route finding in the desert, and particularly in Joshua Tree, is more difficult than on more conventional mountain trails. The footpaths in Joshua Tree aren't always well marked. Many follow dry washes where it's impossible to maintain a conventional trail because of annual washouts. Locating proper exits from washes requires careful attention. A good map (especially the Trails Illustrated *Joshua Tree* map) and a compass or GPS are essential, even on many of the shorter hikes. Pay close attention to your surroundings and watch for footprints of previous hikers.

Hiking in Joshua Tree is most enjoyable in the fall, winter, and spring. From June to August, the temperatures normally exceed 100°F in the shade. In December and January, temperatures sometimes fall below freezing and the park occasionally receives spectacular snow. Some winter days are cold and windy, but the majority are ideal for a brisk walk.

If you venture far from a road, you're likely to enter a designated wilderness area. Wilderness permits aren't required, but if you plan to be out overnight, you must park and sign in at a backcountry registration board. Backcountry camping is free, but you must camp at least a mile from a road and 500 feet from any trail. Be sure to carry adequate water for your entire trip (typically a gallon per day in the cool seasons).

Wildfire has become a serious threat to Joshua Tree National Park—if you spend much time in the park, you'll inevitably pass through burn areas. To some extent, wildfire is a normal and necessary part of the desert ecosystem. Before 1965, however, lightning strikes tended to burn small patches of vegetation. Today, nonnative grasses flourish on the desert floor, fertilized by the nitrogen-rich smog that creeps in from the Los Angeles Basin. By late summer, the dry grasses act as tinder for fearsome brush fires. Catastrophic fires that once occurred every other century now ravage the park twice a decade, threatening to eliminate some of the diverse and unusual plant life that makes Joshua Tree so attractive. As a result, wood fires aren't allowed in the backcountry.

Joshua Tree National Park has so many fine hikes that I've divided them into four chapters. This chapter covers hikes accessed from Park Boulevard, the main thoroughfare between the West and North Entrances; this is the most heavily visited and iconic part of the park. Chapter 16 covers the Black Rock and Covington areas in the western end of the park, which have fewer rock formations but splendid desert vegetation and some of the park's largest Joshua trees; these areas are cut off from the main park and accessed from Highway 62 near Yucca Valley. Chapter 17 covers hikes accessed from Indian Cove, which features amazing rock formations and a huge and popular campground; it's cut off from the main park by the Wonderland of Rocks and is accessed from Highway 62 between Joshua Tree and Twentynine Palms. Chapter 18 covers the vast eastern end of the park, including the popular trails near the Cottonwood campground by the Eagle Mountains, the lonely Pinto Basin, and the remote Coxcomb Mountains; most of

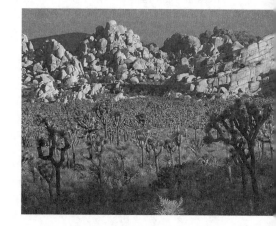

Joshua trees at dawn from Ryan Campground

these hikes are accessed from the South Entrance off the 10 Freeway or by driving through the Pinto Basin from Park Boulevard.

Patty Furbush's *On Foot in Joshua Tree National Park* is recommended for frequent park visitors who want to investigate even more possibilities, including abandoned mines and secluded peaks.

Nomad Ventures, a knowledgeable and well-equipped outfitter, is conveniently located at the corner of Highway 62 and Park Boulevard near the Joshua Tree Visitor Center.

trip 15.1   Maze and Window Rock Loop

see maps on pgs. 358 & 379

Distance	6.5 miles (loop)
Hiking Time	4 hours
Elevation Gain	1,100'
Difficulty	Moderate
Best Times	October–April
Agency	Joshua Tree National Park
Recommended Map	Trails Illustrated *Joshua Tree* or USGS *Indian Cove* 7.5' (only the Trails Illustrated map shows this new trail)
Permit	Joshua Tree National Park entry fee required (see page 355)

DIRECTIONS From the West Entrance Station of Joshua Tree National Park, drive 1.8 miles into the park on Park Boulevard to an unsigned dirt parking area on the left (north) side of the road next to mile marker 24.

Visitors driving through the West Entrance of Joshua Tree are treated to views of outrageously jagged hills on the skyline. The Maze Loop explores some of these peaks and canyons, offering a taste of the outlandish rocks and plants that make Joshua Tree National Park famous. The hike travels through the Mojave Desert environment, presents some spectacular views, and passes the unusual Window Rock. The signage has improved, but the trail still has a wild feel. This is among my favorite moderate trails in the park.

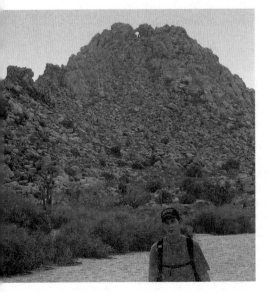

From the parking area, a dirt path leads away from the road. In 40 yards, reach a four-way junction by an old gravel pit. You'll return to this point via the Maze Loop (South Access) Trail at the end of the trip. Go straight on the signed North View Trail. In 100 yards, come to a second junction. The obscure North Canyon Trail turns left, but you stay right for the North View Trail. In another 100 yards, come to yet a third junction. The shorter but less-scenic Maze Loop (North Access) turns right up the wash, but this trip turns left onto the North View Trail.

Continuing along the rocky mountainside, hike another 1.4 miles and climb some switchbacks to reach a saddle. Here, the Copper Mountain View sign marks the first of two

Window Rock

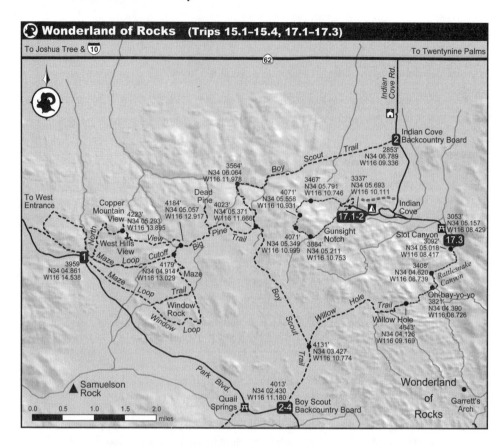

Wonderland of Rocks (Trips 15.1–15.4, 17.1–17.3)

To Joshua Tree & 10

62

To Twentynine Palms

Indian Cove Rd.

Indian Cove
Backcountry Board

2853'
N34 06.789
W116 09.336

Scout Trail

Boy

3564'
N34 06.064
W116 11.978

3467'
N34 05.791
W116 10.746

3337'
N34 05.693
W116 10.111

To West
Entrance

Dead
Pine

4071'
N34 05.558
W116 10.931

Indian
Cove

3053'
N34 05.157
W116 08.429

Copper
Mountain
View

4184'
N34 05.057
W116 12.917

4023'
N34 05.371
W116 11.666

17.1-2

4223'
N34 05.293
W116 13.895

North

Pine Trail

Gunsight
Notch

Slot Canyon

17.3

3092'
N34 05.018
W116 08.417

West Hills
View

View

Big

4071'
N34 05.349
W116 10.999

3884'
N34 05.211
W116 10.753

Cutoff

3408'
N34 04.620
W116 08.739

Rattlesnake
Canyon

3959'
N34 04.861
W116 14.538

1

Maze

Loop

4179'
N34 04.914
W116 13.029

Maze
Trail

Maze
Loop

Window
Rock

Willow

Hole

Trail

Oh-bay-yo-yo
3821'
N34 04.390
W116 08.726

Window Loop

Boy

Willow Hole
4843'
N34 04.126
W116 09.169

Scout

Park Blvd.

4131'
N34 03.427
W116 10.774

Samuelson
Rock

Quail
Springs

4013'
N34 02.430
W116 11.180

Boy Scout
Backcountry Board

2-4

Wonderland

of

Rocks

Garrett's
Arch

0.0   0.5   1.0   1.5   2.0
miles

optional side jaunts that lead to some of the best vistas on the trip. To take it, follow the spur north 0.2 mile until reaching the peak. Copper Mountain is visible across the desert to the north. Continue on the North View Trail 0.3 mile to the second spur, signed WESTERN HILLS VIEW. The trail remains on the high slopes for some time, and then drops steeply into a sandy dry wash. Follow it downstream a short way; then, when reaching a junction with a second wash, turn right and proceed up the second wash. In 40 yards, stay left where the wash forks. Look for cairns or footprints marking this potentially confusing section of trail.

The sandy trail leads into a grove of Joshua trees and reaches a signed junction with the Big Pine Trail, 1.3 miles from the Western Hills View turnoff. You can turn left here and cross the desert 1.7 miles to the Boy Scout Trail (see Trip 15.2), but this trip veers right on the Maze Loop Trail. The Big Pine was a mighty pinyon, now deceased.

In 0.2 mile, the North View Trail ends at the signed Maze Loop Trail. The unsigned northern branch veers right to shortcut back to the trailhead and bypass the best sights, but you continue straight into the Maze, an area of large boulders and interesting rock formations. Watch for large nolinas, more distant relatives of the Mojave yuccas and Joshua trees you've seen along the trail. In 1.0 mile, reach a major wash at the base of Window Rock. Look up at the top of the formation for the prominent thunderbird-shaped window. The signed Window Loop continues straight to curve around the south side of Window Rock, but you turn right into the wash to stay on the Maze Loop, which is a mile shorter and has better views.

In 0.8 mile, a sign marks where you meet the other end of the Window Rock Loop. Turn right and follow the Maze Loop 1.5 miles back to the trailhead.

| trip 15.2 | **Boy Scout Trail** |

Distance	8 miles (one-way)
Hiking Time	4 hours
Elevation Gain/Loss	Negligible/1,300'
Difficulty	Moderate
Trail Use	Suitable for backpacking
Best Times	October–April
Agency	Joshua Tree National Park
Recommended Map	Trails Illustrated *Joshua Tree* or USGS *Indian Cove* 7.5' (start and end of trail have been rerouted since the 1995 edition of the *Indian Cove* map)
Permit	Joshua Tree National Park entry fee required (see page 355)

DIRECTIONS Arrange one vehicle at the Indian Cove backcountry board in Indian Cove and a second one at the Keys West backcountry board in the main park. The two trailheads are only 8 miles apart, but they involve a half-hour drive because they're separated by the nearly impenetrable Wonderland of Rocks.

To reach Indian Cove from Highway 62, drive 8.8 miles east from Park Boulevard in the town of Joshua Tree; then turn south onto Indian Cove Road, 0.4 mile east of mile marker 062 SBD 27.00. Pass the entrance station in 1.1 miles and park at the backcountry board, on the right side of the road 0.5 mile beyond.

To reach the other end, return to Park Boulevard in Joshua Tree and turn left (south). Pass the West Entrance Station and reset your odometer. In 6.4 miles, reach the large paved parking area for the Keys West backcountry board on the north side of the road (0.8 mile east of mile marker 20).

The popular Boy Scout Trail connects the main park to Indian Cove, following the western edge of the outlandish Wonderland of Rocks. It treats the hiker to Joshua tree forests, massive granite boulder piles, yuccas, cacti, and scenic washes. The hike is long enough that it's preferable to do one-way rather than out-and-back. Or better yet, combine

Dawn from the Boy Scout Trail

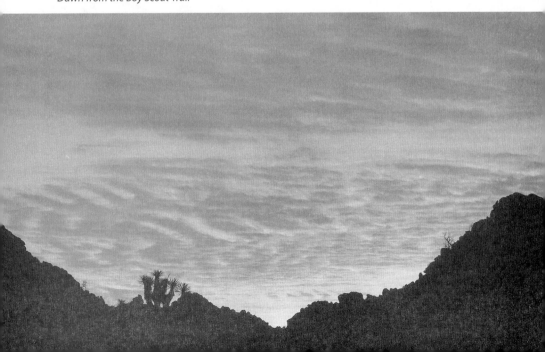

the Boy Scout Trail with Willow Hole and Rattlesnake Canyon (see Trip 15.4) to make the best challenging loop hike anywhere in the park. The Wonderland of Rocks is a day-use area, but camping is allowed on the west side of the Boy Scout Trail. There are excellent sites in the sandy wash about halfway down the trail, but beware of flash flooding anytime thunderstorms threaten the desert.

From the Boy Scout backcountry board, follow the broad trail north across the Joshua tree–studded desert toward the largest granite boulder pile on this side of the Wonderland (Peak 4,602'). Beware of the impressive hedgehog cactus in the middle of the trail. In 1.2 miles, come to a junction on the far side of the boulder pile. The Willow Hole Trail leads right (see Trips 15.3 and 15.4), but the Boy Scout Trail continues to the left across the desert. After another 2.5 miles of easy walking, enter a dry wash and soon come to a signed fork. The Big Pine Trail leads west toward the Maze Loop (see Trip 15.1), but the Boy Scout Trail follows the wash downstream. There is good camping for small parties along this stretch of the wash.

In 0.2 mile, reach a sand-filled tank (a barrier across the wash once used by ranchers to create a small pond). In another 0.2 mile, the trail leaves the wash to the northwest before the wash drops into a steep boulder-filled ravine. Adventuresome travelers may navigate the ravine, but it's much easier to follow the trail as it crosses a low ridge and switchbacks down into a second dry wash. This soon turns right (east) and rejoins the original wash 1.3 miles from where you left it.

The trail continues in and alongside the wash another 0.9 mile before the canyon opens up. It then leads 1.6 miles straight across the gently sloping desert to the Indian Cove backcountry board.

trip 15.3   Willow Hole

Distance	7 miles (out-and-back)
Hiking Time	4 hours
Elevation Gain	200'
Difficulty	Moderate
Best Times	October–April
Agency	Joshua Tree National Park
Recommended Map	Trails Illustrated *Joshua Tree* or USGS *Indian Cove* 7.5' (the start of the trail has been rerouted since the 1995 edition of the Indian Cove map)
Permit	Joshua Tree National Park entry fee required (see page 355)

see maps on pgs. 358, 364, & 379

DIRECTIONS From Highway 62 in Joshua Tree, turn south onto Park Boulevard. Pass the West Entrance Station and reset your odometer. In 6.4 miles, reach the large paved parking area for the Keys West backcountry board on the north side of the road (0.8 mile east of mile marker 20).

The Wonderland of Rocks is an intricate maze and obstacle course whose gigantic monzogranite boulder piles stymie most travelers. One of the few easy ways in is the Willow Hole Trail, which follows a broad sandy wash into this clearing tucked away in the heart of the Wonderland. There is no overnight camping in the Wonderland of Rocks, so make this a day trip.

From the Boy Scout backcountry board, follow the broad trail north across the Joshua tree–studded desert toward the largest granite boulder pile on this side of the Wonderland (Peak 4,602'). In 1.2 miles, come to a junction on the far side of the boulder pile. Turn right (northeast) and follow an old jeep road that eventually enters a wash in 1.6 miles. Follow the wash downstream, passing two washes coming in from the right. Stone walls begin to squeeze the wash into a narrow corridor. In another 0.7 mile, arrive at Willow Hole.

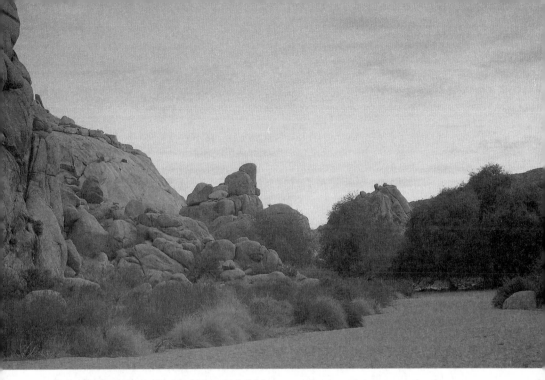

Willow Hole

In the wet season, deep pools of water may be found here. The vegetation is far lusher than elsewhere in this part of the Mojave Desert. This is a pleasant place to have lunch and explore the rock formations. When you've had enough, return the way you came. Alternatively, with a shuttle, continue down the Boy Scout Trail to Indian Cove (see Trip 15.2) or continue down the wash through the Wonderland for 1.5 amazing but difficult boulder-strewn miles to Rattlesnake Canyon (see Trip 15.4).

trip 15.4   Wonderland Traverse

Distance	6 miles (one-way)
Hiking Time	6 hours
Elevation Gain/Loss	Negligible/1,300'
Difficulty	Strenuous
Best Times	October–April
Agency	Joshua Tree National Park
Required Map	Trails Illustrated *Joshua Tree* or USGS *Indian Cove* 7.5' (start and end of Boy Scout Trail have been rerouted since the 1995 edition of the *Indian Cove* map)
Permit	Joshua Tree National Park entry fee required (see page 355)

see maps on pgs. 358, 364, & 379

DIRECTIONS Unless you plan to do a loop hike, arrange one vehicle at the Rattlesnake Canyon Picnic Area in Indian Cove and a second one at the Boy Scout backcountry board in the main park. The shuttle arrangements involve a half-hour drive even though the two trailheads are only a few miles apart because they're separated by the Wonderland of Rocks.

To reach Indian Cove from Highway 62, drive 8.8 miles east from Park Boulevard in the town of Joshua Tree; then turn south onto Indian Cove Road, 0.4 mile east of mile marker 062 SBD 27.00. Pass the entrance station in 1.1 miles and the backcountry board in another 0.5 mile; then continue 1.4 miles to the campground. Turn left (east) and pass through the campsites to reach the picnic area at Rattlesnake Canyon in another 1.3 miles.

To reach the Boy Scout Trailhead, return to Park Boulevard in Joshua Tree and turn left (south). Pass the West Entrance Station and reset your odometer. In 6.4 miles, reach the large paved parking area for the Keys West backcountry board on the north side of the road, 0.8 mile east of mile marker 20.

Travel through the Wonderland of Rocks is arduous, involving constant up-and-down climbing on gigantic granite boulders. It's seldom possible to see more than 100 yards ahead of you and there are few landmarks, so simply describing a route in most parts of the Wonderland is nearly impossible. A rare exception is Wonderland Traverse, which follows a well-defined wash full of jumbo rocks between Willow Hole and Rattlesnake Canyon. Even though this stretch is only 1.5 miles long, it will take hours of challenging scrambling to get through. This is no place for inexperienced hikers, especially those traveling alone. An interesting attraction on this hike is the valley of Oh-bay-yo-yo, where locals have built and maintained a fascinating "fortress" beneath an overhanging boulder. The Wonderland of Rocks is a day-use area; no camping is allowed.

This trip can be done as a one-way hike, or as a loop in conjunction with the Boy Scout Trail (see the variation following). The traverse is best done downhill because washes converge rather than diverge, making navigation much easier.

From the Boy Scout backcountry board, follow the Boy Scout Trail 1.2 miles to the Willow Hole junction; then hike 2.3 miles on an old dirt road and downstream through a wash until the wash seems to end at Willow Hole (see Trip 15.3).

At the big trees in Willow Hole, look ahead for the path. The easiest way is straight forward over a small rise and down the other side. The path to the left is choked with vegetation. The path into a narrow alcove to the right looks promising, but emerges atop a band of cliffs. If you find yourself scrambling on difficult boulders, you haven't found the right path. Beyond the rise, cross a clearing and drop down between two rock piles into a wash. From here on, all travel should be downhill. You may find occasional cairns marking the route.

Boulder-hop down the wash. It soon veers left (take care not to miss this turn and start walking uphill), then back right. The next stretch is choked with huge boulders and is slow, complicated going. The wash opens up again at a grassy clearing 0.7 mile from Willow Hole, and shortly merges with another wash on the right (south). Oh-bay-yo-yo can

Aerial view of the Wonderland of Rocks

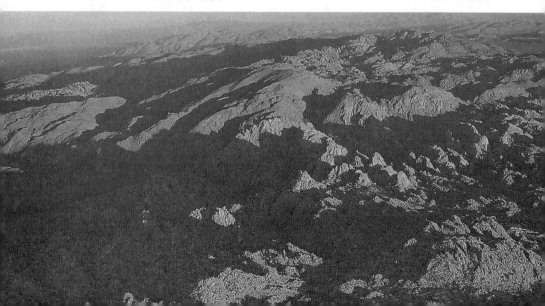

be found in the clearing to the left beneath a huge boulder. Visitors sometimes stock the fortress with supplies. Please take good care of this special spot.

Beyond the confluence, the wash turns left (north) and abruptly descends 0.4 mile over huge boulders and dry waterfalls into the heart of Rattlesnake Canyon. This is one of the few weaknesses in the south wall of the canyon; farther east are sheer cliffs. Turn right (east-northeast) and follow the refreshingly easy path on the floor of Rattlesnake Canyon for 0.5 mile until it bends left. This is a fine place to admire the geology of the park. The light-colored White Tank monzogranite of the Wonderland abuts the brownish Pinto gneiss on the flank of Queen Mountain, making an interesting contrast.

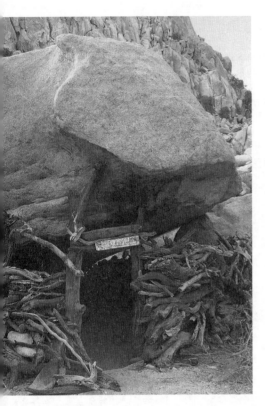

Oh-bay-yo-yo

Shortly beyond, reach a series of potholes marking the top of a rare slot canyon. It's worthwhile to peer over the top, but descending into the canyon here would involve a tricky rappel. Instead, backtrack to the sandy area above the potholes and look for a path to scramble up left to a notch. Descend through the notch past a number of oak trees, and then walk down slabs, taking care to stay left, until you reach easy terrain and can veer right back toward the base of the slot canyon. More interesting potholes are found at the base, some of which may shelter frogs or killer bees.

The final stretch involves some more boulder-hopping. The wash veers right, then left again before reaching the broad flat bottom. On the way you pass granite boulders peppered with enormous pinkish feldspar crystals. Look for a path out of the wash to the left leading to the Rattlesnake Canyon Picnic Area.

VARIATION

This trip can be done as a challenging but magnificent loop starting at the Indian Cove backcountry board; this loop is my favorite trip in Joshua Tree National Park. This option is 14 miles with 1,500 feet of elevation gain and takes about 10 hours. Start early, because you'll navigate the Wonderland at the end of the trip—this is not a place to get stranded after dark.

From the Indian Cove backcountry board, hike up the Boy Scout Trail 6.8 miles to the Willow Hole Trail (see Trip 15.2); then turn left and join the route described above. Unless you've left a second vehicle at the Rattlesnake Canyon Picnic Area, follow the paved road 1.3 miles back to the Indian Cove Campground; then turn right and walk 1.4 miles down Indian Cove Road to the backcountry board.

trip 15.5   **Barker Dam Nature Trail**

Distance	1.5 miles (loop)
Hiking Time	1 hour
Elevation Gain	100'
Difficulty	Easy
Trail Use	Good for kids
Best Times	October–April
Agency	Joshua Tree National Park
Optional Map	Trails Illustrated *Joshua Tree* or USGS *Indian Cove* 7.5'
Permit	Joshua Tree National Park entry fee required (see page 355)

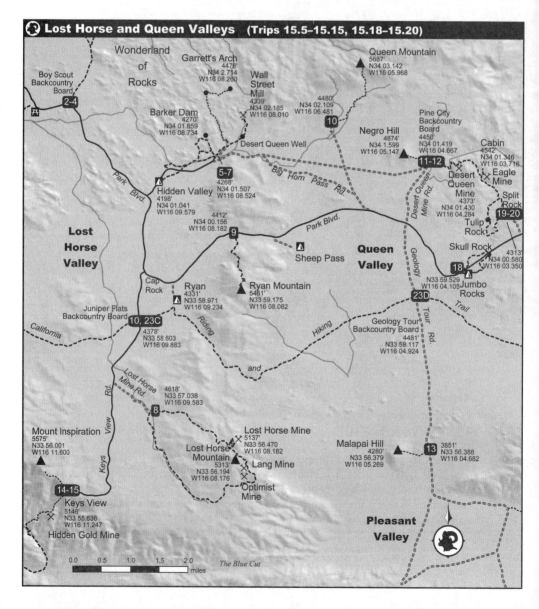

Lost Horse and Queen Valleys (Trips 15.5–15.15, 15.18–15.20)

DIRECTIONS From the main Park Boulevard through Joshua Tree National Park, immediately east of Hidden Valley Campground and 0.2 mile east of mile marker 17, turn north onto a paved road, following signs for Barker Dam. Follow this road 1.6 miles to its end at the Barker Dam parking area.

You can also walk to the trailhead from the Hidden Valley Campground. Look for a trailhead marker near campsite 36—the trail begins across the road about 50 yards beyond this marker. This adds 1.2 miles in each direction.

A century ago, Joshua Tree National Park was wet enough to support limited cattle ranching. Ranchers dug wells and built reservoirs to obtain vital water. Barker Dam, built by the Barker & Shay Cattle Company, is the largest of these efforts. The nature trail past the dam at the edge of the Wonderland of Rocks offers some of the most varied and interesting scenery and vegetation of any short walk in the park. This trip can be combined with the adjacent Wall Street Mill (Trip 15.7) to make a pleasant half-day jaunt.

From the parking area, walk north on the broad trail. In 100 yards, stay left at a junction; the right fork goes to Wall Street Mill. In 0.1 mile, reach the start of the loop trail. Stay right to take the loop counterclockwise. Numerous interpretive signs along the path identify local flora and explain their struggle for survival under the harsh desert conditions.

The loop trail leads through a narrow corridor and opens into a valley. During the wet season, a good-sized lake forms behind Barker Dam, nestled beneath the dramatic cliffs of the Wonderland of Rocks. The murky and uninviting water is a precious resource for park wildlife, so don't try swimming here.

The trail passes along the south side of the large dam and then enters another valley full of Joshua trees and yuccas. Hike south to another junction. The path straight ahead is a shortcut back to Hidden Valley Campground. Follow it a few yards to a large rock on the left covered in petroglyphs. Unfortunately, most of the artwork has been vandalized. Return to the junction and turn east for a short jaunt back to the start of the loop.

trip 15.6   **Garrett's Arch**

Distance	4.2 miles (out-and-back)
Hiking Time	3.5 hours
Elevation Gain	300'
Difficulty	Moderate
Trail Use	Good for kids
Best Times	October–April, day use only
Agency	Joshua Tree National Park
Recommended Map	Trails Illustrated *Joshua Tree* or USGS *Indian Cove* 7.5'
Permit	Joshua Tree National Park entry fee required (see page 355)

DIRECTIONS From the main Park Boulevard through Joshua Tree National Park, immediately east of the Hidden Valley Campground and 0.2 mile east of mile marker 17, turn north onto a paved road, following signs for Barker Dam. Follow this road 1.5 miles. Just before its end at the Barker Dam parking area, turn right onto good dirt Queen Valley Road. Proceed 0.1 mile; then veer left onto an unnamed road and follow it 0.3 mile to the parking area at the end.

This trip takes you deep into the Wonderland of Rocks in search of the elusive Garrett's Arch. Named for park ranger Gary Garrett, who discovered it, it's believed to be the largest natural arch in the park. The journey is as rewarding as the destination, taking you along a series of washes between the magnificent granite domes of the Wonderland. In late spring, the blooming cacti make the trip even more appealing. If you hope to climb into the arch itself, bring a rope and light rack to 0.75 inch. There is no marked trail and the going is slow, although for most of the distance a well-worn climber's path eases your travel. Keen-eyed explorers may discover pictographs along the way. The arch is hidden until you reach its base, and navigation requires a GPS, an excellent sense of direction, or previous familiarity with the Wonderland. Watch the landmarks carefully so that you can find your way out on the return journey.

From the parking area, take the broad, signed path northeast toward the Wall Street Mill. In 100 yards, turn left at an unsigned junction and go north 0.1 mile to the ruins of the Wonderland Ranch, built by the Ohlson family, who prospected in the area. Turn left and thread your way west past scrub oaks for 100 yards to gain the Wonderland Wash; remember this junction so you can locate it on your return.

Turn right and hike north along Wonderland Wash. The path is reasonably good because of the large number of rock climbers who come this way to test their mettle on the Wonderland's incredible granite walls. In addition to scrub oak and pinyon pines, the wash is lined with Mojave yuccas (with curling threads along the blades) and nolinas (no threads), as well as diverse species of cactus. In the spring, beavertail and hedgehog cactus both produce striking magenta blooms. Mojave mound cactus displays exquisite red flowers.

In 0.5 mile, watch for Walrus Rock on the right side of the wash, with an eye socket and angular nose. In another 0.2 mile, Foolproof Tower on the left is recognized by its overhanging cap. The canyon soon opens into Wonderland Valley, ringed by striking rock formations. The two prominent Astrodomes to the northwest stand 250 feet tall and offer perfect face climbing for those skilled enough to attempt the routes. However, this trip continues north on a poorly defined path. In 0.2 mile, cross an east–west wash. In another 0.2 mile, reach the base of the Freak Brothers Domes on the right. These three domes have amusing overhanging noses and are an essential landmark on this trip.

The next rock north of the Freak Brothers is the Weenie. Hike north 0.1 mile until you can turn right and soon join a wash heading east along the north side of the Weenie. Follow this wash between large formations known as Disneyland Dome on the left and Fat Freddie's Cat on the right. In 0.1 mile, reach the Red Obelisk, a short but prominent tower immediately to the left of your wash.

Aerial view from north of route through Wonderland of Rocks to Garrett's Arch

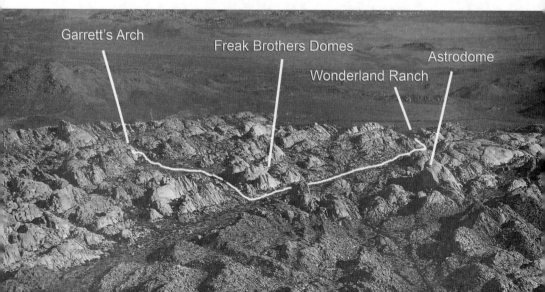

Just beyond this landmark, the wash opens up again into a basin. Look east-northeast for a formation with a sloping apron 0.3 mile away on the far side of the basin. Garrett's Arch is hidden on this formation. Pick a path across the cactus-studded basin and along the base of the formation until you can see Garrett's Arch. Reaching the base of the arch requires scrambling up the third-class slab, which will deter anyone with poor balance or a fear of heights. The final 30-foot pitch into the arch is fifth-class, so most hikers will be content to stop at the base.

trip 15.7	**Wall Street Mill**

see map on p. 364

Distance	1.4 miles (out-and-back)
Hiking Time	1 hour
Elevation Gain	100'
Difficulty	Easy
Trail Use	Good for kids
Best Times	October–April
Agency	Joshua Tree National Park
Recommended Map	Trails Illustrated *Joshua Tree* or USGS *Indian Cove* 7.5'
Permit	Joshua Tree National Park entry fee required (see page 355)

DIRECTIONS From the main Park Boulevard through Joshua Tree National Park, immediately east of Hidden Valley Campground and 0.2 mile east of mile marker 17, turn north onto a paved road, following signs for Barker Dam. Follow this road 1.5 miles. Just before its end at the Barker Dam parking area, turn right onto good dirt Queen Valley Road. Proceed 0.1 mile; then veer left onto an unnamed road and follow it 0.3 mile to the parking area at the end.

Bill Keys built the Wall Street Mill in 1930 to process gold ore. The ore was carted to the top of the mill, then dumped through a crusher and smashed into sand by two great stamps. The sand was mixed with water and mercury; the gold adhered to the mercury,

Wall Street Mill

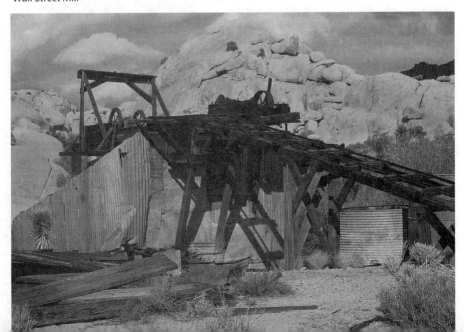

while the worthless gravel washed away. Keys ceased operations in 1966 and the mill was placed on the National Register of Historic Places. This is one of the better preserved examples of early-20th-century mining technology. A short hike through the desert brings you to inspect the structure.

From the parking area, take the broad, signed trail northeast toward Wall Street Mill. In 100 yards, pass two unsigned side trails on the left leading to ruins of the Wonderland Ranch and a rusted car. The main trail (an old dirt road) then passes the Desert Queen Well, where a creaky old windmill once raised water from the ground for mill operations. Beyond, a stone marks the spot where Keys killed Worth Bagley in a 1943 shootout over a land dispute. After five years in jail, Keys was found not guilty on the grounds of self-defense. The path enters a wash and soon arrives at Wall Street Mill.

Explore the site, being mindful around the old structures. Return the way you came.

trip 15.8   Lost Horse Mine and Mountain

Distance	4 miles (out-and-back), 6 miles (loop)
Hiking Time	2–3 hours
Elevation Gain	500'/1,000'
Difficulty	Moderate
Trail Use	Good for kids
Best Times	October–April
Agency	Joshua Tree National Park
Recommended Map	Trails Illustrated *Joshua Tree* or USGS *Keys View* 7.5'
Permit	Joshua Tree National Park entry fee required (see page 355)

see map on p. 364

DIRECTIONS From the main Park Boulevard through Joshua Tree National Park, 0.8 mile east of mile marker 16, turn south onto Keys View Road. In 2.5 miles, turn left at a signed dirt road to Lost Horse Mine. The road ends in 1 mile at a parking area with an outhouse. This road is open for day use only.

The Lost Horse Mine was one of the few highly profitable gold mines in Southern California, yielding 10,000 ounces of gold between 1894 and 1931. The following story of the mine was related by William Keys, a long-time resident of the area. Johnny Lang, a cattle rancher, explored the area when his horse vanished one night. He learned of the mine from a prospector and bought the rights to the mine for $1,000, naming it Lost Horse. Five years later, J. D. Ryan joined the partnership and hauled in a massive steam-powered 10-stamp mill. The mill crushed the ore from the mine; the resulting powder was mixed with water to form a slurry. The slurry was treated with mercury to separate the gold from the debris. The amalgam was smelted to separate the gold and mercury; the mercury was reused, while the gold was shipped in 200-pound bricks to Banning. To power the steam mill, Ryan ran

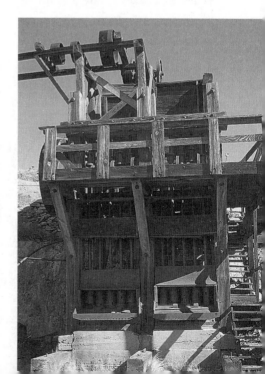

Lost Horse Mine Mill

a pipeline 3.5 miles from the well at his ranch and up 750 feet to the mine. The hills around the mine are still sparsely vegetated because so many trees were cut to generate the steam. According to Keys, Ryan caught Lang stealing gold from the night shift and forced Lang to sell out. Lang later retrieved some of the bullion that he had secreted away near the mine, but he died of exposure along Keys View Road in the winter of 1925, and was buried by Keys near the Lost Horse Mine turnoff. As you hike this popular trail to the mine, imagine this Wild West drama unfolding and take care that your hiking partner doesn't double-cross you.

In May 2009, the Lost Horse Fire started under suspicious circumstances and burned through this area. Thankfully, firefighters stopped it before Lost Horse Mine.

The wide trail, formerly a wagon road, begins at the east end of the parking area. It starts up the wash, but promptly veers left at a sign. Many of the junipers, Mojave yuccas, and nolinas that are common throughout this area were burned in the Lost Horse Fire. The trail tends east beneath a hill strewn with volcanic rocks. For an interesting detour, scramble up to the top of the hill to find five- and six-sided basalt columns naturally formed as the magma cooled and then split apart. One has to travel to Devils Postpile in the Sierra Nevada to find an equally good example of basalt columns.

The trail then gradually climbs to the southeast. In 1 mile, it crosses a low ridge and views open up to the east; soon after, the Lost Horse Mine comes into view. In another mile, reach a trail and an old roadbed forking left toward the mine.

The mill is fenced off. The shaft formerly reached a depth of 500 feet, with lateral tunnels branching every 100 feet. As the wooden frame decayed and the tunnels began to collapse, a sinkhole began to form. The Park Service has plugged the shaft and shored up the mill, but stay clear of the fence for your safety. You can also explore the foundations of the old cabins and the old cyanide settling tanks. Return the way you came.

VARIATION

To climb Lost Horse Mountain, continue southeast up the right fork of the main trail to the saddle at the end of the valley. At the saddle, turn right and hike cross-country up to the top of the ridge. There are three small bumps of nearly equal height on the top of the ridge; the farthest one is the highest and is home to the summit register. The summit offers panoramic views, including Lost Horse Valley and San Gorgonio and San Jacinto to the west, Ryan Mountain to the north, and black Malapai Hill in Pleasant Valley to the east. This excursion adds 1 mile and 300 feet of elevation gain to your adventure.

ALTERNATIVE FINISH

For an even better trip that's just 2 miles longer, make a loop rather than retracing your steps. Continue southeast up the right fork of the main trail to a saddle in 0.2 mile, where you have a good view of Malapai Hill's basalt slopes. (This saddle is the departure point for the Lost Horse Mountain variation described above.) Descend the steep and rugged remains of a former mining road into a beautiful system of ridges and gullies. In 0.5 mile, reach the remains of Lang Mine.

Follow the trail as it climbs onto a ridge and then turns west along the south flank of Lost Horse Mountain. In another 0.5 mile, pass a chimney at the site of the former Optimist Mine. The deep mine shaft can be found above a large pile of tailings. It isn't fenced, so treat it with healthy respect.

In another 1.3 miles, the trail crosses a dry wash. The trail generally follows the wash, sometimes along the side and sometimes straight down the sandy center, through a secluded valley full of Joshua trees. In 2.2 miles, reach the dirt road at an unmarked junction, which is difficult to identify. Turn right (east) and hike up the road 0.1 mile to the trailhead where you began.

trip 15.9   Ryan Mountain

see
map on
p. 364

Distance	3 miles (out-and-back)
Hiking Time	2 hours
Elevation Gain	1,000'
Difficulty	Moderate
Best Times	October–April
Agency	Joshua Tree National Park
Recommended Maps	Trails Illustrated *Joshua Tree* or USGS *Indian Cove* and *Keys View* 7.5'
Permit	Joshua Tree National Park entry fee required (see page 355)

DIRECTIONS From the main Park Boulevard through Joshua Tree National Park at mile marker 13, park at the large signed Ryan Mountain Trailhead parking lot, on the south side of the road.

J. D. and Thomas Ryan, owners of the lucrative Lost Horse Mine, built a homestead around 1900, and the bright red adobe walls are still visible. The mountain overlooking their homestead has come to be known as Ryan Mountain. At 5,461 feet, it's one of the tallest peaks in Joshua Tree National Park. Ryan Mountain offers perhaps the best panoramic view in the park. In the distance, the tall summits of San Jacinto and San Gorgonio, capped with snow in the winter and spring, rise above the scenic features of Joshua Tree.

From the signed trailhead on the south side of the parking area, walk south past huge boulders. The wide and well-built trail soon begins climbing steadily and continues at a nearly constant grade all the way to the summit. Many rock steps are built into the mountainside. In 0.2 mile, pass a signed junction with a trail on the left coming in from Sheep Pass Group Campground (near site 1). As the trail rounds the corner of the mountain, the enormous Saddle Rocks come into view. Look for climbers on the longest technical routes in the park. Eventually, the trail crosses a small wash and follows the east side of the mountain before it ends at a sign and huge rock pile on the summit. After enjoying the views, return the way you came.

Ryan Mountain

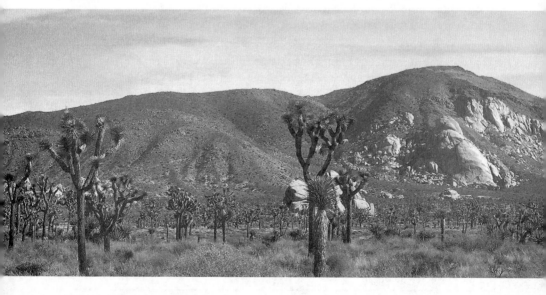

trip 15.10   Queen Mountain

Distance	4 miles (out-and-back)
Hiking Time	3 hours
Elevation Gain	1,200'
Difficulty	Moderate
Best Times	October–March
Agency	Joshua Tree National Park
Required Map	Trails Illustrated *Joshua Tree* or USGS *Queen Mountain* 7.5'
Permit	Joshua Tree National Park entry fee required (see page 355)

see map on p. 364

DIRECTIONS From Park Boulevard through Joshua Tree National Park, 0.4 mile east of mile marker 11, turn north onto good dirt Big Horn Pass Road. Drive north, staying right at a fork in 0.4 mile; then continue straight at a four-way junction, arriving at the road's end 1.8 miles from the paved road.

Queen Mountain (5,687') is the second-tallest summit in Joshua Tree National Park and one of the most fun scrambles in the park. This cross-country adventure features a walk along a sandy wash, followed by a scramble up a rocky gully to the summit rocks. Queen Mountain offers grand views over Queen Valley, the Wonderland of Rocks, and out to the high ridges of San Gorgonio and San Jacinto. Queen Mountain is in a day-use area; no camping is allowed.

From the parking area, look north toward the mountain to identify your route. The two highest points are separated by a prominent saddle on the ridge. The true summit is the one to the left of the saddle. A rocky gully leads to the saddle—this is your route. Also, closely note where you're leaving your vehicle. You'll be returning cross-country to this spot and may not be able to see the vehicle until you're very close. A GPS can be helpful if you're not an experienced desert navigator.

Hike due east across the desert 0.25 mile to the second wash. A trail once led in this direction, but few traces remain. Turn left at the wash and follow it northeast. Watch for old man prickly pear and cholla cacti. Climb some rock slabs as you pass between two low hills; then continue northeast up the wash. Look for another wash, strewn with light-colored rocks, coming straight down from the south face of the peak. When you come close to this wash, depart from the wash you've been following and walk up the left (west) side toward the main gully coming down from the notch. Hike up the gully or along a dirt use trail on the left side of the gully. Pass some huge prickly pear cacti along the way.

At the saddle atop the gully is a flat sandy clearing. The true high point is a slab to the west (left), partially hidden behind a large rock outcrop. You may find a faint path marked with cairns passing around the south side of the outcrop, then leading up the huge slab to the summit.

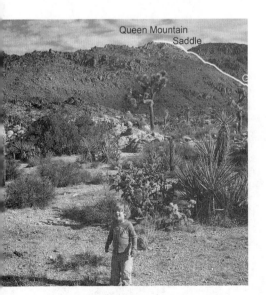

Queen Mountain Saddle

Queen Mountain approach

Return the way you came, taking care to exit the wash at the right place to reach the road's end. There are some low hills to the west of the parking area.

trip 15.11 Desert Queen Mine

Distance	1 mile (out-and-back)
Hiking Time	30 minutes
Elevation Gain	300'
Difficulty	Easy
Trail Use	Good for kids
Best Times	October–April
Agency	Joshua Tree National Park
Recommended Map	Trails Illustrated *Joshua Tree* or USGS *Queen Mountain* 7.5'
Permit	Joshua Tree National Park entry fee required (see page 355)

see map on p. 364

DIRECTIONS From the main Park Boulevard through Joshua Tree National Park, 0.1 mile east of mile marker 10 and directly opposite the Geology Tour Road, turn north onto good dirt Desert Queen Mine Road and proceed 1.3 miles to the parking area at the Pine City backcountry board.

M ost gold miners in California toiled hard to extract a meager existence from marginally productive veins. The owners of the Desert Queen Mine were some of the rare few to make substantial profits. According to the U.S. Bureau of Mines, 3,845 ounces of gold were extracted from the mine between 1895 and 1961. Nevertheless, owning the mine was no stroke of luck. Frank James discovered gold here in 1894, but his time to enjoy it was short. Jim McHaney took over the mine after his henchman shot James "in self-defense" under suspicious circumstances. But Jim's mining career was terminated in 1900 when he was arrested in San Bernardino for counterfeiting. In subsequent years, the mine changed hands under other unfortunate circumstances. In 1976, the mine was placed on the National Register of Historic Places. This short hike tours the site and invites you to imagine the heady heyday of the gold rush. The National Park Service has covered most of the shafts for safety. Nevertheless, keep a close eye on children so that they don't wander into trouble.

Desert Queen Mine

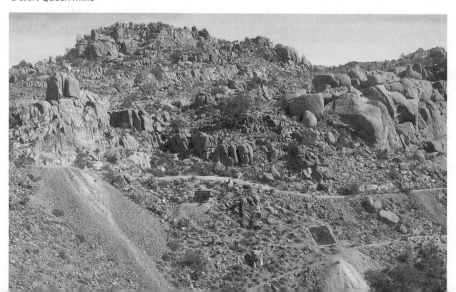

Begin hiking east from the parking area on a dirt road. In 0.2 mile, near the low stone walls of a ruined structure, turn left and descend the old mining road into Desert Queen Wash. Continue up the mining road to reach some covered mine shafts and historic mining equipment. It's worth the walk farther up the road/trail onto the ridge, which is riddled with many more shafts.

VARIATIONS———

Two other trails depart from the Pine City backcountry board. The Pine City Trail is a 4-mile out-and-back hike with 300 feet of elevation gain. The mining operation at Pine City is long gone and has nothing to see, but the trail passes some interesting rocks and desert plants.

The Lucky Boy Loop is a more compelling loop, also 4 miles with 300 feet of elevation gain. It follows a wash and trail and passes shafts from the Elton Mine, which was active but unprofitable in the 1930s.

---

trip 15.12　Negro Hill

Distance	1.2 miles (out-and-back)
Hiking Time	1 hour
Elevation Gain	400'
Difficulty	Easy
Best Times	October–April
Agency	Joshua Tree National Park
Recommended Maps	Trails Illustrated *Joshua Tree* or USGS *Queen Mountain* 7.5'
Permit	Joshua Tree National Park entry fee required (see page 355)

see map on p. 364

DIRECTIONS From the main Park Boulevard through Joshua Tree National Park, 0.1 mile east of mile marker 10 and directly opposite Geology Tour Road, turn north onto good dirt Desert Queen Mine Road and proceed 1.3 miles to the parking area at the Pine City backcountry board.

Negro Hill (4,875') is an unprepossessing dark-colored bump in Queen Valley that offers some of the best panoramic views in all of the park. The cross-country walk up the dirt slopes traverses a splendid cactus garden. While the ascent isn't difficult, hikers must have good balance and exercise caution due to the abundance of prickly plants.

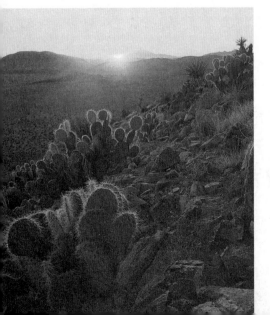

From the Pine City backcountry board, look northwest and identify the nearby Negro Hill. Pick your favorite path to the top; all are feasible. Walk 0.3 mile across Queen Valley to the base of the hill; then climb another 0.3 mile up the moderately steep slope. The hillside is covered with Mojave yucca and many species of cactus, including cholla, pancake prickly pear, and hedgehog. It's also a great place to find the somewhat uncommon cushion foxtail cactus.

Beware of pancake prickly pear cactus on Negro Hill when descending at sunset!

The high point is near the northern end of the mountain, recognizable by the large pancake prickly pear cactus. From the top, you can enjoy 360-degree views over Queen Valley to Queen Mountain, the corner of the Wonderland of Rocks, San Gorgonio and San Jacinto, and Ryan Mountain.

If you go for the sunset, be sure to descend before it becomes too dark. Picking a cross-country path through the cactus is difficult in the dark. If in doubt, head due south to a dirt road; then turn left and follow it back to your vehicle.

trip 15.13 Malapai Hill

Distance	1.5 miles (out-and-back)
Hiking Time	1.5 hours
Elevation Gain	500'
Difficulty	Moderate
Trail Use	Good for kids
Best Times	October–March
Agency	Joshua Tree National Park
Recommended Map	Trails Illustrated *Joshua Tree* or USGS *Malapai Hill* 7.5'
Permit	Joshua Tree National Park entry fee required (see page 355)

see map on p. 364

DIRECTIONS From Park Boulevard through Joshua Tree National Park, 0.1 mile east of mile marker 10, turn south onto the dirt Geology Tour Road. This road is listed as a 4WD route but is usually passable to Malapai Hill in a standard on-road vehicle. At the start of the road, look for a small box containing a pamphlet about the sights along the Geology Tour Road; these are sold on the honor system for 25¢ and are well worth the investment. Drive south 4.4 miles to marker 7, and park off the road.

Malapai Hill is a black double-humped basalt mound, the remnant of a recent intrusion of magma into the monzogranite. The hike to the summit of the hill from the Geology Tour Road is shorter than it looks, and is a fun excuse to get out of the car and put your hands on some geology.

Malapai Hill

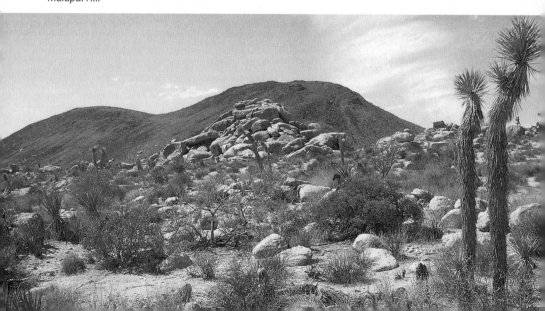

The right (northern) hump of Malapai Hill is the high point. From the parking area, head straight across the desert toward the summit. A large monzogranite rock pile blocks your way and it's slightly easier to bypass on the left (south). Watch out for the plentiful cactus. Ascend the hill any way you like, either on the steep dirt or up the piles of basalt talus. From the top, enjoy the panoramic views over Queen Valley. Lost Horse and Ryan Mountains are to the west. The Hexie Mountains are to the east, and the Little San Bernardino Mountains are to the south.

On the west side, you can find a few five- and six-sided basalt columns. Test your compass on the black rocks. Some are magnetite and will deflect the needle.

trip 15.14 Mount Inspiration

Distance	1.5 miles (out-and-back)
Hiking Time	1.5 hours
Elevation Gain	700'
Difficulty	Easy
Trail Use	Good for kids
Best Times	October–April
Agency	Joshua Tree National Park
Optional Map	Trails Illustrated *Joshua Tree* or USGS *Keys View* 7.5'
Permit	Joshua Tree National Park entry fee required (see page 355)

see map on p. 364

DIRECTIONS From the main Park Boulevard through Joshua Tree National Park, 0.8 mile east of mile marker 16, turn south onto Keys View Road. Proceed 5.5 miles to the parking area at the end of the road.

Keys View, atop the Little San Bernardino Mountains, is a popular automobile destination for park visitors, offering overlooks of the Coachella Valley. Hikers willing to venture up the short but steep trail to Mount Inspiration are rewarded with even better panoramic views on a clear day. Those who are observant, quiet, and lucky might even

Nolina at sunset

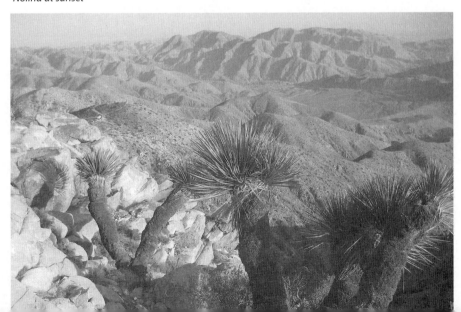

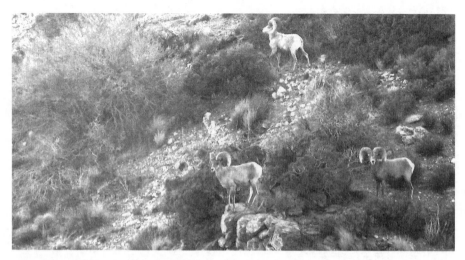

Bighorn sheep below Mount Inspiration

catch sight of the elusive desert bighorn sheep. Mount Inspiration is one of the park's major summits that stand at more than 5,000 feet.

Take the unsigned trail from the northwest side of the parking area up the steep hill to the north. The trail is rocky and sometimes poorly defined. After passing numerous junipers and yuccas, reach the top of the hill marked with a large cairn. Descend the trail northwest to a saddle, then up to a second rocky hill, Point 5,559'. This is a satisfying summit with grand views, but purists will want to continue on over a third minor bump to the Inspiration benchmark, the true high point.

The views from the top on a clear day include the Coachella Valley and Salton Sea to the south, San Jacinto and San Gorgonio towering to the west, and the valleys, hills, and rock formations of Joshua Tree to the north. Sunrise and sunset are especially good times. Unfortunately, smog from the Los Angeles Basin tends to blow eastward, obscuring the views as much as half of the time.

trip 15.15   **Mount Inspiration from the Coachella Valley**

see map on p. 364

Distance	14 miles (out-and-back)
Hiking Time	9 hours
Elevation Gain	4,600'
Difficulty	Strenuous
Best Times	October–April
Agency	Joshua Tree National Park
Required Map	Trails Illustrated *Joshua Tree* or USGS *Keys View* 7.5'

DIRECTIONS From the 10 Freeway (I-10), take Exit 131 for Ramon Road. Drive east on the north side of the freeway for 4.5 miles, and turn left onto Thousand Palms Road. Proceed nearly 5 miles to its end at Dillon Road. Two minor roads continue on the opposite side of Dillon Road—take the right road, which starts off as poor pavement and eventually becomes good dirt. Stay on the main road as you pass many spurs. In 4 miles, reach a junction about a mile east of Fan Hill. A dirt road leads south and a fainter old jeep road leads north. Park here. If you reach the end of the main road at an aqueduct service area littered with unbelievable quantities of shotgun shells and broken glass, you've gone 0.25 mile too far.

A ny mountaineer who spends enough time in the Joshua Tree area will inevitably start to wonder about the steep south wall of the Little San Bernardino Mountains. From the Keys View overlook, an intricate maze of ridges and canyons seems to spiral down into the desert below. One of the classic cross-country adventures in this area is to climb Mount Inspiration the hard way, from the Coachella Valley. This demanding trip visits an old mine site and offers rugged, desolate beauty. Watch for bighorn sheep, which are known to haunt these seldom-visited slopes.

Maps of this area are incomplete. The majority of miles on this trip follow an old mining road to a point just beneath Hidden Gold Mine. The Trails Illustrated map doesn't show the road at all, and the *Keys View* topo represents the road as a trail ending long before the mine. Both maps place the mine too low in the canyon.

From the parking area, hike north on an old dirt mining road. In 250 feet, pass a post marking the road closure at the wilderness boundary. Follow the road as it hugs the east edge of a huge alluvial fan covered with creosote bushes. In about 3 miles, the road veers right (east) into a narrower canyon and soon passes a cable and rock barrier marking the former wilderness boundary. In another 0.8 mile, the road swings left into the first canyon on the north. Continue 1.1 miles to the end of the road. The road deteriorates near the end and can become indistinct.

Continue hiking cross-country up the canyon, staying right at a fork. The canyon narrows and turns back to the left. At the next fork (**N33° 55.265' W116° 11.708'; 3,850'**), veer right up a tributary canyon. The upper reaches of this canyon become unpleasantly steep and loose; the thought of carrying heavy loads of ore down this canyon gives one pause. Pass scattered beams, then a shallow excavation, and then the partially collapsed site of two adits.

Scramble up a short distance to the ridge, which soon becomes easier. The desert scrub gives way to junipers. You may find traces of a prospector's trail leading up the ridge. As you climb, breathtaking panoramas open up beneath you extending from the Salton Sea past the Santa Rosa and San Jacinto Mountains to San Gorgonio. After 1,100 feet of climbing, pop over the lip to the Keys View overlook, where you may startle tourists who have driven to the site. At this point, you've traveled 6 miles and climbed 4,000 feet.

You might choose to turn back here and retrace your steps. For the complete mountaineering experience, continue to the top of Mount Inspiration. From the west end of the

Morning light from Keys View, with San Jacinto on the horizon

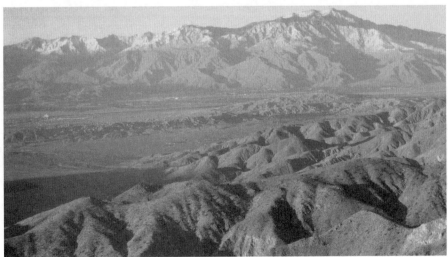

parking lot, follow a climber's trail up the hill, down to a saddle, and up again. Skirt the north edge of the next bump, climb Point 5,558', and continue to a third bump, which is the true peak. A benchmark reading "Inspiration" can be found atop the bouldery summit.

Return the way you came, or follow the ridge descending south from Point 5,558'. The ridge splits and any of the branches can be negotiated, but steep drop-offs near the bottom of all of the ridges require some route finding to circumvent. The mining road can be found just below the ridges.

---

trip 15.16   **Mount Minerva Hoyt**

Distance	7 miles (out-and-back)
Hiking Time	5 hours
Elevation Gain	1,900'
Difficulty	Strenuous
Best Times	October–April
Agency	Joshua Tree National Park
Required Map	Trails Illustrated *Joshua Tree* or USGS *Indian Cove* 7.5'
Permit	Joshua Tree National Park entry fee required (see page 355)

DIRECTIONS From the West Entrance Station of Joshua Tree National Park, drive 5.8 miles into the park on Park Boulevard to the Quail Springs Picnic Area, on the right (south) side of the road near mile marker 20.

As mentioned in the chapter introduction, Joshua Tree National Park owes its existence to Minerva Hoyt, a Pasadena socialite and conservationist who lobbied FDR to give the area National Monument status in 1936. In 2013, the U.S. Board on Geographic Names bestowed her name upon a summit in the center of the park to commemorate her efforts.

The mountain can be approached by cross-country routes from the north or the east. This trip describes the northern approach, which is more strenuous, but shorter and more interesting. This route crosses Johnny Lang Canyon and passes Lang Mine. After Lang sold out of the Lost Horse Mine (see Trip 15.8), he moved to this scenic canyon and continued his prospecting.

Minerva Hoyt climbers' route, bypassing Lang Mine

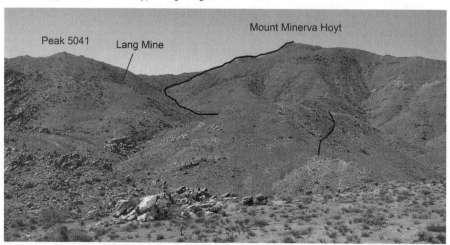

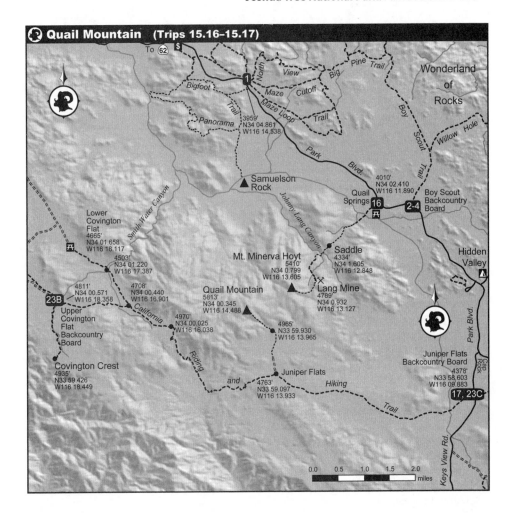

From the picnic area, look south and identify Mount Minerva Hoyt, labeled on topographic maps as Peak 5,405'. You'll reach the summit from the saddle just left of the peak. Head south from the picnic area on a good unsigned trail leading to a wash emerging from a rocky ravine. Follow the wash, dodging brush and scrambling over boulders in the narrow ravine, until it widens into a valley. Continue south up the valley to a low saddle.

Drop 200 feet down from the saddle into Johnny Lang Canyon; then pick a path up the other side. A prominent gully descends from the saddle between Mount Minerva Hoyt and Peak 5,041'. As you head up toward this saddle, you'll pass the trace of an old road/trail used by Lang. Soon you'll see his mine on the north slope of Peak 5,041'. It's worth a detour up the steep slope to peer down the shaft through a massive grate installed by the Park Service.

From Lang Mine, the easiest route is to continue up to the summit of Peak 5,041', then turn right and drop slightly to the saddle before you finish the climb up Mount Minerva Hoyt. If you skipped the mine, just continue up the gully until you feel like turning right and ascending the slopes to the summit.

If you're still looking for more adventure, consider continuing southwest for a mile to Quail Mountain, the park's highest point (see Trip 15.17).

trip 15.17   Quail Mountain

Distance	13 miles (out-and-back)
Hiking Time	7 hours
Elevation Gain	1,800'
Difficulty	Strenuous
Trail Use	Suitable for backpacking
Best Times	October–April
Agency	Joshua Tree National Park
Required Maps	Trails Illustrated *Joshua Tree* or USGS *Keys View* and *Indian Cove* 7.5'
Permit	Joshua Tree National Park entry fee required (see page 355)

see map on previous page

DIRECTIONS From the main Park Boulevard through Joshua Tree National Park, 0.8 mile east of mile marker 16, turn south onto Keys View Road. In 1.1 miles, turn right onto Juniper Flats Road and park at the signed Juniper Flats Trailhead, on your right.

Quail Mountain (5,813') is the highest point in Joshua Tree National Park. The mountain is at the southeast end of a long and complex ridge separating Covington Flats from the main part of Joshua Tree National Park. It's situated far from any roads, and there's a lengthy approach across Lost Horse Valley.

Follow the California Riding and Hiking Trail west through healthy stands of Joshua trees. In 1.7 miles, pass a turnoff to the south for the Stubbe Spring Loop; then in another 1.9 miles, pass another turnoff to the south for the other end of the loop. In an additional 1 mile, reach a dirt road (closed) crossing the trail at the aptly named Juniper Flats.

Turn right (north) onto the road and follow it 0.5 mile to the end. Two peaks are visible to the northwest. The true summit is the rightmost, farther one. Take a good look so you can identify it later, before you enter more complicated terrain ahead. Also, identify landmarks at the end of the road so you can find your way back. Hike across the flats toward the peak, and climb either the southeast ridge or the canyon immediately south of the ridge. This is a good area to watch for wildlife.

You may notice some pieces of aircraft wreckage near the summit. In 1999, two civilian T-28s crashed into the west side of the mountain near the 5,300-foot level when clouds obscured the peak.

The summit offers panoramic views on a clear day. Four other major high points in the park (Eureka Peak to the west, Inspiration Point to the southeast, Ryan Mountain to the east, and Queen Mountain to the northeast) are all visible. On the horizon are the highest points in three more distant ranges: San Gorgonio in the San Bernardino Mountains, San Jacinto in the San Jacinto Mountains, and Toro Peak in the Santa Rosas. After enjoying the view, return the way you came.

trip 15.18   Skull Rock Nature Trail

Distance	1.7 miles (loop)
Hiking Time	1 hour
Elevation Gain	200'
Difficulty	Easy
Trail Use	Good for kids
Best Times	October–April
Agency	Joshua Tree National Park
Recommended Map	Trails Illustrated *Joshua Tree* or USGS *Malapai Hill* 7.5'
Permit	Joshua Tree National Park entry fee required (see page 355)

see map on p. 364

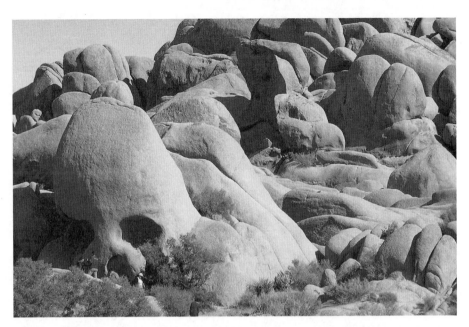

Skull Rock draws throngs of visitors.

DIRECTIONS From the main Park Boulevard through Joshua Tree National Park, 0.7 mile east of mile marker 9, park directly opposite the entrance to Jumbo Rocks Campground. If no space is available on the side of the road, look for additional parking on the campground road.

The Skull Rock Nature Trail tours the outstanding geology of the Jumbo Rocks area and passes interpretive signs describing the uniquely adapted desert vegetation. It can be reached from one of three trailheads: the one described above across from the Jumbo Rocks Campground entrance, from Skull Rock itself 0.6 mile farther east along Park Boulevard, or from the Jumbo Rocks Campground across from site 93.

This trip assumes a clockwise loop starting at the campground entrance, crossing the road at Skull Rock, continuing to the campground, and returning by way of the campground road. Rock formations along the way tempt curious hikers to explore and scramble. It's easy to accidentally stray from this trail, so backtrack if you find yourself off route.

The signed trail starts on the north side of the road and wanders through a granite boulder field before entering a sandy wash. Squeeze past rocks in the wash and reach a small dam (locally known as a tank), where ranchers once collected water. The tank has long since filled with sand. Exit the wash just beyond, and cross the road at Skull Rock, 0.8 mile from the start. Skull Rock is a fine example of *tafoni,* a technical term for concave hollows common on rocks in the park. Geologists believe these hollows formed underground when decaying plant matter released acids that weakened the adjacent rock. Subsequently, the topsoil and weakened granite eroded away, leaving the pitted boulders.

Hike back on the south side of the road through the Jumbo Rocks. Watch for dikes of aplite that protrude like teeth from the softer granite. Interpretive signs identify plants such as junipers, pinyon pines, Mojave yuccas, creosote bushes, and jojoba. Many of these plants were used by Native Americans for medicinal purposes and science is just beginning to rediscover their benefits. In 0.5 mile, reach the campground road. Turn right and walk 0.4 mile up the road to where you began the loop.

trip 15.19 **Split Rock**

Distance	2 miles (loop)
Hiking Time	1.5 hours
Elevation Gain	500'
Difficulty	Easy
Trail Use	Good for kids
Best Times	October–April
Agency	Joshua Tree National Park
Recommended Map	Trails Illustrated *Joshua Tree* or USGS *Queen Mountain* 7.5'
Permit	Joshua Tree National Park entry fee required (see page 355)

see map on p. 364

DIRECTIONS From the main Park Boulevard through Joshua Tree National Park east of Jumbo Rocks Campground, 0.1 mile east of mile marker 7, turn north at a sign for Split Rock. Follow the good dirt road 0.5 mile to the Split Rock Picnic Area, at the end.

The Split Rock loop is an enjoyable ramble among Joshua Tree's humongous monzo-granite boulders. Rock climbers flock to this area, and it's likely that you'll see them clinging to the walls on a pleasant day. The terrain is complicated, and the trail isn't always marked as well as it could be, so this trip is not recommended for inexperienced navigators.

From the Split Rock picnic area, hike north on a poorly defined trail around the left side of a house-sized boulder. The back side of the overhanging rock forms a cave, with a small tunnel at the rear that young explorers love to crawl through. Continue north and descend into a valley dotted with Mojave yuccas. Split Rock is visible to the right, with the sky peeking through a narrow fissure in the upper portion.

In 0.3 mile, the trail abruptly bends to the left at a sign indicating SPLIT ROCK in both directions. A narrower trail on the right leads to the Eagle Cliffs (see Trip 15.20). Follow the trail to the left, which leads southwest and then south. In another 0.6 mile, reach another clump of huge granite boulders. Look to your right for a formation aptly named Tulip Rock.

The trail continues south 0.3 mile, then abruptly turns left and meanders through the boulders and cliffs back toward the picnic area. Pass another vista of Tulip Rock; then enter a wash leading through a gap between the rocks. If you look back just before you enter the wash, you may see a rock crag with a "window" and another smaller formation with an arch.

Posts mark the exit from the wash and the path back to the southwest side of the Split Rock picnic area.

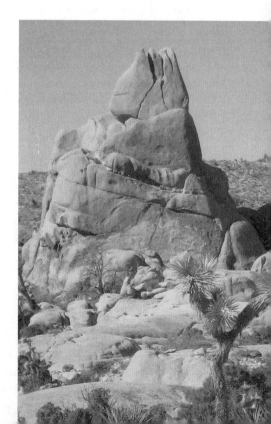

Tulip Rock

trip 15.20   Eagle Cliffs and Mine

see map on p. 364

Distance	3 miles (one-way or out-and-back)
Hiking Time	2 hours
Elevation Gain	900'
Difficulty	Moderate
Trail Use	Good for kids
Best Times	October–April
Agency	Joshua Tree National Park
Required Map	Trails Illustrated *Joshua Tree* or USGS *Queen Mountain* 7.5'
Permit	Joshua Tree National Park entry fee required (see page 355)

DIRECTIONS This hike can be done either as a one-way traverse from the Split Rock Picnic Area to the Pine City backcountry board or as an out-and-back from either trailhead. To reach the Pine City Trailhead from Park Boulevard, 0.1 mile east of mile marker 10, turn north onto good dirt Desert Queen Mine Road and proceed 1.3 miles to the signed parking area, where you can leave a car or bicycle.

To reach Split Rock, return to Park Boulevard and continue east 3 miles to a point 0.1 mile east of mile marker 7. Turn left (north) at a sign for Split Rock. Follow the good dirt road 0.5 mile to the Split Rock Picnic Area, at the end.

The Eagle Cliffs are a beautiful area of granite and rich desert vegetation. A fascinating cabin is built into the rocks high up on the ridge beside the small Eagle Mine. This short but action-packed one-way hike tours the Split Rock area, the Eagle Cliffs, and the Desert Queen Mine, using an unmaintained trail that's rugged and occasionally faint. If you don't want to arrange a shuttle, you can begin from either end. The hike from Split Rock is slightly shorter and easier to follow, but the hike from the Pine City board is less strenuous.

This hike has many features to keep kids interested, but the steep climbs and numerous cacti and sharp rocks may be hard on kids younger than about 7. Don't confuse the Eagle Cliffs in the center of the park with the Eagle Mountain at the eastern end of the park.

From the Split Rock picnic area, hike north on a poorly defined trail around the left side of a house-sized boulder. The back side of the overhanging rock forms a cave, with a small tunnel at the rear that young explorers love to crawl through. Continue north and descend into a valley dotted with Mojave yuccas. Split Rock is visible to the right, with the sky peeking through a narrow fissure in the upper portion. Look at the ridge to the northwest and identify the prominent gully leading up to an obelisk-shaped rock on the skyline. This landmark will be your guide on the climb. The *Queen Mountain* topo omits the Eagle Cliffs Trail, but the gully is southwest of Peak 4,793'.

In 0.3 mile, the main trail abruptly bends to the left at a sign indicating SPLIT ROCK

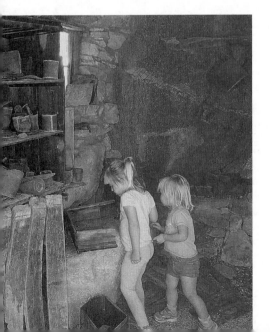

Cabin at Eagle Mine: Please leave historical artifacts undisturbed so that future visitors may enjoy them as well.

to the left and back from where you came. Take an unsigned and unmaintained trail on the right, which leads north-northwest to the base of the gully. Travel becomes more difficult as you climb the gully and the trail is obscure in places, but continue up to the crest beside a pinyon pine, 0.7 mile from the Split Rock Trail and not far from the obelisk. Cat's claw, nolina, and various cactus including pancake prickly pear, silver cholla, Engelmann's hedgehog, and barrel cactus enliven the trip as you ascend.

Hike down the north side of the ridge 25 yards to a pile of tailings beside a small adit. The trail forks here. The right trail leads north, briefly regaining the ridge and reaching another tailings pile in 0.2 mile. The grated Eagle Mine shaft is partially concealed by a live oak beside the tailings. The site was located in 1895 by Robert Muir and was worked by various miners over the years. A remarkable cabin can be found built into the cliff just north of the mine. It was built sometime after 1890 and is one of the best-preserved historical structures in the park. Take care not to disturb the cabin or remove any artifacts; they become mere junk without their historical context.

If you're descending to the Pine City Trailhead, return to the fork below the ridgeline and take the other path down into a bowl, then down into a second valley. William Keys used to pack ore down this trail by burro in the 1930s and process it at the Wall Street Mill to extract $35 of gold from each ton of hard-won ore.

In 0.4 mile, the trail turns left onto the remains of an abandoned mining road. From here, you can look back up to the obelisk on the ridge. Follow the road 0.4 mile to the Desert Queen Mine, an extensive cluster of shafts on the ridgeline. The trail turns south and descends into a canyon, where you'll find several more shafts and abandoned mining equipment. In 0.3 mile, cross the Desert Queen Wash. Follow the old mining road back up to the northwest and out to the backcountry board in 0.4 mile.

trip 15.21 Arch Rock Nature Trail

Distance	0.3 mile (loop)
Hiking Time	15 minutes
Elevation Gain	50'
Difficulty	Easy
Trail Use	Good for kids
Best Times	October–April
Agency	Joshua Tree National Park
Optional Map	USGS *Malapai Hill* 7.5'
Permit	Joshua Tree National Park entry fee required (see page 355)

DIRECTIONS From Highway 62 in the town of Twentynine Palms, turn south onto Utah Trail. Drive through the North Entrance Station of Joshua Tree National Park and continue to the junction with Pinto Basin Road, a total of 8.8 miles from Highway 62. Turn left and proceed 2.7 miles to the White Tank Campground. Turn left again onto a dirt road, and park near site 9 at the signed Arch Rock Trailhead.

Arches and natural bridges are formed when more rapid erosion takes place on the lower parts on a rock. These formations are common in sandstone but rare in granite. Arch Rock is one of these unusual granite arches. A short nature trail explains the arch and many of the park's other prominent geological features. Arch Rock is located halfway along the loop trail.

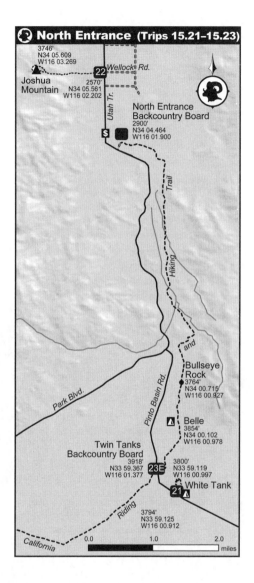

North Entrance (Trips 15.21–15.23)

3746'
N34 05.609
W116 03.269

Joshua
Mountain

2570'
N34 05.561
W116 02.202

Wellock Rd.

22

Utah Tr.

North Entrance
Backcountry Board
2900'
N34 04.464
W116 01.900

S

Hiking and Riding Trail

Bullseye
Rock
3764'
N34 00.715
W116 00.927

Belle
3854'
N34 00.102
W116 00.978

Twin Tanks
Backcountry Board
3918'
N33 59.367
W116 01.377

23E

3800'
N33 59.119
W116 00.997

21

White Tank

Park Blvd.

Pinto Basin Rd.

3794'
N33 59.125
W116 00.912

California

0.0   1.0   2.0
miles

A century ago, Joshua Tree had a climate wet enough to support limited ranching. Ranchers built small dams called tanks across washes to retain rainwater for their cattle. The White Tank Campground and the entire White Tank monzogranite rock formation are named for one of these tanks, which is located just beyond Arch Rock. For a visit to White Tank, follow an alley south past the arch and along the base of a vertical-walled boulder. Then turn left and descend through a tunnel under a large boulder to the wash, where you can see the White Tank. This tank, like most, has filled with sand over the decades.

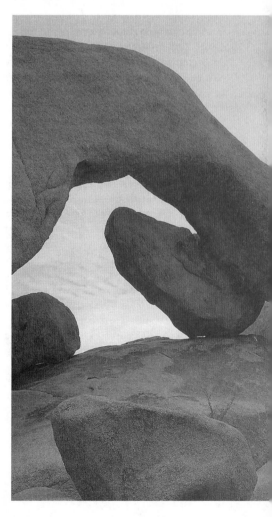

Arch Rock

see map on previous page

trip 15.22 Joshua Mountain

Distance	2.8 miles (out-and-back)
Hiking Time	3 hours
Elevation Gain	1,200'
Difficulty	Moderate
Best Times	October–April
Agency	Joshua Tree National Park
Recommended Map	Trails Illustrated *Joshua Tree* or USGS *Queen Mountain* 7.5'
Permit	Joshua Tree National Park entry fee required (see page 355)

DIRECTIONS From Highway 62 east of downtown Twentynine Palms, turn south onto Utah Trail. Pass the Oasis Visitor Center in 0.5 mile, and continue another 2.5 miles to an intersection with Wellock Road. Park on the shoulder of the road. Alternatively, if you're coming from the south, exit the North Entrance Station and continue 1.0 mile to the aforementioned intersection.

Joshua Mountain would be an insignificant hill on the flank of Queen Mountain were it not for the enormous granite block with a gigantic overhanging corner on its summit. The mountain is also known as Indian Head because imaginative travelers driving south from Twentynine Palms can make out the chiseled profile of a stern face watching over the desert. Joshua Mountain is a short and fun cross-country hike that passes a great variety of cacti, climbs a wash, and then circles the base of the summit to an easier scramble up the back side. Children who like rock scrambling will enjoy the route, but it's not recommended for those who are unsteady on their feet or uncomfortable with heights.

From the parking area, look west to identify the prominent stone summit and the gully that leads straight up to the summit cliffs. Hike across the desert toward the base of the gully. This section of the Mojave is rich with desert plant life. Along the way you'll see Mojave yuccas, silver chollas, pencil chollas, beavertail, hedgehog, barrel, and pincushion cacti. Shortly before you reach the base of the gully, cross a wide, deep wash.

Ascend the gully. For the first part, it's easiest to stay on the slopes to the left, avoiding the larger boulders choking the center. A faint climber's trail may be seen for part of the way. Later, the bottom of the gully becomes easier, though there's plenty of easy boulder-hopping. The gully levels out beneath the summit cliffs, 1 mile from the start.

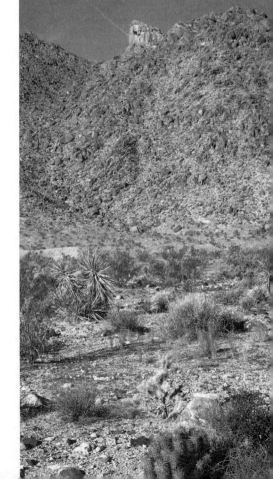

Granite peak of Joshua Mountain above the approach gully

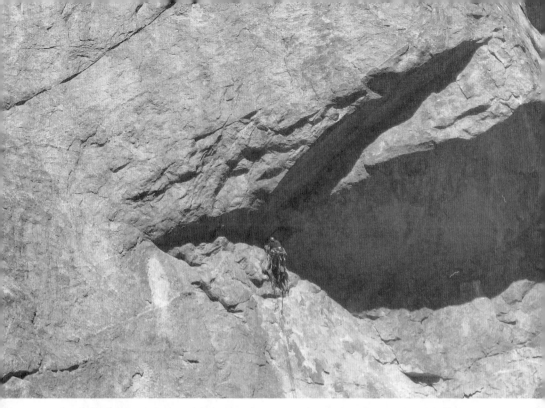

Rock climbers on Joshua Mountain

The cliffs ahead are climbable only by expert rock climbers. You may see intrepid climbers testing their skills on the huge overhanging chin of Indian Head. The gully forks beneath the cliffs; the right fork passes around the east side of the mountain, while the left fork climbs and loops around the west side. Take either fork and work your way around to the north side of the mountain, where more gradual slopes lead up a huge granite slab to the summit. Consider ascending one way and descending the other. You must do a bit of rock scrambling shortly before you reach the top of Joshua Mountain. Take care with children because of the sheer drop off the edge of the summit.

trip 15.23 **California Riding and Hiking Trail**

Distance	37 miles (one-way)
Hiking Time	2–5 days
Elevation Gain	2,500'
Difficulty	Moderate–strenuous backpack
Trail Use	Suitable for backpacking, suitable for equestrians
Best Times	October–April
Agency	Joshua Tree National Park
Required Maps	Trails Illustrated *Joshua Tree* or USGS *Yucca Valley South, Joshua Tree South, East Deception Canyon, Keys View, Malapai Hill,* and *Queen Mountain* 7.5'
Permit	Joshua Tree National Park entry fee required (see page 355)

DIRECTIONS This lengthy hike is divided into five segments. The driving directions for each trailhead are as follows:

(A) Black Rock Campground From Highway 62 in Yucca Valley, 0.4 mile east of mile marker 062 SBD 12.00, turn south onto Joshua Lane directly opposite Highway 247. Joshua Lane veers east and then back south. At a T-junction in 4.4 miles, turn right and then immediately left onto Black Rock Canyon Road and drive into the campground. Shortly after entering the campground, look for the Black Rock backcountry board on the east side of the road. The road is divided here, and the sign can be difficult to see. If you reach the ranger station, you've gone too far.

(B) Upper Covington Flat From Highway 62, 0.2 mile east of mile marker 062 SBD 15.00, turn south at the traffic light onto La Contenta Road. In 1 mile, the road turns to good dirt. In another 2.9 miles, veer left at a sign for Covington Flats. The Park Service recommends 4WD for this road, but it's usually passable by low-clearance vehicles. In 6 miles, the road forks—stay right, as the left fork goes to the desolate Lower Covington Flat picnic area. In another 1.8 miles, turn left at a junction; the right fork goes to Eureka Peak. Finally, in another 1.9 miles, reach the Upper Covington Flat parking area, at the end of the road.

(C) Keys View Road From the main Park Boulevard through Joshua Tree National Park, 0.8 mile east of mile marker 16, turn south onto Keys View Road. In 1.1 miles, turn right onto Juniper Flats Road and park at the signed Juniper Flats Trailhead, on your right.

(D) Geology Tour Road From the main Park Boulevard through Joshua Tree National Park, 0.1 mile east of mile marker 10, turn south onto the dirt Geology Tour Road. The first part of this road is normally passable by low-clearance vehicles. In 1.5 miles, park at the backcountry board.

(E) Twin Tanks At the Pinto Wye, 4.6 miles south of the North Entrance Station, turn onto Pinto Basin Road. Go 2.2 miles to the Twin Tanks parking area, on the west side of the road.

North Entrance From Highway 62 in Twentynine Palms, turn south onto Utah Trail. Drive 4 miles to the North Entrance Station of Joshua Tree National Park. Then continue 0.4 mile. Turn east on an unmarked dirt road, and go 0.2 mile to the parking area at the North Entrance backcountry board. Alternatively, from Park Boulevard 0.6 mile north of mile marker 1, turn east on the aforementioned dirt road.

The California Riding and Hiking Trails Act was passed in 1945 to establish a trail system spanning the entire state. The ambitious project was never completed, and much of it fell into disuse. However, several segments of the California Riding and Hiking Trail (CRHT) still exist, and the 37-mile part through Joshua Tree National Park offers a grand tour of the main park. There's nothing like crossing the park on foot to gain an intimate appreciation of the topography and desert life of this region. This trip can be done as a long backpacking trip or as some combination of five shorter sections. There is no water along the way, so it's helpful to cache water ahead of time near some of the road crossings. The trail is not always clearly marked and is most suitable for experienced backcountry hikers. If you only have time for a shorter trip, the first two segments are recommended because they traverse the wildest country and the most diverse scenery.

| trip 15.23 | **SEGMENT A: Black Rock Campground to Upper Covington Flat** |

Distance	7.5 miles (one-way)
Hiking Time	4 hours
Elevation Gain	800'
Recommended Maps	Trails Illustrated *Joshua Tree* or USGS *Yucca Valley South* and *Joshua Tree South 7.5'*

see map on p. 394

The first part of this trail has especially diverse and interesting desert plant life. It passes a complex warren of trails that are shown on the Trails Illustrated map but not on the USGS topos, so route finding requires care. From the backcountry board, the sandy trail leads east and then south through a forest of Joshua trees for 0.2 mile to a signed junction. Follow the CRHT east out of the wash. Look for Mojave yuccas, silver chollas, and junipers. The yuccas bloom impressively in the spring. In 1.1 miles, reach a second signed junction with the Fault Trail, which veers off to the right. In another 0.3 mile, reach a wash and look for another junction with the Short Loop going south up the wash. Beyond, reach an area that burned in the 2006 Covington Fire. Charred Joshua trees litter the melancholy hillside.

The trail enters a sandy wash and passes two more signed junctions leading south to the Cliff Trail. In another 1.3 miles, the wash forks. Stay on the left fork. (You may see footprints from people who accidentally took the right fork; this leads to the Bigfoot Trail, which is shown on the Trails Illustrated map, but which has nearly vanished into the desert.) Then, 1.4 miles later, the wash begins to emerge from the canyon you've been following. In 0.4 mile, the Eureka Peak Trail cuts off to the right. In another 0.2 mile, reach a dirt road leading west to Eureka Peak. Stay on the CRHT paralleling the road east toward Upper Covington Flat. Soon, reach a road junction. The northeast fork descends to Lower Covington Flat and Yucca Valley, while the CRHT follows alongside the southeast fork toward the Upper Covington Flat Trailhead. The trail gradually descends through the valley full of healthy Joshua trees, heading toward a low pass between the hills to the east. Look to the right for the Upper Covington Flat parking area. If the trail becomes faint and you start following a wash down to the north, you're going the wrong way.

Covington fire burn area

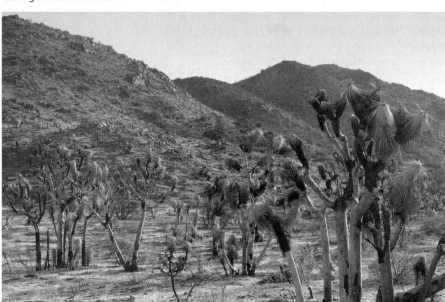

trip 15.23   SEGMENT B: Upper Covington Flat to Keys View Road

Distance	11 miles (one-way)
Hiking Time	6 hours
Elevation Gain	1,100'
Recommended Maps	Trails Illustrated *Joshua Tree* or USGS *Joshua Tree South, East Deception Canyon,* and *Keys View* 7.5'

See maps on pgs. 379, 385, & 394

This is the most remote section of the trail, passing through seldom-visited country behind Quail Mountain. It features some of the largest Joshua trees and prickly pear cacti in the park. It also offers an opportunity for a side trip up Quail Mountain, the highest point in the park. The trail can be hard to follow in places and is unsuitable for inexperienced hikers.

Two trails depart from the parking area in Upper Covington Flat: the signed Covington Crest Trail leads south (see Trip 16.5), while you should take the unmarked CRHT leading east. Note that the 1994 revision of the *Joshua Tree South* 7.5' map shows the trails diverging east of the road's end; this is no longer accurate. In less than 0.1 mile, look on the right side of the trail for the decomposing hulk of what was once the largest Joshua tree in the park. On the left side, another enormous tree still stands.

In 0.6 mile, cross a low saddle and descend into a lonely valley. Cross two washes and come to a signed junction in another 1.1 miles. The trail to the left returns to Lower Covington Flat, while the trail to the right climbs southeast up the valley for 1 mile. This valley is littered with the carcasses of burned Joshua trees and chollas. The complex mass of Quail Mountain looms to the east.

Continue to the right and after reaching another broad saddle, the trail descends into the next valley to the south. Enormous treelike pancake prickly pear cacti grow alongside the trail, along with fine groves of Joshua trees and Mojave yuccas. After rounding the south end of Quail Mountain, 2 miles down the valley, the trail turns east and begins climbing again. It crosses a saddle and, in 2 miles, comes to a dirt road (now closed) in Juniper Flats.

From this point, you can make a 3-mile round-trip north to climb Quail Mountain (see Trip 15.17), but, the CRHT continues east. In 1 mile, it passes the Stubbe Spring Loop Trail leading south, and then in 1.9 more miles passes a second junction to the south with the other end of the loop. There is no reliable source of water at the spring, and to protect wildlife, the Park Service prohibits camping near water sources. Beyond, Ryan Mountain is visible to the east and Lost Horse Mine comes into view as a black speck on a hill south of Ryan Mountain (see Trip 15.8). As you finish the last 1.7 miles through Lost Horse Valley to Keys View Road, you pass through yet another healthy Joshua tree forest and enjoy views of landmarks including Cap Rock and the Headstone.

If you complete this trip in the early evening, consider a short drive up to Keys View to catch the sunset over the park.

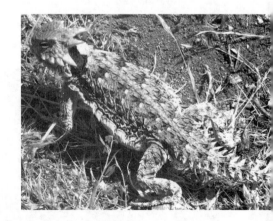

Horned lizard, commonly known as a "horny toad"

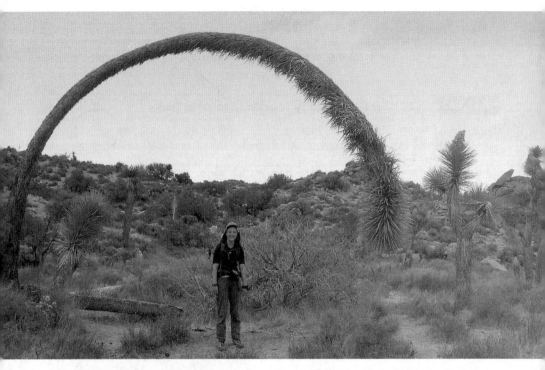

Rainbow Joshua tree along the CRHT

trip 15.23	SEGMENT C: **Keys View Road to Geology Tour Road**

Distance	6.5 miles (one-way)
Hiking Time	3 hours
Elevation Gain	400'
Recommended Maps	Trails Illustrated *Joshua Tree* or
	USGS *Keys View* and *Malapai Hill* 7.5'

see
maps on
pgs. 364
& 379

This stretch of trail leads past Ryan Campground and through a low pass hidden between Ryan and Lost Horse Mountains, then descends across the broad Queen Valley. It's well marked throughout.

The eastbound trail begins 0.1 mile north of the Juniper Flats parking area, on Keys View Road, and leads through the vast Joshua tree forest of Lost Horse Valley. In 0.8 mile, it reaches the south end of Ryan Campground. Watch for rock climbers on Headstone Rock, which is crookedly balanced atop an inselberg at the far end of the campground. Day hikers can start from the campground to shorten the trip, but backpackers must start at the backcountry board at Juniper Flats.

The trail then turns right and leads east toward the low point to just south of Ryan Mountain. As you climb, junipers begin to appear. In places, the path follows an old pipe used to carry water during the mining days. Beyond Ryan Campground 1.9 miles, cross the broad saddle and descend into Queen Valley. In 0.4 mile, watch for the foundation of an old miner's cabin on the left (north) side of the trail. It's easy to miss, but stone markers along the edge of an old pathway provide a clue that you're close. The mature pancake prickly pear growing inside hints at the age of the ruins.

The remainder of the hike leads mostly downhill through another great forest of Joshua trees in Queen Valley, crossing the occasional dry wash en route.

---

trip 15.23   **SEGMENT D: Geology Tour Road to Twin Tanks**

see
map on
p. 364

Distance	4.3 miles (one-way)
Hiking Time	2 hours
Elevation Gain	100'
Recommended Map	Trails Illustrated *Joshua Tree* or USGS *Malapai Hill* 7.5'

This is the shortest and easiest section of the trail. The obvious trail leads mostly downhill across the valley between Jumbo Rocks Campground and the Hexie Mountains. The hills in this part of the park are mostly ancient gneiss, accentuated with the occasional granite outcrop. Thin dikes of light-colored aplite crisscross the desert and in several places they cross the trail.

In about a mile, the trail leads past the south face of Crown Prince Lookout, a granite formation where a World War II airplane warning station was once perched. The rocks near here offer some of the only sheltered camping in the sandy desert. Views from the trail extend back to Ryan and Queen Mountains. San Jacinto can be seen over the shoulder of Lost Horse Mountain, and at times Toro Peak can be seen behind the Little San Bernardino Mountains. Soon views open up into the enormous Pinto Basin to the east. When the trail reaches the paved Pinto Basin Road, the Twin Tanks parking lot can be seen 0.2 mile north along a spur trail.

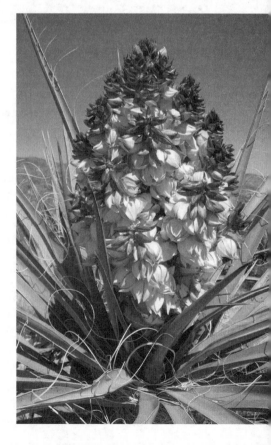

Mojave yucca in bloom

see
map on
p. 385

trip 15.23   **SEGMENT E: Twin Tanks to North Entrance**

Distance	7.1 miles (one-way)
Hiking Time	3.5 hours
Elevation Gain	100'
Recommended Map	Trails Illustrated *Joshua Tree* or USGS *Malapai Hill* and *Queen Mountain* 7.5'.

This section of the trail parallels the paved road and is almost entirely downhill. The trail is set just far enough back from the road so that vehicles are occasionally seen and seldom heard. The first part passes beside a field of house-sized granite boulders. The northern stretch becomes harder to follow in places as it descends along a series of washes.

The trail crosses the paved Pinto Basin Road 0.2 mile south of the Twin Tanks backcountry board. In 1.1 miles, it passes along the east edge of Belle Campground. In 0.7 mile, look for Bullseye Rock, the northernmost boulder along the route. The rock is visible to the east immediately after passing a pile of boulders close to the trail.

In another 0.6 mile, the trail crosses a paved mining road near Pinto Wye. It becomes fainter as it crosses a wash and climbs the rise around the east side of a hill. Beyond, the trail drops into a maze of washes. The vegetation here includes Mojave yuccas, silver and pencil chollas, and bladderpods. The elevation here is lower than most of the park, so it's a good place to see early wildflowers in March. If the trail has been obliterated by winter storms, just hike north between the road and hills, watching for wooden posts marking the route. In 4 miles, just beyond where the paved road turns left, the trail also turns left, leading generally toward the stone summit of Joshua Mountain. In another 0.7 mile, reach the North Entrance backcountry board marking the end of the trail.

Bullseye Rock

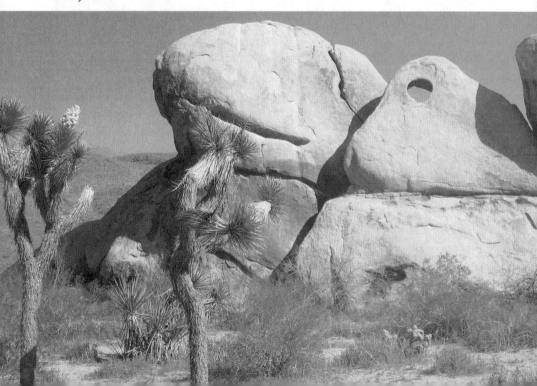

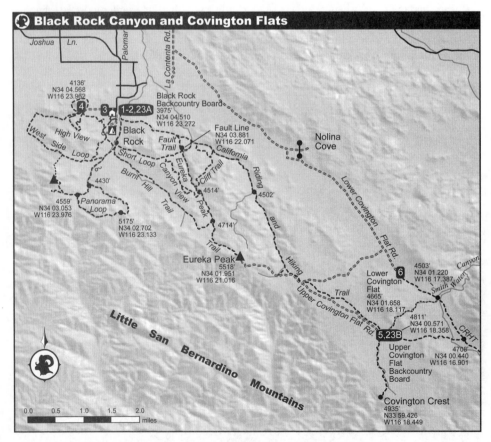

Joshua Tree National Park: Black Rock and Covington

This chapter covers the western end of the park, including the Black Rock and Covington areas. See Chapter 15 for an overview of Joshua Tree National Park. This area has no roads connecting it to the main park, although intrepid hikers can follow the California Riding and Hiking Trail (see pages 388–393 for the five segments of Trip 15.23) across the mountains. (Segments 15.23A and 15.23B are shown on the map below.)

Black Rock lacks the park's famous rock formations but compensates with particularly lush desert vegetation. It's particularly enjoyable in the spring when the desert blooms. The Black Rock Campground is unusual because it has water and accepts reservations. Black Rock is accessed from Joshua Lane in Yucca Valley.

Black Rock Canyon and Covington Flats

Joshua Ln.

Palomar

La Contenta Rd.

4136'
N34 04.568
W116 23.962

4   **3**   **1-2,23A**

Black Rock
Backcountry Board
3975'
N34 04.510
W116 23.272

Black Rock

West Side Loop

High View

Short Loop

Fault Trail

Burnt Hill Trail

4430'

4559'
N34 03.053
W116 23.976

Panorama Loop

5175'
N34 02.702
W116 23.133

Eureka Canyon View Trail

Eureka Peak

Cliff Trail

4514'

4714'

Fault Line
N34 03.881
W116 22.071

California Riding and Hiking Trail

4502'

Nolina Cove

Lower Covington Flat Rd.

Eureka Peak
5518'
N34 01.951
W116 21.016

Hiking Trail

Upper Covington Flat Rd

Lower Covington Flat
4665'
N34 01.658
W116 18.117

4503'
N34 01.220
W116 17.387

6

Smith Water Canyon

4811'
N34 00.571
W116 18.358

5.23B

Upper Covington Flat Backcountry Board

4708'
N34 00.440
W116 16.901

CRHT

Covington Crest
4935'
N33 59.426
W116 18.449

Little San Bernardino Mountains

0.0   0.5   1.0   1.5   2.0
miles

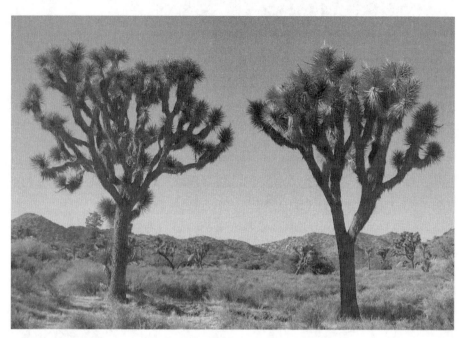

Black Rock and Covington are renowned for their lush desert vegetation.

Covington is notable for enormous Joshua trees, perhaps the largest in the park. This lightly visited area is accessed from Highway 62 just east of Yucca Valley via a long, graded dirt road.

trip 16.1   Black Rock Canyon Panorama Loop

Distance	6.5 miles (semiloop)
Hiking Time	4 hours
Elevation Gain	1,200'
Difficulty	Moderate
Trail Use	Suitable for equestrians
Best Times	October–April
Agency	Joshua Tree National Park
Required Map	Trails Illustrated *Joshua Tree* or USGS *Yucca Valley South* 7.5'
Permit	Joshua Tree National Park entry fee required (see page 355)

see map opposite

DIRECTIONS From Highway 62 in Yucca Valley, turn south onto Joshua Lane at the BLACK ROCK CAMPGROUND sign, opposite where Highway 247 intersects Highway 62, 0.4 mile east of mile marker 062 SBD 12.00. Follow Joshua Lane as it winds east, then back south, and then reaches a T-junction in 4.4 miles. Turn right and then immediately left onto Black Rock Canyon Road, which leads into the campground. The trailhead is at the Black Rock backcountry board, on the east side of the road shortly past the entrance. The road is divided, and the trail can be hard to see.

Black Rock Canyon is located near the western edge of Joshua Tree National Park and is connected to the main park only by way of a long and strenuous footpath. While it lacks the outlandish rock formations characteristic of the main park, Black Rock makes up

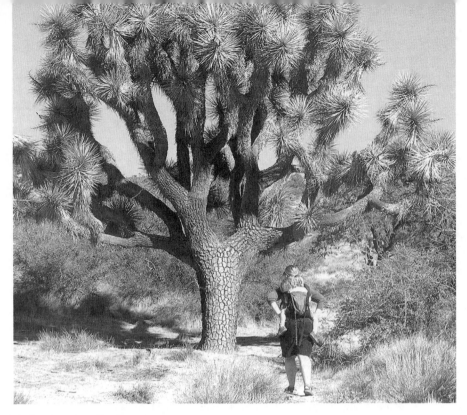

Joshua tree along Panorama Loop

for this with an exceptionally lush and beautiful assortment of prickly desert vegetation, including junipers, Mojave yucca, silver cholla cactus, and, of course, Joshua trees.

An extensive but poorly marked trail network fans out from Black Rock Campground. The trails aren't shown on USGS topographic maps and can be difficult to follow at times, so you should have a good sense of direction if you venture out in this area.

The Panorama Loop is my favorite moderate hike in this area. It explores a series of washes before climbing to a ridgeline with a splendid view and then returning via another wash system.

From the Black Rock backcountry board, walk east 0.1 mile; then enter a sandy wash leading south. Pass signed trails on the left to the California Riding and Hiking Trail (CRHT) and Short Loop; then reach a four-way junction in 0.6 mile. The Burnt Hill Trail goes left and a connector to the West Side Loop and campground goes right, but this trip continues south along the main wash into Black Rock Canyon.

In 0.3 mile, pass an unmarked wash on the right where you may find footprints leading to connect with the West Side Loop. In 0.4 mile, the canyon narrows and you pass Black Rock Spring. In 0.2 mile, reach a signed junction where the loop splits. Navigation is easier if you follow the right fork to make a counterclockwise loop. In 0.4 mile, pass a sign on the right pointing to Warren Point. In 1.1 miles, reach the ridge. In 0.3 mile, reach the high point on the ridge, where the views are truly panoramic. The steep, sandy trail veers left (north) down the ridge, then northwest down the canyon. In 1.2 miles, return to the split in the loop. Hike north down the wash and return to the trailhead.

VARIATION

To make a detour to Warren Point, follow the signed trail west up the wash. Soon you'll see Warren Point ahead and to the right; it's the only rocky summit in the vicinity. In 0.3 mile, turn right at a signed fork and follow the trail up to the east ridge of Warren Point, reaching the summit in another 0.4 mile. There are great views of San Jacinto and San Gorgonio and the Little San Bernardino Mountains from the top. This enjoyable excursion adds 500 feet of elevation gain and 1.4 miles of hiking.

---

trip 16.2   Eureka Peak

see map on p. 394

Distance	4.5 miles (one-way), 9 miles (loop)
Hiking Time	3–6 hours
Elevation Gain	1,800'
Difficulty	Strenuous
Trail Use	Suitable for backpacking
Best Times	October–April
Agency	Joshua Tree National Park
Required Maps	Trails Illustrated *Joshua Tree* or USGS *Yucca Valley South* and *Joshua Tree South* 7.5'
Permit	Joshua Tree National Park entry fee required (see page 355)

DIRECTIONS From Highway 62 in Yucca Valley, turn south onto Joshua Lane at the BLACK ROCK CAMPGROUND sign, opposite where Highway 247 intersects Highway 62, 0.4 mile east of mile marker 062 SBD 12.00. Follow Joshua Lane as it winds east, then back south, and then reaches a T-junction in 4.4 miles. Turn right and then immediately left onto Black Rock Canyon Road, which leads into the campground. The trailhead is at the Black Rock backcountry board, on the east side of the road shortly past the entrance. The road is divided, and the trail can be hard to see.

If you plan to do this as a one-way hike, arrange to be picked up at the top near Upper Covington Flat, which is accessed via a long dirt road. The road is usually (but not always) passable by low-clearance passenger vehicles. From Highway 62 between Yucca Valley and Joshua Tree, 0.2 mile east of mile marker 062 SBD 15.00, turn south onto La Contenta Road. In 1 mile, the road becomes good dirt. In another 1.9 miles, veer left at a sign for Covington Flats. Cross the park boundary (no fee station) and through an area recovering from a catastrophic fire triggered by lightning in the summer of 2006. In 6 miles, bear right at a junction; then in 1.8 miles, turn right at another junction. Proceed 1.4 miles to the end of the road on a hilltop 0.1 mile south of Eureka Peak.

Eureka Peak (5,518') is one of the major summits above 5,000 feet in Joshua Tree National Park. It's accessed by a trail from Black Rock Campground and by a road from Upper Covington Flat. This trip can be done as a one-way hike with a shuttle or as a loop trip from Black Rock Campground. The peak itself is unimpressive, save for its views of San Gorgonio, but the journey is rewarding. The trail explores beautiful washes and ridges lushly blanketed by yuccas and cacti.

This trip is described in the uphill direction from Black Rock Campground, but you can also do the hike downhill from the peak. A maze of other trails runs through this area; they're usually marked, but be sure to carry a map and navigation equipment.

From the backcountry board at the trailhead, hike east and then south up a wash 0.2 mile through a forest of Joshua trees. Take a signed turnoff for the California Riding and Hiking Trail leading east out of the wash. Admire the diverse plant life, including silver cholla cacti, Mojave yuccas, and junipers amidst the Joshua trees. In another 1.1 miles, reach a second signed junction. Turn right (south) on the Fault Trail; the California Riding and Hiking Trail continues left.

The Fault Trail climbs gradually for 0.3 mile, and then steeply ascends a low ridge with views of a wide wash beyond. From this ridge, it's worth making a detour left (east) for 150 feet. Just before you reach a small hill, look for a foot-wide crevice between two rocks near a stand of nolinas. Geologists believe this crevice formed during the 1992 Landers earthquake, which tore the hill asunder. Most of the gap has been filled in by erosion, but the line may be faintly seen continuing down the hill.

Continue 0.1 mile down off the ridge to the end of the Fault Trail and a signed junction with the Short Loop Trail. Turn left and walk a few yards to a second sign for the Eureka Peak Trail, which goes south up a broad, sandy wash.

Follow the Eureka Peak Trail all the way up the wash. The wash has some dramatic sections with sheer walls. Several signs point out other trails climbing out along the way. In 0.8 mile, the Cliff Trail exits up a narrow defile on the left. Just 0.2 mile beyond, the Canyon View Trail exits to the right. In another 0.1 mile, the wash forks, and a confusing wooden marker seems to indicate EP in both directions. Stay right in the main wash. The left fork follows a very faint path through a system of washes to the Bigfoot Trail; few traces remain, and the route is not recommended for casual hiking (although the trail is shown on the Trails Illustrated map). In another 0.6 mile, the Burnt Hill Trail exits to the right. The Eureka Peak Trail continues over a saddle at the head of the wash, reaching another junction in 0.9 mile with the south end of the Bigfoot Trail. Continue 0.2 mile up to the summit of Eureka Peak. If you left a vehicle near the summit, your trip is essentially finished.

ALTERNATIVE FINISH

There are many ways to return to Black Rock on foot. You can retrace your steps. You can descend the dirt road 0.8 mile toward Upper Covington Flat, then join the California Riding and Hiking Trail (see Trip 15.23) and follow it back to Black Rock. Or you can return via any of the other trails that branch off the Eureka Peak Trail. The Burnt Hill Trail is especially recommended; the distance is scarcely longer and it traverses a beautiful valley full of Joshua trees.

San Gorgonio Mountain from Eureka Peak

trip 16.3	**West Side Loop**

see map on p. 394

Distance	4.5 miles (loop)
Hiking Time	2.5 hours
Elevation Gain	900'
Difficulty	Easy
Trail Use	Suitable for equestrians
Best Times	October–April
Agency	Joshua Tree National Park
Recommended Map	Trails Illustrated *Joshua Tree* or USGS *Yucca Valley South* 7.5'
Permit	Joshua Tree National Park entry fee required (see page 355)

DIRECTIONS From Highway 62 in Yucca Valley, turn south onto Joshua Lane at the BLACK ROCK CAMPGROUND sign, opposite where Highway 247 intersects Highway 62, 0.4 mile east of mile marker 062 SBD 12.00. Follow Joshua Lane as it winds east, then back south, and then reaches a T-junction in 4.4 miles. Turn right and then immediately left onto Black Rock Canyon Road, which leads into the campground. Park at the ranger station.

The West Side Loop, which circles the hills to the southwest of Black Rock Campground, is the newest addition to the extensive network of trails from Black Rock Campground. While it lacks some of the diversity and splendor of the Panorama Loop (Trip 16.1), it's none-theless quite enjoyable and worthy of a hike if you're a repeat visitor. The entire area is rich with Joshua trees, Mojave yuccas, nolinas, junipers, pinyon pines, and many species of cactus.

Walk west from the ranger station toward the low hills. At the edge of the campground, slightly south of the ranger station, find the sign marking the beginning of the West Side Loop Trail. Walk west 100 yards to another sign for the West Side Loop where the trail

San Jacinto's north face from the West Side Loop

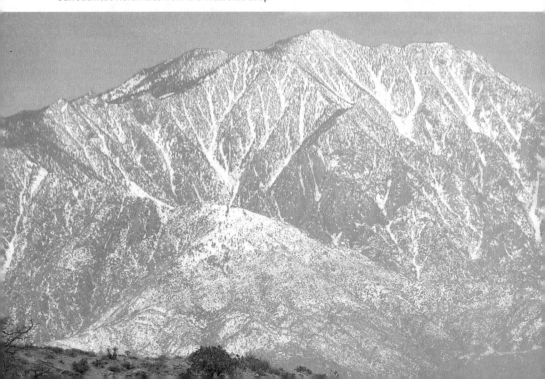

forks. This description assumes a clockwise circuit with most of the elevation gain near the beginning, so turn left (south).

Hike along the back of the campground. Pass a junction with an old trail coming in from site 30 and join a dirt road. Follow the road as it veers left near a water tank; then immediately turn right onto a trail. In 0.4 mile from the start, reach a junction where a sign indicates the West Side Loop to the right.

Follow the trail along the edge of the hills for 0.6 mile. At another signed junction in a wash, a horse trail leads down, but the West Side Loop goes up another 0.6 mile to a low saddle in the hills. Use trails lead north and south from the saddle into the hills. The trail south follows the crest of the hills to Warren Point (see Trip 16.1). But the West Side Loop continues west, undulating as it crosses a number of minor gullies before dropping steeply into Little Long Canyon. Good views of San Jacinto and San Gorgonio loom beyond the desert slopes.

In 0.6 mile, reach the bottom of the wash, which is marked with another sign for the West Side Loop. Turn right and walk down the wash 0.3 mile to a junction with another wash. The Little Long Canyon hiking corridor leads 1.1 miles up this second wash, but our loop continues downhill (north). In 0.4 mile, exit the wash to the right. In another 0.1 mile, reach a junction. The Boundary Trail West goes left (west), but our loop stays right and climbs eastward toward a second low saddle. Cross the saddle in 0.5 mile; then pass two junctions with the High View Nature Trail (Trip 16.4). In 0.9 mile, arrive back at the signpost at the edge of Black Rock Campground.

---

trip 16.4   High View Nature Trail

Distance	1.4 miles (loop)
Hiking Time	1 hour
Elevation Gain	400'
Difficulty	Easy
Trail Use	Good for kids
Best Times	October–April
Agency	Joshua Tree National Park
Recommended Map	Trails Illustrated *Joshua Tree* or USGS *Yucca Valley South* 7.5'
Permit	Joshua Tree National Park entry fee required (see page 355)

see map on p. 394

DIRECTIONS From Highway 62 in Yucca Valley, turn south onto Joshua Lane at the BLACK ROCK CAMPGROUND sign, opposite where Highway 247 intersects Highway 62, 0.4 mile east of mile marker 062 SBD 12.00. Follow Joshua Lane as it winds east, then back south, and then reaches a T-junction in 4.4 miles. Turn right and then immediately left onto Black Rock Canyon Road, which leads to the campground. Enter the campground and stop at the ranger station to request an interpretive pamphlet for the nature trail. Then return to the campground exit and turn left (west) at a sign for Horse Camp. Proceed 0.7 mile to the end of the road.

This aptly named nature trail makes a loop around the rich Joshua tree woodland southwest of Black Rock Campground. Twenty-three interpretive markers along the path introduce the visitor to the botany and geology of the park. Ask at the Black Rock ranger station for a brochure explaining the markers. Supplies were limited at this writing. This trail can also be reached from Black Rock Campground on foot by following the West Side Loop for 0.5 mile (see Trip 16.3).

Follow the trail south from the parking area. At an immediate indistinct fork, stay left on the main trail to make a clockwise loop. Cross the West Side Loop Trail in 0.1 mile; then climb 0.5 mile up the steep hill to the south for an excellent view and a summit register.

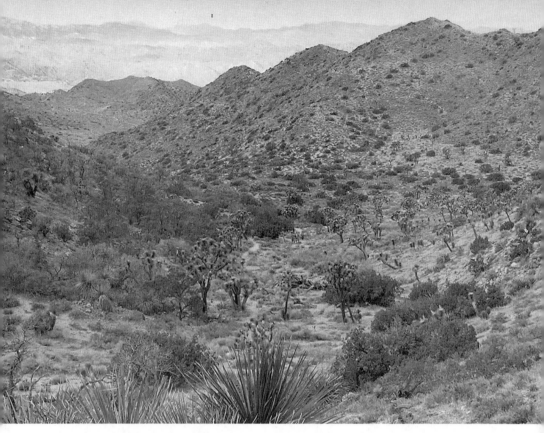

Joshua trees on the High View Nature Trail

San Gorgonio is the massive mountain to the west. Enjoy the gnarled old nolinas standing near the peak.

Continue down to a saddle south of the summit. An unmarked trail leads south from this saddle up to the highest hills, but the nature trail turns right and descends into a small valley full of Joshua trees, junipers, and pinyon pines. In 0.7 mile, cross the West Side Loop Trail again; then arrive back at the trailhead.

VARIATION

If you're looking for more, consider the unmarked South Park Peak Trail on the north side of the parking area. This trail makes a 0.7-mile loop and gains 250 feet to the small peak overlooking Yucca Valley.

trip 16.5 **Covington Crest**

Distance	3 miles (out-and-back)
Hiking Time	2 hours
Elevation Gain	100'
Difficulty	Easy
Trail Use	Suitable for equestrians
Best Times	October–April
Agency	Joshua Tree National Park
Recommended Maps	Trails Illustrated *Joshua Tree* or USGS *Joshua Tree South* and *East Deception Canyon* 7.5'

see map on p. 394

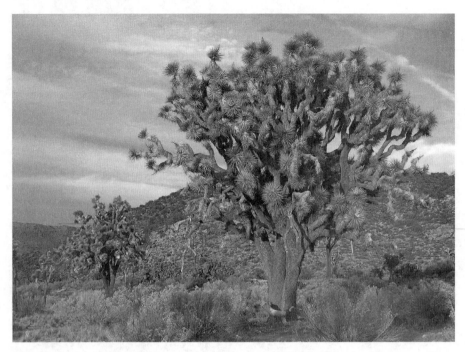

Gigantic Joshua tree at Upper Covington Flat

DIRECTIONS Covington Flats is accessed via a long dirt road. The road is usually, but not always, passable by low-clearance passenger vehicles. From Highway 62 between Yucca Valley and Joshua Tree, 0.2 mile east of mile marker 062 SBD 15.00, turn south onto La Contenta Road. In 1 mile, the road becomes good dirt. In another 1.9 miles, veer left at a sign for Covington Flats. Cross the park boundary (no fee station) and through an area recovering from a catastrophic fire triggered by lightning in the summer of 2006. In 6 miles, stay right at a junction; then in 1.8 miles, turn sharply left at another junction. Proceed 1.9 miles to the end of the road at Upper Covington Flat.

Covington Flats is a rarely visited gem in the crown of Joshua Tree National Park, offering seclusion among some of the park's largest Joshua trees. The short Covington Crest Trail leads past some of these trees to the lip of the Little San Bernardino Mountains, where unfathomable canyons twist down into the Coachella Valley below. This trip is especially enjoyable near sunset on a partially cloudy day, when you can watch the sky light up in rich red splendor as the sun retires behind San Jacinto.

Two trails depart from the Upper Covington Flat parking area. One trail is marked Covington Crest and leads south. The unmarked trail leads east along the California Riding and Hiking Trail (see Trip 15.23). It's worth taking a 0.1-mile jaunt along the eastern trail to see some of the park's largest Joshua trees up close. Along the way look for the remains of what once was the park's largest Joshua tree. Nearby is another gigantic multiarmed behemoth.

Return and take the signed Covington Crest Trail. The path is narrow but reasonably well defined. It leads 1.6 miles to an overlook at the edge of the valley with fantastic views of the Santa Rosa Mountains, San Jacinto, and the Little San Bernardinos. For an even better view, walk 0.3 mile northwest along the lip to a nearby hill with a single prominent tree. After enjoying the scenery, return to the parking area.

trip 16.6 **Covington Loop**

Distance	6 miles (semiloop)
Hiking Time	3–4 hours
Elevation Gain	800'
Difficulty	Moderate
Best Times	October–April
Agency	Joshua Tree National Park
Recommended Map	Trails Illustrated *Joshua Tree* or USGS *Joshua Tree South* 7.5'

see map on p. 394

DIRECTIONS Covington Flats is accessed via a long dirt road. This road is usually, but not always, passable by low-clearance passenger vehicles. From Highway 62 between Yucca Valley and Joshua Tree, 0.2 mile east of mile marker 062 SBD 15.00, turn south on La Contenta Road. In 1 mile, the road becomes good dirt. In another 1.9 miles, veer left at a sign for Covington Flats. Cross the park boundary (no fee station) and through an area recovering from a catastrophic fire. In 6 miles, stay left at a junction. In 0.6 mile, reach the Lower Covington Flats Picnic Area.

This clockwise loop offers a diversity of scenery in a lightly visited corner of the park. It begins with a trek through the fire-ravaged Lower Covington Flat, then climbs a ridge to the magnificent Upper Covington Flat. It then returns cross-country through an attractive canyon where Native Americans once made their home. The trip is particularly appealing to groups with children, who will enjoy the boulder-hopping down the canyon.

From the parking area, follow the signed trail south toward Lower Covington Flat through an area decimated by a series of fires. The trail soon begins a descent, briefly passing through areas that survived the infernos. Cross some minor washes; then, in 1.0 mile, reach the major Smith Water wash. You'll return to this point after the cross-country section of the hike. Follow trail markers across the wash. Continue another 1.0 mile to a signed junction with the California Riding and Hiking Trail.

Make a hard right turn onto the trail to Upper Covington Flat. Cross two more minor washes and scale the ridge. As you exit the burn area, you can enjoy the diverse desert flora including pinyon pines, junipers, Mojave yuccas, nolinas, and prickly pear cactus. Upon cresting the ridge, the magnificent Joshua tree forest of Covington Flats comes into view. Some of the largest trees in the park can be found in this valley.

In 1.7 miles, immediately before you reach the Covington Flats backcountry board, turn right down the prominent Smith Water Wash that leads northeast into a canyon. There is no trail through the canyon, but you have only one path to follow. Descend a small dry waterfall near the top of the canyon, and pick your way around boulders, fallen trees, and brush. Children will particularly enjoy this section. Near the bottom of the canyon, descend a series of three more easy dry waterfalls. The last one is the tallest, but can be descended easily by staying to the right. Covington Spring is usually dry, but water sometimes runs through the canyon in the springtime. Below the last waterfall, careful observers may see bedrock mortars and other signs that Native Americans inhabited this area in times of greater rainfall.

The wash soon meets the Lower Covington Flat trail, 1.5 miles from the backcountry board. Turn left and retrace your steps the last mile to where you left your vehicle.

VARIATION

The National Park Service describes an alternative version of this loop in which you walk back along the road between the Upper and Lower Covington Trailheads. This involves 4.6 miles of walking along dirt roads and misses the fun scrambling, but it might be preferable for those who prefer flatter walking.

chapter 17

Joshua Tree National Park: Indian Cove

This chapter covers the popular Indian Cove area of Joshua Tree National Park (see Chapter 15 for an overview of the park). Indian Cove has no roads connecting it to the main park because it's surrounded by the rugged Wonderland of Rocks, but hikers can make the connection via the Boy Scout Trail or challenging cross-country routes through the Wonderland.

Indian Cove draws throngs of rock climbers to play on the granite blocks. It's about 1,000 feet lower than the rest of the park and somewhat sheltered from the wind, so it can be warmer in the winter. The campground has more than 100 gorgeous sites, mostly nestled beside interesting rock formations, as well as huge group sites that draw youth groups.

Because of the terrain, hiking options tend to be short, difficult, or both. Most visitors will enjoy scrambling through the rock formations as well as taking longer hikes.

trip 17.1　　Indian Cove Nature Trail

Distance	0.6 mile (loop)
Hiking Time	30 minutes
Elevation Gain	100'
Difficulty	Easy
Trail Use	Good for kids
Best Times	September–April
Agency	Joshua Tree National Park
Map	None
Permit	Joshua Tree National Park entry fee required (see page 355)

see map on p. 358

DIRECTIONS From Highway 62, 0.4 mile east of mile marker 062 SBD 27.00, turn south onto Indian Cove Road. Drive past the entrance station and past a dirt road leading west to the group campsites—a total of 3 miles from Highway 62. At the main campground, turn right and drive all the way west through the maze of campsites to the end of the road, just beyond campsite 90. Park near the signed start of the Indian Cove Nature Trail. Alternatively, the trail can be accessed from the west end of the group campsites.

This short nature trail at the west end of the Indian Cove Campground is a good place to take a stroll and learn about the plant

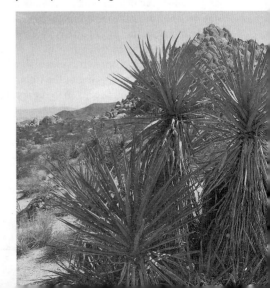

Mojave yucca at Indian Cove

and animal life of this unusual corner of the Mojave Desert. The trail circles through the desert and along a sandy wash. In the creek, it threads past desert willows. Above, look for pencil and silver cholla cacti, Mojave yuccas, desert almonds, creosote, and jojoba bushes.

trip 17.2   Gunsight Loop

see map on p. 358

Distance	3 miles (loop)
Hiking Time	2.5 hours
Elevation Gain	800'
Difficulty	Moderate, with extensive boulder scrambling
Best Times	October–March
Agency	Joshua Tree National Park
Recommended Map	Trails Illustrated *Joshua Tree* or USGS *Indian Cove* 7.5'
Permit	Joshua Tree National Park entry fee required (see page 355)

DIRECTIONS From Highway 62, 0.4 mile east of mile marker 062 SBD 27.00, turn south onto Indian Cove Road. Drive past the entrance station and past a dirt road leading west to the group campsites—a total of 3 miles from Highway 62. At the main campground, turn right and drive all the way west through the maze of campsites to the end of the road, just beyond campsite 90. Park near the signed start of the Indian Cove Nature Trail.

The Wonderland of Rocks casts a siren's spell to curious explorers. The otherworldly boulders, buttresses, and towers of monzogranite are a marvel to discover, but are a challenge to both movement and navigation. More than one hiker has become lost overnight, and the body of a stray hiker took years to discover. Gunsight Loop samples the pleasures of the Wonderland. This relatively short hike requires challenging boulder scrambling that is unsuitable for young children or those with less-than-excellent balance. Rock climbers would rate the route third-class, meaning there's hands-on climbing but no rope is required. Nobody should stray into the Wonderland without good cross-country navigation skills, and a compass or GPS receiver. The Wonderland of Rocks is a day-use area; no camping is allowed.

Gunsight Notch

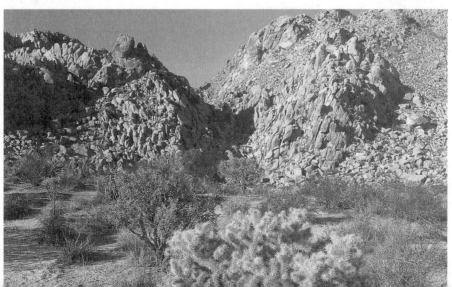

The Wonderland of Rocks forms a forbidding ridge south of Indian Cove, separating the cove from the rest of Joshua Tree National Park. From the parking area, look southwest to the obvious low point in the ridge. This is Gunsight Notch. This cross-country route climbs the boulder-filled canyon through the notch into a small valley on the other side; it then curves right and descends through the next canyon to the west via dry waterfalls before returning through a wash.

Walk south past the nature trail a few yards and look for traces of an old dirt road. Follow it a short distance as it heads toward Gunsight Notch; soon the road veers left and you make a beeline for the canyon. Watch for the silver and pencil chollas and the cat's claw acacias that threaten unwary hikers.

The canyon is full of huge boulders. Pick your favorite route; if one path is blocked with overhanging rocks, you can usually find another more moderate way nearby. After the most difficult lower stretch, the canyon momentarily opens into a small wash before closing in again. Continue up the main canyon and cross over Gunsight Notch into a sandy wash, 0.6 mile from the start.

The walking is now much easier. Go 0.3 mile and round a bend into a valley. The wash forks. The main branch continues southwest and eventually emerges from the Wonderland near the Boy Scout Trail. This loop, however, takes the right (west) fork, which soon becomes partially choked with rocks and bushes. Follow the wash as it climbs and curves right before it gains a crest and enters another small flat valley in another 0.3 mile.

Hike across the valley and through another wash, veering right around the rocks to aim for the lowest point to the north. You may find some cairns along the way, but the walking is mostly cross-country. In 0.3 mile, come to the top of a canyon descending to the northeast. Look for the wash at the bottom among the rocky buttresses. The first part of the descent to a small flat area is moderate, but the canyon soon plunges steeply into the desert below. The climbing is generally easier than Gunsight Notch, but the two cruxes involve descending dry waterfalls.

In 0.5 mile, emerge from the canyon at the sandy wash. Follow the wash, avoiding copious cat's claws. In 0.6 mile, come to a junction with the Indian Cove Nature Trail wash. Turn right and walk upstream 100 feet to rocky steps exiting on the left that lead 0.2 mile back to the trailhead.

trip 17.3   Rattlesnake Canyon

see map on p. 358

Distance	2.5 miles (out-and-back)
Hiking Time	2 hours
Elevation Gain	400'
Difficulty	Moderate
Best Times	October–April
Agency	Joshua Tree National Park
Recommended Map	Trails Illustrated *Joshua Tree* or USGS *Indian Cove* 7.5'
Permit	Joshua Tree National Park entry fee required (see page 355)

DIRECTIONS From Highway 62, 0.4 mile east of mile marker 062 SBD 27.00, turn south onto Indian Cove Road. Drive past the entrance station and past a dirt road leading west to the group campsites—a total of 3 miles from Highway 62. At the main campground, turn left (east) to pass through the campsites and, in 0.8 mile, bear right (south) to reach the picnic area at Rattlesnake Canyon, 0.3 mile farther.

The Wonderland of Rocks is a fascinating but formidable barrier to travel in Joshua Tree National Park. Rattlesnake Canyon climbs into the Wonderland from the picnic area

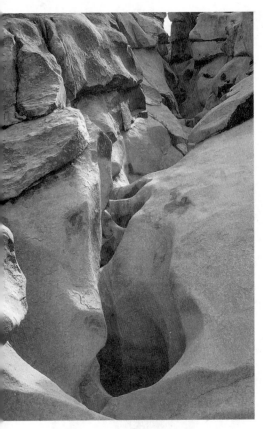

The slot in Rattlesnake Canyon

east of Indian Cove Campground. It treats the hiker to a number of remarkable geological formations, including a rare slot canyon carved through the monzogranite. Although this hike is short, it involves plenty of boulder-hopping and easy rock scrambling, so it's not suited for those who are unsure of foot. However, it's a fun romp for carefully supervised children. The Wonderland of Rocks is a day-use area; no camping is allowed.

From the picnic area, hike down into the wash and turn right to follow it upstream into the mouth of a canyon. You'll soon encounter easy boulder-hopping. Look for the granite boulders sprinkled with enormous pinkish feldspar crystals. In 0.3 mile, the main canyon turns abruptly left. Look for a steep rise, where the creek has carved an unusual slot canyon. It's interesting to explore potholes at the canyon bottom, which hold life-sustaining water for desert wildlife; you may encounter frogs or killer bees in the pools.

Bypass the slot canyon by moving right (west) past the cliffs and scrambling up past several oak trees to a notch. Beyond the notch, descend back to the sandy floor of Rattlesnake Canyon. If no water is running, it's interesting to walk back to the top of the slot and peer down the impressive drop-off.

The canyon continues south. The ancient brownish Pinto gneiss forming the slopes of Queen Mountain to the east stands in vivid contrast to the much younger White Tank monzogranite rock that forms most of the Wonderland.

Soon, the canyon turns sharply to the right. You can follow it a half mile or more before you turn around and retracing your steps. Beware of snakes in the aptly named Rattlesnake Canyon, especially when passing near brush.

---

trip 17.4   **Fortynine Palms Oasis**

Distance	3 miles (out-and-back)
Hiking Time	2 hours
Elevation Gain	600'
Difficulty	Easy
Trail Use	Good for kids
Best Times	October–April
Agency	Joshua Tree National Park
Recommended Map	Trails Illustrated *Joshua Tree* or USGS *Queen Mountain* 7.5'

see map on next page

DIRECTIONS From Highway 62, 0.2 mile east of mile marker 062 SBD 29.00, turn south onto Canyon Road. Follow it south and then west 1.7 miles to the trailhead, at the end.

The Fortynine Palms Oasis is one of five palm oases scattered about Joshua Tree National Park. (The other oases include Mara, Cottonwood, Lost Palms, and Munsen.) The attractive location, nestled in a steep-walled canyon, and its relatively easy access make this a very popular hike. If you come on a pleasant weekend, expect to have plenty of company. If you have time for a longer hike, the Lost Palms Oasis (see Trip 18.5) is even more spectacular and has more interesting cacti and rock formations along the route.

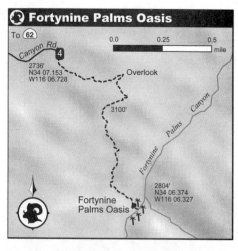

The well-built trail climbs a series of steps to reach a ridge. Just before you reach the ridge, look for a vista point on the left with great views over the town of Twentynine Palms. Several other minor paths branch off the main trail, but they tend to lead to difficult boulder-hopping, so stay on the main trail.

The top of the ridge marks the halfway point. From here, you can glimpse part of the oasis in Fortynine Palms Canyon to the south. The trail descends past creosote and brittlebushes and barrel cacti into the canyon. Arrive at the oasis, where a flat rock shaded by palms makes a perfect lunch stop. Notice how many of the California fan palms are missing their lower fronds. A series of fires over the years have burned the trunks clean without killing the trees.

The Park Service asks hikers to stop at the end of the trail so as to avoid disturbing the wildlife that depend on the oasis.

Fortynine Palms Oasis

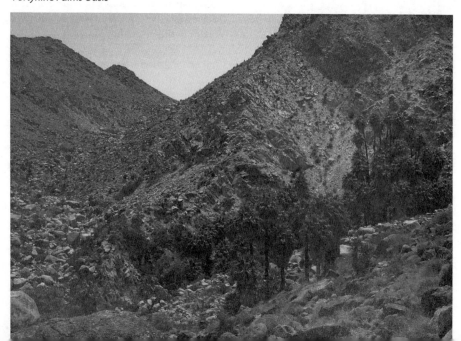

chapter 18

Joshua Tree National Park: East

This chapter covers the vast eastern side of Joshua Tree National Park. See Chapter 15 for an overview of the park.

The most heavily used area in this end of the park is the Cottonwood Campground. Note that the campground is near the South Entrance, not the East Entrance, although the Pinto Basin Road links Cottonwood to Park Boulevard. If you take this road, be sure to stop for a brief walk through the Cholla Cactus Garden.

Other hikes in this part of the park are more obscure, and you're likely to find solitude on them. Several are accessed from the Pinto Basin; others are accessed from the 10 Freeway south of the park. The rugged and challenging Coxcomb Mountains stand in the northeast corner of the park and are accessed from Highway 62.

The Pinto Basin is part of the Colorado Desert, which is lower, hotter, and drier than the Mojave. The plant life is naturally different. Some of the notable species include barrel and teddy bear cholla cactus and ocotillo.

Bighorn carcass in Munsen Canyon (see Trip 18.7)

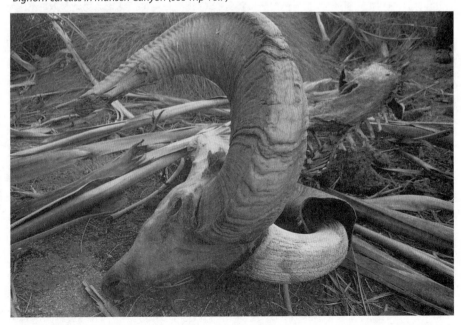

trip 18.1 Pinto Mountain

Distance	9 miles (out-and-back)
Hiking Time	6 hours
Elevation Gain	2,700'
Difficulty	Strenuous
Best Times	October–April
Agency	Joshua Tree National Park
Required Map	Trails Illustrated *Joshua Tree* or USGS *Pinto Mountain* 7.5'
Permit	Joshua Tree National Park entry fee required (see page 355)

DIRECTIONS Park at the Turkey Flats backcountry board on Pinto Basin Road. This well-marked parking area is 14 miles northwest of the Cottonwood Ranger Station and 16 miles southeast of the Pinto Wye on Park Boulevard. If you're coming from the 10 Freeway (I-10) and aren't planning to visit other parts of the park, the Cottonwood Entrance is the most direct.

Pinto Mountain (3,985'), overlooking the sprawling Pinto Basin, is sure to provide a classic desert mountaineering experience and impressive summit views. The lightly visited basin in the eastern side of the park is also a promising place to spot wildlife, especially at dawn and in the evening. Consider bringing a sleeping bag and ground pad to bivouac on the summit and enjoy the sunrise. Note that a free self-issue wilderness permit is required at the trailhead kiosk for overnight travel. Pinto Basin is part of the Colorado Desert and is about 10 degrees warmer than the higher Mojave Desert in the western park, so go on a cool day.

The trip begins at the large Turkey Flats backcountry board. An early rancher attempted to raise poultry here; the venture failed but the name remained. From the backcountry board, look north-northeast at Pinto Mountain and pick out your route. The peak has two summits; the one to the right is more conical and looks slightly higher, but the one on the left is

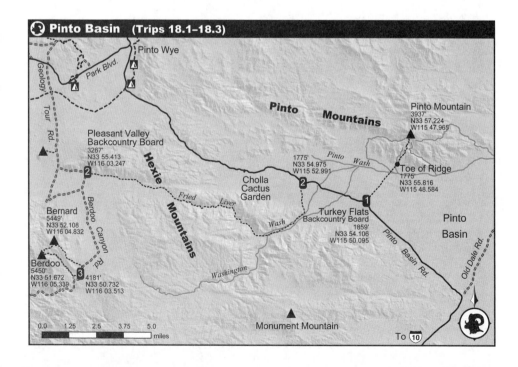

Pinto Basin (Trips 18.1–18.3)

Pinto Wye

Geology Tour Rd.

Park Blvd.

Pleasant Valley
Backcountry Board
3267'
N33 55.413
W116 03.247

Pinto
Mountains

Pinto Mountain
3937'
N33 57.224
W115 47.965

1775'
N33 54.975
W115 52.991

Pinto Wash

Toe of Ridge
1775'
N33 55.816
W115 48.584

Hexie Mountains

Fried Liver

Cholla
Cactus
Garden

Bernard
5449'
N33 52.108
W116 04.832

Berdoo Canyon Rd.

Wash

Turkey Flats
Backcountry Board
1859'
N33 54.106
W115 50.095

Pinto
Basin

Pinto Basin Rd.

Old Dale Rd.

Berdoo
5450'
N33 51.672
W116 05.339

4181'
N33 50.732
W116 03.513

Washington

0.0 1.25 2.5 3.75 5.0
miles

Monument Mountain

To 10

actually tallest. Identify a narrow and well-defined ridge directly below the summit rising out of the desert. The ridge is immediately right of a prominent wash. Although the peak can be climbed by any number of washes and ridges, this ridge is the easiest and most direct way up.

Pick a path across the sandy creosote-studded Pinto Basin aiming directly for the toe of the ridge. Look back to identify a landmark on the mountain behind you to guide your return journey. You'll pass over a low sand dune, honeycombed with countless burrows used by the wildlife to escape the desert sun. Watch for the elusive desert tortoise and the dune-dwelling Mojave fringe-toed lizard. Drop down into a system of dry washes on the floor of the basin; then climb to the toe of the ridge, 2.5 miles from the start.

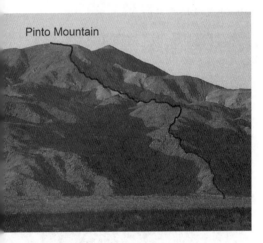

Pinto Mountain

The no-nonsense climb now heads directly up the ridge. You may find bits of use trail formed by two- and four-footed mountain climbers. Barrel cactus favor these dry, well-drained slopes; you'll also encounter cholla, foxtail pincushion cactus, ocotillo, and nolina as you ascend. Be alert for rattlesnakes. Reach the top of a small bump on the ridge; then stay on the ridge over several more bumps before you make the final steep climb to the summit, marked with an enormous cairn. Retrace the same ridge on your descent—it's easy to get drawn onto the more convoluted ridge to the east.

Pinto Mountain South Ridge route

trip 18.2   Fried Liver Wash

Distance	15 miles (one-way)
Hiking Time	8 hours
Elevation Loss	1,500'
Difficulty	Strenuous
Trail Use	Suitable for backpacking
Best Times	October–April
Agency	Joshua Tree National Park
Recommended Maps	Trails Illustrated *Joshua Tree* or USGS *Pinto Mountain, Washington Wash,* and *Fried Liver Wash* 7.5'
Permit	Joshua Tree National Park entry fee required (see page 355)

DIRECTIONS This is a one-way trip requiring a 45-minute car shuttle. Park one vehicle at the endpoint, on the shoulder of Pinto Basin Road where Fried Liver Wash intersects the road. This point is west of mile marker 13 and is most easily recognized by the line of smoke trees in the wash (see map opposite for GPS coordinates). If you're heading eastbound and you pass a sign reading FRIED LIVER WASH, you've gone slightly too far despite the sign suggesting that you're in the right place.

Return to the Pinto Wye, 13 miles northeast on Pinto Basin Road. Turn left and take Park Boulevard 5 miles west to the Geology Tour Road. This road is listed as a 4WD route but is often passable to the trailhead in an ordinary passenger car. At the start of the road, look for a small box containing a pamphlet about the sights along the Geology Tour Road; these are sold on the honor system for 25¢ and are well worth the investment. Follow the dirt road south 7 miles to the Pleasant Valley backcountry board.

Fried Liver Wash cuts a long canyon through the heart of the remote Hexie Mountains. Who could help but want to visit a place with a name like this? The wash is especially attractive in April after a wet winter, when it's a great place to admire desert wildflowers. There is no defined trail; the hike simply follows the wash. Cross-country navigation skills are required, and you're likely to have the place to yourself. This trip can be done as a day hike or overnight trip. If you're staying overnight, no wilderness permit is required. However, you must sign in at the backcountry board, camp at least a mile from the road, and carry plenty of water.

From the Pleasant Valley backcountry board, hike east along the faint remains of an old mining road. The Hexie Mountains to the north are formed from dark varnished gneiss pushed up by the northern branch of the Blue Cut fault. They're dotted with numerous old prospects and decorated with beautiful barrel cactus and Mojave yuccas. To the south is a playa, or dry lakebed. Notice how the plant life in the salty soil is much different than that in other parts of the desert. The lake occasionally fills after a heavy rain.

Hiking east, the road/trail becomes indistinct at times. It may become easier to walk in the wash. In 2.7 miles, cross a barbed-wire fence; then, in another 0.5 mile, pass the ruins of an old stone cabin. Continue west-southwest, staying south of the hills. In another 1.7 miles, reach the east end of Pleasant Valley where Fried Liver Wash abruptly narrows and enters a canyon.

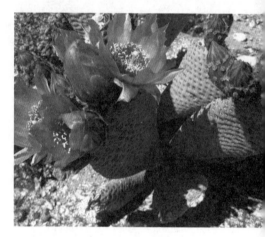

Beavertail cactus produces splendid magenta flowers.

Meander down Fried Liver Wash 5.6 miles through the heart of the Hexie Mountains to the intersection with Washington Wash where the canyon broadens. Continue downstream 2 miles until you reach the east end of the Hexie Mountains and the wash opens up onto a broad alluvial fan. The wash repeatedly forks; stay left at each major fork and head directly north to reach the Pinto Basin Roads.

---

trip 18.3   **Bernard and Little Berdoo Peaks**

Distance	6 miles (loop)
Hiking Time	4 hours
Elevation Gain	2,200'
Difficulty	Strenuous
Best Times	October–April
Agency	Joshua Tree National Park
Recommended Map	Trails Illustrated *Joshua Tree* or USGS *Rockhouse Canyon* 7.5'
Permit	Joshua Tree National Park entry fee required (see page 355)

see map on p. 410

DIRECTIONS From Park Boulevard through Joshua Tree National Park, 0.1 mile east of mile marker 10, turn south onto the dirt Geology Tour Road. This road is listed as a 4WD route, but is often passable to the trailhead in an ordinary passenger car. At the start of the road, look for a small box containing a pamphlet about the sights along the Geology Tour Road; these are sold on the honor system for 25¢ and are well worth the investment. Follow the road south 7.9 miles to the junction with Berdoo

Canyon Road. Turn left (south) and take Berdoo Canyon Road 5.0 miles, passing a dry wash and a ridge shortly before you find parking on the side of the road.

If you have a high-clearance 4WD vehicle, you can continue down the dramatic Berdoo Canyon Road to Dillon Road in the Coachella Valley after the hike. The road follows a sandy wash, which is impassable and at risk of flash flooding during a heavy rain. Ask about road conditions at the entrance station; the road may be damaged after a good winter's precipitation.

This trip is a cross-country adventure into the remote backcountry to visit two of the park's 5,000-plus-foot summits. It features a good variety of terrain and plant life, fine views, and a high chance of solitude. Each peak has its own merits: Little Berdoo offers the best views, while Bernard is the more attractive rocky summit. You can save half a mile and a few hundred feet of elevation by climbing just one of the peaks. The summits aren't visible from the trailhead, and some navigation skill is required. If you become lost, you can always get out by hiking east until you reach Berdoo Canyon Road.

Leave your vehicle and pick a path westward, crossing several small drainages, to reach a major dry wash in 0.5 mile (**N33° 50.639′ W116° 03.866′; 4,056′**). Turn right and follow the wash upstream into the mountains, passing several side washes along the way. In 1.5 miles, the wash narrows and passes between rock walls, then splits (**N33° 51.606′ W116° 04.713′; 4,637′**). The right fork leads to Bernard Peak, but this trip takes the left fork to Little Berdoo. Follow the wash until it becomes indistinct. The true summit is hard to identify from below, but continue in the same direction you'd been traveling and gain the ridge; then head for the high point, 0.7 mile from the fork. From Little Berdoo, you can enjoy dramatic views over the labyrinthine canyons of the Little San Bernardino Mountains to San Jacinto, Toro Peak, and the Salton Sea.

Look northeast and pick out Bernard Peak's rocky pyramid 0.7 mile away. Take the path of least resistance along the ridge; you may encounter some use trails along the way. The summit plateau burned recently, wiping out magnificent stands of yuccas and nolinas. Scramble up the easy rocks to the summit.

You have at least two options to return. You may hike south into the canyon to rejoin the major dry wash in 0.6 mile and then retrace your steps. Or you may follow the southeast ridge of Bernard for 1.1 miles over one minor bump to a saddle (**N33° 51.459′ W116° 04.174′; 4,698′**) before a prominent bump. This ridge is notable for a fine grove of Joshua trees, Mojave yuccas, and nolinas. From the saddle, descend east-southeast into a wash that leads back to the Berdoo Canyon Road in 1 mile. Turn right and follow the road 0.4 mile to your vehicle.

Bernard Peak summit ridge

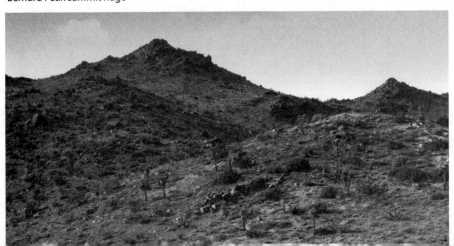

trip 18.4   **Mastodon Peak Loop**

Distance	2.6 miles (loop)
Hiking Time	1.5 hours
Elevation Gain	400'
Difficulty	Easy, but some scrambling on the summit rocks
Trail Use	Good for kids
Best Times	October–March
Agency	Joshua Tree National Park
Recommended Map	Trails Illustrated *Joshua Tree* or USGS *Cottonwood Spring* 7.5'
Permit	Joshua Tree National Park entry fee required (see page 355)

DIRECTIONS From the 10 Freeway, 32 miles east of Indio, take Exit 168 north for Cottonwood Springs Road into Joshua Tree National Park. Drive 7.2 miles to the Cottonwood Visitor Center, where you pay your park admission fee. Turn right (east) and proceed 1.1 miles to the Cottonwood Spring Trailhead parking area, at the end of the road.

This short loop hike in the southeastern part of Joshua Tree National Park treats you to an oasis, traces of an ancient Cahuilla Indian village, fun scrambling up the rocky summit of Mastodon Peak, ruins of two old mines, and a signed nature trail, all in less than a league of walking.

From the trailhead, descend southeast into the Cottonwood Spring Oasis. The Cahuilla Indians once inhabited this lush and shady site; in the late 1800s it became popular among miners seeking precious water. The California fan palms that now occupy the oasis were introduced after 1920.

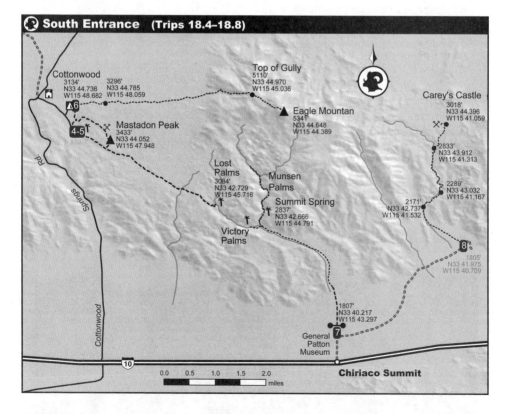

South Entrance   (Trips 18.4–18.8)

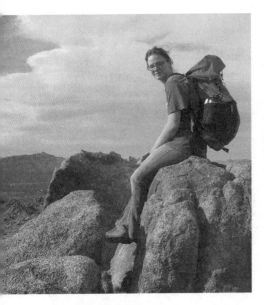

Mastodon Peak

Continue southeast to a signed junction at 0.6 mile. Turn left (north) and follow the trail 0.3 mile to another signed junction at the base of the rocky Mastodon Peak. Can you find the vantage point from which prospectors imagined the mountain to be an enormous elephant head? Turn right and circle around the peak 0.1 mile until you find a faint trail scrambling up the east side of the mountain. The climb to the summit is steep and exposed, but it's not difficult. Enjoy the far-reaching views from the summit extending over the Salton Sea to the Santa Rosa Mountains and San Jacinto.

Return to the junction at the base of the peak and continue north. Pass ruins of the Mastodon Mine, which was worked by the Hulsey family from 1934 to 1971. Be careful around old mines; the shafts and timbers are notoriously unstable.

After passing the mine, the trail wanders in and out of a wash for a mile until arriving at another trail junction near the foundations of the old Winona Mill, a gold mill worked by George Hulsey in the 1920s. The Cottonwood Campground is to the right, but your path continues straight, following a signed nature trail another 0.4 mile until it returns to the parking area.

trip 18.5 Lost Palms Oasis

Distance	7.5 miles (out-and-back)
Hiking Time	4 hours
Elevation Gain	700'
Difficulty	Moderate
Best Times	October–March
Agency	Joshua Tree National Park
Recommended Map	Trails Illustrated *Joshua Tree* or USGS *Cottonwood Spring* 7.5'
Permit	Joshua Tree National Park entry fee required (see page 355)

DIRECTIONS From the 10 Freeway, 32 miles east of Indio, take Exit 168 north for Cottonwood Springs Road into Joshua Tree National Park. Drive 7.2 miles to the Cottonwood Visitor Center, where you pay your park admission fee. Turn right (east) and proceed 1.1 miles to the Cottonwood Spring Trailhead parking area, at the end of the road.

The Lost Palms Oasis hike showcases Joshua Tree National Park at its best. You'll hike across cactus-covered hills on a clearly marked and well-kept trail. The oasis, hidden in a deep canyon studded with trademark Joshua Tree quartz monzonite, is home to the largest stand of California fan palms in the park. Lost Palms is in a day-use area; no camping is allowed.

From the trailhead, descend southeast into the Cottonwood Spring Oasis. This oasis was once home to the Cahuilla Indians. The bean pods from the thorny mesquite tree were a major food source for the Indians. Look for deep mortars in the granite boulders where the women ground the beans into flour.

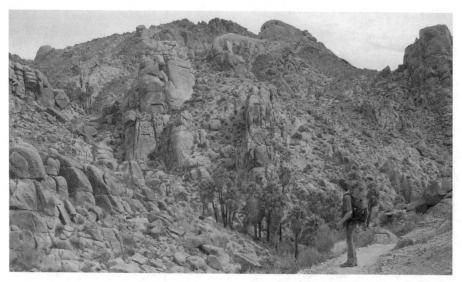

Lost Palms Oasis

Continue southeast to a signed junction at 0.6 mile. The left fork leads to Mastodon Peak (see Trip 18.4), but you should take the right fork, following the arrow for Lost Palms Oasis. The hike will take you across the flat desert past countless cholla cacti, yuccas, and ocotillos, then in and out of dry washes in the badlands before you reach another signed trail junction at the canyon rim, 3.5 miles from the start.

The official trail ends at an overlook of Lost Palms Oasis. Look for a smaller collection of palms in an upper side canyon. An optional trail makes a steep and rocky descent into the oasis on the canyon floor. Your efforts are rewarded at the bottom of the canyon when you stand among the largest collection of fan palm trees in Joshua Tree National Park. Once you're finished basking at the oasis, you can return via the same trail. Alternatively, if you're feeling adventurous, you can choose to take a short detour to Mastodon Peak. This adds 2 miles to your day but offers fun rock-scrambling, spectacular views, and a taste of mining history.

VARIATION

Highly motivated hikers can continue 0.8 mile down the boulder-filled gorge from Lost Palms Oasis to visit Victory Palms, a collection of three mature trees and several pups.

---

trip 18.6 ## Eagle Mountain

Distance	10 miles (out-and-back)
Hiking Time	7 hours
Elevation Gain	2,500'
Difficulty	Strenuous
Best Times	October–April
Agency	Joshua Tree National Park
Required Maps	Trails Illustrated *Joshua Tree* or USGS *Cottonwood Spring, Porcupine Wash,* and *Hayfield* 7.5'
Permit	Joshua Tree National Park entry fee required (see page 355)

see map on p. 414

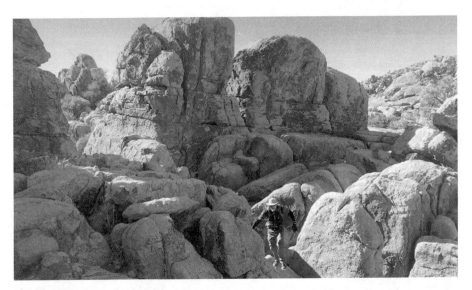

Boulder piles on Eagle Mountain

DIRECTIONS From the 10 Freeway, 32 miles east of Indio, take Exit 168 north on Cottonwood Springs Road into Joshua Tree National Park. Drive 7.2 miles to the Cottonwood Visitor Center, where you pay your admission fee. Turn right (east) and proceed 0.7 mile; then turn left onto the road to the Cottonwood Campground and park by the restroom at Loop B.

Eagle Mountain (5,350') is a delightful desert cross-country adventure. The climb treats you to lush desert vegetation and the distinctive reddish Eagle Mountain quartz monzonite boulders. As the summit is the highest point in the eastern side of the park, the views from the top are magnificent. The hike requires basic cross-country navigational skills and vigorous rock-hopping, but no difficult scrambling.

From the Cottonwood Campground near site 17B, the mountain is located due (magnetic) east and appears rather unimposing behind a line of low hills. Walk across the desert on a bearing of 83 degrees to a gap in the hills where you can pick up a shallow wash. Follow this wash through the hills until it splits on the far side, 0.8 mile from the campground. The creosote bushes near the start give way to Mojave yucca, nolina, and many species of cactus including silver and pencil cholla, hedgehog, pancake prickly pear, and shy but lovely foxtail cactus.

Identify the prominent canyon splitting Eagle Mountain's western slope. Strike out cross-country on a bearing of 90 degrees for the mouth of the canyon. Take advantage of washbeds when you can to avoid vegetation and minimize your impact on the desert.

Most hikers pick a path directly up the steep canyon, and something of a use trail has developed, but the terrain isn't difficult, and any ridge or gully will eventually get you up. From the top of the canyon, the summit comes into view 0.7 mile away on a heading of 130 degrees. Don't be misled by the closer and lower peak due south. Drop down 100 feet into a lush basin and then continue up to the top.

From the summit of Eagle Mountain, views are particularly striking to the south toward the Salton Sea over the jumbled rocks concealing the Munsen Palms Oasis. As you turn to the right, you'll see the Santa Rosa Mountains, the Desert Divide, San Jacinto, and San Gorgonio. The western peaks of Joshua Tree rise beyond the Pinto Basin. Turning north and east, you may pick out the rocky masses of the Sheephole and Coxcomb Mountains and the lonely desert ranges near the Colorado River.

see
map on
p. 414

trip 18.7   Munsen Palms

Distance	8 miles (out-and-back)
Hiking Time	6 hours
Elevation Gain	1,200'
Difficulty	Strenuous
Best Times	October–April
Agency	Joshua Tree National Park
Recommended Maps	Trails Illustrated *Joshua Tree* or USGS *Cottonwood Spring* and *Hayfield* 7.5'

DIRECTIONS From the 10 Freeway, 36 miles east of Indio, take Exit 173 for Chiriaco Summit. Head north off the exit onto Summit Road and turn right onto Chiriaco Road. In 0.1 mile, turn left (north) onto a dirt road along the eastern edge of The General Patton Memorial Museum. Follow it north 0.5 mile to a junction with a major dirt road; then continue north 0.1 mile to a parking area at a sign for Joshua Tree National Park. If the berm at the junction is too high for a low-clearance vehicle to overcome, parking at the junction is an option. (This is a unique hike for pilots, who land at Chiriaco Summit airport and hike directly from the airfield.)

The Munsen Palms are the most remote and obscure palm oasis in Joshua Tree National Park. More than 100 trees are spread out in small clumps along 2 miles of Munsen Canyon. Reaching this beautiful canyon requires extensive and often difficult scrambling up car-sized boulders. Wear long pants and be prepared to dodge all manner of spiky desert life. Munsen Canyon is day use only to protect the herd of bighorn sheep that roam its confines. You're likely to see the remains of sheep—they are protected, so please leave them undisturbed.

From the parking area, head north on an abandoned dirt track past stands of teddy bear cholla, ocotillo, and creosote bushes. In 0.3 mile, cross a power-line service road. In another 0.6 mile, the track fades into a broad wash as it enters the mouth of Lost Palms Canyon. The walking is easy in the gently sloping sandy wash, which is mostly vegetated with smoke trees, palo verde, and desert willows. Watch for jackrabbits darting between the trees.

In another 2.5 miles, reach the first opening on the right. This is the mouth of Munsen Canyon, and can be difficult to recognize because it's completely choked with boulders. Some abandoned 2-inch pipe leads up the canyon, left over from an ill-fated mining attempt. If you reach Victory Palms (three lonely trees with a few pups), you've gone 0.2 mile too far.

Rock-hopping gets easier approaching Summit Springs.

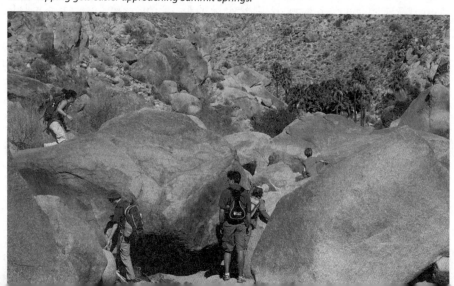

Ascend Munsen Canyon to Summit Springs, the first and arguably most attractive of the oases in Munsen Canyon. This 0.4-mile stretch involves challenging boulder-scrambling and route-finding, and it would be extremely difficult with a heavy pack.

This trip turns around here, but curious explorers may continue up the canyon for about 2 hours to see more of the Munsen Palms. The terrain is less difficult, but you'll still have to overcome numerous obstacles and thread past plenty of cat's claw and other vegetation. Watch for Mojave yucca, nolina, and barrel cactus on the relatively easy hike to the second oasis. The third oasis has small clusters of trees spread out over a longer section of the canyon. When the canyon narrows, you can make a tricky ascent of a jumbled dry waterfall. Just before you reach a lone palm in Munsen Canyon, look up a side canyon on the right for a scenic grove of palms. After some more unpleasant bushwhacking, you can reach a fifth compact oasis. Just above this point, you can scramble up another side canyon on the right to find yet another grove.

trip 18.8   Carey's Castle

Distance	8 miles (out-and-back)
Hiking Time	6 hours
Elevation Gain	1,200'
Difficulty	Moderate
Best Times	October–April
Agency	Joshua Tree National Park
Recommended Map	Trails Illustrated *Joshua Tree* or USGS *Hayfield* 7.5'

see map on p. 414

DIRECTIONS From the 10 Freeway, 36 miles east of Indio, take Exit 173 for Chiriaco Summit. Head north off the exit onto Summit Road and turn right onto Chiriaco Road. In 0.1 mile, turn left (north) onto a dirt road along the eastern edge of The General Patton Memorial Museum. In 0.5 mile, turn right (east) at a T-junction onto a graded dirt service road that follows the buried Colorado River Aqueduct. Drive 3.4 miles to a dirt turnout on the left side of the road. If you're at MWD service hatch 128.16, you're 0.1 mile short of the trailhead. If the road bends sharply right at the base of the mountain, you've gone 0.1 mile too far.

A prospector named Carey worked a mine in the remote Eagle Mountains in the 1940s. Near his mine, he built his "castle," a one-room dwelling under an overhanging boulder.

Carey's Castle

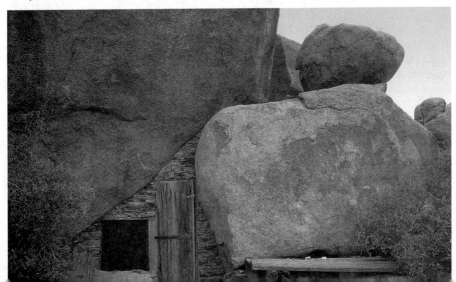

Now within the border of Joshua Tree National Park at the head of Red Butte Wash, Carey's Castle has become a legendary destination for adventurous hikers. Getting to the castle involves 4 miles of spectacular cross-country travel up the twisty wash. The mountains are full of outlandish rock formations and exotic desert vegetation; they're especially attractive when the desert bursts into bloom after the winter storms. Solid navigational skills are necessary to locate the hidden site; a GPS receiver is handy, but good old-fashioned route-finding is perfectly sufficient.

From the parking area, a trace trail leads over a small hump into a wash. This is one of the braids of Red Butte Wash, which gently slopes up northwest into the Eagle Mountains. The main part of the wash is about 0.2 mile farther west. The vegetation is most impressive here, and features ocotillos, palo verdes, smoke bushes, and many species of cacti. Identify the mouth of the biggest canyon to the northwest and pick a path up the wash toward it. Eventually, the wash you're in will merge into the wider sandy bottom of Red Butte Wash, where you're likely to see footprints or cairns left by prior explorers.

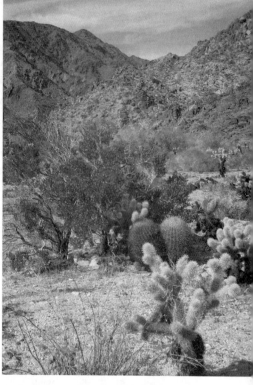

Lush desert vegetation near Red Butte Wash

Another large canyon opens up from the left (west), but stay in Red Butte Wash as it turns north. In 1.3 miles, the wash forks. The left fork goes up what appears to be the largest canyon, while the right fork turns a corner and heads toward huge cliffs of light-tan granite that stand in contrast to the reddish-brown rock you've been passing. Turn right. In 0.5 mile, at the first break in the canyon's north wall, veer left and continue up the sandy wash. Soon, find yourself occasionally hopping over the polished granite boulders on the canyon floor. In 0.3 mile, stay left again at another fork. As you gain elevation, the canyon walls become shorter. Watch for brittlebushes, desert lavenders, and Mojave yuccas. In 1.1 miles, the wash forks again. The main branch leads left, but this hike veers right. Soon, the wash is choked with boulders. Pick a path up the rocks to the sand beyond. In 0.7 mile, the wash opens into a small valley strewn with huge boulders. At the top of the valley, look for a faint trace of trail that was once an old mining road.

Carey's Castle is to the right, hidden on the north side of an enormous boulder. You can open the wooden door and inspect the premises, which includes windows, shelves, a table, and bedsprings. Walls of stones and mortar fill the gaps between the boulders. Be careful to leave the place exactly as you found it so that others can enjoy the same adventure. Dates on magazines found in a cave nearby suggest that Carey lived here in the 1940s.

The mine shaft is located 0.1 mile from the castle. Follow the faint trail/road, as it leads west and then veers south. Look for a metal grate sealing the top of the shaft. Pieces of a rotting wooden ladder can still be seen leading down into the deep hole.

Return the way you came. Navigation is easy—just hike down the wash. If you stay in the main part of the wash, you may emerge at the dirt road a few hundred yards west of your vehicle; if so, turn left and make the short jaunt back.

trip 18.9 Spectre Point

Distance	13 miles (semiloop)
Hiking Time	9–12 hours
Elevation Gain	3,200'–4,000' (depending on the number of peaks)
Difficulty	Strenuous
Best Times	October–April
Agency	Joshua Tree National Park
Required Map	Trails Illustrated *Joshua Tree* or USGS *Cadiz Valley SW* 7.5'

DIRECTIONS From Highway 62 about 40 miles east of Twentynine Palms, park at a turnout on the south side of the road, 0.8 mile east of mile marker 72.

While driving on lonely desert highways, mountain climbers sometimes pass imposing jagged desert peaks and wonder what they'd be like to climb. The Coxcomb Mountains, located in the remote northeast corner of Joshua Tree National Park, are emblematic of such mysterious summits. The crest of the Coxcombs is a triple-peaked massif. The highest peak is called Spectre Point. The northern peak is called Aqua (or Tensor), and has a USGS benchmark. And the most difficult summit to climb is called Dyadic. These challenging cross-country climbs belong on the must-do list of any serious desert mountaineer. The northern Coxcomb Mountains are in a day-use area; no camping is allowed.

This hike can be done as a semiloop. It begins with a long but easy walk across the desert along an old road to the base of the northern Coxcomb Mountains. Then the route makes a beeline up a steep and boulder-filled series of canyons to the summit plateau. Spectre and Aqua are both rated class two. Dyadic involves fourth-class climbing on crumbling weathered granite, so a 100-foot rope and some slings are recommended if you choose to climb that summit. Bag as many of the peaks as you desire; then explore an alternate descent that's longer but arguably easier before you return on the old road.

From the parking area, a sandy jeep road (now gated and closed to vehicles) leads south through the creosote-studded desert. After passing some rock mounds, it veers left (southeast) toward the distinctive low saddle between the high parts of the dramatic

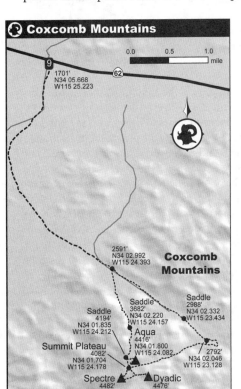

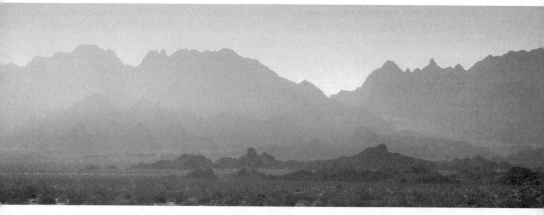

The Coxcomb Mountains

Coxcomb Mountains. In 3.6 miles, the jeep road drops into the broad wash leading toward the saddle. Continue up 0.2 mile. Look for a prominent gully to the south leading to a broad gap immediately left of the highest rocks. Leave the main wash and head south up an easy side wash to the base of the gully, which is rocky but easier than it looks. Climb to the top, and then follow a wash that continues up the valley beyond. At the top of the valley, it's easiest to stay left as you climb to another saddle. You've now traveled 1.0 difficult mile since leaving the main wash.

Descend into the canyon beyond and turn right. Hike up the canyon, staying left at several forks, to a point just below the pinyon-clad Aqua Peak; continue up the canyon to a saddle on the right (west) side of Aqua 0.6 mile from the last saddle. There are great views from here into the Pinto Basin.

South of this saddle, and slightly obscured from view, is the summit plateau. If you plan to climb Aqua Peak, turn left (east) and follow the easy ridge to the 4,416-foot summit. Climbing Aqua is also worthwhile because it offers good views to help you plan your path to the other summits. Otherwise, go south to the plateau. From the plateau, Aqua is located to the north, Spectre to the southwest, and Dyadic to the east, all within a quarter mile but hard to distinctly identify until you start to climb out of the hole. The easiest climb to Spectre is via the north face or northeast ridge. Dyadic has a challenging Class 3+ summit fin that's best accessed by any of several options from the south side. Descending the north face isn't recommended; it involves very loose downclimbing and some precarious rappels. All of the summits have awesome views of the rugged Coxcomb Mountains and desolate Pinto Basin.

You can return the way you came, but an enjoyable loop option is to follow the drainage east from the summit plateau. The wash drops down a step, then becomes wide and sandy, then descends a dry waterfall in the narrows, then becomes easy again. After 1.0 mile of boulder-hopping, the wash dumps into a main northwest- to southeast-trending wash. You may find signs of a shortcut use trail that leads north 100 yards over a low ridge, into the wash leading northwest. If you miss the shortcut, continue into this main wash, turn left, and follow its serpentine path northwest to where you may see a cairn marking the other end of the shortcut. In any event, continue 0.4 mile northwest to the distinctive saddle that you approached early in the trip; then 1.4 miles down, rejoin the jeep road where it exits the left side of the wash. Finally, follow this road 3.6 easy downhill miles back to the highway.

chapter 19

Mojave National Preserve

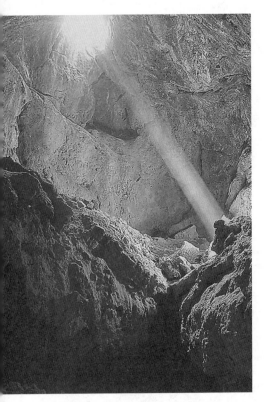

Sun streams through a skylight at the Lava Tube (see Trip 19.9).

The vast Mojave National Preserve was established by Congress in 1994 to protect 1.6 million acres of pristine desert in eastern California. Located between Joshua Tree and Death Valley National Parks, this area receives scant attention compared with its better-known neighbors, but the scenery is no less varied and remarkable. The area includes sand dunes, limestone caverns, volcanic craters, granite peaks, Joshua tree forests, and petroglyphs. Street-legal four-wheeling enthusiasts trace the historic Mojave Road, where Army contractors once hauled their goods by wagon across the harsh desert. Settlements here are few and far between, and you must be prepared to handle any unforeseen difficulties on your own.

Mojave National Preserve possesses a rich and complex geologic history. The area was once submerged under a warm sea. The seabed accumulated expansive deposits of carbonate sediment, the skeletal remains of invertebrate shellfish. About 140 million years ago, during the Cretaceous period, collisions along the San Andreas Fault forced California upward out of the sea. The Mojave Desert was thrust upward to form a huge plateau, and the gradual process of erosion carried away much of the now-exposed seabed sediment. More-recent tectonic activity pushed up many of the chains of mountains that border the Mojave Desert. Until relatively recently, the area received far more rainfall and resembled Africa's verdant savannas; herds of mastodons, rhinoceros, and camels roamed the great plains and their fossils can still be seen. At the end of the last Ice Age, about 10,000 years ago, rainfall patterns changed and the desert as we now know it came into existence. The great rivers and lakes dried up, but their traces can still be found in the landscape. Meanwhile, recent volcanic activity has left a chain of cinder cones and lava flows across the desert.

Native Americans carried on a precarious existence in this difficult environment. The Mojave and Chemehuevi were the predominant tribes in the area, but their numbers were estimated at only about 1,000 spread over the enormous desert. The Spanish were the first

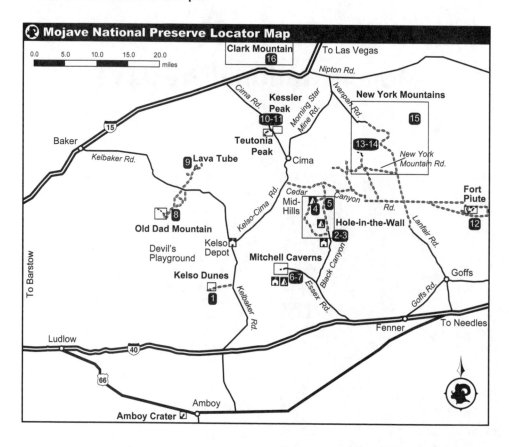

Mojave National Preserve Locator Map

Europeans to visit the area. In 1776, Francisco Garcés, a Franciscan priest, tirelessly explored the desert borderlands of far northern New Spain to find Indian souls to convert to Catholicism. From the Colorado River, he crossed what is now the Mojave National Preserve, following Piute Creek and then passing the New York and Providence Mountains and the Kelso Dunes before reaching the Mojave River near Barstow. The American trapper Jedediah Smith took a similar route 50 years later, but he had such a bad experience with hostile Indians and hunger that few others dared follow. Finally, in 1857, the War Department commissioned Edward Beale to build a wagon road along the 35th parallel across northern New Mexico and Arizona. In a marginally successful experiment, Beale imported camels to work the road, but the outbreak of civil war doomed the experiment to the dust heap of history. Forts were established a day's journey apart, but the Mojave Road's heyday was short-lived.

Wagon traffic trickled off in the 1880s and 1890s after the completion of the transcontinental railroad and rerouting of mail along the safer Bradshaw Trail. By the turn of the 20th century, miners and ranchers were well established in the area, but farming proved unprofitable in all but the wettest years. In the mid-20th century, the region began drawing recreational users. Unfortunately, off-road vehicle use, vandalism, and poaching led to the destruction of archaeological sites and the loss of the desert tortoise and other threatened desert life. The establishment of the Mojave National Preserve seeks to safeguard the park's myriad natural treasures—unique geologic features, wildlife habitats, native ecosystems, and more—for today's visitors and those to come.

Tourism in the area took off in the 1930s when Jack Mitchell began guiding visitors by lantern light through a spectacular pair of limestone caverns. He sold the area to the state of California in 1954. Now ranger-led tours of the Mitchell Caverns are offered in the Providence Mountains State Recreation Area, a state park within the National Preserve.

The Mitchell Caverns and the famous Kelso Dunes are not to be missed, but much of the charm of the Mojave National Preserve comes from exploring the back roads and lesser-visited trails. Distances are great and services are few in the eastern Mojave. Fill up with gas in Baker, Barstow, or Needles before you visit. (In a pinch, some of the most expensive gas in California can also be found in Fenner, on the 40 Freeway.) Wireless coverage is spotty, so bring a reliable vehicle and come prepared to take care of yourself if you stray from the beaten path. A satellite locator beacon such as the SPOT could summon help in an emergency. A high-clearance 4WD vehicle is helpful for exploring the back roads, though most of the hikes in this chapter can be reached in an ordinary passenger vehicle. Dirt roads can become impassable after rain, and AAA may not cover towing on dirt roads. Carry a good map, extra food, and plenty of water. Temperatures are also widely variable, and fluctuations between day and night can be extreme. The summers are almost unbearably hot in the desert, while the winters bring snow to the taller peaks.

One of the best ways to enjoy the Mojave National Preserve is to make a several-day visit during the cooler months. Although there are established campgrounds at Hole-in-the-Wall, Mid Hills, and Mitchell Caverns, there's also a long tradition of free camping in the open desert. Camping by your vehicle is allowed alongside dirt roads in any site that has traditionally been used for the purpose. (Look for beaten ground with a fire ring; many such areas are indicated on the Tom Harrison map.) Bring your own firewood and tinder; gathering is prohibited.

Visitor information is available at the Kelso Depot, a magnificent Union Pacific railroad station that has recently been renovated by the Park Service. Another visitor center is located near the Hole-in-the-Wall Campground. Information is also available at the Preserve Headquarters in Barstow. At this writing, there are no entrance fees and no permits required except for large groups and special events such as weddings. Well-behaved dogs on leash are welcome on the trails.

Street-legal 4WD vehicles can still trace the Old Mojave Road from the Colorado River to Soda Dry Lake. Those interested in the two-day excursion along this footnote of history will appreciate Dennis Casebier's excellent *Mojave Road Guide*.

Michael Digonnet's comprehensive *Hiking the Mojave Desert* is recommended for frequent preserve visitors interested in exploring mines, obscure peaks, and other hidden treasures in the area.

trip 19.1   Kelso Dunes

Distance	3 miles (out-and-back)
Hiking Time	3 hours
Elevation Gain	500'
Difficulty	Moderate
Trail Use	Dogs allowed, good for kids
Best Times	October–April
Agency	Mojave National Preserve
Optional Map	Trails Illustrated *Mojave National Preserve* or USGS *Kelso Dunes* 7.5'

see map on next page

DIRECTIONS From the 40 Freeway (I-40), 28 miles east of Ludlow and 65 miles west of Needles, take Exit 78 for Kelbaker Road. Go 16 miles north to the signed Kelso Dunes turnoff. Alternatively, from Kelso Depot, go 7 miles south to the same turnoff. Follow the excellent dirt road west 2.8 miles to the signed trailhead and outhouse.

The Kelso Dunes—the second-largest and third-highest sand dunes in North America—are the highlight of many visits to Mojave National Preserve. Winds pick up the fine sands from the Mojave River Sink and carry them across the Devils Playground. Eddies formed by the Granite and Providence Mountains cause the winds to drop their loads, creating the Kelso Dunes. Although this trip to the top of the highest dune is relatively short, the climb up loose sand can be exhausting. It's easy for groups to split up before the final climb because the route is in view all the way and because there are plenty of smaller hills to enjoy along the way. Primitive camping is also available another 1 mile west by a lonely windswept tree; there is no camping at the trailhead.

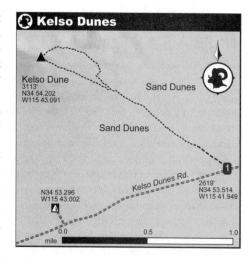

The Kelso Dunes are also known as "booming dunes" because under the right conditions they emit a sound like low thunder. The phenomenon is found only in relatively few dunes in the world and is an active subject of scientific investigation. The best way for you to investigate it yourself is to slide down the steep face of the biggest dune!

From the signed trailhead, follow the well-defined trail northwest through the creosote bushes. Soon, the sands begin. Unless a recent sandstorm has obliterated the tracks, footprints clearly lead toward the highest dune. In 1 mile, veer right and head for a point just left of the saddle between the two biggest dunes. This route avoids climbing the steepest sections of sand. Once you reach the ridge, turn left and climb a spectacular razorback ridge of sand to the summit. There are fine views of the Granite Mountains to the south, the rugged limestone-cliffed Providence Mountains to the east, and the Devils Playground to the north.

Return by descending straight down the face of the dune and walking directly back to the trailhead, rejoining the main trail in about 0.4 mile.

Kelso Dunes summit

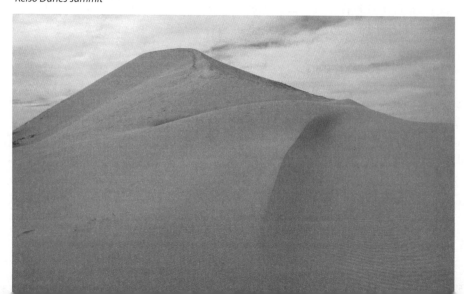

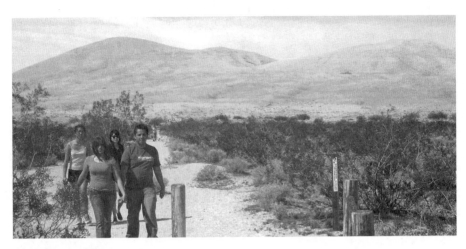

Kelso Dunes Trailhead

trip 19.2   **Hole-in-the-Wall**

see
map on
next
page

Distance	1.5 miles (loop)
Hiking Time	1 hour
Elevation Gain	200'
Difficulty	Easy
Trail Use	Dogs allowed, good for kids
Best Times	September–May
Agency	Mojave National Preserve
Optional Map	Trails Illustrated *Mojave National Preserve* or USGS *Columbia Mountain* 7.5'

DIRECTIONS From the 40 Freeway, 50 miles east of Ludlow and 43 miles west of Needles, take Exit 100 for Essex Road. Drive north 10 miles to a junction; then bear right onto Black Canyon Road and continue another 10 miles. Turn left onto a good dirt road at a signed junction for the Hole-in-the-Wall Visitor Center, and park at the visitor center.

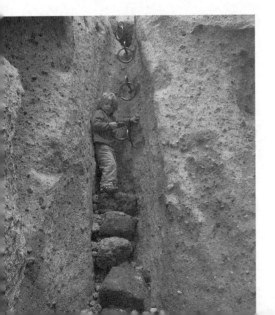

A volcanic eruption 18 million years ago in the Mojave Desert emitted dense blasts of superheated ash. The ash, dust, and volcanic gas from the eruption compacted and cemented together as it cooled, forming what is known as volcanic tuff. This popular loop hike explores the narrow Banshee Canyon that snakes through the fascinating and colorful rock formation. Gas trapped in the ash created pockets in the tuff. The hike descends a short vertical section in the narrow slot canyon; metal rings have been set in the rock to provide holds. A person of ordinary physical ability can negotiate the rings, but young children may need a boost and some hikers

Rings Trail

may find the slot claustrophobic. Dogs must be lifted or pushed up the two narrow chutes where the rings are located.

VARIATION

Hole-in-the-Wall is located next to a popular campground. A quarter-mile nature trail leads from the south end of the campground to the visitor center. This is a worthwhile walk for those staying at the campground, and it's a good way to learn to identify the cacti, yuccas, and bushes common to the eastern Mojave Desert.

From the trail marker at the visitor center parking area, curve east and then south around the base of the volcanic formation, passing close by Wild Horse Canyon Road. As the trail passes prominent boulders at the southern end of the loop, look carefully for several small petroglyphs. Skin oils can stain the rock art, so please don't touch the petroglyphs. The trail continues through a lush desert landscape of Mojave yuccas, buckhorn chollas, and barrel cacti. As the trail curves northward, pass near a backcountry campsite

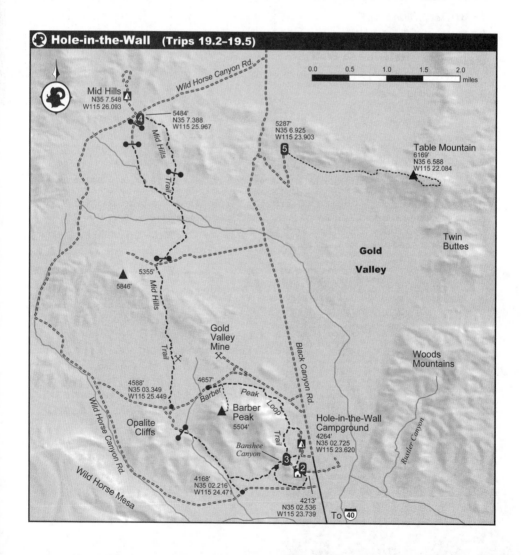

Hole-in-the-Wall (Trips 19.2–19.5)

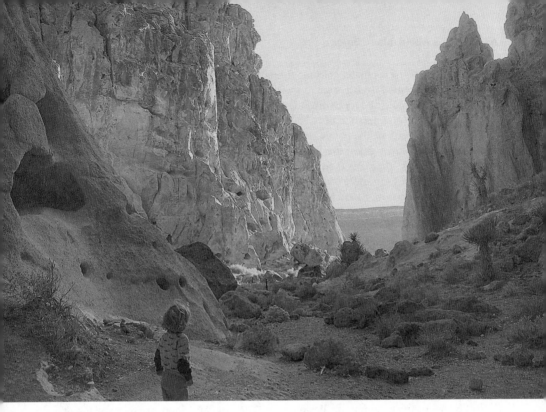

Banshee Canyon

on a spur road and through a cattle gate; then come to a junction with the Mid Hills Trail/ Barber Peak Loop (see Trips 19.3–4).

This trip follows the right fork into spectacular Banshee Canyon. Take a few minutes to explore the many holes in the wall. A trail marker indicates the narrowing of the canyon and the approach to the vertical slots. Climb the rocks leading to the two chutes, and use the metal rings for handholds and footholds. Continue up the rocks to reach a picnic area. A short side trail to the right leads to an overlook into Banshee Canyon. When you're done, follow the dirt road 0.2 mile back to the visitor center.

trip 19.3 Barber Peak Loop

Distance	5 miles (loop)
Hiking Time	3 hours
Elevation Gain	800'
Difficulty	Moderate
Trail Use	Dogs allowed
Best Times	October–April
Agency	Mojave National Preserve
Recommended Map	Trails Illustrated *Mojave National Preserve* or USGS *Columbia Mountain 7.5'*

DIRECTIONS From the 40 Freeway, 50 miles east of Ludlow and 43 miles west of Needles, take Exit 100 for Essex Road. Drive north 10 miles to a junction; then bear right onto Black Canyon Road and continue another 10 miles. Turn left onto a good dirt road at a signed junction for the Hole-in-the-Wall Visitor Center. Follow the road 0.6 mile to its end at a picnic area, passing the visitor center along the way.

Barber Peak is the dramatic volcanic formation overlooking the popular Hole-in-the-Wall Campground. Constructed in spring 2008, the Barber Peak Loop Trail circles the peak and offers a moderate hike conveniently located beside the campground and ranger station. It follows a combination of old dirt roads and newly constructed trail.

From the west end of the picnic area above Banshee Canyon, find the signed Barber Peak Loop Trail to the right of the Rings Loop Trail. Follow this footpath north along the base of Barber Peak's dramatic orange and brown cliffs. These cliffs are composed of Wild Horse Mesa Tuff, a form of volcanic ash welded together during the eruption of Woods Mountain. Air pockets in the ash produced the shallow caves and arches. The trail traverses a natural garden of Mojave yucca and buckhorn cholla, barrel, pancake prickly pear, and hedgehog cactus. In 0.5 mile, reach the stark edge of the 2005 Hackberry Fire burn area. Descend to a cattle fence in 0.2 mile. A path on the right follows the fenceline 0.2 mile back to the north end of the Hole-in-the-Wall Campground, but our loop passes through the gate. Be sure to close it behind you lest cattle pay a visit to the campground.

Curve around the rhyolite cliffs forming the northeast side of Barber Peak and pass a second gate in another 0.5 mile. Descend some stone steps. In 0.4 mile, cross a jeep track by a water tank. Just beyond, turn left at a trail marker. Continue 0.8 mile and then merge onto another dirt road.

Follow the road-trail west, continuing to circle the mountain. In 0.6 mile, stay left at a fork and reach a marker for the Mid Hills Trail (see Trip 19.4). Stay left at a second fork in another 0.1 mile. Continue 0.4 mile to the end of the road, where the trail resumes, leading south through a wash. The white walls of volcanic tuff to your right are called the Opalite Cliffs because of the uncommon silicate mineral they contain. Soon, arrive at the top of a waterfall in a narrow canyon. Ranchers had built a small dam to store water in the canyon, but the reservoir has completely filled with sand. Just before the waterfall, the trail cuts left and up to bypass the obstacle. Pass a gate at the top of the trail and descend into the valley below. This section of the desert is richly vegetated with cacti and Mojave yucca. Something about this area is especially favorable for yuccas. The world's tallest Mojave yucca used to stand 27 feet tall here until it toppled in 2008, and several other yuccas in the areas may be contenders for champion status.

Reach a trail junction 1.0 mile from the end of the road. The right fork leads 0.25 mile to a trailhead on Wild Horse Canyon Road, but this loop turns left. In 0.7 mile, reach a fork at the mouth of Banshee Canyon. Stay left and enter the spectacular canyon (see Trip 19.2). Climb two short steep slots using metal rings driven into the rock, and emerge back at the picnic area where you began.

VARIATION

Barber Peak itself can be climbed from most directions if you carefully search for weaknesses in the cliffs. The easiest route to the summit begins at the extreme northern point on the Barber Peak Loop Trail. Look south toward the peak and pick out a path that completely avoids the cliff bands. At the top, turn right and walk 0.1 mile to the high point. The side trip to the summit is 0.5 mile with 850 feet of elevation gain. Cows have left evidence of climbing most of the way to the top, but none have signed in at the summit register.

see map on p. 428

trip 19.4   Mid Hills to Hole-in-the-Wall

Distance	8 miles (one-way)
Hiking Time	4 hours
Elevation Gain/Loss	600'/1,800'
Difficulty	Moderate
Trail Use	Dogs allowed, suitable for equestrians
Best Times	October–April
Agency	Mojave National Preserve
Recommended Map	Trails Illustrated *Mojave National Preserve* or USGS *Columbia Mountain* 7.5' (trails not shown)

DIRECTIONS This trip requires a 9-mile car shuttle. From the 40 Freeway, 50 miles east of Ludlow and 43 miles west of Needles, take Exit 100 for Essex Road. Drive north 10 miles to a junction; then bear right onto Black Canyon Road and continue another 10 miles. Turn left onto a good dirt road at a signed junction for the Hole-in-the-Wall Visitor Center. Follow the road 0.6 mile to its end at a picnic area, passing the visitor center along the way. Leave one vehicle here.

Return to Black Canyon Road and continue north 6.7 miles on this road, which soon becomes graded dirt. Turn left onto graded dirt Wild Horse Canyon Road, and go 2.0 miles west to the signed entrance to Mid Hills Campground. Park at the signed Mid Hills Trailhead, on the south side of the road opposite the campground.

The Mid Hills to Hole-in-the-Wall Trail is the longest hiking trail in Mojave National Preserve. It was once notable for its splendid desert vegetation, much of which was incinerated when a lightning strike ignited the Hackberry Fire in 2005. Most of the trail is within a cattle grazing allotment. The Barber Peak Trail (see Trip 19.3) is now the more interesting option in the area, but this one-way hike is also worth a visit if you're staying at one of the campgrounds and can persuade a friend to pick you up at the far end. Spring is best, when you might catch a terrific wildflower display. Carsonite posts clearly mark the northern part of the route, but the occasionally faint southern end is marked with cairns so more attention is required to stay on route. The trail is closed to mountain bikes, but biking the road is another option to close a loop.

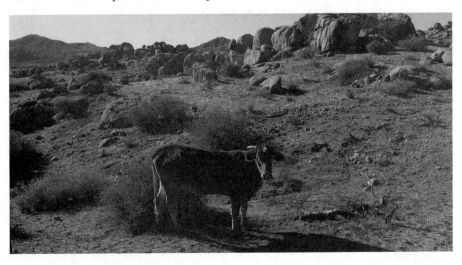

Cattle share the Mid Hills Trail.

From the trailhead, look for a gated dirt road on the right and the signed main trail on the left. Start walking up the main trail, which climbs 0.4 mile onto a hill from which you can gaze out over Round Valley toward Table Mountain. Four miles to the northeast is Government Holes, a rare reliable water source in this arid land. Cattle ranching began here in the 1860s and homesteaders arrived in the 1910s. During that unusually wet decade, farming looked promising, but when the weather became drier, life became desperate. Ranchers and farmers came into conflict over the few sources of water and fertile ground. In 1925, J. W. Robinson and Matt Burts had one of the last shootouts of the Old West at Government Holes, each emptying his revolver and dying in the gunfight.

Descend south through the hills. Some Utah junipers have escaped the fire, while others are ghostly skeletons. In the spring, watch for wildflowers and for the western tent caterpillar webs in the desert almond. In 0.8 mile, pass through a gate. In another 0.6 mile, come to a signed junction by an old jeep track where the trail joins a wash.

VARIATION

The lightly used path to the right, marked by more carbonite signposts, leads north back up the wash to the trailhead. It passes through two gates around a well and then becomes the dirt road that eventually reaches the gate by the trailhead. This path can be used to make a 3.4-mile loop from Mid Hills with 500 feet of elevation gain.

Follow the wash south 0.2 mile; then exit right at a post and continue 1.0 mile up the gradual slope to a gate by another ranching road. Your path soon merges with an old road and passes interesting granite boulders. In 0.4 mile, cross a saddle between Peak 5,846' and a subsidiary summit. Descend 0.6 mile; when the road veers left, continue south on the fainter trail.

In 1.4 miles, join the Barber Peak Loop at a well-marked junction near the Opalite Cliffs. Turn right and follow an old road out of the burn area and into the lush canyon. In 0.6 mile, the road ends at a dry waterfall and a trail cuts left past a gate to bypass the obstacle. The next section features exquisite desert vegetation, including massive Mojave yuccas that grow to the stature of Joshua trees. In 0.8 mile, stay left where a signed spur on the right cuts down to Wild Horse Road. In 0.7 mile, stay left again at another signed junction and enter Banshee Canyon. Ascend the striking canyon and climb the rings to reach the Hole-in-the-Wall Trailhead in 0.2 mile.

trip 19.5   Table Mountain

Distance	4 miles (out-and-back, from high-clearance trailhead)
Hiking Time	2.5 hours
Elevation Gain	1,100'
Difficulty	Moderate
Trail Use	Dogs allowed
Best Times	October–May
Agency	Mojave National Preserve
Recommended Maps	Trails Illustrated *Mojave National Preserve* or USGS *Columbia Mountain* and *Woods Mountain* 7.5'

see map on p. 428

DIRECTIONS From the 40 Freeway, 50 miles east of Ludlow and 43 miles west of Needles, take Exit 100 for Essex Road. Drive north 10 miles to a junction; then bear right onto Black Canyon Road and continue another 10 miles to a signed road on the left for the Hole-in-the-Wall Visitor Center. Reset your odometer and continue 5.1 miles up Black Canyon Road to an obscure dirt road on the right, possibly hidden by the high berm. (This point can also be reached by driving south from Wild Horse

Canyon Road for 1.5 miles.) Low-clearance vehicles should park here and may have a challenge simply crossing the berm. High-clearance vehicles can take this poor road 0.6 mile, and turn left. Follow this even worse road with paint-scratching bushes, exiting left onto jeep tracks when the road becomes a wash, and park at its end in 0.6 mile beside a windmill.

Eighteen million years ago, magma and superheated gases burst through the surface of the Earth, forming a trapdoor volcano now known as Woods Mountain. Between this eruption and two that followed, Woods Mountain ejected at least 30 times as much material as Mount St. Helens blew out in 1980. The dramatic rock formations around Hole-in-the-Wall are remnants of this mighty eruption. Table Mountain is another of these prominent formations, a sheer-walled mesa of basalt overlaying older granitic rocks.

This cross-country trip takes you to the flat-topped summit of the aptly named mountain, exploiting one of the few breaks in the cliffs. This area burned in the 2005 Hackberry Fire. The pinyon pines that once graced the area are now eerie skeletons, but the smaller shrubs have begun the cycle of regeneration. You're likely to encounter cottontails darting between the bushes.

If you're starting from the low-clearance trailhead on Black Canyon Road, hike to the windmill mentioned in the driving directions. You can either follow the roads 1.2 miles, or cut the distance in half by hiking east up over the side of a hill and the northeast down to the windmill.

From the windmill, walk southeast along a cattle fence for 0.6 mile until you pass the toe of a bouldery ridge. Duck under the fence and make a beeline for a shallow bowl on the right side of the ridge, another 0.6 mile. Pick the easiest path up this bowl and continue in the same direction until Table Mountain comes into view again. Turn left and work your way up onto the ridgeline, where you can follow an easy grassy path east toward the

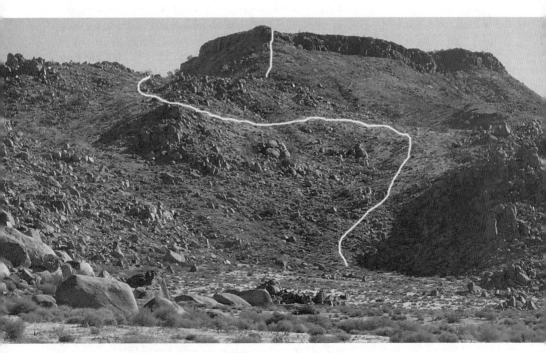

Table Mountain summit route

summit. The final stretch up steep dirt can be tiring but requires no rock scrambling. Watch for columnar basalt formations in the cliffs. Emerge near a post marking the high point of Table Mountain.

If you have time, it's well worth making a 1-mile circuit around the mesa to enjoy the ever-changing views. Gold Valley and Round Valley contain private inholdings within Mojave National Preserve, and it's amazing to see how many ranchers are holding out against long odds in the unforgiving desert.

If you enjoy boulder scrambling, you might return along the ridge. Stay south of the crest to avoid the toughest obstacles.

trip 19.6   Mitchell Caverns

Distance	1 mile (out-and-back)
Hiking Time	1.5 hours
Elevation Gain	100'
Difficulty	Easy
Trail Use	Good for kids
Best Times	September–May
Agency	Providence Mountains State Recreation Area
Optional Map	Trails Illustrated *Mojave National Preserve* or USGS *Fountain Peak* 7.5'
Permit	California State Parks admission fee required (see website below)

DIRECTIONS From the 40 Freeway, 50 miles east of Ludlow and 43 miles west of Needles, take Exit 100 for Essex Road. Drive north 10 miles to a junction. Stay left and continue another 6 miles to park at the Providence Mountains State Recreation Area Ranger Station.

Mitchell Caverns is a spectacular system of limestone caves in the Providence Mountains. Visitors to the caverns will see stalactites, stalagmites, shields, draperies, soda straws, and other rare and beautiful formations. Cavern tours last 1.5 hours; call ahead at 760-928-2586 for reservations and times. The caves are 65°F year-round, but the half-mile trail to them can be sizzling in the summer or icy in the winter. A six-site campground with no facilities for RVs or large groups is located across from the ranger station.

Mitchell Caverns was closed in 2011 during the California state budget crisis, and its unattended visitor center was vandalized soon after. The park finally reopened in 2017 after years of delays. See www.parks.ca.gov/?page_id=615 for more information.

The Providence Mountains were once part of an ancient seabed. Around 250 million years ago, vast layers of shells accumulated on the sea floor and were compressed to form limestone. More recently, the limestone was thrust upward and partially covered with volcanic rhyolite; the mountains now consist of an upper core of rhyolite and a lower layer of limestone. Some 12 million years ago, when there was significantly more rainfall in the area, mildly acidic rainwater percolated down and dissolved the limestone, forming chambers which the Chemehuevi Indians call "Eyes of the Mountains." Businessman and prospector Jack Mitchell purchased the area in 1932 and developed the caverns as a tourist

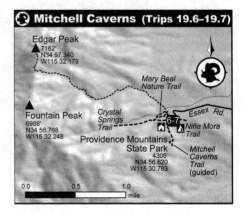

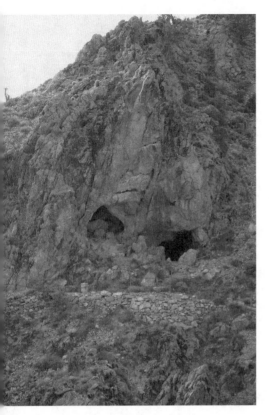

Entrance to Mitchell Caverns

attraction, offering full-day tours by lantern. He had a flair for drama and his tours involved crawling through narrow tunnels and visiting features that he called "The Queen's Chamber" and "The Bottomless Pit." The state of California acquired the caverns in 1954 and further "improved" them for easier travel; young children will have no difficulty with the walk. Now the Providence Mountains State Recreation Area is a state park within the boundaries of the Mojave National Preserve. The ranger-led tours are less romantic than Mitchell's, but far more factually accurate.

If you have additional time before or after a tour, several short and enjoyable trails start at Mitchell Caverns parking area.

(1) Mary Beal Nature Trail (0.5 mile) Starting at the north end of the parking lot, this trail loops through a wonderful variety of cacti and other desert plants. Obtain a booklet at the trailhead or ranger station describing the numbered attractions. The trail is named for an amateur naturalist who spent half a century exploring the area and collecting botanical specimens.

(2) Niña Mora Trail (0.5 mile) Starting at the east end of the campground, this trail follows a ridge covered with cacti and yuccas past the grave of Niña Mora, the infant daughter of a Mexican miner who worked the mines here a century ago. The trail leads to a viewpoint above the Clipper Valley.

(3) Crystal Springs Trail (1.2 miles, 600' elevation gain) The trail starts adjacent to the Mitchell Caverns Trail near the ranger station, steeply climbs through areas of cacti, junipers, and pinyon pines into the volcanic rhyolite formations of the upper Providence Mountains, and reaches a spring in the dramatic Crystal Canyon.

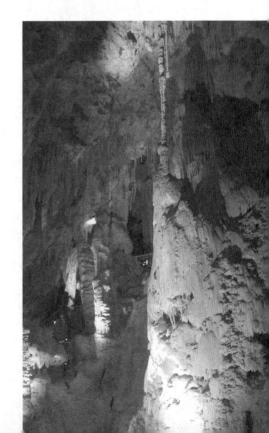

Stalagmites and stalactites in Mitchell Caverns

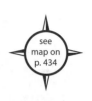

see map on p. 434

trip 19.7	**Edgar Peak**

Distance	4.2 miles (out-and-back)
Hiking Time	8 hours
Elevation Gain	3,000'
Difficulty	Strenuous
Best Times	October–May
Agency	Providence Mountains State Recreation Area
Recommended Map	Trails Illustrated *Mojave National Preserve* or USGS *Fountain Peak* 7.5'
Permit	Day-use fee required ($10)

DIRECTIONS From the 40 Freeway, 50 miles east of Ludlow and 43 miles west of Needles, take Exit 100 for Essex Road. Drive north 10 miles to a junction. Stay left and continue another 6 miles to park at the Providence Mountains State Recreation Area Ranger Station.

The complex and rugged Providence Mountains run 30 miles from south to north, forming a nearly impregnable barrier for early travelers in the Eastern Mojave. Edgar Peak (7,162') is the highest point in the range. Its Jurassic-era rhyolite buttresses are an imposing view from many parts of the park. The mountain is encrusted with the densest garden of cactus found in any hike in this book; if you enjoy desert botany, you'll love the vegetation, but if you dread prickly plants, avoid this trip. Bighorn sheep roam the Providence Mountains, but count yourself lucky if you catch sight of these shy and well-camouflaged creatures. A recent winter snowfall can render the summit rocks icy and impassable. If you're lucky enough to find a cool day in May or June for this hike, you'll be treated to countless cacti in bloom.

Providence Mountains State Recreation Area was closed in 2011 during the California state budget crisis, but the park finally reopened in 2017 after years of delays.

Dodging cactus en route to Edgar Peak

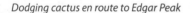

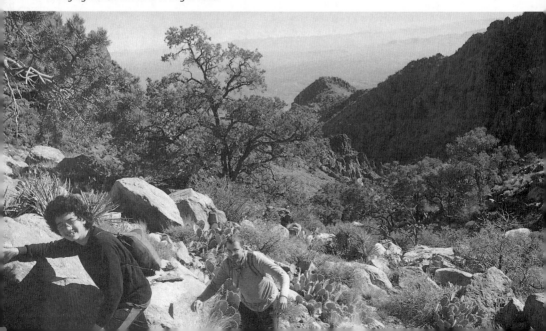

From the north end of the ranger station, follow the signed Mary Beal Nature Trail north. Stay right at an immediate fork. When the trail passes above the state park maintenance shed and begins to veer left, depart the trail and strike out across the desert toward the prominent canyon to the north. Pick a path through the barrel, buckhorn, old man and pancake prickly pear, and hedgehog cactus, and Mojave and blue yucca.

Enter the canyon and follow it upward (west). At first, the bottom of the wash is mostly clear of vegetation and makes for the easiest walking. Around 4,700 feet, pinyon pines, desert agave, and cat's claw acacia join the mix, and sprawling Mojave prickly pear cactus becomes your chief obstacle. Pass through a narrow stretch; then pass two side canyons on the left dropping off Fountain Peak. As the wash becomes more difficult to maneuver, consider climbing onto the slopes to the left. Around 5,700 feet, the cacti subside and you continue up the scree-filled gully to a notch on the ridge 0.3 mile south of Edgar Peak.

Turn right and pick a path to the peak. Some route finding is necessary to avoid Class 3 and harder obstacles. The easiest route initially stays on the east side of the ridge, then follows the rocky ridgeline for a time, and finally climbs an easy gully to the summit.

VARIATION

This peak is on the Desert Peaks Section list and so is Mitchell Point (7,048'), 1.6 miles to the north. Some peak baggers run the ridge between the peaks—which is more complex and time consuming than it might initially appear—and almost invariably descend through rocks and cacti by headlamp. Access to Gilroy Canyon can be problematic; search online for the latest trip reports.

Fountain Peak (6,988') is 0.7 mile to the south. The ridge connecting it to Edgar is also slow going with tricky route-finding and some fourth-class obstacles.

---

trip 19.8 Old Dad Mountain

Distance	5 miles (out-and-back)
Hiking Time	5 hours
Elevation Gain	2,000'
Difficulty	Strenuous
Best Times	October–April
Agency	Mojave National Preserve
Required Map	Trails Illustrated *Mojave National Preserve* or USGS *Old Dad Mountain* 7.5'

DIRECTIONS A 4WD vehicle is recommended because this approach follows sandy and rocky washes. Be prepared to dig yourself out if you get stuck, and carry plenty of water and supplies. The drive is confusing because there are many power-line access road spurs; do it during daylight hours, if possible.

From the 15 Freeway (I-15) in Baker, take Exit 246 for Kelbaker Road and follow it east, then south, 19 miles to unmarked dirt Aiken Mine Road, which crosses Kelbaker Road just south of a line of cinder cones and 0.5 mile south of mile marker 19. The turnout, on the right (east) side of the road at the intersection, is the only large parking area along this part of Kelbaker Road.

Alternatively, from Kelso Depot, follow Kelbaker Road 15 miles north to Aiken Mine Road.

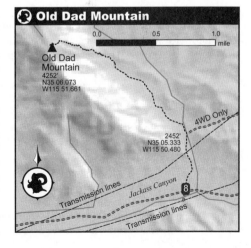

Turn southwest and follow the dirt road 1.6 miles to a T-junction. Turn right and follow the road, which curves around to the south. Eventually, it curves southwest and enters the wash of Jackass Canyon, following a row of three transmission lines. Stay in the main wash rather than taking any of the numerous power-line spur rows. In 5.0 miles from the T-junction, reach a major tributary wash leading north along the southeast side of Old Dad Mountain. Park near this junction; options are limited unless you park in the wash itself.

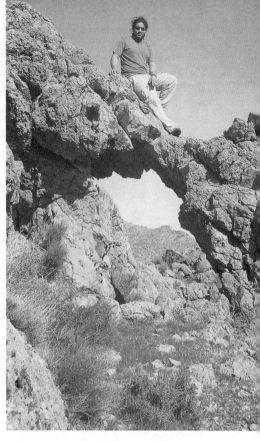

Scrambling up Old Dad Mountain

Old Dad Mountain was named in response to the nearby Old Woman Mountains. Joseph "Old Dad" Wallace was a railroad worker from Kelso who was accused of murdering his fiancée. He fled to the hills and became a miner. This trip is a short but steep and fun climb to the 4,252-foot limestone summit. The mountain hike appears difficult at first, but with careful route-finding, it's possible to stay on Class 2 scrambling. The rock here is highly abrasive and will tear up your flesh and clothes; suitable attire is recommended. Bighorn sheep frequent this area, and lucky visitors may see them. Keep your eye out for fossils in the limestone.

Topo maps show a dirt road leading north up the wash, but no trace remained in 2016. Walk north up the wash. In 0.6 mile, the wash splits and a power-line road exits to the right. (High-clearance 4WD vehicles might be able to get this far.) Take the left fork of the wash and continue 1.2 miles until it turns west and joins the prominent canyon on the east face of Old Dad Mountain.

Identify the steep ridge to the right of this canyon, and climb this ridge to 4,000 feet. This involves fun scrambling up interesting rock, but shouldn't be too difficult as long as you're on-route. Then turn left and hike up gentler slopes to the summit.

From the top, enjoy views of the Devils Playground, Soda Dry Lake, the lava beds, and the Kelso Dunes. On a clear winter day, the snowcapped summits of San Jacinto, San Gorgonio, Mount Charleston, and Telescope Peak are all visible. Return the way you came.

---

trip 19.9   **Lava Tube**

Distance	0.5 mile (out-and-back)
Hiking Time	30 minutes
Elevation Gain	100'
Difficulty	Easy
Trail Use	Good for kids
Best Times	October–April
Agency	Mojave National Preserve
Optional Map	Trails Illustrated *Mojave National Preserve* or USGS *Indian Spring* 7.5'

DIRECTIONS From the 15 Freeway in Baker, take Exit 246 for Kelbaker Road and follow it east, then south, 19 miles to the unmarked Aiken Mine Road, a dirt road that crosses Kelbaker Road just south of a line of cinder cones. The turnout, on the right (east) side of the road at the intersection, is the only large parking area along Kelbaker Road.

Alternatively, from Kelso Depot, follow Kelbaker Road 15 miles north to Aiken Mine Road. Follow the excellent dirt road 4.6 miles northeast to an unmarked fork. Turn left onto a narrow and sandy dirt road, which leads north past a corral and ends at a parking area in 0.3 mile. Be careful of the sand—though it's usually not a problem, passenger cars have become mired here.

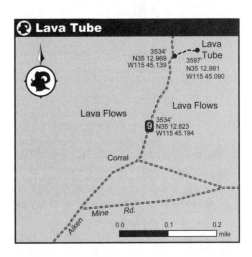

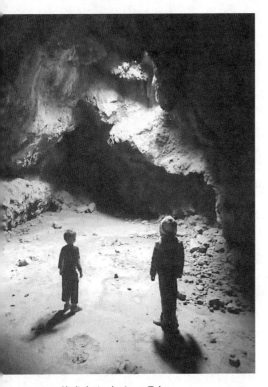

Skylight in the Lava Tube

A mong the many notable geological features of Mojave National Preserve are a chain of cinder cones and lava flows located between Baker and Kelso Depot. In one of the lava beds is a lava tube, which formed when the surface of the lava flow cooled and hardened into a crust while the molten center flowed on. This short trip leads into the tube. Make sure to bring a flashlight and watch your head on the low ceilings.

From the parking area, hike up a closed road north onto the lava flow. In 0.2 mile near the crest of the flow, look for a clearing and trail on the right (east) marked by a metal stake. Follow the trail east 100 yards as it gently climbs through the black lava flow. Pass a pair of sinister-looking "eyes" marking the bottom end of the lava tube, and then reach the gaping main entrance. A sturdy metal ladder was installed in 2008, providing an easy descent to the floor of the lava tube.

Follow a tunnel that leads back toward the eyes and opens up into a large chamber; then return the way you came.

trip 19.10   **Teutonia Peak**

Distance	3.2 miles (out-and-back)
Hiking Time	2 hours
Elevation Gain	700'
Difficulty	Moderate
Trail Use	Dogs allowed
Best Times	October–April
Agency	Mojave National Preserve
Recommended Map	Trails Illustrated *Mojave National Preserve* or USGS *Cima Dome* 7.5'

DIRECTIONS From the 15 Freeway, 25 miles east of Baker, take Exit 272 for Cima Road. Proceed south 11 miles to a small turnout on the right (west) with a trail marker. Alternatively, the trailhead can be reached by driving 6 miles north on Cima Road from Cima.

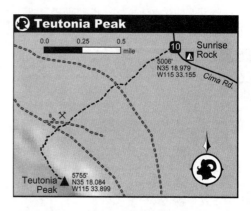

Cima Dome appears unremarkable at first, but careful inspection reveals it to be an unusual formation: a nearly symmetrical hump of monzonite nearly 10 miles in diameter protruding from the desert floor. The igneous dome formed underground from an ancient upwelling of magma. The softer overlying rock eroded away, leaving the dome. Its size is best appreciated from a distance; you get a good view from the 15 Freeway near the Cima Road exit. On its northeast flank, the rocky Teutonia Peak (5,755') breaks the symmetry, and is slightly taller than the center of the dome itself. This hike leads to the peak through one of the largest Joshua tree woodlands in the Mojave Desert.

There is an excellent primitive camping site at Sunrise Rock, 0.1 mile south of the Cima Dome Trailhead. Turn east on a dirt road along the north side of the rock, and pick a site among the junipers and Joshua trees.

The beginning of the trail is marked with a picture of a hiker and an interpretive panel about the Joshua tree forest in the desert woodland, but there is no mention of Teutonia Peak itself. The trail leads southwest directly toward Teutonia Peak. This is a lush region of desert full of Joshua trees, blue yucca, and buckhorn cholla. Occasional exposed granite slabs remind you of the geologic origin of Cima Dome. In 0.5 mile, cross a dirt road. In another 0.5 mile, cross a second network of dirt roads near an old mine. The proper path is marked with trail signs. If you're feeling adventurous, take a 100-yard detour right (west) toward a deep mine shaft that's now fenced off. The trail soon begins to climb, making a few switchbacks before reaching the ridge. As you gain elevation, the Joshua tree forest gives way to junipers and pancake

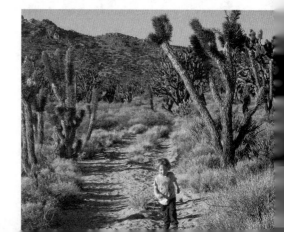

Teutonia Peak Trail

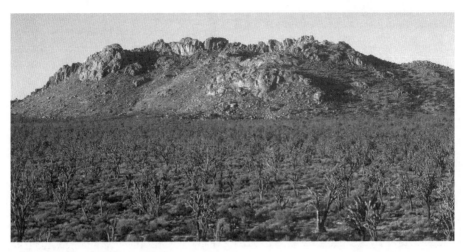

Teutonia Peak from Sunrise Rock

prickly pear cacti. The trail turns left (south-southeast) and follows the ridge just west of its crest. Good views of the gently sloping Cima Dome unfold to the west. At 0.6 mile from the mine, the trail reaches the ridge again at a notch between some of the huge toothlike summit boulders. Here, you can enjoy views to the east of the Ivanpah Mountains and of the jagged New York Mountains to the southeast.

Return the way you came. A fainter trail leads on partway around the boulders to the south, but soon ends. The summit rocks are tricky, and a rope and climbing skills are recommended if you choose to scale them.

trip 19.11 Kessler Peak

see map on next page

Distance	4 miles (out-and-back or loop)
Hiking Time	4 hours
Elevation Gain	1,100'
Difficulty	Moderate
Best Times	October–April
Agency	Mojave National Preserve
Required Map	Trails Illustrated *Mojave National Preserve* or USGS *Cima Dome* 7.5'

DIRECTIONS From the 15 Freeway, take Exit 272 for Cima Road and go south 11 miles to the Teutonia Peak Trailhead; then continue 0.6 mile farther south to unmarked and easily overlooked dirt Kessler Peak Road, on the left. Go north on Kessler Peak Road 1.1 miles, passing two pleasant campsites, to reach the 2WD parking area at a junction (parking here brings the round-trip up to 5.5 miles). If you have a 4WD vehicle, take the right fork and then a left at a junction immediately beyond. In 0.2 mile, reach a junction in a wash. Turn right and take the poor road leading up the sandy wash for 0.5 mile (wide vehicles might get scratched by nearby vegetation). After passing a ridge, find a place to park off the road.

Kessler Peak (6,163') is the high point of the Ivanpah Mountains and, being centrally located, offers unsurpassed views of Mojave National Preserve. The mountain was misnamed for Dan Kistler, a butcher by trade, who was murdered by a Piute.

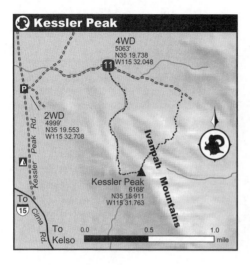

Kessler Peak

4WD
5063'
N35 19.738
W115 32.048

11

2WD
4999'
N35 19.553
W115 32.708

P

Kessler Peak Rd.

Kessler Peak
6168'
N35 18.911
W115 31.763

To
15

Cima Rd.

To
Kelso   0.0   0.5   1.0
                                          mile

Ivanpah Mountains

This moderate climb is a good intro-duction to cross-country desert mountain-eering. Amid the Joshua trees and Utah junipers, watch for an incredible assort-ment of cactus, including grizzly and pan-cake prickly pear cactus, staghorn cholla, Mojave mound, Engelmann's, barrel, and shy pincushion cactus. You'll likely find piles of cholla cactus debris guarding the entrance to pack rat dens. Only about eight parties a year presently sign in to the regis-ter atop the peak.

From the 4WD parking, head south up an alluvial fan, which soon becomes a well-defined wash. In 0.6 mile, stay right where the wash forks below a granite wall. Take the wash as it soon curves left, and in 0.5 mile stay right at another fork. Continue 0.6 mile up the steepening wash to a saddle directly west of the summit. The buildings to the south are Kessler Springs Ranch. Turn left and head up, passing over a false summit to reach the true high point in 0.3 mile.

From here, enjoy the panoramic views. The Ivanpah Mountains run north toward the tow-ering limestone Clark Mountain. Mount Charleston looms in the distance. Turning clockwise, Cima Dome's perfectly round shape is clearly visible. Look for the Kelso Dunes and Devils Playground at the base of the Granite Mountains, with San Jacinto and San Gorgonio visible in the distance on a clear day. The Providence Mountains and Mid Hills form a backbone through the center of the Mojave National Preserve. The New York Mountains and Castle Peaks stand out above Ivanpah Valley.

You can return the way you came, or make a somewhat more strenuous loop by descending the steep and rocky northeast ridge. Pick your way down the slope to a saddle; then pass over or around two minor bumps. Descend an even steeper slope on lichen-encrusted unstable granite boulders. Rather than climbing over the last bump on the ridge, veer left into a wash and follow the wash or the slopes above it northwest and then north until the terrain finally eases and you can reach the road in the wash. Just to the east is another viewpoint of the New York Mountains from the deep notch in the Ivanpah crest, but you can turn left and walk west down the wash to the point where you began.

trip 19.12   **Fort Piute**

Distance	5 miles (out-and-back), 6 miles (loop)
Hiking Time	3–4 hours
Elevation Gain	1,000'
Difficulty	Moderate
Trail Use	Dogs allowed
Best Times	October–April
Agency	Mojave National Preserve
Recommended Maps	Trails Illustrated *Mojave National Preserve* or USGS *Signal Hill* and *Homer Mountain* 7.5'

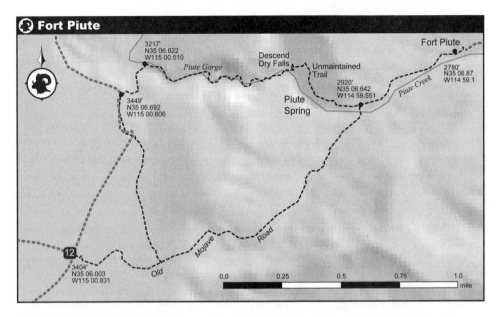

Fort Piute

3217'
N35 06.822
W115 00.510

Piute Gorge

Descend
Dry Falls

Unmaintained
Trail

2920'
N35 06.642
W114 59.551

Fort Piute

2780'
N35 06.87
W114 59.1

Piute Creek

3449'
N35 06.692
W115 00.606

Piute
Spring

3404'
N35 06.003
W115 00.831

12

Mojave Road

Old

0.0   0.25   0.5   0.75   1.0
mile

DIRECTIONS A 4WD vehicle is recommended to reach this trailhead. Always check on road conditions after heavy rains. From the 40 Freeway in Fenner, 57 miles east of Ludlow and 36 miles west of Needles, take Exit 107 for Goffs Road. Drive north 10 miles to the old Goffs Schoolhouse, and then turn left onto Lanfair Road. Drive north 10 miles until the road turns to dirt; then proceed another 5.7 miles to the signed junction with the Cedar Canyon Road. Immediately north of the junction, turn right (east) onto a utility road (you may see an arrow labeled PT&T). Proceed 3.6 miles to an unmarked V-junction. Stay right and continue 5.8 miles across the Lanfair Valley, crossing some sandy washes. Just before you reach the Piute Mountains, turn left onto a dirt road and proceed north 0.5 mile to a wide clearing marked with cairns.

The Mojave Road was once a trade route for Native Americans crossing the desert between the Colorado River and the Pacific Ocean. Before the Civil War, it became a wagon road, and after the war, camps were established a day's travel apart to protect travelers from hostile Indians displaced by white settlers. The camps went into decline in 1883, when the Southern Pacific Railroad was completed farther south of the Mojave Road. Fort Piute is one of these derelict garrisons, located at the base of the Piute Mountains. The area is also noteworthy because of Piute Spring, which flows year-round to support lush vegetation, its waters then sinking back into the desert sands. This hike follows the Mojave Road past some petroglyphs to the fort overlooking the creek, and then offers the option of returning via the spectacular Piute Gorge. Entering the gorge involves some third-class rock scrambling down dry waterfalls.

From the parking area, walk due east past some posts marking the wilderness boundary; vehicles aren't permitted beyond the posts. The path is initially faint, but soon becomes the well-defined Old Mojave Road, which switchbacks up the slope. As you climb, the creosote bushes yield to Mojave yucca, buckhorn cholla, and barrel and hedgehog cacti. In 0.6 mile, reach the crest of the ridge and begin descending the exceedingly rocky road.

After rounding a corner to the left, the canyon bottom comes into view. The Mojave Road descends to the bottom of a dry wash and follows it for some distance, then exits at a clearly marked point on the left side where the wash turns right, 1.1 miles down from the ridge. Immediately after leaving the wash, look for petroglyphs on a boulder beside the trail. Sharp-eyed hikers may notice several more petroglyphs along the route. The Mojave Road descends a band of red rock. Wheel tracks can still be seen gouged into the rock where the wagon teams struggled up the steep hill. In 0.2 mile, arrive at the perennial Piute Creek. Such a reliable source of water is rare in the Mojave Desert.

The trail jogs left upstream and then promptly crosses and climbs the north bank to a junction. Turn right (east) and follow the trail through rich fields of yuccas and cacti overlooking Piute Creek. This area was once a lush riparian zone of cottonwood, willow, and mesquite, which provided vital nourishment to birds, toads, and much desert wildlife. In September 2004, careless visitors triggered a wildfire that burned 12 acres along the creek; the trees are gradually recovering. In 0.6 mile, arrive at the low stone walls, which are all that remains of Fort Piute. Enjoy the exhibits and imagine what a soldier's life might have been like at such a remote outpost. Please don't climb, sit on, or disturb the fragile historic fort walls. After exploring, you may return the way you came.

ALTERNATIVE FINISH

Alternatively, return via the Piute Gorge Loop Trail, the most remote and least maintained trail in the park. **Note:** *This variation is recommended only for experienced hikers carrying a detailed map.*

At the trail junction immediately north of the Piute Creek crossing, an unmaintained trail leads west above the creek. In 0.3 mile, reach a vista atop steep loose cliffs where you can see Piute Spring, clearly identifiable by the lush vegetation below and the barren sandy wash above. (The path stays above the cliff to avoid bushwhacking through the vegetation in the canyon.) The route becomes somewhat difficult to identify here, but is marked with cairns as it switchbacks up and leads 0.2 mile north toward a side canyon entering from the north. The trail descends into this gully, which cuts through red, purple, and brown volcanic rocks. The gully drops into Piute Gorge. This is the crux of the hike, involving climbing down dry waterfalls (third class on unstable rock). Look for paths bypassing some of the falls.

The route turns right (west) and enters the spectacular narrows of Piute Gorge, passing through many-hued volcanic rock formations and threading past house-sized boulders that plummeted off the canyon walls into the creekbed. The route follows the meandering canyon 0.9 mile upstream until the steep walls abruptly end as the creek enters a zone of tan sedimentary rock. A good trail exits on the left side and climbs steeply 0.2 mile up to the road at a parking area.

The other trailhead is 0.9 mile south across the flat desert. You can follow the road or a trail that parallels it for 0.3 mile to a jog in the road overlooking the next ravine. From here, the road and trail diverge. The road leads straight back to your vehicle, while the trail veers up the hill, climbing to meet the Old Mojave Road just below the ridge crest.

---

trip 19.13 ## Caruthers Canyon

Distance	2 miles (out-and-back)
Hiking Time	1 or more hours
Elevation Gain	400'
Difficulty	Easy
Trail Use	Dogs allowed, good for kids
Best Times	October–May
Agency	Mojave National Preserve
Recommended Map	Trails Illustrated *Mojave National Preserve* or USGS *Pinto Valley* and *Ivanpah* 7.5'

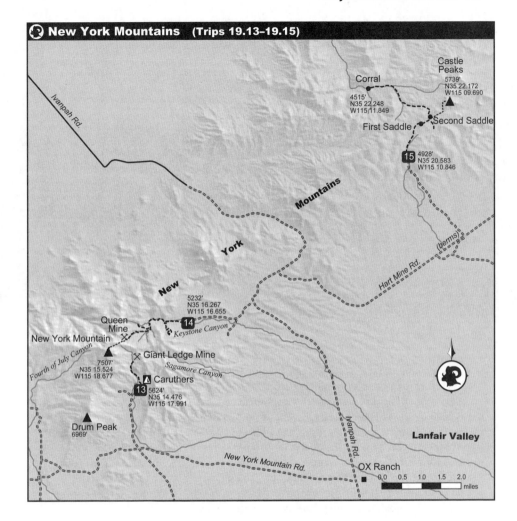

New York Mountains (Trips 19.13–19.15)

Castle Peaks
5739'
N35 22.172
W115 09.690

Corral
4515'
N35 22.248
W115 11.849

First Saddle
Second Saddle

15 4928'
N35 20.583
W115 10.846

Mountains

(berms)

York

Hart Mine Rd.

New

5232'
N35 16.267
W115 16.655

Queen Mine
14 Keystone Canyon

New York Mountain
7507'
N35 15.524
W115 18.677

Fourth of July Canyon

Giant Ledge Mine
Sagamore Canyon

Caruthers
13 5624'
N35 14.476
W115 17.991

Drum Peak
6969'

Ivanpah Rd.

Lanfair Valley

New York Mountain Rd.
OX Ranch

0.0 0.5 1.0 1.5 2.0
miles

Ivanpah Rd.

DIRECTIONS A high-clearance vehicle is recommended to reach this trailhead. From the 40 Freeway in Fenner, 57 miles east of Ludlow and 36 miles west of Needles, take Exit 107 for Goffs Road. Drive north 10 miles to the old Goffs Schoolhouse, and then turn left onto Lanfair Road. Drive north 21 miles to the OX Ranch. The first 10 miles are paved and the remainder is graded dirt, and the road name eventually changes to Ivanpah Road. Then turn left (west) onto graded, occasionally signed dirt New York Mountain Road. Proceed 5.4 miles, and turn right (north) at an unsigned junction onto a fair dirt road and drive 1.8 miles toward the mountains. Along the way, pass an old windmill and water tank; stay straight on the main road, keeping right at forks; and, shortly after you cross a sandy wash, look for a large turnout on the right that makes a good parking spot. You may prefer to park before the wash to avoid getting stuck in the sand.

The New York Mountains, named for their dramatic skyline, are the second highest range in the park and offer refreshingly cool camping and hiking in the remote heart of the Mojave National Preserve. Caruthers Canyon is the most scenic of the canyons penetrating the range. The canyon is misspelled for George Carruthers, who established a homestead here in 1915. Botanists are especially interested in this canyon because it's home

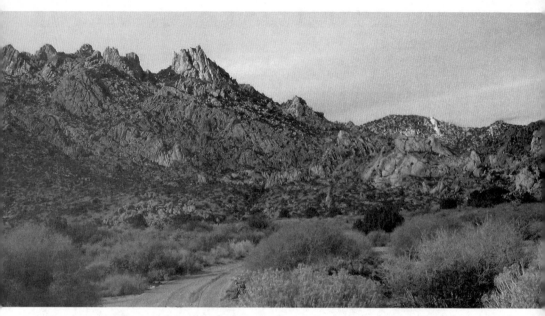

New York Mountains

to a unique mutant of the single-leaf pinyon pine (*Pinus monophylla*) with bundled pairs of needles rather than the normal single needle.

Hike north on the dirt road, which rapidly deteriorates to 4WD only and soon becomes impassable to all vehicles. Numerous fine primitive camping sites are located along the road; a fork to the right (east) leads to one with a picnic table and fire pit. Follow the main road up the canyon beneath the quartz monzonite spires of the New York Mountains. It's worth getting off the trail to wander through the rocks. In 0.6 mile, cross the creekbed. Soon reach the top of a small rise, where you can enjoy fine views back to the south.

The Giant Ledge Mine is just beyond. Established in 1902, it followed a vein of copper. **Note:** *The mine is on private property—please don't trespass.*

---

trip 19.14 **New York Mountain**

see map
on
previous
page

Distance	6 miles (out-and-back)
Hiking Time	6 hours
Elevation Gain	2,200'
Difficulty	Strenuous
Best Times	October–April
Agency	Mojave National Preserve
Required Map	Trails Illustrated *Mojave National Preserve* or USGS *Ivanpah* 7.5'

DIRECTIONS A high-clearance vehicle is strongly recommended. From the 15 Freeway, take Exit 286 for Nipton Road east. In 3.4 miles, turn right (south) onto Ivanpah Road. Go 12 miles to the end of the pavement; then drive another 4.9 miles along the graded dirt road to signed Hart Mine Road. Continue on Ivanpah Road another 1.2 miles to where you can turn right onto an unmarked road leading into Keystone Canyon. Bear left at an immediate fork to stay on the main road. In 0.6 mile, stay right at a Y. In another 1.4 miles, the road ends at a wash by a sign for the Keystone Canyon Trail. A spur to the right leads to parking and camping.

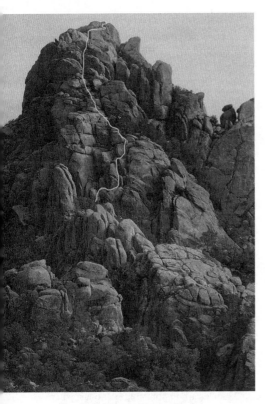

New York Mountain summit route

The New York Mountains are the second-tallest range in the Mojave National Preserve and are prominent from many directions. This trip to the highest point (7,532') in the range involves challenging route-finding and airy scrambling. Every party attempting this hike should have an experienced mountaineer, and some will appreciate bringing a short rope to descend from the summit. Persistent mountaineers are rewarded with outstanding views. The hike up Keystone Canyon also features an abandoned mine and lush desert vegetation. A topographic map and compass or GPS are essential. Note that the USGS map labels the lower north summit as "New York" and the higher southern summit as "New York Two." If you wish to watch the sunset or sunrise from the top, you can find sandy sheltered bivouac sites just below the summit rocks.

The first challenge is to navigate up Keystone Canyon on an abandoned mining road. The road is severely washed out and impassable by normal 4WD vehicles, and enters a wilderness area where vehicles are now prohibited anyway. Hike up the road/trail, which crosses the wash at the trailhead. Colorful rock crags tower over the pinyon–juniper woodland. As you enter the mouth of the canyon in 0.6 mile, watch for another mining road forking to the left. When Keystone Canyon turns sharply left in another 0.7 mile, watch for the narrow mouth of Live Oak Canyon on the right. Soon after, pass another mining road veering right out Keystone Canyon to climb into Live Oak Canyon. The canyon is aptly named for the canyon live oaks in the area. In another 0.1 mile, the canyon divides yet again, with a smaller wash coming down from Keystone Spring to the south, while the main Keystone Canyon turns west and steepens.

At 2.2 miles from the trailhead, the road ends at Queen Mine atop a heap of tailings. Old rails emerge from the partially flooded adit. Remember that exploring abandoned mines is extremely dangerous, and enjoy it from outside. The green rocks in the vicinity get their color from copper oxides.

The next challenge is to gain a saddle between Keystone and Caruthers Canyons at 2,060 meters, or 6,758 feet (**N35° 15.760' W115 18.367'**). This saddle is west of the hill that is west of Peak 2,069 m on the USGS topographic map. The saddle isn't clearly visible from the mine, but you simply continue southwest up the steep wash. In places, you may find bits of trail used by prospectors and hikers. Pass two more adits before you reach the saddle.

From the saddle, you can see for the first time two rocky summits across Caruthers Canyon. The one on the right is New York Mountain, and your next goal is to reach the saddle just right of the mountain. Although you can follow the ridge west and then southwest over the north peak, this route is rocky and circuitous. Instead, make a level traverse to the southwest into Caruthers Canyon, staying below some rock ribs. When you reach the wash in the canyon, follow it up; then climb the steep slope to the saddle. You'll likely find traces of climbers' trails that will ease the ascent.

Your final challenge is finding a path up the imposing granite summit. Two narrow corridors allow passage from east to west through the towering rocks. Avoid the first one, which is choked by oaks, but take the second, southern one. Look for a weakness where you can turn left and climb south up boulders onto the summit ridge. This point (**N35° 15.552' W115° 18.697'**) is beside a pinyon pine and may be marked with cairns. It's well worth finding because alternatives are much more difficult.

The climb is steep at first but soon eases. The crux is the final climb onto the summit. The only nontechnical route is a sloping crack system on the right (west) side. This short third-class pitch is exposed, but the holds are good. After enjoying the summit, return the way you came.

---

trip 19.15   Castle Peaks

Distance	2.2+ miles (out-and-back)
Hiking Time	1+ hours
Elevation Gain	200+'
Difficulty	Easy
Trail Use	Dogs allowed
Best Times	October–April
Agency	Mojave National Preserve
Required Map	Trails Illustrated *Mojave National Preserve* or USGS *Castle Peaks* 7.5'

see map on p. 445

DIRECTIONS A high-clearance vehicle is strongly recommended to reach this remote trailhead. From the 15 Freeway, take Exit 286 east onto Nipton Road. In 3.4 miles, turn right (south) onto Ivanpah Road. Go 12 miles to the end of the pavement, then another 4.9 miles along the graded dirt road to signed Hart Mine Road. Turn left (east) and follow the good dirt road 4.9 miles. When the main road abruptly turns right, stay left on a fair dirt road that crosses several earthen berms. (The Barnwell and Searchlight Railway ran along this route from 1907 to 1924.) In 0.9 mile, reach a four-way junction. Turn left (north) and follow the rutted dirt road north 3.0 miles to its end at a wilderness boundary marker. Immediately before the boundary marker is a large parking area on the right with a fire ring.

Castle Peaks

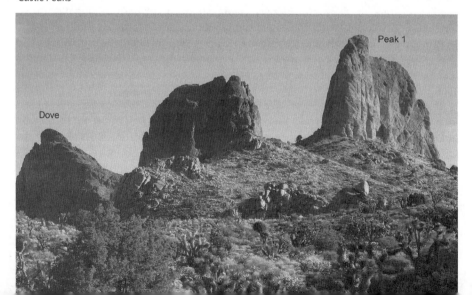

The mysterious volcanic spires of the Castle Peaks can be seen from the 15 Freeway and from the Lanfair Valley. This trip visits the extremely remote mountains, eroded plugs of crumbling Miocene-era volcanic breccia. Half the fun is in simply reaching the trailhead. The trail, a former rancher's jeep track, gently climbs to a good vista point. Intrepid hikers may leave the trail and brave dense stands of cactus to climb to the base of the spires.

Hike north past the wilderness boundary markers along a closed jeep road through a lush forest of Joshua trees, blue yucca, juniper, and buckhorn cholla. In 1.1 miles, reach a low saddle with good views of the Castle Peaks. If you're looking for an easy, kid-friendly hike, this is a good place to have a snack and scramble on the nearby boulder pile before returning the way you came.

For even better views, continue on the jeep track down into a valley and then up to the next saddle, 0.5 mile. The road forks just before the saddle and rejoins on the far side. From here, one could strike out cross-country toward the bases of any of the peaks. The summits themselves involve Class 4 and 5 climbing on unstable breccia and aren't recommended; see summitpost.org for details if you wish to learn more.

VARIATION

Hikers may also continue down the ranch road, which deteriorates into a wash and eventually reaches the corrals of an old grazing allotment. Wildflowers can be very good along this wash. This is a 7.5-mile out-and-back hike with 1,100 feet of elevation gain.

---

trip 19.16 **Clark Mountain**

Distance	2.8 miles (out-and-back)
Hiking Time	4 hours
Elevation Gain	1,500'
Difficulty	Strenuous
Best Times	October–April
Agency	Mojave National Preserve
Required Map	Trails Illustrated *Mojave National Preserve* or USGS *Clark Mountain 7.5'*

see map on next page

DIRECTIONS Note: *The drive requires a high-clearance vehicle and passes through an active mining area. Roads through the mine have been rerouted in the past and might be rerouted again.* From the 15 Freeway in Mountain Pass, take Exit 281 north onto Bailey Road; then make an immediate left onto paved Clark Mountain Road. In 0.9 mile, the road crosses a cattle guard and becomes good dirt. Stay on this road as it threads through the mining property.

In 0.8 mile, stay right at a Y, following the sign for RIGHT OF WAY ACCESS. In another 0.5 mile, veer right and pass through a gate signed PUBLIC ACCESS ROAD; then stay right just beyond. In 0.2 mile, pass a poor dirt power-line road on the left; then, in another 0.2 mile, descend into a wash and make a hard left, which brings you to rocky and sandy stretches where high clearance may be helpful.

In 1.2 miles, veer left at a junction by a 115 kV power line; then, in 0.5 mile, veer right at a Y above a substation. This road leads to a gated FAA radio facility, but you'll turn immediately left onto a lesser-used dirt road (high clearance essential) that descends, veers left to switchback up a hill, and then continues up into a canyon.

In 2.0 miles, come to an easy-to-miss split near a side canyon. The main road continues 0.1 mile to an elaborate picnic area that's the alternate trailhead and a good place to camp, but if you have a 4WD vehicle, turn left up the side canyon and proceed 0.7 mile to the end of the road.

Clark Mountain (approximately 7,907') is the highest point in Mojave National Preserve. This imposing limestone peak has no easy way up; this route requires third-class scrambling and some parties will appreciate having a 25-meter rope along. The mountain lies within the Mesquite Mountains Wilderness and is in the only portion of Mojave

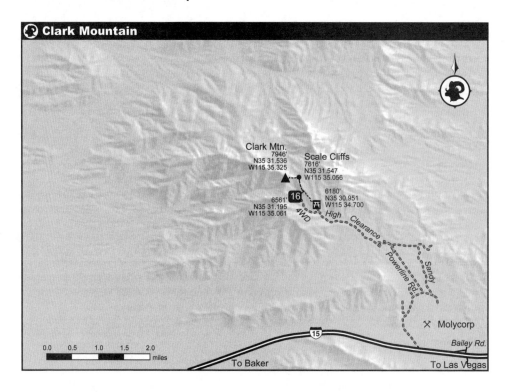

Clark Mountain

Clark Mtn.
7946'
N35 31.536
W115 35.325

Scale Cliffs
7616'
N35 31.547
W115 35.056

6180'
N35 30.951
W115 34.700

6561'
N35 31.195
W115 35.061

High Clearance

4WD

16

Powerline Rd.

Sandy

Molycorp

Bailey Rd.

15

To Baker

To Las Vegas

0.0   0.5   1.0   1.5   2.0
miles

National Preserve north of the 15 Freeway. Rock climbers consider the limestone cliffs on the eastern side of the mountain (east of this route) to be among the best in the world, and a 250-foot overhanging route called Jumbo Love is rated 5.15b—it was the hardest climb in North America when Chris Sharma completed it in 2008.

The Mountain Pass area is also noted for a huge open-pit rare earth mine operated by Molycorp. These metals are found in a handful of sites around the world and are critical components of integrated circuits and some advanced batteries and wind turbines. The rare earth ore is naturally associated with radioactive radium and thorium. The mine was closed in 1998 after a series of wastewater spills contaminated the desert and competition from China made the operation unprofitable. When China became the sole producer, supply was sharply curtailed and prices skyrocketed. Congress determined that the mine should be reopened for national security reasons, and Molycorp invested half a billion dollars to resume operations in 2012. China slashed prices again and Molycorp was forced into bankruptcy in 2015.

From the 6,560-foot upper parking area, pick a path northeast up steep scree slopes to the crest of the ridge. Intersecting the ridge at about 6,900 feet, turn left and continue up steep slopes. The ridge offers imposing views of the cave-riddled limestone amphitheater on the south face of Clark Mountain. The pinyon-juniper woodland is dotted with little-leaf mountain mahogany, old man prickly pear, Mojave mound cactus, and the beautiful Clark Mountain agave, which is smaller than the desert agave found in the Santa Rosa Mountains.

You may find traces of a climber's trail as you pick your way up the scree. At 7,200 feet, reach the base of a band of cliffs on the ridge. Stay just below them on the east side and continue up the slope. At 7,600 feet, just before you reach the skyline ridge, find the first weakness in the cliffs. Scramble up a 50-foot pitch of third-class limestone to a tree where you could set a belay. Then work your way up and right to a notch in the knife-edge ridge, where you turn left. You may find cairns just below the ridgeline as you climb to the 7,800-foot false summit. The bighorn sheep scat indicates that mountaineers aren't the only ones to climb these ledges.

From here, you have impressive views of the limestone buttresses on the north face. Hike west on or just below the ridgeline through a garden of cactus and agave for a quarter mile to reach the true summit.

On the descent, retrace your steps. If you wish, you can bypass the third-class cliff by returning to the notch in the knife-edge ridge and following the fun third-class ridge east a few hundred feet until it ends on easier terrain.

VARIATION

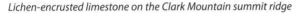

You can start Clark Mountain from the picnic area, which may be preferable if your vehicle lacks the clearance to reach the upper trailhead. This alternative adds 0.4 mile each way and 400 feet of extra climbing in a rugged but beautiful wash. From the picnic area, find the trail beside the fire pit that leads north into the wash. When a dry waterfall blocks the wash, exit right and scramble up very steep scree slopes; then traverse until you can drop back into the wash above the waterfall. Ascend the wash 0.1 mile until it gets brushy; then work your way up steep scree slopes on the left to join the ridge, and follow it up to join the main route.

Lichen-encrusted limestone on the Clark Mountain summit ridge

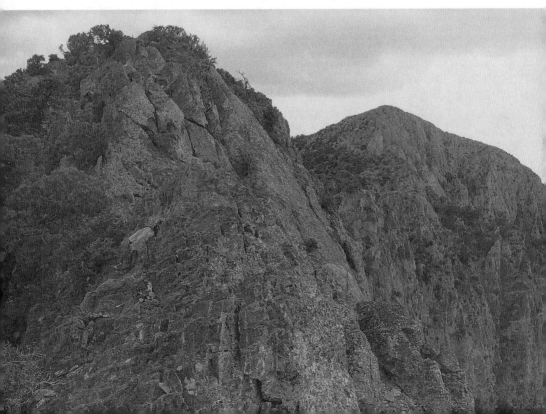

chapter 20

Mojave Trails National Monument

Mojave Trails National Monument, designated by President Obama in 2016, encompasses 1.6 million acres in the Mojave Desert, including 350,000 acres of wilderness. The monument is named to commemorate the series of trails that have crossed this unforgiving land. The Mojave Indian Trail was the earliest known route between the Colorado River and the Pacific Ocean, traveled by Native Americans for untold centuries. The Old Spanish Trail was established in 1829, passing through Afton Canyon. By 1882, the Southern Pacific Railroad tamed this fearful journey. In 1912, the National Old Trails Road was completed, linking the Pacific and Atlantic Oceans by pavement for the first time. This road was redesignated as the famous Route 66 in 1926. General Patton trained more than a million troops here while preparing for the North Africa campaign of World War II. Today, the 40 Freeway spans the region, carrying travelers at such great speed that few have time to see the subtle beauty of the desert.

Monument designation protects much natural and human heritage. Geologically, the monument contains remarkable volcanic formations including Amboy Crater and the Pisgah lava tubes, as well as the Cadiz sand dunes. Paleontologists visit the Cady Mountains for Miocene fossils and the aptly named Trilobite Wilderness. Biologists continue to learn

Cadiz Dunes (see Trip 20.5)   Photo: Bob Wick/Bureau of Land Management

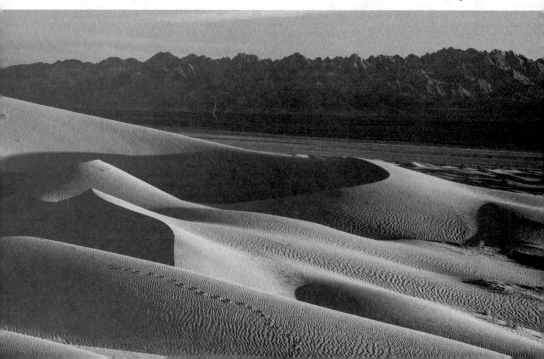

about the remarkable biodiversity at the interface of the Mojave and Colorado Deserts, including the threatened desert tortoise. This life is nourished by subsurface aquifers that date back to the Ice Age when many of the valleys were filled with lakes. Archaeologists trace human presence in the area back at least 10,000 years to the days of these lakes, and later peoples of the Mojave left petroglyphs and other signs of their civilization.

The region has few established hikes as of the time of writing. Several of the notable ones are included in this chapter. Endless possibilities exist for uncharted cross-country exploration—keep your eyes open as you visit!

trip 20.1 Afton Canyon

Distance	3.6 miles (out-and-back)
Hiking Time	2.5 hours
Elevation Gain	200'
Difficulty	Easy
Trail Use	Dogs allowed, good for kids, suitable for equestrians
Best Times	October–April
Agency	BLM Barstow Field Office
Recommended Maps	USGS *Dunn* and *Cave Mountain* 7.5'

DIRECTIONS From the 15 Freeway (I-15), at mile marker 15 SBD 111, 36 miles east of Barstow, take Exit 221 south onto good dirt Afton Road. Shortly bear left at a junction with Old Mojave Road, then left again to pass the Afton Canyon Group Camping Area. In 3.5 miles from the freeway, arrive at Afton Canyon Campground.

This hike follows the Mojave River through the colorful Afton Canyon to a pair of shallow caves. The Mojave River normally flows underground, but impermeable rocks keep the waters on the surface in this region. During the wet season, the river is a dependable source of water here, and it was an important resource to the Native Americans who lived in the region. Over the past two centuries, the river has supported explorers,

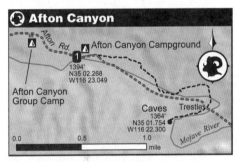

prospectors, and settlers following the Mojave Trail across the vast parched desert. In 1905, railroad tracks were built through the river canyon to link Utah to Los Angeles. The Union Pacific Railroad now operates these tracks. You're likely to get your feet wet, so sandals are recommended. At rare times of heavy flow in the Mojave River, this hike is not advisable.

Afton Canyon was cut during the Ice Age about 19,000 years ago. When the climate was much wetter, a chain of large lakes filled the basins between Barstow and Death Valley. Lake Manix burst its basin and cut the deep canyon that the Mojave River now follows.

Park in the large clearing at the entrance to the Afton Canyon Campground, taking care not to block any campsites. There is an outhouse, but you shouldn't count on water being available here.

From the campground, continue east on foot along the main dirt road that you'd been driving. In 0.2 mile, the road turns right (south) and crosses the Mojave River. At this point, leave the road and begin following the river. The best route varies from season to season and year to year, so use your judgment. You may find sporadic traces of trail along

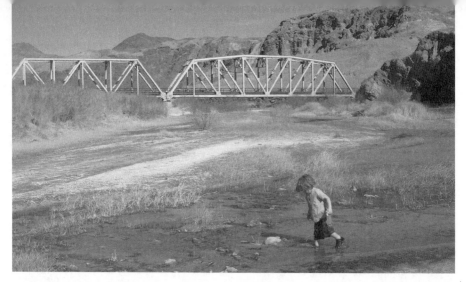

At play in Afton Canyon

the north bank. Depending on the water levels and vegetation, it may be easier to walk on the salt-encrusted sandy riverbed. If neither of these options looks good, you can ford the river and follow the road along the south side.

The walls of the canyon begin to rise. Some are carved from spectacular sedimentary rock tinted red, brown, tan, green, and black. In 1.5 miles, follow the riverbed as it turns right (south) and crosses under a large railroad trestle and recrosses the road. In another 0.4 mile, look for a shallow cave in the mountainside where the river bends back to the left. A second cave can be found just to the east.

Return the way you came. When you reach the trestle, you can follow the road back; this is easier walking and a slightly shorter route, but it receives heavy ATV traffic. If you want a longer hike, however, Afton Canyon continues another 6 miles. Many of the tributary canyons are also interesting, and the unusual geology draws rock hounds seeking specimens.

trip 20.2   Sheephole Mountain

Distance	4.5 miles (out-and-back)
Hiking Time	6 hours
Elevation Gain	2,300'
Difficulty	Strenuous
Best Times	October–April
Agency	BLM Needles Field Office
Required Map	USGS *Dale Lake* 7.5'

DIRECTIONS From Highway 62 in Twentynine Palms, turn north onto Adobe Road. In 2.0 miles, turn right (east) onto Amboy Road. Follow Amboy Road 23 miles to Sheephole Pass. At 0.5 mile, before you reach the microwave relay station at the pass, turn right onto a very sandy dirt road (the last of several before the relay station). Go 0.3 mile to the lip of a deep wash. If you don't have a 4WD vehicle, parking on the shoulder of Amboy Road may be preferable.

Sheephole Mountain is the high point in the Sheephole Valley Wilderness. In many ways, the scramble to the summit is an archetypal desert mountaineering experience. Though short in distance, it's physically grueling because of the unrelenting steep boulders that must be overcome. Wicked cat's claw acacia will snatch at your clothes and exposed skin. Numerous false summits raise and then crush your hopes. As one might expect,

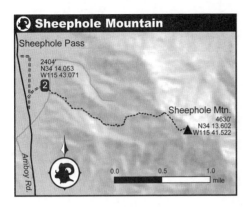

Sheephole Mountain

Sheephole Pass

2404'
N34 14.053
W115 43.071

Sheephole Mtn.
4630'
N34 13.602
W115 41.522

Amboy Rd.

0.0   0.5   1.0
mile

bighorn sheep roam the range and mark their presence with copious scat. The rocky peak offers expansive views across the desolately beautiful desert.

Look east from your vehicle and identify the mouth of a major canyon breaching the steep slopes of the mountain. You may see traces of old mining activity near the canyon mouth. Drop down into a deep and broad dry wash running perpendicular to the canyon mouth. Cross the wash and begin walking up the canyon. In another 0.2 mile, pass the remains of another mine site. Continue southeast up the canyon another 0.7 mile to its head, north of the point marked 1041T on the topographic map.

From here, the climbing begins in earnest. Ascend the left (east) wall of the canyon, which eventually becomes a ridge. Careful route-finding is necessary to pick your way through the granite obstacles; the rock isn't always of the highest quality. At the highest point on the ridge is a steep granite outcrop. Before you reach its difficult slabs, traverse right and continue scrambling up the easiest path you can to the skyline.

Drop down a few feet and turn right (southeast) to hike across the brushy summit plateau. If you head for the high point too soon, you'll get caught up among steep and difficult boulders. The best route is to hike all the way to the southwest side of the summit before turning left and climbing the slabs (Class 2–3). The true high point is marked with a stake, which helps to distinguish it from the numerous false summits you might accidentally climb.

From the top, you can admire the lofty summits of San Gorgonio and San Jacinto, the dry Bristol Lake bed, the cinder cone at Amboy, and the vast expanses of desert wilderness.

trip 20.3   Pisgah Lava Tubes

see map on next page

Distance	2 miles (out-and-back)
Hiking Time	2 hours (plus 2–3 hours for exploring)
Elevation Gain	300'
Difficulty	Moderate
Trail Use	Good for kids
Best Times	October–April
Agency	BLM Barstow Field Office
Optional Maps	USGS *Hector, Sleeping Beauty,* and *Lavic Lake* 7.5'

DIRECTIONS From the 40 Freeway (I-40) east of Barstow, take Exit 33 south onto Hector Road. Shortly come to a T-junction and turn left (east) onto Historic Route 66 (National Trails Highway). Proceed 4.6 miles and turn right (south) onto Pisgah Crater Road. In 1.5 miles, park at a turnout before a gate.

Pisgah Crater is a volcanic cinder cone believed to have formed as recently as 25,000 years ago. A nearby vent emitted a flow of molten rock that formed a large lava field. As the outer shell of lava cooled in the air, an inner layer continued to flow in places, leaving dozens of lava tubes hidden beneath the surface.

This trip visits three of these tubes. It's a truly remarkable destination, and it could easily be spoiled; furthermore, the caves are protected by law. Take special care to protect the area. Remind your hiking partners not to leave trash or deface the rock, and carry out any trash you might discover. Part of this trip crosses private property. Although there is a long tradition of hikers visiting the lava tubes, abusing the land may result in loss of access. A headlamp is essential. A helmet, long pants and sleeves, gloves, and even knee pads will make your explorations more enjoyable. Most of this area is trailless in confusing terrain. To find the lava tubes, it's extremely helpful to bring a GPS or a friend who knows the area. Caving can be a dangerous sport. Be careful while crossing the lava field because tube roofs may collapse.

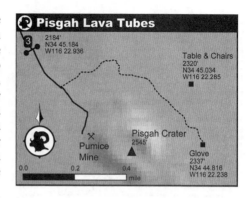

From the parking area, look southeast and identify the black mound of Pisgah Crater. Significant mining operations are taking place on the side of the crater; remain clear of the mine for both safety and to avoid disturbing the landowner. A low ridge extends north from the crater into the lava field. Look for a small ravine at the north end of the ridge. Your first goal is to reach this ravine. One way to do this is to hike up the road 0.2 mile, then turn left and follow the edge of the lava field toward the ravine. Soon you may find a use trail. When the trail vanishes in the lava field, pick a path across the sharp lava toward the Glove tube (see GPS coordinates on map).

The Glove lava tube has an entrance near the south end of a large collapsed chamber. It requires some agility to crawl into the mouth and down a 4-foot drop. Soon the tube becomes taller and one can walk upright for hundreds of feet, passing minor obstacles. Just before the end of the tube is a caving register. At the end, look for the mouth of a narrow tunnel on the left about 5 feet off the ground. Skinny adults can squeeze through this tunnel by crawling on their stomach. Turning around is impossible in several places; if you're too large, your only way out is to crawl backward. Getting stuck here could be serious, so take great care if you choose to explore. The tunnel loops back to the main tube, ending with a 6-foot drop. Retrace your steps.

A second segment of the Glove tube can be entered about 100 feet northeast of the first entrance. Enter through a tight hole near the south end of a second collapsed chamber. The tube initially requires stooping or crawling, but eventually opens into a tunnel through which one could drive a bus. At the end, retrace your steps.

The Table and Chairs tube is located 0.3 mile to the north. This tube features a cavelike mouth in which explorers once established a base camp. At the back of the cave, one can crawl west on hands and knees through a tube for several hundred feet. Look for lava-drip stalactites on the ceiling. The last part is the tightest, but can be negotiated by most adults. Climb up and out to a cairn marking the exit.

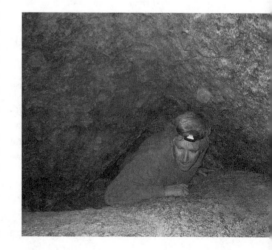

At least 200 other lava tubes have been documented in this area. Take some time to explore before you find your way back to your vehicle.

Tight squeeze in the Glove

trip 20.4   Amboy Crater

Distance	3 miles (out-and-back)
Hiking Time	2 hours
Elevation Gain	400'
Difficulty	Easy
Trail Use	Dogs allowed, good for kids
Best Times	October–April
Agency	BLM Needles Field Office
Optional Map	USGS *Amboy Crater* 7.5'

see map on next page

DIRECTIONS From the 40 Freeway, 28 miles east of Ludlow, take Exit 78 south onto Kelbaker Road and drive 11 miles to a T-junction with Historic Route 66 (National Trails Highway). Turn right (west) and continue 6 miles into Amboy, then 1.7 miles farther to a signed turnoff for Amboy Crater National Natural Landmark. Follow good dirt Crater Road south 0.5 mile to the trailhead parking area. Amboy can also be reached from the south via a scenic drive from Twentynine Palms.

Amboy Crater is a volcanic cone of ash and cinders rising out of a lava flow. It has erupted at least four times; the most recent eruption happened 10,000 years ago. One of the youngest volcanoes in North America, it was designated a National Natural Landmark in 1973.

This short hike leads through the basalt flows and up a breach in the crater wall to the center of the cone. After the winter rains, the fields of purple sand verbena and desert lily along this route are especially photogenic. This trip has enough attractions to keep a child captivated, and the steady stream of freight trains on the Atchison, Topeka and Santa Fe line blowing their whistles at Amboy lend a certain atmosphere that captivates train buffs.

Amboy Crater

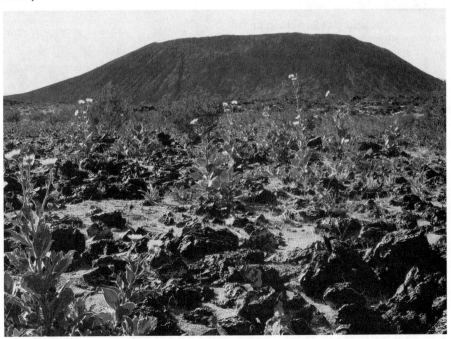

The crater is located on Bureau of Land Management land outside the boundaries of Mojave National Preserve.

Note: *The Twentynine Palms Marine Corps Air Ground Combat Center is immediately west of Amboy Crater. This is an active bombing range. Do not enter the range, and don't touch unexploded stray ammunition.*

Two trails leave from the parking area. At the southeast end, a wheelchair-accessible path leads 100 yards to a shaded viewing platform. The main trail departs from the west end near the outhouses. It snakes through the basalt lava flows along an old jeep track toward the crater, passing some shaded benches en route. Sometimes the path can be faint, but look for footprints and occasional trail markers if you're in doubt. If you examine the lava closely, you may see tiny green crystals of olivine.

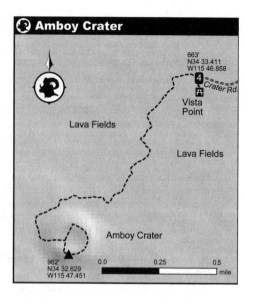

Amboy Crater

663'
N34 33.411
W115 46.858
Crater Rd.
Vista Point
Lava Fields
Lava Fields
Amboy Crater
962'
N34 32.629
W115 47.451
0.0   0.25   0.5
mile

Do not climb the main wall of the crater directly—this contributes to unsightly erosion. Instead, follow the trail as it curves around to the right (west) side and enters the crater via a hidden break. From the center of the crater, consider taking one of the paths up to the rim and circumnavigating the lip of the volcano, which offers good views of the lava flow and the Bristol dry lake to the south. Return the way you came.

trip 20.5   ## Cadiz Dunes

Distance	1 mile (out-and-back)
Hiking Time	30 minutes
Elevation Gain	120'
Difficulty	Easy
Trail Use	Good for kids
Best Times	October–March
Agency	BLM Needles Field Office
Optional Map	*Cadiz Lake NW 7.5'*

DIRECTIONS A high-clearance 4WD vehicle is recommended because of deep sand and ruts. From Highway 62, 0.3 mile east of mile marker 62 SBD 102 (62 miles east of Twentynine Palms), turn north onto graded dirt Cadiz Road at a BLM sign. After 35.6 miles, turn left (southwest) at a CADIZ DUNES WILDERNESS sign onto Cadiz Dunes Road, and follow it 2.8 miles to the parking area at the end.

   If you're coming from the north via Historic Route 66, take Cadiz Road 13.2 miles south from Chambless to Cadiz Dunes Road.

The Cadiz Dunes are as remote as any spot in the Mojave. The dunes were formed by winds carrying sand from the Cadiz Dry Lake, a playa left over from the Ice Age when lakes filled each basin in the area. Once a playground for off-roaders, they've been protected since 1994 as part of the 19,935-acre Cadiz Dunes Wilderness. The dunes are habitat

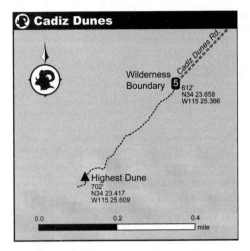

Cadiz Dunes

Wilderness Boundary **5** 612'
N34 23.658
W115 25.366

Cadiz Dunes Rd.

▲ Highest Dune
702'
N34 23.417
W115 25.609

0.0   0.2   0.4
                              mile

for the vulnerable Mojave fringe-toed lizard. Camping is permitted at the trailhead and in the dunes, but avoid windy days! Photographers love the area in morning and evening light. The Old Woman Mountains form a striking backdrop to the northeast.

The tallest cluster of dunes is visible about 0.5 mile from the parking area. The first part of the walk is infested with nonnative tumbleweeds that leave nasty stickers buried in the sand, so you'll be glad to keep your shoes on until you've passed the worst of them.

On your return, you may find the parking area hidden behind dunes. Watch for the dirt road or follow your tracks to navigate back.

Racing to the top of the big dune

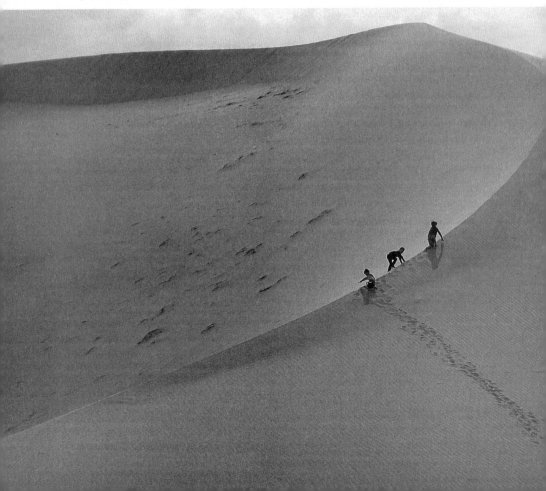

Best Hikes

BIG THREE MOUNTAIN CLIMBS

Mount Baldy Loop (Trip 1.1) 10,064-foot monarch of the San Gabriel Mountains.
San Gorgonio Mountain (Trip 5.1 or 5.14) 11,499-foot crown of the San Bernardino Mountains.
San Jacinto Peak (Trip 9.23 or 9.18) 10,804-foot pinnacle of the San Jacinto Mountains.

MORE GREAT PEAKS

Cucamonga Peak (Trip 1.10) Wilderness experience with magnificent views over the Inland Empire.
Iron Mountain (Trip 1.13) Challenging climb up Big Bad Iron. Don't get stuck-a by yucca!
San Bernardino Peak (Trip 5.9) Inspiring scenery and a historic-survey site.
Tahquitz Peak (Trip 9.14) Granite walls, lodgepole forests, and chickadees make this feel like a trip to the Sierra Nevada.
Cornell Peak (Trip 9.22) Beautiful forest approach to a classic pyramid, with an airy summit block.
Antsell Rock (Trip 10.1) Stimulating summit rocks on the rugged Desert Divide.
Murray Hill (Trip 12.2) Surprisingly vigorous for a low summit, with cactus and panoramic views.
Mopah Point (Trip 13.9) Massive volcanic plug with a devious and exciting route.
New York Mountain (Trip 19.14) Rugged cross-country desert adventure with mining history and a fun summit ridge.
Clark Mountain (Trip 19.16) Towering limestone walls and unique desert vegetation.

BEST MODERATE LOOPS

Los Santos Loop (Trip 8.4) Circle through the Engelmann oaks and spring wildflowers past a vernal pool.
Fern Canyon (Trip 11.13) Palm oases, wall of ferns, cactus-studded ridge.
Ladder and Big Painted Canyons (Trip 13.1) Unique geology: slot canyons, colorful rocks, ladders.
Maze and Window Rock Loop (Trip 15.1) Close encounters with iconic rock formations and yuccas.
Black Rock Canyon Panorama Loop (Trip 16.1) Yuccas, cactus, and great views.
Barber Peak Loop (Trip 19.3) Circumnavigate the dramatic volcanic mesa through a playground of desert vegetation and the gorgeous Banshee Canyon.

BEST OASES

Lower Palm Canyon (Trip 11.12) World's largest California fan palm oasis.
Magnesia Spring Falls (Trip 12.5) Cross-country adventure up a wild canyon with dry falls and many oases.
McCallum Nature Trail (Trip 14.1) Short hike to two oases and a reflecting pond.
Lost Palms Oasis (Trip 18.5) Cross the fiery Joshua Tree badlands to a hidden oasis.

BEST SPRING WILDFLOWERS

Los Santos Loop (Trip 8.4) Some of the Inland Empire's best wildflowers in March and April of a wet year.
Black Rock Canyon Panorama Loop (Trip 16.1) Blooming Joshua trees, Mojave yuccas, cacti, and wildflowers, along with terrific views.

BEST FALL COLORS

Aspen Grove (Trip 5.17) A rare grove of quaking aspens along a creek on San Gorgonio's northeast flank. Visit in October.

BEST BIRD-WATCHING

Sylvan Meadows Loop (Trip 8.2) Diverse birds and gorgeous Engelmann oaks at the Santa Rosa Plateau Ecological Preserve.

Big Morongo Canyon Preserve (Trip 14.4) Birds and bird-watchers flock to this rare wetland between the San Bernardino Mountains and Joshua Tree.

BEST SUNSETS

Sunset Peak (Trip 2.1) After a steep scramble up a firebreak, enjoy a picnic and the golden light on Mount Baldy before you descend the fire road.

Mount Inspiration (Trip 15.14) Brilliant sunsets over San Jacinto on a partly cloudy evening.

BEST MINES

Lost Horse Mine and Mountain (Trip 15.8) Treachery in the desert. A well-preserved 10-stamp mill at a highly profitable gold mine.

Desert Queen Mine (Trip 15.11 or Trip 15.20) Cursed gold brought the owners more grief than fortune.

BEST FULL-MOON HIKES

Museum Trail (Trip 11.3) The desert becomes mysterious by moonlight.

Boy Scout Trail (Trip 15.2) Eerie rock formations in the Wonderland of Rocks.

BEST GEOLOGY TOURS

Owl Canyon (Trip 6.3) Wild colors, dry falls, and even a natural tunnel near the Barstow syncline.

Ladder and Big Painted Canyons (Trip 13.1) Scale a slot canyon using a system of ladders; then descend the brilliant Big Painted Canyon.

Mitchell Caverns (Trip 19.6) Rare and spectacular formations in the limestone caverns.

BEST HOT SPRINGS

Deep Creek Hot Springs (Trip 3.1) Trek across the desert to the Inland Empire's favorite skinny-dipping pool.

BEST HIKES WITH KIDS

Heart Rock (Trip 3.2) Easy walk through the woods to a waterfall and pool with a remarkable rock formation.

Cougar Crest (Trip 4.3) A perennial favorite walk in the woods above Big Bear Lake.

Big Falls (Trip 5.4) Play along Mill Creek en route to the falls.

Vernal Pool (Trip 8.5) Young naturalists can explore the pool from a boardwalk in March of a good rain year.

Kelso Dunes (Trip 19.1) An unforgettable slide down the tallest of the booming dunes.

Hole-in-the-Wall (Trip 19.2) A thrilling climb down a slot into Banshee Canyon, followed by a loop back through areas of yuccas and cacti.

Pisgah Lava Tubes (Trip 20.3) Adventurous kids will enjoy watching their grownups try the tight squeeze. Bring a GPS to find the tubes.

BEST STRENUOUS HIKES

The Three T's (Trip 1.11) A classic hike near Mount Baldy over Timber, Telegraph, and Thunder.

Pines-to-Palms (Trip 11.14) Follow Palm Canyon all the way from Highway 74 to the oasis near Palm Springs. Full spectrum of desert flora arranged by elevation.

Art Smith Trail (Trip 12.7) A gem of the Santa Rosa Mountains, with cacti, oases, and outlandish rocks. Descend the Hahn Buena Vista Trail for fantastic views of San Jacinto.

Boo Hoff Loop (Trip 12.11) Follow an ancient Indian footpath on the slopes of Martinez Mountain with views of the Salton Sea.

Wonderland Traverse (Trip 15.4) Can you find your way through the mazelike Wonderland of Rocks? Rock-hopping on huge boulders, and a visit to a hidden "fortress."

BEST MONSTER HIKES

Nine Baldy Area Peaks (Trip 1.12) All the major summits around Baldy.

Continued on next page

San Antonio Ridge (Trip 1.14) Cross-country romp from Iron Mountain to Mount Baldy along a truly gnarly ridge.

San Gorgonio Nine Peaks Challenge (Trip 5.20) Grand traverse of the San Bernardino Ridge.

Nine Peaks of the Desert Divide (Trip 10.6) Awesome scenery along the Pacific Crest Trail's most rugged stretch south of the Sierra Nevada.

Cactus-to-Clouds (Trip 11.4) Palm Springs to San Jacinto. A Southern California classic, and North America's biggest continuous ascent by trail.

Snow Creek (Trip 11.8) An incredible snow couloir topping out directly on San Jacinto's peak. The toughest hike in this book.

Rabbit Peak from the Salton Sea (Trip 12.19) Only 6,640 feet, but the most strenuous mountain in Southern California. Amazing cacti and agaves.

Three Saints (Trips 1.1, 5.1, and 9.23) San Jacinto, San Gorgonio, and San Antonio (Mount Baldy), in 24 hours or bust!

BEST MOUNTAIN BIKING

Skyline Trail (Trip 4.11) Moderate climb to a moderate flowing ridge run with grand views.

Santa Ana River Trail (Trip 5.16) Gorgeous forest with some narrow and challenging portions.

Simpson Park (Trip 7.19) Well-developed trail system through the hills. Boulders, views, and wildflowers.

Agency Contact Information

BUREAU OF LAND MANAGEMENT (BLM)

blm.gov

Barstow Field Office

2601 Barstow Road
Barstow, CA 92311
760-252-6000

Needles Field Office

1303 S. Highway 95
Needles, CA 92363
760-326-7000

Palm Springs–South Coast Field Office

1201 Bird Center Drive
Palm Springs, CA 92262
760-833-7100

CALIFORNIA STATE PARKS

www.parks.ca.gov

Lake Perris State Recreation Area

www.parks.ca.gov/?page_id=651

17801 Lake Perris Drive
Perris, CA 92571
951-940-5600
Hours: Daily, 6 a.m.–10 p.m.

Mount San Jacinto State Park and State Wilderness

www.parks.ca.gov/?page_id=636

25905 Highway 243
Idyllwild, CA 92549
951-659-2607
Hours: Weekdays, 10 a.m.–4 p.m., weekends,
8 a.m.–4 p.m.
Wilderness/camping permits: tinyurl.com
/msjpermits

Providence Mountains State Recreation Area

www.parks.ca.gov/?page_id=615

38200 Essex Road (16 miles northwest of I-40)
Essex, CA 92332; 760-928-2586

NATIONAL PARK SERVICE

nps.gov

Castle Mountains National Monument

nps.gov/camo

BARSTOW HEADQUARTERS
2701 Barstow Road, south of the 15 Freeway
Barstow, CA 92311
760-252-6100
Hours: Monday–Friday, 8 a.m.–4 p.m.

Joshua Tree National Park

nps.gov/jotr

COTTONWOOD VISITOR CENTER
Pinto Basin Road, 8 miles north of the 10 Freeway
at Cottonwood Spring
Twentynine Palms, CA 92277
760-367-5500
Hours: Daily, 8:30 a.m.–4 p.m.

JOSHUA TREE VISITOR CENTER
6554 Park Blvd., 1 block south of Highway 62
Joshua Tree, CA 92256
760-366-1855
Hours: Daily, 8 a.m.–5 p.m.

OASIS VISITOR CENTER
74485 National Park Drive
(National Park Drive at Utah Trail)
Twentynine Palms, CA 92277
760-367-5500
Hours: Daily, 8:30 a.m.–5 p.m.

Mojave National Preserve

nps.gov/moja

BARSTOW HEADQUARTERS
2701 Barstow Road, south of the 15 Freeway
Barstow, CA 92311
760-252-6100
Hours: Monday–Friday, 8 a.m.–4 p.m.

KELSO DEPOT VISITOR CENTER
Kelbaker Road between the 15 and 40 Freeways
Kelso, CA 92309
760-252-6108
Hours: Thursday–Monday, 10 a.m.–5 p.m.; closed
Tuesday, Wednesday, and December 25

Continued on next page

U.S. FOREST SERVICE (USFS)
www.fs.usda.gov

Angeles National Forest
www.fs.usda.gov/angeles

MOUNT BALDY VISITOR CENTER
Mount Baldy Road, about 10 miles north of the
210 Freeway in Upland
Mount Baldy, CA 91759
909-982-2829
Hours: Saturday–Sunday, 7 a.m.–3:30 p.m.

SAN GABRIEL RIVER RANGER STATION
110 N. Wabash Ave.
Glendora, CA 91741
626-335-1251
Hours: Monday–Friday, 8 a.m.–4:30 p.m.

San Bernardino National Forest
www.fs.usda.gov/sbnf

BARTON FLATS VISITOR CENTER
Highway 38, 18 miles east of the Mill Creek
Visitor Center
Angelus Oaks, CA 92305
909-794-4861
Hours: Open Memorial Day–mid-October;
hours vary

BIG BEAR DISCOVERY CENTER
40971 North Shore Drive (Highway 38)
Fawnskin, CA 92333
909-382-2790
Hours: Monday, Thursday, and Friday, 9 a.m.–
4 p.m.; Saturday–Sunday, 8:30 a.m.–4:30 p.m.;
closed Tuesday–Wednesday

LYTLE CREEK RANGER STATION
1209 Lytle Creek Road
Lytle Creek, CA 92358
909-382-2851
Hours: Monday, Thursday, and Friday–Sunday,
8 a.m.–4:30 p.m.; closed Tuesday–Wednesday

MILL CREEK VISITOR CENTER
34701 Mill Creek Drive (corner of Mill Creek
Road/Highway 38 and Bryant Street)
Mentone, CA 92359
909-382-2882
Hours: Monday, Thursday, and Friday, 8 a.m.–
4:30 p.m.; Saturday–Sunday, 7 a.m.–3:30 p.m.;
closed Tuesday–Wednesday
Wilderness and camping permits: sgwa.org

SAN JACINTO RANGER STATION
54270 Pine Crest Ave. (corner of Highway 243 and
Pine Crest Avenue)
Idyllwild, CA 92549
909-382-2921
Hours: Monday–Tuesday and Friday–Sunday,
8 a.m.–4 p.m. (closed noon–1 p.m.); closed
Wednesday–Thursday
Wilderness and camping permits: fsva.org
/forest-information

Santa Rosa and San Jacinto Mountains National Monument (BLM/USFS)
tinyurl.com/srsjmnm

VISITOR CENTER
51500 Highway 74
Palm Desert, CA 92260
760-862-9984
Winter hours (October 1–May 15): Open daily,
9 a.m.–4 p.m. *Summer hours (May 15–
September 30):* Monday–Tuesday and
Friday–Sunday, 8 a.m.–3 p.m.; closed
Wednesday–Thursday

OTHER

City/County Parks

BIG MORONGO CANYON PRESERVE
bigmorongo.org
11055 East Drive
Morongo Valley, CA 92256
760-363-7190
Hours: Daily, 7:30 a.m.–sunset

**CITY OF CLAREMONT
HUMAN SERVICES DEPARTMENT, CITY PARKS**
tinyurl.com/claremontparks
207 Harvard Ave.
Claremont, CA 91711
909-399-5490

CITY OF HEMET PARKS
tinyurl.com/hemetparks
3777 Industrial Ave.
Hemet, CA 92545
951-765-3712

CITY OF LOMA LINDA PARKS
tinyurl.com/lomalindacaparks
25541 Barton Road
Loma Linda, CA 92354
909-799-2810

CITY OF RIVERSIDE PARKS
riversideca.gov/park_rec
6927 Magnolia Ave.
Riverside, CA 92506
951-826-2000

CITY OF YUCAIPA PARKS AND RECREATION
yucaipa.org/recreation/parks
34272 Yucaipa Blvd.
Yucaipa, CA 92399
909-797-2489

CRAFTON HILLS OPEN SPACE CONSERVANCY
chosc.org
PO Box 1475
Yucaipa, CA 92399

MORENO VALLEY PARKS
tinyurl.com/morenovalleyparks
14177 Frederick St.
Moreno Valley, CA 92552
951-413-3000

RIVERSIDE COUNTY REGIONAL PARK AND OPEN-SPACE DISTRICT
rivcoparks.org
4600 Crestmore Road
Jurupa Valley, CA 92509
800-234-7275, 951-955-4310

SAN BERNARDINO COUNTY REGIONAL PARKS
sbcounty.gov/parks
777 E. Rialto Ave.
San Bernardino, CA 92415
909-387-2757

SAN BERNARDINO COUNTY SPECIAL DISTRICTS, PARKS AND RECREATION
specialdistricts.org/index.aspx?page=80
157 W. Fifth St.
San Bernardino, CA 92415
909-387-6076

SYCAMORE CANYON WILDERNESS PARK, AMEAL MOORE NATURE CENTER
mysycamorecanyon.com
400 Central Ave.
Riverside, CA 92507
951-826-2596
Hours: Thursday–Sunday, 9 a.m.–5 p.m.

Natural Areas and Preserves

COACHELLA VALLEY PRESERVE
coachellavalleypreserve.org
29200 Thousand Palms Canyon Road
Thousand Palms, CA 92276
760-343-2733
Hours: Trails open daily, sunrise–sunset; visitor
  center open May–September (hours vary)

HEAPS PEAK ARBORETUM
heapspeakarboretum.com
Rim of the World Scenic Byway (Highway 18),
  just southeast of Lake Arrowhead
Skyforest, CA 92385
Hours: Daily, sunrise–sunset

IDYLLWILD NATURE CENTER
rivcoparks.org/education/idyllwild-nature-center
25225 Highway 243
Idyllwild, CA 92549
951-659-3850
Hours: Wednesday–Sunday, 9 a.m.–4 p.m.; closed
  all major holidays

INDIAN CANYONS
tahquitzcanyon.com
38500 S. Palm Canyon Drive
Palm Springs, CA 92264
760-323-6018
Hours, October 1–July 4: Daily, 8 a.m.–5 p.m.
  Hours, July 5–September 30: Friday–Sunday,
  8 a.m.–5 p.m.

THE LIVING DESERT ZOO AND GARDENS
livingdesert.org
47900 Portola Drive
Palm Desert, CA 92260
760-346-5694
Hours, October 1–July 4: Daily, 7:30 a.m.–5 p.m.; no
  new hikers allowed on the trail past 3:30 p.m.
  Hours, July 5–September 30: Friday–Sunday,
  7:30 a.m.–1:30 p.m.

REDLANDS CONSERVANCY
redlandsconservancy.org
PO Box 855
Redlands, CA 92373
909-389-7810

SANTA ROSA PLATEAU ECOLOGICAL RESERVE
tinyurl.com/srpreserve
39400 Clinton Keith Road
Murrieta, CA 92562
951-677-6951
Hours: Daily, sunrise–sunset

TAHQUITZ CANYON
tahquitzcanyon.com
500 W. Mesquite Ave.
Palm Springs, CA 92264
760-416-7044
Hours, October 1–July 4: Daily, 8 a.m.–5 p.m.
  Hours, July 5–September 30: Friday–Sunday,
  8 a.m.–5 p.m. No new hikers allowed on the
  trail past 3:30 p.m.

THE WILDLANDS CONSERVANCY
wildlandsconservancy.org

Oak Glen Preserve
39611 Oak Glen Road
Oak Glen, CA 92399; 909-797-8507
Hours, April–October: Daily, 8 a.m.–5 p.m. *Hours,
  November–March:* Daily, 8 a.m.–4:30 p.m.

Pioneertown Mountains Preserve
51010 Pipes Canyon Road
Pioneertown, CA 92268
760-369-7105
Hours: Daily, sunrise–sunset

Whitewater Preserve
9160 Whitewater Canyon Road
Whitewater, CA 92282
760-325-7222
Hours: Daily, 8 a.m.–5 p.m. except Thanksgiving,
  December 25, and January 1

Activity Groups

Hiking with an organized group is a great way to visit new places, learn new skills, and make new friends. Southern California has a variety of local and regional hiking groups. Here's a sampling.

COACHELLA VALLEY HIKING CLUB The CVHC is the largest hiking group in the California desert, offering more than 150 hikes a year in the desert and surrounding mountains. Nonmembers are welcome to participate. For more information, visit cvhikingclub.net.

DESERT TRAILS HIKING CLUB Desert Trails organizes hikes from October to June around the Coachella Valley and nearby mountains. Nonmembers are welcome but are charged a $5 guest fee. For more information, visit deserttrailshiking.com.

MEETUP.COM This website lists a vast number of group activities for many interests. Look under "Outdoors & Adventure" for your area.

OUTDOORS CLUB Volunteers for this web-based club lead outdoor activities of many types in Southern California. The first three activities are free for nonmembers. Visit outdoorsclub.org.

SIERRA CLUB The Angeles Chapter of the Sierra Club organizes more than 4,000 outings of all sorts each year in Southern California. Most are open to nonmembers. For more information, visit angeles.sierraclub.org.

The U.S. Forest Service (USFS) and Bureau of Land Management are chronically underfunded and have few staff to patrol or maintain their respective trails. Much of that work has been undertaken by volunteer groups such as the ones listed below. Aside from the satisfaction of performing a valuable service, joining one of these groups is a great way to spend time outside and meet other hikers.

> **FOREST SERVICE VOLUNTEER ASSOCIATION** fsva.org
>
> **FRIENDS OF THE DESERT MOUNTAINS** desertmountains.org
>
> **SAN GABRIEL MOUNTAINS TRAILBUILDERS** sgmtrailbuilders.org
>
> **SAN GORGONIO WILDERNESS ASSOCIATION** sgwa.org

Managing agencies such as the USFS also organize hikes from time to time; many of these trips include expert commentary by naturalists. Check with the ranger stations or visitor centers listed in Appendix B for more information.

References

HIKING

Ferranti, Philip, with Hank Koenig. *140 Great Hikes In and Near Palm Springs.* 6th edition. Boulder: Colorado Mountain Club, 2014.

Furbush, Patty. *On Foot in Joshua Tree National Park.* 5th edition. Moose, WY: M. I. Adventure Publications, 2005.

Randall, Laura. *Five-Star Trails: Palm Springs.* Birmingham, AL: Menasha Ridge Press, 2016.

Robinson, John W., and David Harris. *San Bernardino Mountain Trails: 100 Hikes in Southern California.* 7th edition. Birmingham, AL: Wilderness Press, 2016.

Schad, Jerry. *Afoot & Afield Los Angeles County.* 3rd edition. Birmingham, AL: Wilderness Press, 2009.

Schad, Jerry, and David Harris. *101 Hikes in Southern California.* 3rd edition. Birmingham, AL: Wilderness Press, 2013.

BACKCOUNTRY ROADS

Massey, Peter. *Backcountry Adventures Southern California: The Ultimate Guide to the Backcountry for Anyone with a Sport Utility Vehicle.* Castle Rock, CO: Adler Publishing Company, 2006.

NATURE

Croissant, Ann, and Gerald Croissant, with Shirley DeBraal. *Wildflowers of the San Gabriel Mountains.* Las Vegas: Stephens Press, 2007.

Hickman, James C. *The Jepson Manual: Higher Plants of California.* Berkeley: University of California Press, 1993.

Ingram, Stephen. *Cacti, Agaves, and Yuccas of California and Nevada.* Los Olivos, CA: Cachuma Press, 2008.

Knute, Adrienne. *Plants of the East Mojave: Mojave National Preserve.* Rev. edition. Barstow, CA: Mojave River Valley Museum, 2003.

Lanner, Ronald M. *Conifers of California.* Los Olivos, CA: Cachuma Press, 1999.

Mackay, Pam. *Mojave Desert Wildflowers.* Guilford, CT: Falcon Press, 2013.

Mackay, Pam, and Timothy Thomas. *Southern California Mountain Wildflowers: A Field Guide to Wildflowers Above 5,000 Feet: San Bernardino, San Gabriel, and San Jacinto Ranges.* Guilford, CT: Falcon Press, 2016.

Munz, Philip A. *Introduction to California Desert Wildflowers.* Berkeley: University of California Press, 2004.

Pavlik, Bruce M., Pamela Muick, and Sharon Johnson. *Oaks of California.* Los Olivos, CA: Cachuma Press, 1993.

Quinn, Ronald D., and Sterling C. Keeley, with Marianne D. Wallace. *Introduction to California Chaparral.* Berkeley: University of California Press, 2006.

Trent, D. D., and Richard W. Hazlett. *Joshua Tree National Park Geology.* Joshua Tree, CA: Joshua Tree National Park Association, 2002.

Continued on next page

HISTORY

Olander, Ann, and Farley Olander. *Call of the Mountains: The Beauty and Legacy of Southern California's San Jacinto, San Bernardino and San Gabriel Mountains.* Las Vegas: Stephens Press, 2005.

Robinson, John W. *The San Bernardinos: The Mountain Country from Cajon Pass to Oak Glen, Two Centuries of Changing Use.* 5th edition. Arcadia, CA: Big Santa Anita Historical Society, 2001.

Robinson, John W. *The San Gabriels: Southern California Mountain Country.* San Marino, CA: Golden West Books, 1977.

Robinson, John W. *San Gorgonio: A Wilderness Preserved.* San Gorgonio, CA: San Gorgonio Volunteer Association, 1991.

Robinson, John W. and Bruce D. Risher. *The San Jacintos.* Arcadia, CA: Big Santa Anita Historical Society, 1993.

Aerial view of the Coachella Valley, with San Jacinto, San Antonio, and San Gorgonio on the skyline
Photo courtesy of Desert Map and Aerial Photo, Palm Desert, California

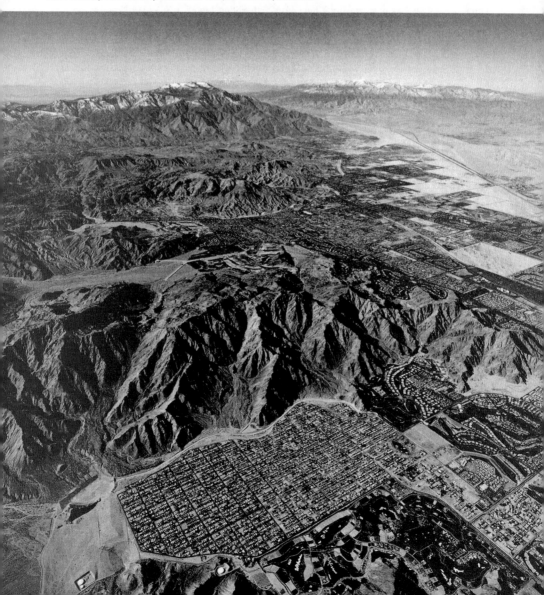

Index

Note: Page numbers followed by *m* indicate a map.

About the Author

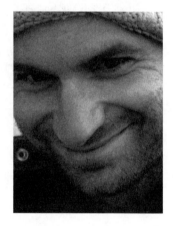

David Harris is a professor of engineering at Harvey Mudd College in Claremont, California. He is the author or coauthor of six hiking guidebooks and five engineering textbooks. David grew up rambling around the Desolation Wilderness as a toddler in his father's pack and later roamed the High Sierra as a Boy Scout. As a Sierra Club trip leader, he organized mountaineering trips throughout the Sierra Nevada. Since 1999, he has been exploring the mountains and deserts of Southern California.

David's other books for Wilderness Press are *101 Hikes in Southern California* (with Jerry Schad), *Afoot & Afield Orange County* (with Jerry Schad), *Day & Section Hikes Pacific Crest Trail: Southern California,* and *San Bernardino Mountain Trails* (with John W. Robinson).